Clinical Embryology

Zsolt Peter Nagy • Alex C. Varghese
Ashok Agarwal
Editors

Clinical Embryology

A Practical Guide

Springer

Editors
Zsolt Peter Nagy, MD, PhD,
HCLD (ABB), EMB (ACE)
Scientific and Laboratory Director
Reproductive Biology Associates
Atlanta, GA, USA

Alex C. Varghese, PhD
Senior Embryologist
Montreal Reproductive Centre
Montreal, QC, Canada

Ashok Agarwal, PhD, HCLD (ABB),
EMB (ACE)
Director, Center for Reproductive Medicine
Cleveland Clinic
Cleveland, OH, USA

ISBN 978-1-4614-8375-5 ISBN 978-1-4614-8376-2 (eBook)
DOI 10.1007/978-1-4614-8376-2
Springer New York Heidelberg Dordrecht London

Library of Congress Control Number: 2013951513

Printed on acid-free paper

Springer is part of Springer Science+Business Media (www.springer.com)

Preface

Over 3 decades of our experience with sperm and oocyte preparation for insemination proves that these procedures are everything but trivial. Although they are regarded as routine daily procedures, the selection of applied techniques depending on the conditions and settings can dramatically affect outcomes. Sperm preparation techniques need to be carefully adapted based on semen parameters, such as after surgical procedure from testicular or epididymal sample, or following cryopreservation. Further, it is approached differently again, if patient is affected by a disease condition, such as HIV and may be prepared differently for IUI, IVF, or ICSI. After fertilization, the choice of culture method and conditions can exert a dramatic effect on the physiology and viability of the growing embryo. A profound understanding is necessary for the shifting metabolomic requirements of the embryo and providing adequate conditions that are essential for the most successful outcome. Moreover, proper assessment of embryo viability is essential to provide the highest success rate. In addition to the traditional morphological embryo evaluation, there are several novel techniques developed in recent years (including genetic, proteomic, metabolomic, and time-lapse assessments) that promise advanced and standardized measurement of embryo viability. Supernumerary oocytes and embryos now can be more efficiently cryopreserved using vitrification, where success critically depends on the suitably selected method and procedure, which can be improved by fully understanding how different conditions affect outcome.

The main objective of this textbook was to provide a comprehensive review on the above topics, presenting detailed descriptions on practical approaches, as well to offer theoretical background to give a full scientific aspect. In addition to the well-established procedures, a large number of well-documented novel techniques and approaches are presented by authors, who are pioneers in their field. As a result, this textbook is indispensible resource for all embryologists, postgraduate students in clinical embryology, cryo-biologists and researchers working in assisted reproduction field.

We are thankful to Richard Lansing, executive editor, for his support and advice and Kristopher Spring, Associate Editor and Margaret Burns, publishing manager, for their tireless efforts in reviewing and editing each of the manuscripts. Furthermore, we would like to thank all our outstanding contributors for sharing their knowledge and experience. Finally, we are indebted to our families who have endured many long nights when we were working late on this book.

Atlanta, GA, USA — Zsolt Peter Nagy, MD, PhD
Montreal, QC, Canada — Alex C. Varghese, PhD
Cleveland, OH, USA — Ashok Agarwal, PhD

Contents

Contributors

Ahmed M. Abou-Setta, MD, PhD George & Fay Yee Centre for Healthcare Innovation, University of Manitoba/Winnipeg Regional Health Authority, Winnipeg, MB, Canada

Ashok Agarwal, PhD, HCLD (ABB), EMB (ACE) Director, Center for Reproductive Medicine, Cleveland Clinic, Cleveland, OH, USA

Gautam N. Allahbadia, MD, DNB, FNAMS Rotunda - The Center For Human Reproduction, Bandra, Rotunda Blue Fertility Clinic and Keyhole Surgery Center, Shivaji Park, Rotunda Fertility Clinic and Keyhole Surgery Center, Andheri, Mumbai, India

Belén Aparicio, PhD In Vitro Fertilization Laboratory, IVI Valencia, Valencia, Spain

Amir Arav, DMV, PhD Core Dynamics, Nes Zionna, Israel

Said Assou, PhD CHU Montpellier, Institute for Research in Biotherapy, Hôpital Saint-Eloi, Montpellier, Cedex, France

Baris Ata, MD Department of Obstetrics and Gynecology, Uludag University, Bursa, Turkey

Barry Behr, PhD, HCLD IVF Laboratory, Department of Obstetrics and Gynecology, Stanford School of Medicine, Stanford, CA, USA

Patricia Bernal, DVM Reproductive Biology Associates, Sandy Springs, GA, USA

Edson Borges Jr., MD Fertility—Center for Assisted Fertilization, São Paulo, Brazil

Charles Bormann, PhD Reproductive Endocrinology, Wisconsin Oncofertility Clinic, UW Hospital and Clinics, Madison, WI, USA

L. Botros, MSc Molecular Biometrics, Inc., Norwood, MA, USA

Imène Boumela CHU Montpellier, Institute for Research in Biotherapy, Hôpital Saint-Eloi, Montpellier, Cedex, France

Hakan Cakmak, MD Department of Obstetrics, Gynecology and Reproductive Sciences, Yale-New Haven Hospital, New Haven, CT, USA

Ching-Chien Chang, PhD Reproductive Biology Associates, Atlanta, GA, USA

Alice A. Chen, PhD Auxogyn, Inc., Menlo Park, CA, USA

Ri-Cheng Chian, PhD Department of Obstetrics and Gynecology, Royal Victoria Hospital, Women's Pavilion F, Montreal, QC, Canada

Ana Cobo, PhD IVI Valencia (Sede Central), Plaza de la Policía local, Valencia, Spain

Joe Conaghan, PhD Embryology Laboratories, Pacific Fertility Center, San Francisco, CA, USA

Giovanni Coticchio, BSc, MSc, MMedSc, PhD Biogenesi, Reproductive Medicine Centre, Istituti Clinici Zucchi, Monza, Italy

Hervé Dechaud, MD Department of Gynecology and Obstetrics and Reproductive Medicine, CHU Montpellier, Montpellier, Cedex, France

Thomas Elliott, BSc Reproductive Biology Associates, Atlanta, GA, USA

Sandro C. Esteves, MD, PhD Androfert Center for Male Reproduction, Campinas, São Paulo, Brazil

Arancha Galán, PhD In Vitro Fertilization Laboratory, IVI Valencia, Valencia, Spain

David K. Gardner, PhD Department of Zoology, University of Melbourne, Parkville, VIC, Australia

Nicolás Garrido, PhD Andrology Laboratory and Semen Bank, Instituto Valenciano de Infertilidad (IVI), University of Valencia, Valencia, Spain

Samir Hamamah, MBD, PhD INSERM U 1040, University Hospital of Montpellier, Arnaud de Villeneuve Hospital, Montpellier, Cedex, France

Medical School of Montpellier, University Hospital of Montpellier, Montpellier, Cedex, France

ART/PGD Department, University Hospital of Montpellier, Montpellier, Cedex, France

Sperm Bank (CECOS), University Hospital of Montpellier, Montpellier, Cedex, France

Thorir Hardarson, PhD Fertility Center Scandinavia, Gothenburg, Sweden

Gary Harton, BS, TS (ABB) Department of Molecular Genetics, Reprogenetics, LLC, Livingston, NJ, USA

Aparna Hegde, MD IVF Laboratory, Department of Obstetrics and Gynecology, Stanford School of Medicine, Stanford, CA, USA

Ralf Henkel, PhD Department of Medical Bioscience, University of the Western Cape, Bellville, Cape Town, South Africa

M. Henson, PhD Molecular Biometrics, Inc., Norwood, MA, USA

Jack Huang, MD, PhD Center for Reproductive Medicine, Weill Cornell Medical College, New York Presbyterian Hospital, New York, NY, USA

Robert P.S. Jansen, MD, CREI Sydney IVF, Sydney, Australia

K. Judge, PhD Molecular Biometrics, Inc., Norwood, MA, USA

Jennifer L. Kulp, MD Division of Reproductive Endocrinology and Infertility, Yale University School of Medicine, New Haven, CT, USA

Michelle Lane, BSc, PhD Repromed, Dulwich, Adelaide, SA, Australia

Christine Leary, BSc Hull IVF Unit, East Riding Fertility Services, The Women and Children's Hospital, Hull Royal Infirmary, Hull, UK

Henry J. Leese, BSc, PhD Hull York Medical School, University of Hull, Hull, UK

Don Leigh, PhD (UNSW) Sydney IVF, Sydney, Australia

Juergen Liebermann, PhD, HCLD (ABB) IVF and Embryology Laboratories, Fertility Centers of Illinois, Chicago, IL, USA

Ana S. Lopes, DVM, PhD Reproductive Medicine Unit-Heilig Hart Hospital, Leuven Institute for Fertility and Embryology (LIFE), Leuven, Belgium

Roberta Maggiulli, PhD GENERA Centre for Reproductive Medicine, Clinica Valle Giulia, Rome, Italy

James Marshall, BAppSc (UTS) Sydney IVF, Sydney, Australia

J. Ryan Martin, MD Division of Reproductive Endocrinology and Infertility, Yale University School of Medicine, New Haven, CT, USA

Steven J. McArthur, BSc Sydney IVF, Sydney, Australia

Rubina Merchant, PhD Rotunda - The Center For Human Reproduction, Bandra, Rotunda Blue Fertility Clinic and Keyhole Surgery Center, Shivaji Park, Rotunda Fertility Clinic and Keyhole Surgery Center, Andheri, Mumbai, India

Marcos Meseguer, PhD In Vitro Fertilization Laboratory, IVI Valencia, Valencia, Spain

Devin Monahan, BSc The Ronald O. Perelman and Claudia Cohen Center for Reproductive Medicine, Weill Cornell Medical College, New York, NY, USA

Santiago Munné, PhD Department of Molecular Genetics, Reprogenetics, LLC, Livingston, NJ, USA

Zsolt Peter Nagy, MD, PhD, HCLD (ABB), EMB (ACE) Scientific and Laboratory, Reproductive Biology Associates, Atlanta, GA, USA

Liesl Nel-Themaat, PhD Reproductive Biology Associates, Atlanta, GA, USA

Queenie V. Neri, BSc, MSc The Ronald O. Perelman and Claudia Cohen Center for Reproductive Medicine, Weill Cornell Medical College, New York, NY, USA

Gianpiero D. Palermo, MD, PhD The Ronald O. Perelman and Claudia Cohen Center for Reproductive Medicine, New York, NY, USA

Weill Cornell Medical College, New York, NY, USA

Eleonora Bedin Pasqualotto, MD, PhD Department of Gynecology, University of Caxias do Sul, Caxias do Sul, RS, Brazil

Fabio Firmbach Pasqualotto, MD, PhD Department of Urology, University of Caxias do Sul, Bairro Sao Pelgrino, RS, Brazil

Pasquale Patrizio, MD, MBE, HCLD Department of Obstetrics, Gynecology and Reproductive Sciences, Yale University School of Medicine, Yale Fertility Center, New Haven, CT, USA

Antonio Pellicer, MD Department of Gynecology and Obstetrics, Instituto Valenciano de Infertilidad (IVI), University of Valencia, Valencia, Spain

Thomas B. Pool, PhD, HCLD (ABB) Fertility Center of Antonio, San Antonio, TX, USA

Patrick Quinn, PhD, HCLD Sage IVF, A Cooper Surgicol Company, Redmond, OR, USA

Claude Ranoux, MD, MS INVO Bioscience, Beverly, MA, USA

José Remohí, MD Department of Gynecology and Obstetrics, Instituto Valenciano de Infertilidad (IVI), University of Valencia, Valencia, Spain

Laura Rienzi, MSc GENERA Centre for Reproductive Medicine, Clinica Valle Giulia, Rome, Italy

Laura Romany, PhD In Vitro Fertilization Laboratory, IVI Valencia, Valencia, Spain

P. Roos, PhD Molecular Biometrics, Inc., Norwood, MA, USA

Zev Rosenwaks, MD The Ronald O. Perelman and Claudia Cohen Center for Reproductive Medicine, Weill Cornell Medical College, New York, NY, USA

D. Sakkas, PhD Department of Obstetrics, Gynecology and Reproductive Sciences, Yale University School of Medicine, New Haven, CT, USA

Lucia De Santis, BSc, MSc IVF Unit, Department of Obstetrics and Gynecology, H S. Raffaele, Universita Vita-Salute, Milan, Italy

Peter N. Schlegel, MD Department of Urology, Weill Cornell Medical College, New York Presbyterian/Weill Cornell Hospital, New York, NY, USA

Lynette Scott, PhD Fertility Centers of New England, Reading, MA, USA

Shehua Shen, MD Auxogyn, Inc., Menlo Park, CA, USA

Zeev Shoham, MD Reproductive Medicine and Infertility Unit, Department of Obstetrics and Gynecology, Kaplan Medical Center, Affiliated to the Hadassah Medical School and the Hebrew University in Jerusalem, Ramat Hasharon, Israel

Gary D. Smith, PhD Departments of OB/GYN, Physiology, and Urology, University of Michigan, Ann Arbor, MI, USA

Reproductive Sciences Program, A Taubman Consortium for Stem Cell Therapies, University of Michigan, Ann Arbor, MI, USA

Danielle G. Smith, BMedChem, PhD Leeds Institute of Molecular Medicine, University of Leeds, St James's University Hospital, Leeds, UK

Roger G. Sturmey, BSc, PhD Centre for Cardiovascular and Metabolic Research, Hull York Medical School, University of Hull, Hull, UK

Jason E. Swain, PhD, HCLD Department of Obstetrics and Gynecology, University of Michigan, Ann Arbor, MI, USA

Shuichi Takayama, PhD Department of Biomedical Engineering, Macromolecular, Science and Engineering Program, University of Michigan, Ann Arbor, MI, USA

Takumi Takeuchi, MD, PhD The Ronald O. Perelman and Claudia Cohen Center for Reproductive Medicine, Weill Cornell Medical College, New York, NY, USA

Hugh S. Taylor, MD Section of Reproductive Endocrinology and Infertility, Department of Obstetrics, Gynecology and Reproductive Sciences, Yale University School of Medicine, New Haven, CT, USA

Alberto Tejera IVI, PhD In Vitro Fertilization Laboratory, IVI Valencia, Valencia, Spain

Maria Traversa, BSc, MSc (Med) Sydney IVF, Sydney, Australia

Michael Tucker, PhD IVF and Embryology Laboratories, Shady Grove Fertility, Rockville, MD, USA

Filippo Ubaldi, MD, MSc GENERA Centre for Reproductive Medicine, Clinica Valle Giulia, Rome, Italy

Gábor Vajta, MD, PhD, DSc Vajta Embryology Consulting, Rakosi and Vajta Trust, Brinsmead, QLD, Australia

Alex C. Varghese, PhD Senior Embryologist, Montreal Reproductive Centre, Montreal, QC, Canada

Sidney Verza Jr., BSc, MSc IVF Laboratory, Androfert-Center for Male Reproduction, Campinas, São Paulo, Brazil

Thamara Viloria, PhD IVF Laboratory, Instituto Valenciano de Infertilidad (IVI), University of Valencia, Valencia, Spain

Matts Wikland, PhD Department of Obstetrics and Gynaecology, University of Göteborg, Göteborg, Sweden

Graham Wright, BSc Reproductive Biology Associates, Atlanta, GA, USA

Chapter 1
Journey of Human Gametes In Vitro: 1978–2010

Zeev Shoham

The history of in vitro fertilization (IVF) and embryo transfer (ET) dates back as early as the 1890s when Walter Heape a professor and physician at the University of Cambridge, England, who had been conducting research on reproduction in a number of animal species, reported the first known case of embryo transplantation in rabbits, long before the applications to human fertility were even suggested [1].

In 1932, Aldous Huxley's *Brave New World* was published. In this science fiction novel, Huxley realistically described the technique of IVF as we know it. Two years later Pincus and Enzmann, from the Laboratory of General Physiology at Harvard University, published a paper in the Proceedings of the National Academy of Sciences of the USA, raising the possibility that mammalian eggs can undergo normal development in vitro. However, it was not until 1959 that indisputable evidence of IVF was obtained by Chang [2] who was the first to achieve births in a mammal (a rabbit) by IVF. The newly ovulated eggs were fertilized in vitro by incubation with capacitated sperm in a small Carrel flask for 4 h, thus opening the way to assisted procreation.

Professionals in the fields of microscopy, embryology, and anatomy laid the foundations for future achievements. The recent rapid growth of IVF-ET and related techniques worldwide are further supported by the social and scientific climate which favors their continuation.

Through the years, numerous modifications have been made in the development of IVF-ET in humans: refinement of fertilization and embryo culture media, earlier transfer of the embryo, improvements in equipment, use of a reduced number of spermatozoa in the fertilization dish, and embryo biopsy among others.

Z. Shoham, MD (✉)
Reproductive Medicine and Infertility Unit, Department of Obstetrics and Gynecology, Kaplan Medical Center, Affiliated to the Hadassah Medical School and the Hebrew University in Jerusalem, 35 Levona Street, Ramat Hasharon 47226, Israel
e-mail: zeev@cc.huji.ac.il

Z.P. Nagy et al. (eds.), *Clinical Embryology: A Practical Guide*,
DOI 10.1007/978-1-4614-8376-2_1, © Springer Science+Business Media New York 2013

The purpose of this manuscript is to acknowledge those who initiated new steps in the development of the treatment protocols and techniques that we now use facilitating such simple and promising IVF-ET procedures.

Development of IVF

In 1965, Edwards together with Georgeanna and Jones at Johns Hopkins Hospital in the United States attempted to fertilize human oocytes in vitro [3]. It took another 8 years until the first IVF pregnancy was reported by the Monash research team of Professors Carl Wood and John Leeton in Melbourne, Australia. Unfortunately, this resulted in early miscarriage [4]. Another step toward the goal of IVF was noted by Steptoe and Edwards who published a report on an ectopic pregnancy following transfer of a human embryo at the late morulae/early blastocyst stage [5]. However, a breakthrough and a huge achievement was noted in 1978 when the first ever IVF birth occurred in Oldham, England on July 25, 1978. This birth was the result of the collaborative work of Steptoe and Edwards [6]. Following this achievement, a year later, the first IVF birth was noted in Australia by the joint Victorian Monash-Melbourne team which occurred at Royal Women's Hospital [7], following the announcement of Howard and Georgianna Seegar Jones about the delivery of the first IVF baby in the United States in 1981. This first IVF birth in the United States was achieved with the use of hMG for ovarian stimulation. The improvement of technology leads to the report of Jacqueline Mandelbaum with Dan Szollosi describing the microstructures of the human oocyte, which became known as *oocyte dysmorphia* [8].

To improve the results of the procedure, efforts were made in optimizing the stimulation protocols, improving the culture media, improving aspiration technique and holding of the oocytes, and improving fertilization techniques. The second part of this manuscript will describe the fields which were developed in parallel, enabling the improvement of the pregnancy rate. These fields are as follows:

- Stimulation protocols
- Culture media
- Aspiration technique, handling of the oocyte, and embryo replacement
- Improved fertilization
- Cryopreservation and storage of embryos and oocytes
- Future manipulation of the oocytes and embryos

Stimulation Protocols

Earlier IVF pregnancies were achieved from unstimulated ovulatory cycles and the success rate remained low. It was later on suggested that in order to improve the fertilization and pregnancy rate, it might be possible to aspirate more than one egg, and this can be achieved during a cycle in which the ovary is stimulated by endogenous or exogenous gonadotropins. During the years, several protocols were developed and each of it was tested in relation to the drug influence on the oocytes. Trounson et al. introduced the use of clomiphene citrate and hMG in the treatment protocols [9]. It was later demonstrated that GnRH agonists can be used to eliminate premature luteinization and control ovarian stimulation [10].

It was Porter et al. who were the first to use GnRH agonists in IVF treatment [11]. Three major protocols using GnRH agonist were developed: the long, short, and ultra-short protocols. Several years later following numerous studies, it was found that the long protocol gave the best results in terms of pregnancy rate.

The administration of GnRH agonists resulted in "flare-up" of gonadotropins from the hypophysis. In some women, this resulted in the development of follicular cyst. In order to reduce the scale of gonadotropin section following the administration of GnRH agonist, it was suggested to give GnRH agonist either during the luteal phase, when serum progesterone is high, or under progesterone administration or during the oral contraception pill. Gonen, Jacobson, and Casper pioneered the use of combined oral contraceptives for follicle synchronization and cycle scheduling in IVF [12].

Following the development of the various stimulation protocols, it was noted that there is a possibility that the steroids production during the luteal phase was not optimal, and it was Casper et al. who were the first to describe the use of low-dose hCG for support of the luteal phase in ART cycles [13].

In order to simplify the stimulation protocol and to shorten it, efforts were invested in developing the GnRH antagonist. Frydman was the first to report the use of the GnRH antagonist, Nal-Glue, to prevent premature LH rise and progesterone in controlled ovarian hyperstimulation treatment [14]. This specific drug was not developed further due to the side effects. Following further efforts, the third generation of the GnRH antagonist was developed, and the first established pregnancy using recombinant FSH and GnRH antagonist was reported by Itskovitz-Eldor et al. [15]. The increasing needs in infertility treatment created the needs to develop new sources for gonadotropins. Recombinant FSH became available during the year 1992, and very soon after, pregnancy was established using a recombinant drug for ovarian stimulation [16, 17]. Following the development of the technology to produce recombinant FSH, it became only a matter of time until the recombinant LH and hCG became available. Pregnancy after treatment with three recombinant gonadotropins was reported by Agrawal et al. [18].

The above-mentioned development summarizes 30 years of gradual development in drugs production and methods of administration. Several additional developments were noted when Emperaire et al. publish their observation that the final stage of ovulation induction can be induce by endogenous LH released by the administration of an LHRH agonist after follicular stimulation for IVF [19].

In addition, a new technology was developed which involved in vitro maturation (IVM) of the oocyte, and Chian et al. demonstrated that hCG priming prior to immature oocyte retrieval in women with PCO increases the maturation rate and produces high pregnancy rates of 40% per started cycle [20]. It seems today that the various protocols and the various drugs available for ovarian stimulation enable the treating physicians to individualize treatment to the specific patient.

Culture Media

Optimal culture media which reflects the changing needs of the developing embryo is of importance for success of IVF treatment. The environment of the oviduct/uterus change dramatically as the zygote/embryo travels. The culture media needs to meet the metabolic needs of preimplantation embryos by addressing energetic and amino acid requirements in a stage-specific manner.

The first advanced culture medium was introduced in 1980 [21]. In 1985, Quinn and Warnes published a formula entitled human tubal fluid (HTF) that mimics the in vivo environment to which the embryo is exposed [22]. Gardner introduced sequential media and blastocyst transfer which now greatly assists in the move to single embryo transfer [23, 24].

The development of a completely chemically defined protein-free embryo culture medium and the births of the first batch of babies generated from the fertilization of eggs collected and inseminated in the medium using spermatozoa also prepared in the same protein-free medium in both conventional IVF and intracytoplasmic sperm injection (ICSI) were introduced in 2000 [25], and since then, the medium remained almost the same.

Aspiration Technique and Handling of the Oocyte and Embryo Replacement

Several techniques for oocyte aspiration have been developed to obtain the largest number of mature oocytes with the least risk to the patients causing minimal damage to the ovary. This was started with laparoscopic retrieval introduced by Steptoe and Edwards in 1978, and laparotomy for infertility related conditions [26].

Lenz and Lauritsen examined and proposed the transabdominal transvesical oocyte aspiration using an ultrasound-guided needle [27]. A year later, Gleicher and his group reported the first vaginal egg retrieval using an abdominal ultrasound [28].

Wikland, together with Hamberger and Nilsson in Gothenburg, Sweden, described the possibility of using a vaginal sector scanner (transvesical or transvaginal technique) for oocyte aspiration [29]. At the same time, Strickler et al. [30] described embryo transfer using abdominal ultrasound guidance. This technique gained additional support from the work done by Feichtinger and Kemeter [31] and it remained the main technique for egg collection until today.

Improved Fertilization

In the process of fertilization, it was first reported by Trounson and his group that there is a need for a delay between oocyte collection and insemination to allow oocytes collected to complete maturation [32]. In parallel, the possibility of using the natural environment of the human tube for the process of fertilization and development of the embryo lead to the development of the gamete intrafallopian tube (GIFT) procedure, and it was Asch et al., in 1984, who were the first to report on pregnancy following translaparoscopic GIFT procedure [33].

Much effort was invested trying to improve fertilization when this would not occur naturally when the egg and the sperm where introduced at the Petri dish in the laboratory. These efforts were started when researchers try to fertilize human oocytes by microinjection of a single sperm under the zona pellucida [34] which was followed by the report of a health delivery using the same technique by Ng et al. [35]. Further achievement was noted when pregnancy was obtained from micromanipulation using zona drilling or mechanical partial zona dissection [36]. However, a breakthrough was achieved when Palermo et al. from the group in Brussels reported on the first pregnancy after ICSI [37].

In order to improve fertilization results after repeated IVF failure or at advanced maternal age, it was suggested to use the cytoplasmic transfer technique. This is based on an assumption that a vital molecule, such as ATP or cell cycle-related kinase, or an organelle, such as mitochondria, is deficient at a critical stage in early development.

The technique aims to improve egg and embryo quality by the donation of ooplasm from supposedly fertile oocytes to patients whose cells are of poorer quality. Transfer of anucleate cytoplasm has been used, and Choen et al. [38], was the first to report on a birth after such a procedure.

Development of Cryopreservation and Storage of Embryos and Oocytes

In 1983, the group of investigators at the Monash IVF Centre reported on the first human pregnancy and birth following cryopreservation, thawing, and transfer of an eight-cell embryo. This embryo-freezing technique was developed in Cambridge, England, on cattle, and with minor adaptations, it was adjusted to humans [39]. A few years later, in 1990, Gordyts et al. reported on the first successful human cleavage-stage embryo vitrification followed by a successful delivery [40]. However, until this period of time, there were difficulties to cryopreserved oocytes, and only in 1999, the birth following vitrification of human oocyte was reported by Kuleshova et al. [41]. During the same year, Porcu et al. reported on the first birth from cryopreserved oocytes and testicular sperm [42]. A major development was noted when Bedaiwy et al. reported in 2006 on the successful cryopreservation of intact human ovary with its vascular pedicle [43]. This was followed in 2008 by the announcement of Porcu et al. on cryopreserved oocytes in cancer patients and the first ever birth of healthy twins after oocyte cryopreservation and bilateral ovariectomy [44].

Manipulation of the IVF Procedure and Technique to Solve Various Causes of Infertility

In 1983, the Monash IVF team achieved the first birth in a woman without ovaries by using donor eggs, by creating of artificial menstrual cycles, and by using a special hormonal formula for the first 10 weeks of pregnancy [45]. This came along with the first successful delivery following egg donation [46]. Still at the same year, in vitro maturation and -fertilization of morphologically immature human oocytes in an IVF setup were developed and published [47]. However, it took 11 years until the first live birth as a result of IVM following transvaginal ultrasound-guided oocyte collection was reported. Further development of the technique was reported by Cohen et al. who achieved a blastocyst development from IVM oocyte plus ICSI plus assisted hatching, which was ended in a healthy birth [48].

The role of assisted hatching is still controversial, and the indication for the procedure is not very clear. However, in 1985, Cohen et al. reported in the Lancet about a birth after replacement of hatching blastocyst cryopreserved at the expanded blastocyst stage [49]. It was later on suggested to use this specific technique of assisted zona hatching to breach the zona pellucida and promote the natural process of hatching when the prognosis is poor [50].

A new era in the field of IVF, i.e., preimplantation genetic diagnosis (PGD) was open with the announcement of Handyside et al. first reported on biopsy of human preimplantation embryos and sexing by DNA amplification [51]. This was followed by the report of pregnancies from biopsied human preimplantation embryos sexed by Y-specific DNA amplification [52]. Still in the same field of PGD, Verlinsky was the first to report on the possibility to do a polar body biopsy, transfer the embryo, and achieve pregnancy [53].

Summary

The field of IVF was developed dramatically during the last 30 years and what was considered to be a miracle has become a common practice around the world. The field is still being developed in various directions to find solution to those couples who are infertile, to those who wish to become pregnant at an elder age, beyond the boundaries of nature, and to those who, due to medical reasons, need to delay the time of procreation.

British physiologist Robert Edwards, whose work led to the first "test-tube baby", won the 2010 Nobel prize for medicine or physiology. As many as 4 million babies have been born since the first IVF baby in 1978 as a result of the techniques Edwards developed, together with a now-deceased colleague, Patrick Steptoe.

We can expect further developments in the drug development, reduce the difficulties involved in stimulation of the ovaries moving into natural cycles, and obviously find a way to define the best embryo for replacement which might give the patients the highest chance to become pregnant.

References

1. History of IVF—the milestones. 2010. www.IVF-Worldwide.com/ivf-history.html. Accessed 20 Nov 2010.
2. Chang MC. Fertilization of rabbit ova in vitro. Nature. 1959;184 Suppl 7:466–7.
3. Edwards RG, Donahue RP, Baramki TA, Jones Jr HW. Preliminary attempts to fertilize human oocytes matured in vitro. Am J Obstet Gynecol. 1966;15(96):192–200.
4. De Kretzer D, Dennis P, Hudson B, et al. Transfer of a human zygote. Lancet. 1973;2:728–9.
5. Steptoe PC, Edwards RG. Reimplantation of a human embryo with subsequent tubal pregnancy. Lancet. 1976;1:880–2.
6. Steptoe PC, Edwards RG. Birth after the reimplantation of a human embryo. Lancet. 1978;2:366.
7. Lopata A, Johnston IW, Hoult IJ, Speirs AI. Pregnancy following intrauterine implantation of an embryo obtained by in vitro fertilization of a preovulatory egg. Fertil Steril. 1980;33:117–20.
8. Szollosi D, Mandelbaum J, Plachot M, Salat-Baroux J, Cohen J. Ultrastructure of the human preovulatory oocyte. J In Vitro Fert Embryo Transf. 1986;3:232–42.
9. Trounson AO, Leeton JF, Wood C, Webb J, Wood J. Pregnancies in humans by fertilization in vitro and embryo transfer in the controlled ovulatory cycle. Science. 1981;8(212):681–2.
10. Fleming R, Adam AH, Barlow DH, Black WP, MacNaughton MC, Coutts JR. A new systematic treatment for infertile women with abnormal hormone profiles. Br J Obstet Gynaecol. 1982;89:80–3.
11. Porter RN, Smith W, Craft IL, Abdulwahid NA, Jacobs HS. Induction of ovulation for in-vitro fertilisation using buserelin and gonadotropins. Lancet. 1984;2:1284–5.
12. Gonen Y, Jacobson W, Casper RF. Gonadotropin suppression with oral contraceptives before in vitro fertilization. Fertil Steril. 1990;53:282–7.
13. Casper RF, Wilson E, Collins JA, Brown SF, Parker JA. Enhancement of human implantation by exogenous chorionic gonadotropin. Lancet. 1983;2:1191.
14. Frydman R, Cornel C, de Ziegler D, Taieb J, Spitz IM, Bouchard P. Prevention of premature luteinizing hormone and progesterone rise with a gonadotropin-releasing hormone antagonist, Nal-Glu, in controlled ovarian hyperstimulation. Fertil Steril. 1991;56:923–7.
15. Itskovitz-Eldor J, Kol S, Mannaerts B, Coelingh Bennink H. First established pregnancy after controlled ovarian hyperstimulation with recombinant follicle stimulating hormone and the gonadotrophin-releasing hormone antagonist ganirelix (Org 37462). Hum Reprod. 1998;13: 294–5.
16. Germond M, Dessole S, Senn A, Loumaye E, Howles C, Beltrami V. Successful in-vitro fertilisation and embryo transfer after treatment with recombinant human FSH. Lancet. 1992; 339:1170.
17. Devroey P, van Steirteghem A, Mannaerts B, Bennink HC. Successful in-vitro fertilisation and embryo transfer after treatment with recombinant human FSH. Lancet. 1992;339:1170.
18. Agrawal R, West C, Conway GS, Page ML, Jacobs HS. Pregnancy after treatment with three recombinant gonadotropins. Lancet. 1997;349:29–30.
19. Emperaire JC, Ruffié A, Audebert AJ. Ovulation induction by endogenous LH released by the administration of an LHRH agonist after follicular stimulation for in vitro fertilization. J Gynecol Obstet Biol Reprod (Paris). 1992;21:489–94.
20. Chian RC, Gülekli B, Buckett WM, Tan SL. Priming with human chorionic gonadotrophin before retrieval of immature oocytes in women with infertility due to the polycystic ovary syndrome. N Engl J Med. 1999;341:1624–6.
21. Mohr LR, Trounson AO. The use of fluorescein diacetate to assess embryo viability in the mouse. J Reprod Fertil. 1980;58:189–96.
22. Quinn P, Kerin JF, Warnes GM. Improved pregnancy rate in human in vitro fertilization with the use of a medium based on the composition of human tubal fluid. Fertil Steril. 1985;44:493–8.
23. Gardner DK, Schoolcraft WB, Wagley L, Schlenker T, Stevens J, Hesla J. A prospective randomized trial of blastocyst culture and transfer in in-vitro fertilization. Hum Reprod. 1998; 13:3434–40.

24. Jones GM, Trounson AO, Gardner DK, Kausche A, Lolatgis N, Wood C. Evolution of a culture protocol for successful blastocyst development and pregnancy. Hum Reprod. 1998;13:169–77.
25. Ali J, Shahata MA, Al-Natsha SD. Formulation of a protein-free medium for human assisted reproduction. Hum Reprod. 2000;15:145–56.
26. Roh SI, Dodds WG, Park JM, Awadalla SG, Friedman CI, Kim MH. In vitro fertilization with concurrent pelvic reconstructive surgery. Fertil Steril. 1988;49:96–9.
27. Lenz S, Lauritsen JG. Ultrasonically guided percutaneous aspiration of human follicles under local anesthesia: a new method of collecting oocytes for in vitro fertilization. Fertil Steril. 1982;38:673–7.
28. Gleicher N, Friberg J, Fullan N, Giglia RV, Mayden K, Kesky T, Siegel I. EGG retrieval for in vitro fertilisation by sonographically controlled vaginal culdocentesis. Lancet. 1983;2:508–9.
29. Wikland M, Enk L, Hamberger L. Transvesical and transvaginal approaches for the aspiration of follicles by use of ultrasound. Ann N Y Acad Sci. 1985;442:182–94.
30. Strickler RC, Christianson C, Crane JP, Curato A, Knight AB, Yang V. Ultrasound guidance for human embryo transfer. Fertil Steril. 1985;43:54–61.
31. Feichtinger W, Kemeter P. Transvaginal sector scan sonography for needle guided transvaginal follicle aspiration and other applications in gynecologic routine and research. Fertil Steril. 1986;45(5):722–5.
32. Trounson AO, Mohr LR, Wood C, Leeton JF. Effect of delayed insemination on in-vitro fertilization, culture and transfer of human embryos. J Reprod Fertil. 1982;64:285–94.
33. Asch RH, Ellsworth LR, Balmaceda JP, Wong PC. Pregnancy after translaparoscopic gamete intrafallopian transfer. Lancet. 1984;2:1034–5.
34. Laws-King A, Trounson A, Sathananthan H, Kola I. Fertilization of human oocytes by microinjection of a single spermatozoon under the zona pellucida. Fertil Steril. 1987;48:637–42.
35. Ng SC, Bongso A, Ratnam SS, Sathananthan H, Chan CL, Wong PC, Hagglund L, Anandakumar C, Wong YC, Goh VH. Pregnancy after transfer of sperm under zona. Lancet. 1988;2:790.
36. Cohen J, Malter H, Fehilly C, Wright G, Elsner C, Kort H, Massey J. Implantation of embryos after partial opening of oocyte zona pellucida to facilitate sperm penetration. Lancet. 1988;2:162.
37. Palermo G, Joris H, Devroey P, Van Steirteghem AC. Pregnancies after intracytoplasmic injection of single spermatozoon into an oocyte. Lancet. 1992;4(340):17–8.
38. Cohen J, Scott R, Schimmel T, Levron J, Willadsen S. Birth of infant after transfer of anucleate donor oocyte cytoplasm into recipient eggs. Lancet. 1997;350:186–7.
39. Trounson A, Mohr L. Human pregnancy following cryopreservation, thawing and transfer of an eight-cell embryo. Nature. 1983;305:707–9.
40. Gordts S, Roziers P, Campo R, Noto V. Survival and pregnancy outcome after ultrarapid freezing of human embryos. Fertil Steril. 1990;53:469–72.
41. Kuleshova L, Gianaroli L, Magli C, et al. Birth following vitrification of a small number of human oocytes: case report. Hum Reprod. 1999;14:3077–9.
42. Porcu E, Fabbri R, Petracchi S, Ciotti PM, Flamigni C. Ongoing pregnancy after intracytoplasmic injection of testicular spermatozoa into cryopreserved human oocytes. Am J Obstet Gynecol. 1999;180:1044–5.
43. Bedaiwy MA, Hussein MR, Biscotti C, Falcone T. Cryopreservation of intact human ovary with its vascular pedicle. Hum Reprod. 2006;21:3258–69.
44. Porcu E, Venturoli S, Damiano G, Ciotti PM, Notarangelo L, Paradisi R, Moscarini M, Ambrosini G. Healthy twins delivered after oocyte cryopreservation and bilateral ovariectomy for ovarian cancer. Reprod Biomed Online. 2008;17:265–7.
45. Trounson A, Leeton J, Besanko M, Wood C, Conti A. Pregnancy established in an infertile patient after transfer of a donated embryo fertilised in vitro. Br Med J (Clin Res Ed). 1983;286(6368):835–8.
46. Buster JE, Bustillo M, Thorneycroft IH, Simon JA, Boyers SP, Marshall JR, Louw JA, Seed RW, Seed RG. Non-surgical transfer of in vivo fertilised donated ova to five infertile women: report of two pregnancies. Lancet. 1983;23(2):223–4.

47. Veeck LL, Wortham Jr JW, Witmyer J, Sandow BA, Acosta AA, Garcia JE, Jones GS, Jones Jr HW. Maturation and fertilization of morphologically immature human oocytes in a program of in vitro fertilization. Fertil Steril. 1983;39:594–602.
48. Barnes FL, Crombie A, Gardner DK, et al. Blastocyst development and birth after in-vitro maturation of human primary oocytes, intracytoplasmic sperm injection and assisted hatching. Hum Reprod. 1995;10:3243–7.
49. Cohen J, Simons RF, Fehilly CB, Fishel SB, Edwards RG, Hewitt J, Rowlant GF, Steptoe PC, Webster JM. Birth after replacement of hatching blastocyst cryopreserved at expanded blastocyst stage. Lancet. 1985;1:647.
50. Cohen J, Alikani M, Trowbridge J, Rosenwaks Z. Implantation enhancement by selective assisted hatching using zona drilling of human embryos with poor prognosis. Hum Reprod. 1992;7:685–91.
51. Handyside AH, Pattinson JK, Penketh RJ, Delhanty JD, Winston RM, Tuddenham EG. Biopsy of human preimplantation embryos and sexing by DNA amplification. Lancet. 1989;18(1):347–9.
52. Handyside AH, Kontogianni EH, Hardy K, Winston RM. Pregnancies from biopsied human preimplantation embryos sexed by Y-specific DNA amplification. Nature. 1990;19(344):768–70.
53. Verlinsky Y, Ginsberg N, Lifchez A, Valle J, Moise J, Strom CM. Analysis of the first polar body: preconception genetic diagnosis. Hum Reprod. 1990;5:826–9.

Part I
Sperm Processing Methods

Chapter 2
Sperm Processing for IVF

Ralf Henkel

Introduction

The birth of Louise Brown, the first human who was born on 25 July 1978 after the application of assisted reproduction techniques hallmarks the advent of the era of assisted reproductive technology (ART) in the human [1]. The first in vitro fertilization (IVF) cases, including that of Louise Brown, were performed to treat female tubal infertility. Subsequently, the demand for assisted reproduction techniques grew dramatically with the increasing number of men showing poor semen quality. Hence, scientists and clinicians were prompted to develop a wide array of different laboratory techniques focusing on the selection and enrichment of motile and functionally competent spermatozoa from the ejaculate. Since our understanding of the fertilization process and various sperm functions also extended significantly and the percentage of andrological cases with even poorer semen quality increased rapidly, the initial simple sperm separation techniques were not sufficient enough anymore, and new improved sperm separation techniques had to be developed.

Spermatozoa are not only the smallest but also the most polarized cell in the body (sperm head and a flagellum) that even fulfill their physiological functions, fertilization of oocytes, outside the body in a different individual, the female genital tract. Thus, the male germ cell is a very specialized and in certain aspects very sensitive cell. The latter is based on the sperm cell's special composition of its plasma membrane with an extraordinary high amount of poly-unsaturated fatty acids, particularly docosahexanoic acid with six double bonds in the molecule [2]. This feature is the foundation of the high membrane fluidity which is essential in maintaining the extreme polarization of the sperm and is required for normal sperm function [3]. Together with the sperm cell's lack of intrinsic reactive oxygen

R. Henkel, PhD (✉)
Department of Medical Bioscience, University of the Western Cape,
Modderdam Road, Bellville, Western Cape Province, Cape Town 7535, South Africa
e-mail: rhenkel@uwc.ac.za

Z.P. Nagy et al. (eds.), *Clinical Embryology: A Practical Guide*,
DOI 10.1007/978-1-4614-8376-2_2,

species (ROS)-scavenging systems due to a lack of cytoplasm, which is harboring repair mechanisms in any other cell, this renders the male germ cell extremely susceptible to oxidative stress by ROS [4] impairing the membrane function and resulting in loss of fertilizing potential [5, 6], serious damage of the DNA [7, 8] or even cell death.

In vivo, after normal ejaculation for sexual intercourse, spermatozoa depend on scavenging systems provided by the seminal plasma, which is the biological fluid that contains more antioxidant substances than any other physiological fluid does. The most important natural antioxidants in seminal plasma seem to be vitamin C and E [9, 10], superoxide dismutase [11], uric acid [12], glutathione [13], or the polyamine spermine that acts directly as a free radical scavenger [14]. If these protective substances are removed by means of any sperm separation technique, this can cause severe damage to the sperm cell and its membranes since sperm functions like motility or acrosome reaction are basically membrane functions. This damage is set by ROS either by the sperm cells themselves or leukocytes [15–17], which produce about 1,000 times more ROS than spermatozoa [18, 19].

On the other hand, even the extreme polarization of the male germ cell can be a direct target of damage through excessive centrifugation, resuspension, and vortexing of semen samples [15 16 20] as the mechanical stress imposed on the sperm can be harmful to the cell and its functions leading not only to decreased percentages of motile and vital sperm but also to a reduced mitochondrial membrane potential, which is essential for normal sperm function [21–23].

Sperm Processing Methods

In vivo, separation of motile sperm most capable of fertilizing oocytes from immotile sperm, debris, seminal plasma, and leukocytes is taking place in the female genital tract by active migration through the cervical mucus [24]. Yet, this process does not only separate motile and potentially fertile sperm, but it also prepares and enables male germ cells for the fertilization process by means of fundamental physiological changes called capacitation. In turn, the capacitation process involves, among others, changes in the motility pattern, metabolism, and the removal of cholesterol from the plasma membrane leading changed fluidity of the sperm plasma membrane, eventually enabling the sperm to undergo acrosome reaction and thus penetrate and fertilize oocytes [25–29].

The first sperm separation methods that were developed only comprised of one or two washing procedures to eliminate seminal plasma with subsequent resuspension of the male germ cells [30]. Following these first reports on human sperm processing, more sophisticated methods were developed in order to obtain sufficient amounts of motile, functionally competent spermatozoa for IVF, one of them being a swim-up procedure from a washed cell pellet.

Except for the first washing procedures, modern sperm processing techniques can be differentiated in migration, filtration, and density-gradient centrifugation. While for all migration techniques (conventional swim-up and migration-sedimentation), the sperm cells' most obvious feature, self-propelled movement, is an essential prerequisite; the separation principle in the filtration and density-gradient centrifugation techniques is based on a combination of the sperms' own motility and their adherence to filtration matrices and the retention at phase borders, respectively.

Apart from possible financial considerations, sperm physiology and the physiology of the fertilization process have to be taken into account for any method of assisted reproduction in order to better select functional sperm or better protect and "preserve" sperm functions from damages caused by the separation process.

Criteria for a "good" sperm selection are as follows:

- Elimination of seminal plasma, decapacitation factors, and debris
- Elimination/reduction of dysfunctional and ROS-producing sperm
- Elimination/reduction of leukocytes
- Elimination/reduction of bacteria
- Enrichment of functional sperm in terms of motility, DNA integrity, acrosome reaction, and normal sperm morphology
- Cost-effectiveness
- Easy and quick to perform
- Allow processing of larger volumes of ejaculates

However, since none of the different methods available meets all the criteria, it is mandatory for every Andrology laboratory/IVF unit to be able to perform a variety of different sperm separation methods having the individual circumstances of the patients as first priority in mind.

Liquefaction of Ejaculates and Viscous Ejaculates

An essential requirement for any sperm preparation method to be performed is that the semen is liquid. Normally, human semen liquefies after 15–30 min, and these ejaculates can directly be subjected to a sperm processing technique. In the laboratory, semen liquefaction is normally performed by placing the semen sample for 30 min into an incubator at 37°C. However, if the ejaculate does not liquefy after 60 min, which can be the case in about 10% of infertile patients [31], seminal viscosity remains high and can severely interfere with sperm motility resulting in poor yield of motile sperm after sperm separation.

Semen viscosity, which is sometimes referred to as "consistency," can be tested by means of gently aspirating a semen sample into a Pasteur pipette and then allowing the ejaculate dropping out. Normally, the seminal fluid is running out in discrete drops. Threads longer than about 2 cm are indicative of high viscosity and poor liquefaction, i.e., viscosipathy [32]. Since such ejaculates cannot well be processed, liquefaction can be achieved by enzymatic digestion using bromelain (1 mg/mL) [32] or a small spatula tip of approx. 2–5 mg crystalline α(alpha)-chymotrypsin to be mixed into the semen and incubated for 15–30 min at room temperature [33].

However, one still has to consider that these enzymes might be harmful to the sperm or oocyte and have to be removed by washing procedures as soon as possible. Alternatively, viscous semen can also be mixed with IVF medium in order to decrease its viscosity.

NB: Recommendations to force viscous seminal fluid through 18 or 23 gauge needles should be refrained from since such procedure can severely damage sperm.

Swim-Up

Since the introduction of the so-called conventional swim-up procedure by Mahadevan and Baker [34], this method has been successfully used in many IVF units around the world with excellent fertilization rates and is still in use for all techniques in assisted reproduction including intrauterine insemination (IUI) and IVF. This method is simple and cheap and does not require sophisticated equipment or highly specialized skills.

Procedure

Typically, 1 mL of the liquefied semen is mixed with 4 mL of IVF medium containing 10 mg/mL serum albumin or 10% inactivated serum and centrifuged for 10 min at 300×*g*. Then, the supernatant is carefully taken off with a pipette and discarded. For this step, it is essential that the surface of the pellet is not disturbed or that parts of the pellet are sucked into the pipette as this would result in a decreased yield and motility in the sperm suspension. Subsequently, fresh medium is layered very carefully by letting 0.5–1 mL slowly rinse down the inner surface of the test tube tilted at an angle of about 45° on top of the pellet and incubated for 30–60 min at 37°C in an incubator. After this incubation period, the test tube is taken out of the incubator, and the medium is carefully aspirated into a pipette again without disturbing the pellet which can become quite soft during the incubation period. Ideally, sperm fractions with >90% motility can be obtained using this technique.

NB: Considering that the success of the swim-up technique strongly depends on the initial motility in the ejaculate and the size and quality of the surface of the pellet obtained after the centrifugation step, the yield of this technique is rather limited. Therefore, it is advisable to run two or three or more tubes from one semen sample at the same time in order to increase the yield. Since the use of medium that does not contain macromolecules like albumin is detrimental to spermatozoa, it is not advisable to use unsupplemented medium as it might result in sperm sticking to the surface of the test tube leading to a lower yield and motility.

Advantages/Disadvantages of the Technique

Normally, this sperm selection method recovers a very clean fraction of highly motile sperm that can directly be used for insemination in IVF or for IUI. For the latter, it is important that not more than 0.5 mL of the isolated sperm fraction after swim-up is inseminated into the uterus as higher volumes might leak out.

With regard to the quality of the ejaculates, the conventional swim-up technique is rather restricted to good quality ejaculates with high sperm concentration and good motility. With regard to the application of the swim-up for artificial insemination, it is not only important to know that the yield is rather low but also that sperm can be massively damaged by ROS because of the close cell-to-cell contact during the centrifugation step. This is particularly the case in patients with male genital tract infections. If, despite good motility and sperm count in the ejaculate, the expected sperm concentration is less than 10^6/mL after the swim-up, one should consider the effect of ROS.

Migration-Sedimentation

The migration-sedimentation technique, which was originally developed by Tea et al. [35], is a more sophisticated method of sperm processing. Like the swim-up technique, it is based on the sperm cells' own motility, yet combined with a sedimentation step. However, special, commercially available "Tea-Jondet tubes" have to be used. Contrary to the conventional swim-up method, sperm swim up directly from the liquefied semen sample into the supernatant medium, deposit, and accumulate into the inner cone of the tube. Since such a migration technique directly from the semen is the gentlest method of sperm processing, several modifications have been developed, which are even used for ICSI [36–38].

Procedure

In order to process semen for IVF using the migration-sedimentation technique, the "Tea-Jondet tubes" are filled up with 1–2 mL IVF medium supplemented with 10 mg/mL serum albumin or 10% inactivated serum. The overlaying medium must not be too high above the edge of the inner cone. Then, approx. 0.5 mL of liquefied semen is placed in the outer ring around the cone carefully paying attention that no ejaculate is running into the inner cone. After incubating the tubes for 1–2 h at 37°C, the supernatant medium, including the medium in the inner cone, is carefully aspirated with a Pasteur pipette without aspirating remnants of the ejaculate. Typically, sperm fractions with motility rates of more than 90% can be obtained and after adjustment of sperm concentration directly used for insemination.

For the use in ICSI, the whole liquefied ejaculate (or part of it) of the respective patients is centrifuged for 10–15 min at 300×*g*, and the supernatant except for about 0.3–0.5 mL which contains the sperm is discarded. This "concentrated" ejaculate is filled into the "Tea-Jondet tubes" as described above and incubated. In order to obtain higher numbers of motile sperm, processing can be carried out in duplicate.

NB: Like in the swim-up method, the success of isolating motile sperm using migration-sedimentation is dependent on initial quality of the ejaculate. For its application in ICSI, it is, however, important that the semen must *not* be diluted with medium for centrifugation. The seminal plasma is then still able to have at least some protection against oxidative stress.

Advantages/Disadvantages of the Technique

Migration-sedimentation is one of the gentlest methods of processing sperm and usually results in a very clean fraction of highly motile, functional sperm.

Considering the very low recovery rate in its original protocol, this method is rather restricted to higher quality ejaculates. The technique is also a bit more expensive than the conventional swim-up and requires advanced skills.

Glass Wool Filtration

Using a different approach Paulson and Polakoski [39] succeeded to separate motile from immotile sperm by means of densely packed glass wool fibers. The principle for the separation of motile spermatozoa from immotile, debris and leukocytes is not only rested in the self-propelled movement of the sperm cells but also on a filtration effect of the glass wool fibers, for which both are responsible, a mechanical retention of the bigger particles in the ejaculate as well as the adhesion of these particles to the surface of the glass fibers [40]. Hence, the kind of glass wool used plays a cardinal role in the success of this technique, and it is not possible to use any kind of glass wool for sperm processing [41]. This adhesion and filtration process is a feature of glass wool filtration that may contribute to the selection of spermatozoa with matured nuclei, i.e., with good chromatin condensation [42].

Recently, Grunewald et al. [43] developed a glass wool, which chemically activated to bind annexin V to the surface of the glass wool fibers. Annexin V binds to externalized phosphatidyl serine and is an indicator of apoptotic cells [44, 45]. While the conventional glass wool filtration is in routine use in many IVF centers, clinical data supporting the efficiency of this new molecularly activated glass wool remains to be seen.

Procedure

Useful glass wool is available from Manville Fiber Glass Corp. (code 112; Denver, CO) or glass wool columns from TransMIT (SpermFertil®; Giessen, Germany). While from the former, 15–30 mg of glass wool has to be loosely packed in a Pasteur pipette or small syringe, the latter are sterile, ready-to-use glass wool columns. In order to eliminate loose glass particles, both columns have to be flushed carefully with at least 2 mL sterile IVF medium. Subsequently, the glass wool column must be put on a new sterile test tube and filled with 1–3 mL *liquefied* fresh semen. Filtration should take place in an incubator at 37°C with occasional visual control in order to avoid the column falling dry. Immediately after the semen has passed through the glass wool, the column is washed with 0.5 mL fresh IVF medium. Finally, the filtrated semen will be diluted in the ratio 1:5 with fresh IVF medium and centrifuged for 10 min at 300×*g*. The supernatant will then have to be carefully discarded and the pellet resuspended in fresh IVF medium. For better washing of sperm, this procedure can be repeated. This sperm suspension can then be used for insemination after adjusting sperm concentration.

NB: As high concentrations of "particles" might block the column and prevent semen from being filtrated properly, the amount of semen used depends on sperm and debris concentration. Therefore, in cases of high "particle" concentrations, the ejaculate can be divided on 2–3 glass wool columns for filtration and the filtrates eventually be combined. For gentle sperm processing using glass wool filtration, it is fundamentally important that the sperm separation takes place first. Only afterward, washing of sperm should take place.

Advantages/Disadvantages of the Technique

Principally, glass wool filtration is an easy to perform technique, which results in the recovery of spermatozoa with good motility. Since the whole ejaculate can be filtrated, ejaculates from patients with oligozoospermia can be processed. In addition, the technique eliminates up to 90% of leukocytes contaminating the semen and therefore reduces ROS significantly [46]. As a disadvantage, it can be brought bear that the filtration does not result in as clean fractions as the swim-up procedure does. There is always some debris or immotile sperm that pass through the mesh.

Density-Gradient Centrifugation with Different Media

Density-gradient centrifugation is another method for gentle sperm separation. Its principle is based on the ability of motile sperm cells to penetrate concentration boundaries in direction of the centrifugation force. This penetration is quicker the faster sperm swim; thus, highly progressively swimming sperm are reaching the bottom of a centrifuging test tube quicker than immotile or poorly motile sperm, which are retained at the boundaries of interphases.

The first reports employing density-gradient centrifugation to isolate progressively motile human spermatozoa date back to 1981 and 1983 [47, 48]. Initially, Percoll®, a medium containing polyvinylpyrrolidone-coated silica particles, was used to create media with different densities. Since 1996, however, Percoll® has been withdrawn from the market for use in assisted reproduction because of its possible risk of being contaminated with endotoxins [49, 50]. Yet, other density media have emerged from the market with good results in separating highly motile sperm, competent for fertilization. These new density media are based on silane-coated silica particles and have been proven to have very low toxicity. The most commonly used new density media are SilSelect® (FertiPro N.V., Beernem, Belgium), SupraSperm® (MediCult, Jyllinge, Denmark), PureSperm® (NidaCon International AB, Mölndal, Sweden), or ISolate® (Irvine Scientific, Santa Ana, CA, USA).

Like for glass wool filtration, the selection of nuclear matured sperm in terms of chromatin condensation has been described for density-gradient centrifugation [51, 52]. Moreover, while recent studies showed that processing of sperm with PureSperm® resulted in significantly lower percentages of sperm exhibiting DNA damage and extended survival rate [53, 54], older studies using Percoll® rather revealed adverse effects on the sperm DNA [55, 56]. Moreover, for the high motility fraction of density gradient prepared spermatozoa lower percentages of sperm with externalized phosphatidyl serine and disrupted mitochondrial membrane potential have been described [57].

Procedure

There are two different kinds of density gradients that can be performed, the continuous or the discontinuous. Nowadays, most labs are using the discontinuous gradient employing a two-step gradient consisting of 40% (45%) and 80% (90%) density medium. These density gradients can either be bought ready to use or can be made from high-concentration stock solutions. Depending on the product used, the two-step gradient is prepared by *carefully* overlaying 1–2 mL of the high-density solution (80%/90%) with 1–2 mL of the low-density solution (40%/45%). A distinct phase border between the two layers must be visible. After the gradient is equilibrated in 5% CO_2 at 37°C in an incubator, 1 mL of the liquefied and thoroughly mixed semen sample is *carefully* dispensed on top of the prepared gradient. Again, a distinct phase border should be visible. Subsequently, the gradient is centrifuged for 20–30 min at 300–400×*g*.

After this centrifugation step, the soft pellet can be obtained in two ways. Firstly, by carefully aspirating the pellet with a Pasteur pipette. By applying this procedure, nothing of the overlaying layers should be aspirated. Secondly, the top layers of the gradient can be removed and discarded first, and then the pellet can be aspirated and placed into a clean test tube. This sample has then to be resuspended in 3–5 mL fresh sperm preparation or IVF medium and centrifuged 10 min at 300–400×*g* again. This procedure has to be repeated twice. After adjusting sperm concentration, the finally resulting sperm suspension can be used for insemination.

NB: Overloading the gradient with either too much volume or a too high number of "particles" (spermatozoa and/or debris) will result in poor sperm separation. On the other hand, in cases of oligozoospermia or asthenozoospermia, more than one test tube can be prepared in order to obtain a sufficient number of competent sperm for fertilization.

Advantages/Disadvantages of the Technique

Normally, density gradient centrifugation results in a good and clean fraction of highly motile spermatozoa with good recovery. Even ejaculates with low sperm counts from patients with oligozoospermia can be processed. The possibility to process the full volume of the ejaculate increases the yield. Considering that the technique eliminates leukocytes to a large extent, ROS are significantly reduced.

The formation of good interphases between the different media gradients is essential for the quality of the sperm separation and needs special attention during the preparation. After the density-gradient centrifugation the "soft pellet" containing the high-quality sperm has to be washed in order to eliminate the density medium. Thus, an additional centrifugation step is required.

References

1. Edwards RG, Steptoe PC, Purdy JM. Establishing full term human pregnancies using cleaving embryos grown *in vitro*. Br J Obstet Gynaecol. 1980;87:737–56.
2. Zalata AA, Christophe AB, Depuydt CE, et al. The fatty acid composition of phospholipids of spermatozoa from infertile patients. Mol Hum Reprod. 1998;4:111–8.
3. Khosrowbeygi A, Zarghami N. Fatty acid composition of human spermatozoa and seminal plasma levels of oxidative stress biomarkers in subfertile males. Prostaglandins Leukot Essent Fatty Acids. 2007;77:117–21.
4. Aitken RJ, Clarkson JS, Fishel S. Generation of reactive oxygen species, lipid peroxidation, and human sperm function. Biol Reprod. 1989;40:183–97.
5. Aitken RJ, Clarkson JS. Significance of reactive oxygen species and antioxidants in defining the efficacy of sperm preparation techniques. J Androl. 1988;9:367–76.
6. Vigil P, Wöhler C, Bustos-Obregón E, et al. Assessment of sperm function in fertile and infertile men. Andrologia. 1994;26:55–60.
7. Lopes S, Jurisicova A, Sun JG, et al. Reactive oxygen species: potential cause for DNA fragmentation in human spermatozoa. Hum Reprod. 1998;13:896–900.
8. Henkel R, Hajimohammad M, Stalf T, et al. Influence of deoxyribonucleic acid damage on fertilization and pregnancy. Fertil Steril. 2004;81:965–72.
9. Chow CK. Vitamin E and oxidative stress. Free Radic Biol Med. 1991;11:215–32.

10. Niki E. Action of ascorbic acid as scavenger of active and stable oxygen radicals. Am J Clin Nutr. 1991;54:1119S–24.
11. Kobayashi T, Miyazaki T, Natori M, et al. Protective role of superoxide dismutase in human sperm motility: superoxide dismutase activity and lipid peroxide in human seminal plasma and spermatozoa. Hum Reprod. 1991;6:987–91.
12. Grootveldt M, Halliwell B. Measurement of allantoin and uric acid in human body fluids. Biochem J. 1987;242:803–8.
13. Li TK. The glutathione and thiol content of mammalian spermatozoa and seminal plasma. Biol Reprod. 1975;12:641–6.
14. Ha HC, Sirisoma NS, Kuppusamy P, et al. The natural polyamine spermine functions directly as a free radical scavenger. Proc Natl Acad Sci USA. 1998;95:11140–5.
15. Alvarez JG, Lasso JL, Blasco L, et al. Centrifugation of human spermatozoa induces sublethal damage; separation of human spermatozoa from seminal plasma by a dextran swim-up procedure without centrifugation extends their motile life. Hum Reprod. 1993;8:1087–92.
16. Agarwal A, Ikemoto I, Loughlin KR. Effect of sperm washing on levels of reactive oxygen species in semen. Arch Androl. 1994;33:157–62.
17. Henkel R, Kierspel E, Stalf T, et al. Effect of reactive oxygen species produced by spermatozoa and leukocytes on sperm functions in non-leukocytospermic patients. Fertil Steril. 2005;83:635–42.
18. Ford WCL. The role of oxygen free radicals in the pathology of human spermatozoa: implications of IVF. In: Matson PL, Lieberman BA, editors. Clinical IVF forum; current views in assisted reproduction. Manchester: Manchester University Press; 1990. p. 123–39.
19. de Lamirande E, Gagnon C. Capacitation-associated production of superoxide anion by human spermatozoa. Free Radic Biol Med. 1995;18:487–95.
20. Mortimer D. Sperm preparation techniques and iatrogenic failures of in vitro fertilization. Hum Reprod. 1991;6:173–6.
21. Marchetti C, Obert G, Deffosez A, et al. Study of mitochondrial membrane potential, reactive oxygen species, DNA fragmentation and cell viability by flow cytometry in human sperm. Hum Reprod. 2002;17:1257–65.
22. Meseguer M, Garrido N, Martinez-Conejero JA, et al. Relationship between standard semen parameters, calcium, cholesterol contents, and mitochondrial activity in ejaculated spermatozoa from fertile and infertile males. J Assist Reprod Genet. 2004;21:445–51.
23. Henkel R, Fransman WO, Hipler UC, Wiegand C, Schreiber G, Menkveld R, Weitz F, Fisher D. Typha capensis (Rohrb.)N.E.Br. (bulrush) extract scavenges free radicals, inhibits collagenase activity and affects human sperm motility and mitochondrial membrane potential in vitro – A pilot study. Andrologia. 2011 Jul 6. doi: 10.1111/j.1439-0272.2011.01179.x. [Epub ahead of print].
24. Mortimer D. Sperm Transport in the Human Female Reproductive Tract. In: Finn CA, editor. Oxford Reviews of Reproductive Biology, vol. 5. Oxford: Oxford University Press; 1989. p. 30.
25. Yanagimachi R, Bhattacharyya A. Acrosome-reacted guinea pig spermatozoa become fusion competent in the presence of extracellular potassium ions. J Exp Zool. 1988;248(3):354–60.
26. Harrison RAP. Capacitation mechanisms, and the role of capacitation as seen in eutherian mammals. Reprod Fertil Dev. 1996;8:581–894.
27. de Lamirande E, Leclerc P, Gagnon C. Capacitation as a regulatory event that primes spermatozoa for the acrosome reaction and fertilization. Mol Hum Reprod. 1997;3:175–94.
28. Mortimer ST, Swan MA, Mortimer D. Effect of seminal plasma on capacitation and hyperactivation in human spermatozoa. Hum Reprod. 1998;13:2139–46.
29. De Jonge C. Biological basis for human capacitation. Hum Reprod Update. 2005;11:205–14.
30. Lopata A, Brown JB, Leeton JF, et al. In vitro fertilization of preovulatory oocytes and embryo transfer in infertile patients treated with clomiphene and human chorionic gonadotropin. Fertil Steril. 1978;30:27–35.
31. Jequier AM. Male Infertility. Carlton, Australia: A Guide for the Clinician. Blackwell Science Pty Ltd.; 2000.

32. World Health Organization. Laboratory Manual for the Examination of Human Semen and Sperm–Cervical Mucus Interaction. New York: Cambridge University Press; 1999.
33. Köhn FM, Schuppe HC, Jung A, et al. Das Spermiogramm—Praktische Anleitungen. 2. Auflage, CD-ROM, Justus-Liebig-Universität, Gieβen. 2002. www.agma.med.uni-giessen.de/spermiogramm
34. Mahadevan M, Baker G. Assessment and preparation of semen for in vitro fertilization. In: Wood C, Trounson A, editors. Clinical in vitro fertilization. Berlin: Springer; 1984. p. 83–97.
35. Tea NT, Jondet M, Scholler R. A migration-gravity sedimentation method for collecting motile spermatozoa from human semen. In: Harrison RF, Bonnar J, Thompson W, editors. In vitro fertilization, embryo transfer and early pregnancy. Lancaster: MTP; 1984. p. 117–20.
36. Sanchez R, Stalf T, Khanaga O, et al. Sperm selection methods for intracytoplasmic sperm injection (ICSI) in andrological patients. J Assist Reprod Genet. 1996;13:110–5.
37. Zavos PM, Abou-Abdallah M, Aslanis P, et al. Use of the multi-ZSC one-step standardized swim-up method: recovery of high-quality spermatozoa for intrauterine insemination or other forms of assisted reproductive technologies. Fertil Steril. 2000;74:834–5.
38. Hinting A, Lunardhi H. Better sperm selection for intracytoplasmic sperm injection with the side migration technique. Andrologia. 2001;33:343–6.
39. Paulson JD, Polakoski KL. A glass wool column procedure for removing extraneous material from the human ejaculate. Fertil Steril. 1977;28:178–81.
40. Sanchez R, Concha M, Ichikawa T, et al. Glass wool filtration reduces reactive oxygen species by elimination of leukocytes in oligozoospermic patients with leukocytospermia. J Assist Reprod Genet. 1996;13:489–94.
41. Henkel RR, Schill WB. Sperm preparation for ART. Reprod Biol Endocrinol. 2003;1:108.
42. Henkel R, Franken DR, Lombard CJ, et al. The selective capacity of glass wool filtration for normal chromatin condensed human spermatozoa: a possible therapeutic modality for male factor cases? J Assist Reprod Genet. 1994;11:395–400.
43. Grunewald S, Miska W, Miska G, et al. Molecular glass wool filtration as a new tool for sperm preparation. Hum Reprod. 2007;22:1405–12.
44. Oosterhuis GJ, Mulder AB, Kalsbeek-Batenburg E, et al. Measuring apoptosis in human spermatozoa: a biological assay for semen quality? Fertil Steril. 2000;74:245–50.
45. Said T, Agarwal A, Grunewald S, et al. Selection of nonapoptotic spermatozoa as a new tool for enhancing assisted reproduction outcomes: an in vitro model. Biol Reprod. 2006;74:530–7.
46. Henkel R, Ichikawa T, Sanchez R, et al. Differentiation of ejaculates in which reactive oxygen species are generated by spermatozoa or leukocytes. Andrologia. 1997;29:295–301.
47. Gorus FK, Pipeleers DG. A rapid method for the fractionation of human spermatozoa according to their progressive motility. Fertil Steril. 1981;35:662–5.
48. Arcidiacono A, Walt H, Campana A, et al. The use of Percoll gradients for the preparation of subpopulations of human spermatozoa. Int J Androl. 1983;6:433–45.
49. Pharmacia Biotech. Important notice: Percoll® not to be used in assisted reproduction technologies in humans. Pharmacia Biotech Inc., Piscataway, NJ, Dec 12, 1996.
50. Strehler E, Baccetti B, Sterzik K, et al. Detrimental effects of polyvinylpyrrolidone on the ultrastructure of spermatozoa (Notulae seminologicae 13). Hum Reprod. 1998;13:120–3.
51. Hammadeh ME, Kühnen A, Amer AS, et al. Comparison of sperm preparation methods: effect on chromatin and morphology recovery rates and their consequences on the clinical outcome after in vitro fertilization embryo transfer. Int J Androl. 2001;24:360–8.
52. Zini A, Gabriel MS, Zhang X. The histone to protamine ratio in human spermatozoa: comparative study of whole and processed semen. Fertil Steril. 2007;87:217–9.
53. Morrell JM, Moffatt O, Sakkas D, et al. Reduced senescence and retained nuclear DNA integrity in human spermatozoa prepared by density gradient centrifugation. J Assist Reprod Genet. 2004;21:217–22.
54. Ricci G, Perticarari S, Boscolo R, et al. Semen preparation methods and sperm apoptosis: swim-up versus gradient-density centrifugation technique. Fertil Steril. 2009;91:632–8.

55. Zini A, Mak V, Phang D, et al. Potential adverse effect of semen processing on human sperm deoxyribonucleic acid integrity. Fertil Steril. 1999;72:496–9.
56. Zini A, Nam RK, Mak V, et al. Influence of initial semen quality on the integrity of human sperm DNA following semen processing. Fertil Steril. 2000;74:824–7.
57. Barroso G, Taylor S, Morshedi M, et al. Mitochondrial membrane potential integrity and plasma membrane translocation of phosphatidylserine as early apoptotic markers: a comparison of two different sperm subpopulations. Fertil Steril. 2006;85:149–54.

Chapter 3
PESA/TESA/TESE Sperm Processing

Sandro C. Esteves and Sidney Verza Jr.

Two major breakthroughs occurred in the area of male infertility only 2–3 years apart [1–3]. The first was the development of intracytoplasmic sperm injection (ICSI) for the treatment of male factor infertility due to severely abnormal semen quality [1]. The second was the extension of ICSI to azoospermic males and the demonstration that spermatozoa derived from either the epididymis or the testis were capable of normal fertilization and pregnancy [2, 3]. In the case of azoospermia, two totally different clinical situations exist, i.e., obstructive and nonobstructive azoospermia (NOA). In obstructive azoospermia (OA), spermatogenesis is normal, but a mechanical blockage exists in the genital tract, somewhere between the epididymis and the ejaculatory duct, or the epididymis and vas deferens are totally or partially absent. Causes of OA are acquired or congenital. Acquired OA may be due to vasectomy; failure of vasectomy reversal; postinfectious diseases; surgical procedures in the scrotal, inguinal, pelvic, or abdominal regions; and trauma. Congenital causes of OA include cystic fibrosis, congenital absence of the vas deferens (CAVD), ejaculatory duct or prostatic cysts, and Young's syndrome [4]. NOA comprises a spectrum of testicular histopathology resulting from various causes that include environmental toxins, medications, genetic and congenital abnormalities, varicocele, trauma, endocrinologic disorders, and idiopathic. Sperm can be easily obtained from men with OA whereas individuals exhibiting NOA have historically been the infertile men most difficult to treat [4, 5].

Several sperm retrieval methods have been developed to collect epididymal and testicular sperm in azoospermic men. It is out of our scope to discuss which technique is best to surgically retrieve sperm. As a general rule, either percutaneous

S.C. Esteves, MD, PhD (✉)
Androfert-Center for Male Reproduction, Campinas, São Paulo, Brazil
e-mail: s.esteves@androfert.com.br

S. Verza Jr., BSc, MSc
IVF Laboratory, Androfert-Center for Male Reproduction, Campinas, São Paulo, Brazil
e-mail: labfiv@androfert.com.br

Z.P. Nagy et al. (eds.), *Clinical Embryology: A Practical Guide*,
DOI 10.1007/978-1-4614-8376-2_3, © Springer Science+Business Media New York 2013

Table 3.1 Glossary of terms in sperm processing

ICSI. Intracytoplasmic sperm injection: a procedure in which a single spermatozoon is injected into the oocyte cytoplasm

Azoospermia. Absence of spermatozoa in the microscopic examination of the seminal fluid after centrifugation on at least two separate occasions

PESA. Percutaneous epididymal sperm aspiration: a procedure in which a needle is inserted into the epididymis to retrieve spermatozoa for use in an ICSI procedure

MESA. Microsurgical epididymal sperm aspiration: a microsurgical procedure used to aspirate spermatozoa directly from the epididymal tubules for use in an ICSI procedure

TESA. Testicular sperm aspiration: a procedure in which a needle is inserted into the testis in order to retrieve spermatozoa for use in an ICSI procedure

TESE. Testicular sperm extraction: operative removal of testicular tissue in an attempt to collect sperm for use in an ICSI procedure

Micro-TESE. Microdissection testicular sperm extraction: a microsurgical procedure used to dissect the seminiferous tubules within the testis in an attempt to identify areas of sperm production and extract spermatozoa for use in an ICSI procedure

Sperm processing. Laboratory techniques used to remove contaminants (cellular debris, microorganisms, red blood cells, etc.) and to select the best quality spermatozoa to be used in conjunction to assisted reproduction technology

Cryopreservation. The freezing process for storage of gametes or gonadal tissue at ultra-low temperature

(PESA) [6] or microsurgical epididymal sperm aspiration (MESA) [2] can be successfully used to retrieve sperm from the epididymis in men with OA. Testicular sperm aspiration (TESA) can be used to retrieve sperm from the testes either in men with OA who fail PESA or in those with NOA [6, 7]. Testicular sperm extraction (TESE) using single or multiple open biopsies [8–10] and, more recently, microsurgery (micro-TESE) are indicated for men with NOA [11–13] (Table 3.1).

Processing of surgically retrieved spermatozoa differs from the commonly used methods for processing ejaculates. Sperm processing should not only ease the selection of the best quality spermatozoa for ICSI but also optimize their fertilizing ability, whenever possible. The laboratory has a crucial role in the handling of these often compromised specimens, particularly in the cases of NOA and after the freeze–thawing process. In order to achieve their goals, laboratory personnel should (1) receive the best quality surgically retrieved specimen possible, with minimal or no contaminants such as red blood cells and noxious microorganisms, (2) minimize the iatrogenic cellular damage during sperm processing by mastering technical skills and controlling several factors, including centrifugation force and duration, exposure to ultraviolet light and temperature variation, laboratory air quality conditions, dilution and washing steps, quality of reagents, culture media, and disposable materials, and (3) improve the sperm fertilizing potential, if possible, by using stimulants or selecting viable sperm for ICSI when only immotile spermatozoa is available. In this chapter, our aims are to provide a step-by-step laboratory description of the commonly used methods for PESA/TESA/TESE sperm processing and identification of viable immotile sperm for ICSI, as well as to present our group's clinical results of ICSI using testicular and epididymal sperm. Finally, we critically discuss the tips and pitfalls of sperm processing techniques for surgically retrieved specimens.

Step-by-Step Protocol of the Laboratory Procedures

Materials, Equipments, Reagents, and IVF Laboratory Setup

Operating Room

- Sterile surgical gloves and syringes (1, 20 mL).
- 0.7 × 25 (22 G), 0.45 × 13 (26 G), and 1.2 × 40-mm (18 G; for TESA/TESE only) disposable needles.
- 2% Lidocaine hydrochloride solution.
- Heating block for test tubes (e.g.: Fisher, USA).
- Syringe holder (for TESA only, see Fig. 3.1).
- Operating microscope (e.g.: DF Vasconcelos, Brazil; for micro-TESE only).
- Microsurgery instruments (e.g.: ASSI, USA; for micro-TESE only).

IVF Laboratory

- 50 × 09-mm (e.g.: #351006, Falcon, USA) and 60 × 15-mm single well Petri dishes (e.g.: cat.#353037, Falcon, USA; for TESA/TESE only).
- Disposable serological pipettes (5.0 mL; e.g.: cat.#4051 Costar or cat.#356543 Falcon, USA).
- Pipettor 1–200 μL (e.g.: Gilson, France) and sterile tips (cat.#4804, Corning, USA).
- Pipetting device (e.g.: Pipette-aid, Drummond Scientific, USA).
- 6-mL sterile centrifuge polystyrene tubes with caps (e.g.: cat.#352003, Falcon, USA).
- 0.7 × 25-mm needles and tuberculin syringes (e.g.: BD, USA; for TESA/TESE only).
- Fine point permanent marker pen (e.g.: Sharpie, Sandford, USA).
- Injection micropipettes (e.g.: cat.#MIC-50-35; Humagen, USA).
- Laminar flow cabinet (e.g.: Veco, Brazil).
- Warming plates (e.g.: Tokai-heat, Japan).
- Stereomicroscope (e.g.: Leica GZ7, Switzerland).
- Centrifuge (e.g.: model 225; Fisher Scientific, USA).
- Inverted microscope (e.g.: Eclipse E400, Nikon, Japan) equipped with Hoffman modulation contrast and electrohydraulic micromanipulators (e.g.: Narishighe, Japan).

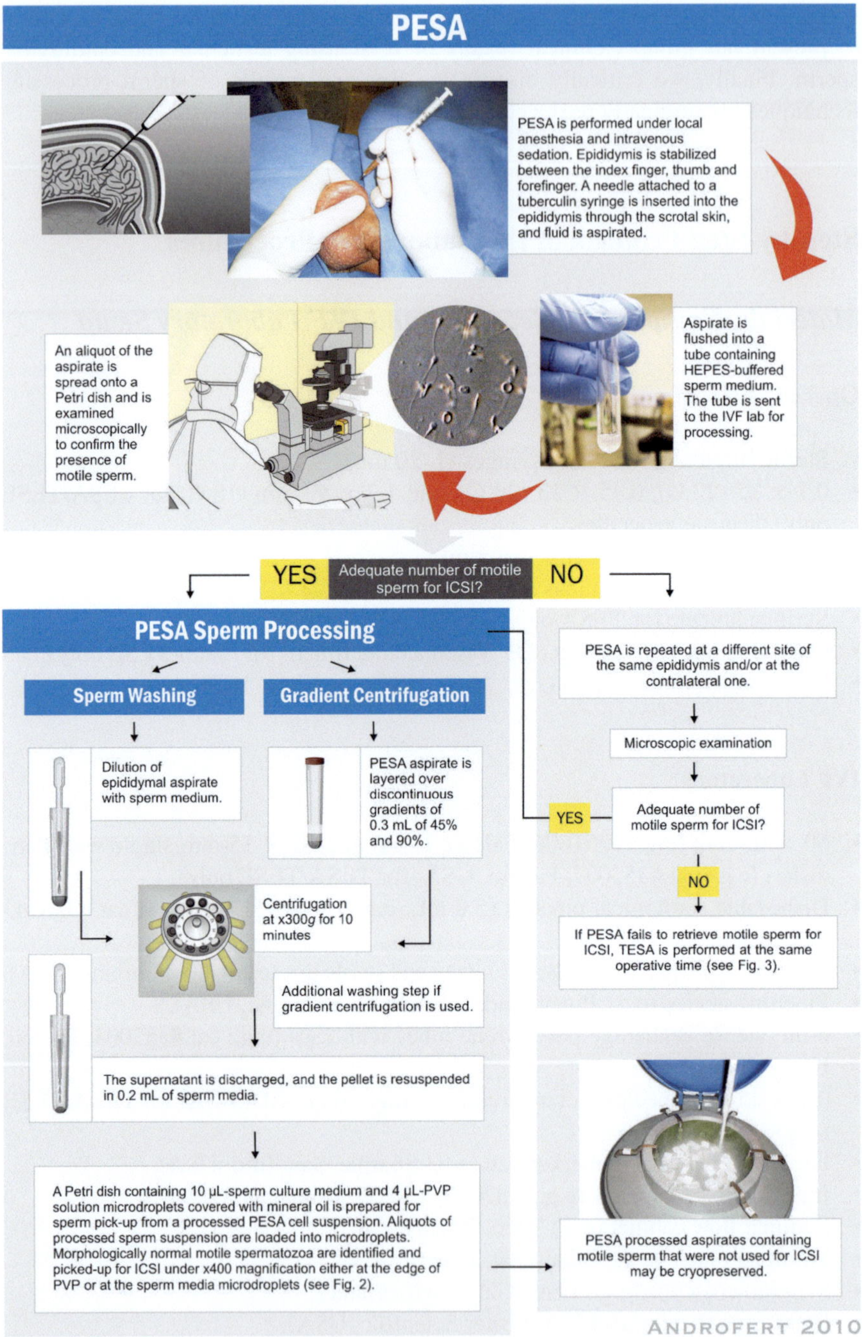

Fig. 3.1 PESA sperm processing. Flow chart illustrates PESA steps from the surgical procedure to the processing of epididymal aspirates for ICSI

- HEPES-buffered Human Tubal Fluid (e.g.: modified HTF culture medium, cat.#90126, Irvine Scientific, USA) and human serum albumin (e.g.: HSA, cat.#9988, Irvine Scientific, USA).
- Mineral oil (e.g.: #9305, Irvine Scientific, USA).
- PVP solution (e.g.: cat.#10111, Vitrolife, Sweden).
- Colloidal density gradient (e.g.: Isolate®, cat.#99264, Irvine Scientific, USA).

Laboratory Setup

Note: Use sterile handling conditions under a laminar flow cabinet or clean room environment during all laboratory steps.

- Prepare a 10 (for PESA) or 20 mL (TESA/TESE) HEPES-buffered protein-supplemented (5% HSA) sperm culture medium, and keep it at 37°C.
- Transfer a 5 mL aliquot of the prepared sperm culture medium to a 6-mL polystyrene tube and send it to the operating room (sperm media is used to flush the aspirating system before aspiration and to incubate epididymal aspirates or testicular specimens upon collection).
- Place two 50 × 09-mm Petri dishes on a warm surface (37°C) inside the laboratory workstation (for PESA only).
- Prepare four 2-well dishes by transferring 0.5 and 1.0 mL sperm medium aliquots to the inner- and outer-dish wells, respectively (for TESA/TESE only). Place two of them onto a warm surface (37°C) inside the workstation, and send the others to the operating room (for TESE only).
- Mount two tuberculin syringes connected with a 22-gauge needle (to be used as tools for mincing and squeezing seminiferous tubules in TESA/TESE processing).

PESA Sperm Processing

Surgical Technique

Note: PESA is performed under local anesthesia (at the spermatic cord level) in association with intravenous anaesthesia using propofol either at the day of oocyte retrieval or the day before.

- A 10 mL solution of 2% lidocaine is injected around the spermatic cord near the external inguinal ring upon patient unconsciousness is achieved. The epididymis is stabilized between the index finger, thumb, and forefinger while the testis is held with the palm of the hand.
- A 26-gauge needle attached to a 1-mL tuberculin syringe is inserted into the epididymis through the scrotal skin. Loupe-magnification is used to avoid injuring small vessels seen through the skin (Fig. 3.1).

- Negative pressure is created, and the tip of the needle is gently moved in and out within the epididymis until fluid enters the syringe. The amount of epididymal fluid obtained during aspiration is often minimal (~0.1 mL), except in cases of CAVD in which 0.3–1.0 mL may be aspirated.
- The needle is withdrawn from the epididymis, and the aspirate is flushed into a 0.5–1.0 mL 37°C sperm medium.
- The tube containing the epididymal aspirate is transferred to the IVF lab next door. PESA is repeated at a different site of the same epididymis (from cauda to caput) and/or at the contralateral one until adequate number of motile sperm is retrieved. If PESA fails to retrieve motile sperm for ICSI, TESA is performed at the same operative time (Fig. 3.1).

Sperm Processing

- Homogenize epididymal aspirate and sperm medium to avoid sperm agglutination (epididymal spermatozoa tend to agglutinate fast). Keep aspirate-containing tubes capped at 37°C.
- Place a 10–20 μL sperm suspension aliquot onto a Petri dish, and spread it as thin as possible using a micropipette tip. Examine the fluid under the inverted microscope (×400 magnification) to confirm the presence of motile sperm. Inform the surgeon promptly if an adequate number of motile sperm is available for ICSI. This step should take no more than 2–3 min to allow the surgeon to decide on continuing or finishing the surgical retrieval. If more PESA specimens are taken, pool samples of similar quality together for processing. If PESA fails and TESA specimens are obtained, process specimens according to the "TESA processing protocol" (see section "TESA Sperm Processing" and Fig. 3.2).
- Upon finishing surgical retrieval, identify aspirate-containing tube(s) according to the epididymis side and site of aspiration, as well as to the presence of motile sperm. Make a decision upon the processing method to be used, i.e., simple washing or two-layer discontinuous mini-gradient centrifugation, based on a gross estimate of sperm density and motility. Use gradient centrifugation when the specimen contains high density of motile sperm, particularly if contaminated with red blood cells, cellular debris, and immotile sperm. Otherwise, use simple washing.
- For density gradient centrifugation, layer an aliquot of the PESA aspirate up to 0.5 mL over 0.3 mL gradients of 45 and 90%, respectively, and centrifuge at 300 × *g* for 10 min. Resuspend the pellet in 1.5 mL fresh sperm medium and repeat centrifugation. Remove the supernatant carefully, leaving about 0.2 mL of medium above the pellet. Resuspend the pellet and keep at 37°C until use.
- For simple washing, dilute epididymal aspirate with fresh sperm medium to a final volume of 1.5–2.0 mL. Centrifuge the mixture at 300 × *g* for 10 min, discharge the supernatant, and then resuspend the pellet in 0.2 mL of sperm medium. When a processed PESA sample is still contaminated with an excessive number

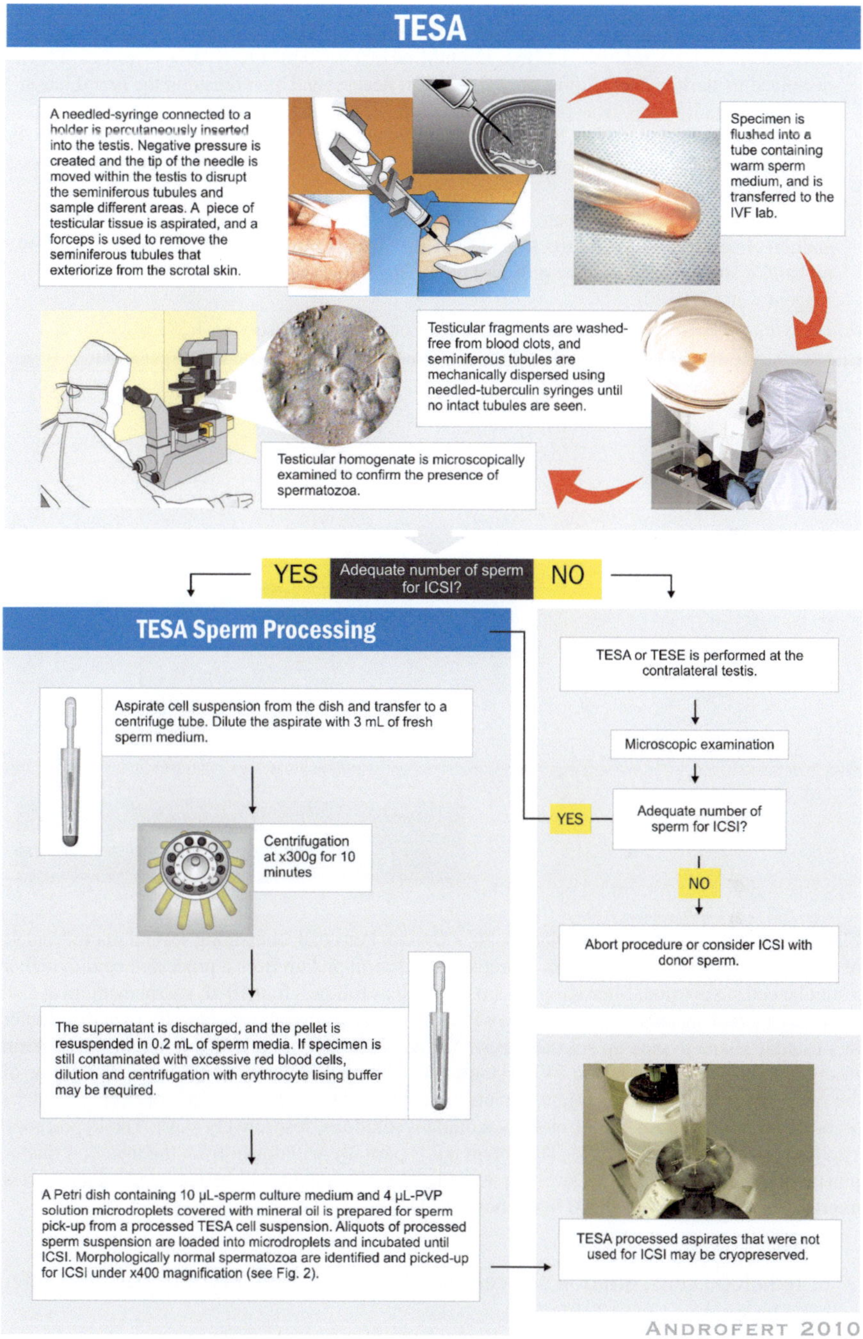

Fig. 3.2 TESA sperm processing. Flow chart illustrates TESA steps from the surgical procedure to the processing of testicular specimens for ICSI

Table 3.2 Solutions for washing samples

Erythrocyte lysis buffer solution (ELBS): 155 mM NH_4Cl + 10 mM $KHCO_3$ + 2 mM EDTA dissolved in sterile water. Adjust the pH to 7.2, if necessary. Upon finishing the first dilution and centrifugation step, resuspend the pellet with 2.0 mL of ELBS and keep the mixture at room temperature for 10 min. Then, centrifuge the sample at 300 × *g* for 5 min, discharge the supernatant, and resuspend the pellet in 0.2 mL of fresh HEPES-buffered protein-supplemented sperm medium [33]
Hyposmotic solution (HOS): Prepare a 150 mOsm/kg HOS solution by dissolving 7.35 mg sodium citrate and 13.51 mg fructose in 1 mL sterile reagent water [21]. Alternatively, a 139 mOsm/kg HOS solution can be prepared by mixing 1 mL sperm medium to 1 mL sterile reagent water [19, 20]
Pentoxifylline solution (PF): Prepare a 5-mM solution of PF by dissolving 1.391 mg pentoxifylline (Sigma cat. No. P-1784) in 1 mL of HEPES-buffered culture medium

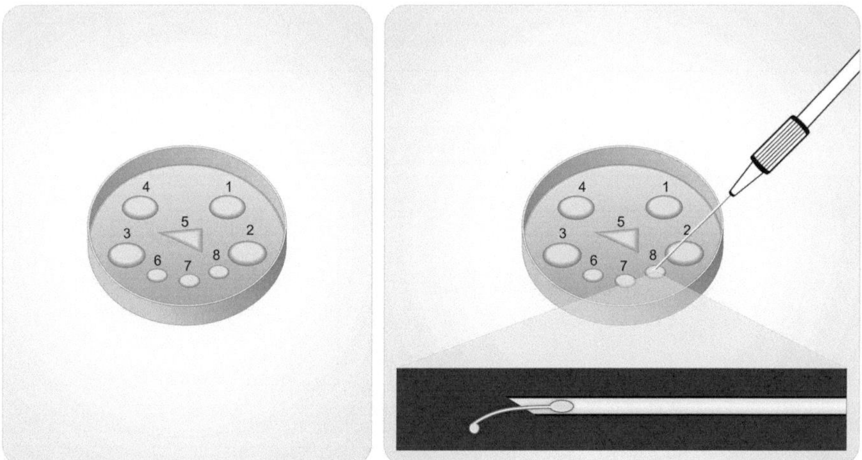

Fig. 3.3 Preparation of microdroplets. A 50 × 09-mm Petri dish containing several microdroplets of culture medium under mineral oil is prepared for sperm pickup from a processed epididymal or testicular cell suspension. Microdroplets are prepared as follows: four 10 μL sperm medium at dish periphery to load specimens (numbered 1–4), one 4 μL polyvinylpyrrolidone (PVP) at dish center in a triangle shape to pick up selected sperm for ICSI (number 5), and two to three 10 μL sperm medium at dish center below the PVP triangle for washing (numbered 6–8). Alternatively, one of the sperm medium-containing microdroplets (e.g., number 8) or the peripheric ones (1–4) may be replaced with the hyposmotic or motility stimulant solutions, respectively (*left*). The hyposmotic swelling test is illustrated (*right*). The sperm tail is partially withdrawn from the injection micropipette into the HOS droplet. A swelling at the level of the tail tip may be seen under the inverted microscope with contrast at ×400 magnification

of red blood cells, dilution and centrifugation with 2 mL erythrocyte lysis buffer may be required (see Table 3.2).

- Prepare a Petri dish containing a series of microdrops under mineral oil for sperm pickup from a processed epididymal cell suspension (Fig. 3.3).
- Load gently a 1 μL sperm suspension aliquot at the center of the polyvinylpyrrolidone (PVP) microdroplet if the suspension contains motile sperm with

progressive motility. After 5–20 min incubation period, morphologically normal motile spermatozoa can be identified and picked up for ICSI with the injection micropipette under ×400 magnification at the edge of the PVP droplet. If progressive motility is low or absent and/or the sample is contaminated with cellular debris, load 1–4 μL sperm suspension aliquot at each 10 μL peripheral microdroplet of HEPES-buffered culture medium to facilitate search and selection of motile sperm. First, aspirate a small volume of PVP into the injection micropipette to improve control during sperm pickup and to avoid blowing air bubbles during ejection of selected sperm into the PVP droplet.

- After finishing sperm pickup from the PESA-processed sample, wash the injection micropipette free of any debris in the PVP droplet.
- Make a final morphologic sperm assessment under ×800 magnification in the group of preselected spermatozoa before ICSI. Immobilize, aspirate into the micropipette, and inject selected sperm into the cytoplasm of metaphase II oocytes.
- Consider cryopreservation of leftover PESA-processed aspirates containing motile sperm that were not used for ICSI. Freezing can be carried out using the fast liquid nitrogen vapor method [14] (Fig. 3.1).

TESA Sperm Processing

Surgical Technique

Note: TESA is performed under local anesthesia, as described in the "PESA protocol," in association with intravenous anaesthesia using propofol either at the day of oocyte retrieval or the day before.

- After anesthetic blockade of the spermatic cord, the epididymis is stabilized between the index finger, thumb, and forefinger while the anterior scrotal skin is stretched.
- A 18-gauge needle attached to a 20-mL syringe is connected to a syringe holder and is inserted through the stretched scrotal skin into the anteromedial or anterolateral portion of the superior testicular pole, in an oblique angle towards the medium and lower poles (Fig. 3.2). Loupe-magnification is used to avoid small vessels seen through the skin.
- Negative pressure is created by pulling the syringe holder while the tip of the needle is moved in and out within the testis in an oblique plane to disrupt the seminiferous tubules and sample different areas. When a small piece of testicular tissue is aspirated, the needle is gently withdrawn from the testis while the negative pressure is maintained. A pair of microsurgery forceps is used to grab the seminiferous tubules that exteriorize from the scrotal skin, thus aiding in the removal of the specimen (see Fig. 3.2).

- The specimen is flushed into a tube containing 0.5–1.0 mL warm sperm medium and is transferred to the IVF lab. TESA or TESE may be performed at the contralateral testis if insufficient number of sperm is retrieved for ICSI.

Sperm Processing

- Discharge TESA aspirate to the outer-dish well. Under stereomicroscopy, identify seminiferous tubules and remove blood clots using the needled tuberculin syringes.
- Transfer seminiferous tubules to the inner-dish well containing fresh sperm medium. Perform a mechanical dispersion of the tubules by mincing repeatedly using both needled tuberculin syringes (use one to hold tubules in place at the bottom of the dish and the other to squeeze and open them). Repeat this step until no intact tubules are seen (see Fig. 3.2).
- Examine the homogenate to confirm the presence of sperm using the inverted microscope at ×400 magnification. Inform the surgeon promptly if an adequate number of sperm for ICSI is available. This step should take no more than 10 min because the patient is kept under anesthesia until a decision of continuing or finishing the surgical retrieval is made. If other TESA specimens are taken, carry out the initial processing steps described above. If TESE specimens are obtained, perform processing according to the "TESE sperm processing protocol" (see section "TESE Sperm Processing" and Fig. 3.4).
- Aspirate and transfer the cell suspension from the inner-well dish to a sterile centrifuge tube. Dilute the aspirate with 3 mL of fresh sperm medium and wash it at 300 × *g* for 7 min. Discharge the supernatant and resuspend the pellet in 0.2 mL of sperm medium. When a processed TESA specimen is still contaminated with an excessive number of red blood cells, dilution and centrifugation with erythrocyte lysis buffer may be required (see Table 3.2).
- Prepare a Petri dish as described in the "PESA protocol" for sperm pickup from a processed testicular cell suspension (see Fig. 3.3).
- Load 1–2 μL sperm suspension aliquot at each 10 μL peripheral microdroplet of HEPES-buffered culture medium to facilitate sperm search and pickup. Proceed to sperm selection and ICSI, as described in the "PESA protocol," and consider cryopreservation of leftover testicular aspirates. Dishes with microdroplets containing TESA-processed sperm can be incubated up to 48 h before ICSI at room temperature in an attempt to improve testicular sperm motility.

TESE Sperm Processing

Micro-TESE Surgical Technique

Note: TESE is performed under local anesthesia, as described in the "PESA protocol," in association with intravenous anaesthesia using propofol either at the day of

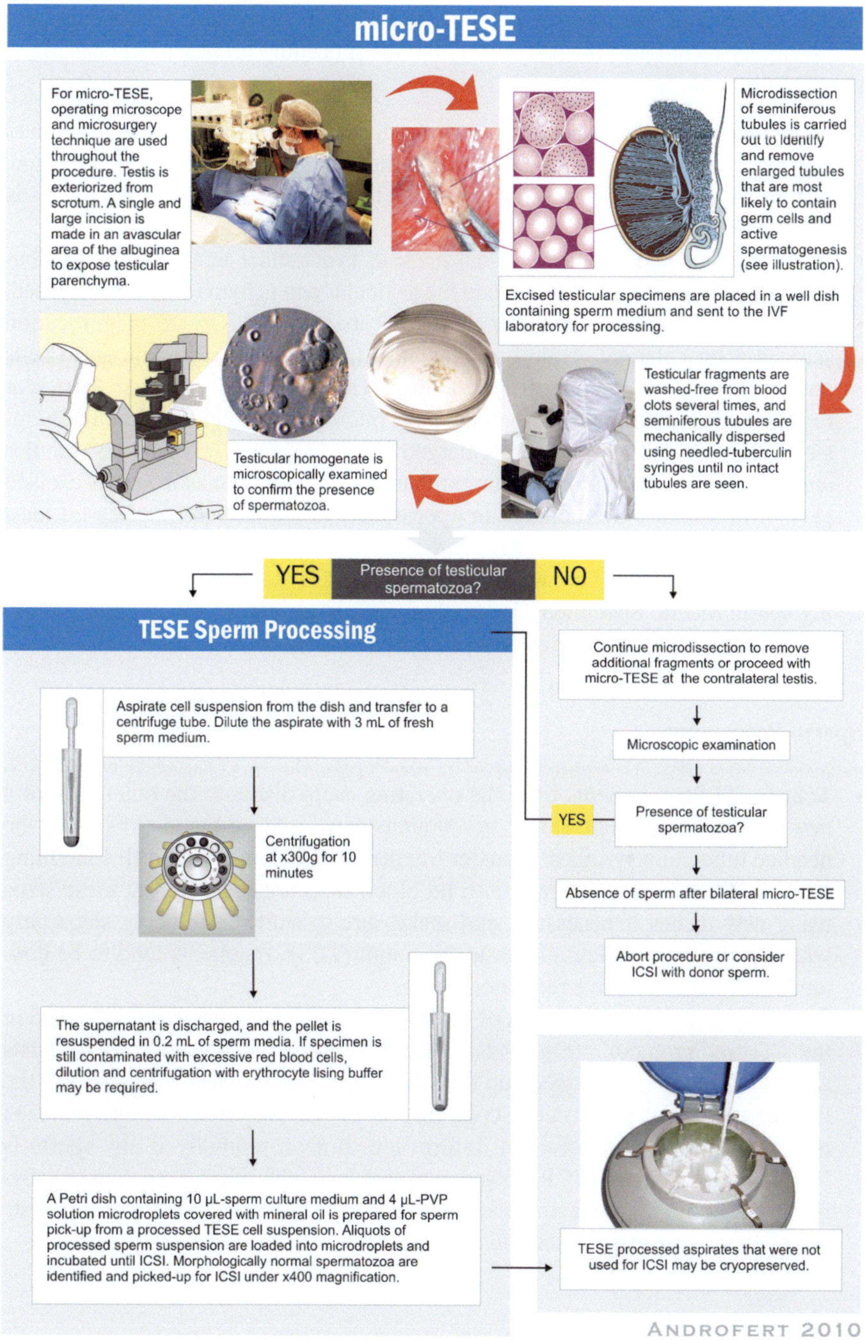

Fig. 3.4 TESE sperm processing. Flow chart illustrates TESE steps from the surgical procedure using micro-TESE for the extraction of testicular parenchyma to the processing of testicular specimens for ICSI

oocyte retrieval or the day before. For micro-TESE, operating microscope and microsurgery technique are used throughout the procedure, as previously described [5, 11] (Fig. 3.4).

- After anesthetic blockade of spermatic cord, the anterior scrotal skin is stretched and the skin and tunica vaginalis are infiltrated with 2 mL of 2% lidocaine. A transverse 2-cm incision is made through the anesthetized layers, and the testis is exteriorized.
- A single, large, midportion incision is made in an avascular area of the tunica albuginea under 6–8× magnification, and the testicular parenchyma is widely exposed.
- Dissection of the testicular parenchyma is carried out at ×16–25 magnification searching for enlarged seminiferous tubules (more likely to contain germ cells and eventually normal sperm production). The superficial and deep testicular regions may be examined, if necessary, and microsurgical-guided testicular biopsies are performed by removing enlarged tubules (Fig. 3.4). If enlarged tubules are not seen, then any tubule different than the remaining ones in size is excised [11]. If all tubules are identical in appearance, random microbiopsies (at least three at each testicular pole) are performed.
- Each excised testicular tissue specimen is placed at the outer-well dish containing sperm media. Specimens are washed grossly to remove blood clots and are sent to the IVF laboratory for processing.

Sperm Processing

- Transfer TESE fragments from the operating room dishes to the outer-well of a new dish in the IVF lab. Under stereomicroscopy, remove blood clots using the needled tuberculin syringes. Transfer fragments to the inner-well dish containing fresh medium and wash again until no blood clots are seen. Repeat these steps using new dishes if necessary, and make sure to start the mincing steps only when erythrocyte contamination is minimum (TESE fragments tend to be contaminated with excessive red blood cells).
- Perform mechanical dispersion of the tubules, and follow the steps described in the "TESA protocol" (Fig. 3.4). Two laboratory technicians/embryologists should work together to speed up the sperm searching process (one mincing the tubules under the stereomicroscope and the other searching for spermatozoa under the inverted microscope). Inform the surgeon promptly if any sperm is found to allow him to decide upon continuing testicular microdissection or moving to the contralateral testis. If other TESE specimens are taken, carry out the initial processing steps described above.

Cryo-Thawed Epididymal/Testicular Sperm Processing

Epididymal and testicular spermatozoa may be cryopreserved using protocols routinely used for ejaculated sperm [15, 16]. After thawing, removal of cryoprotectant is carried out by simple washing, as described in the "TESA sperm processing protocol." If only immotile spermatozoa are seen, a method for selecting viable sperm for ICSI may be used.

Methods for Selecting Viable Immotile Sperm for ICSI

It has been observed that conventional seminal parameters have little or no influence in ICSI outcomes, except when only immotile spermatozoa are available [17, 18]. In certain cases, only immotile spermatozoa are obtained after fresh or cryo-thawed PESA/TESA/TESE processing. Different strategies are described to differentiate live immotile spermatozoa from dead ones, thus aiding in the selection of viable gametes for ICSI.

Hyposmotic Swelling Test (HOST) [19–21]

- Using the microinjection pipette, pick up morphologically normal immotile spermatozoa from the sperm medium droplet and transfer to PVP.
- Aspirate a single spermatozoon head-first into the pipette.
- Move the pipette to the hyposmotic solution (HOS) microdrop (see Fig. 3.3 and Table 3.2), and release only the sperm tail into the HOS solution. Keep it for 5–10 s and observe if a tail tip swelling occurs (sperm tail swelling is often minimal and is a marker of viability in fresh specimens, but may not be suitable for testing cryopreserved ones [21]).
- If tail swelling is seen, aspirate the cell back to the pipette and release it in a drop of fresh medium to allow osmotic re-equilibration (tail swelling often disappears in 5–20 s). If tail swelling is not seen, discharge spermatozoon into the HOS solution.
- Transfer the viable selected spermatozoon to the PVP drop. Repeat these steps until sufficient number of viable sperm is selected for ICSI.

Sperm Tail Flexibility Test (STFT) [22, 23]

- Using the microinjection pipette, pick up morphologically normal immotile spermatozoa from sperm microdroplet (see Fig. 3.3) and transfer to PVP solution.
- Align spermatozoa near the PVP droplet edge.
- Touch sperm tail with the tip of the microinjection pipette, and force the tail to move up and down. Tail is considered flexible when it moves independently of the sperm head (sperm tail flexibility is considered a marker of sperm viability [22, 23]). If tail remains rigid upon touching and sperm head and tail move together as a unit, the spermatozoon is then considered nonviable for ICSI.
- Repeat these steps until sufficient number of viable sperm is selected for ICSI.

Motility Stimulant Sperm Challenge (MSC) [24–26]

Note: Example given using a 5-mM pentoxifylline (PF) solution (see Table 3.2).

- Load a 4 μL aliquot of fresh or cryopreserved PESA/TESA/TESE sperm suspension into the motility stimulant solution microdroplet, and incubate for 20 min (see Fig. 3.3).
- Examine the specimen microscopically searching for moving sperm. In cases of positive MSC, slight noticeable tail twitching is often seen (in rare occasions, vigorous twisting may be observed).
- Pick up motile sperm using the microinjection pipette, and transfer to a fresh microdroplet of sperm medium. Repeat this step 3–4× to wash out any residual PF solution (PF was shown to be embryotoxic in animal studies [27], but is apparently safe if used only on sperm [26]).
- Keep selected spermatozoa in culture or place them into a PVP droplet for sperm selection and immobilization before ICSI.
- Repeat these steps until sufficient number of viable sperm is selected for ICSI to be carried out.

Expert Commentary

PESA and TESA are effective surgical sperm retrieval methods for men with OA regardless of the cause (Table 3.3). However, the adoption of strict criteria to determine that the azoospermia is indeed obstructive is crucial for obtaining a high

Table 3.3 Sperm retrieval rates (SRR) of PESA and TESA in obstructive azoospermia (AO), according to the number of aspiration attempts and the cause of azoospermia

	Presence of motile sperm by PESA; *N* (%)	Cumulative successful retrieval rate; *N* (%)
By retrieval attempt; *N* (%)—130 (100.0%)		
First PESA attempt	66/130 (50.8)	–
Second PESA attempt	29/64 (45.3)	95/130 (73.1)
Third PESA attempt	10/35 (28.6)	105/130 (80.7)
Fourth PESA attempt	7/25 (28.0)	112/130 (86.1)
Rescue TESA after failed PESA	16/18 (88.9)	128/130 (98.4)
By subtype of OA; *N* (%)—142 (100.0%)[a]		
Congenital—30 (23.1%)	21/30 (70.0)	30/30 (100.0)[a]
Vasectomy/failed reversal—64 (49.2%)	40/64 (62.5)	61/64 (95.3)[a]
Postinfection/trauma/iatrogenic—48 (36.9%)	31/36 (81.6)	48/48 (100.0)[a]
Overall SRR; *N* (%)	92/130 (70.8)	139/142 (97.9)[a]

Source: Androfert, Center for Male Reproduction

Congenital: includes cases of CAVD (congenital absence of vas deferens) and ejaculatory duct obstruction (EDO)

[a]PESA + TESA: In 12 cases of postinfectious OA, TESA was performed as the first choice due to intense epididymis fibrosis

Table 3.4 ICSI outcomes using fresh epididymal or testicular spermatozoa retrieved from men with AO

	Epididymal	Testicular	Combined[a]
Number of cycles; N = 136	93	14	29
Female age in years; mean ± SD	32.6 ± 5.3	32.1 ± 5.4	31.6 ± 7.4
2PN fertilization rate (%)	66.0	56.6	59.8
Cleavage rate (%)	99.4	95.7	98.5
Top-quality embryo rate for transfer[b] (%)	51.9	48.9	51.3
Cycles with embryo transfer; N (%)	88 (94.6)	14 (100.0)	29 (100.0)
Number of embryos transferred; mean	2.8	3.3	2.6
Clinical pregnancy rate per transfer; N (%)	45/88 (51.1)	7/14 (50.0)	13/29 (44.8)
Miscarriage rate; N (%)	11/45 (24.4)	1/7 (14.3)	3/13 (23.1)
Live birth rate per transfer; N (%)	34/88 (38.6)	6/14 (42.8)	10/29 (34.5)

Source: Androfert, Center for Male Reproduction

Values expressed as means for fertilization, cleavage, and embryo quality rates

[a]Oocytes were microinjected with epididymal or testicular spermatozoa retrieved from the same patient in the treatment cycle

[b]7–9 Blastomeres of similar size, and grades I or II cytoplasmic fragmentation on the day of embryo transfer (day 3)

successful retrieval rate in the range of 90–100%. Using PESA, our approach is to perform the first aspiration at the epididymis corpus, and proceed to the caput if necessary as aspirates from the cauda are usually rich in poor-quality senescent spermatozoa, debris, and macrophages. Based on our findings, motile spermatozoa is obtained in 73% of the cases after the first or second aspiration. TESA is required as a rescue procedure after a failed PESA in approximately 14% of the individuals (Table 3.3). Most cases of PESA failures are not necessarily technical failures because immotile spermatozoa are found. However, in certain cases of epididymis fibrosis due to multiple PESA attempts or postinfection, PESA may be ineffective. In these cases, PESA can be attempted at the contralateral epididymis or TESA can be applied (Table 3.3). Routinely, procedures are performed under local anesthesia, with or without intravenous sedation, and at the same day of oocyte retrieval. Patients are discharged 1 h later and can return to normal activities in the same day. Oral analgesics are prescribed but pain complaint is minimal. The most common complication is fibrosis at the aspiration site. Other potential complications include hematoma, bleeding, and infection, but are rare [8]. Some authors advocate that MESA allows the collection of larger and cleaner quantities of sperm than PESA, but this debate is trivial. In our series of 142 men with OA, cumulative successful retrieval rate after PESA and/or TESA was 97.9% (Table 3.3), and an adequate number of motile sperm for cryopreservation was obtained in approximately 31% (35/112) of the cases. Clinical outcomes of ICSI using PESA- or TESA-derived spermatozoa are similar in OA (Table 3.4), and results are comparable to those obtained with ejaculated sperm [28] (Table 3.5). Although the cryopreservation rate after PESA is not high, repeated aspirations can be carried out in men with OA at

Table 3.5 ICSI outcomes using spermatozoa derived from ejaculates and retrieved from the epididymis or the testis in men with obstructive and nonobstructive azoospermia

	Ejaculated sperm (N = 220)	Surgically retrieved sperm from azoospermic men (N = 93)		P value
		AO (N = 39)	NOA (N = 54)	
2PN fertilization rate (%)	70.0^{a}	73.6^{b}	52.2^{c}	$<0.05^{c \times a, b}$
Cleavage rate (%)	91.0^{a}	94.8^{b}	77.7^{c}	$<0.05^{c \times a, b}$
Top-quality embryo rate* (%)	48.5^{a}	46.3^{b}	35.7^{c}	$<0.05^{c \times a, b}$
Clinical pregnancy rate (%)	43^{a}	53^{b}	26^{c}	$<0.05^{c \times a, b}$
Miscarriage rate (%)	13	20	14	NS

Adapted from Verza and Esteves [28], with permission

Values expressed as means for fertilization, cleavage, and embryo quality rates. One-way ANOVA was used to compare clinical and laboratorial variables between groups, and the chi-square test was used to compare pregnancy and miscarriage rates. $P < 0.05$ was considered significant; *NS* not significant; Superscripts alphabets indicate pairwise group comparisons

OA obstructive azoospermia; *NOA* nonobstructive azoospermia

*7–9 Blastomeres of similar size, and grades I or II cytoplasm fragmentation on the day of embryo transfer (day 3)

lower cost and morbidity than MESA. In rare circumstances, we perform MESA in men presenting coagulopathies.

When gradient centrifugation is chosen for PESA sperm processing, we recommend that part of the sample is spared and processed by simple washing. The reason is the unpredictability of gradient centrifugation to recover motile sperm in such cases. If recovery is less than desired, we can rely on the washed sample to select motile sperm for ICSI. Due to the relatively low sperm yields in PESA and TESA, it is important to use low volumes of media during sperm processing and wash the sample only once. Centrifugation force and time should be carefully controlled to avoid jeopardizing the often compromised sperm motility.

For NOA, TESE, with or without magnification, is clearly the preferred approach. Efficiency of TESA for retrieving spermatozoa in NOA is only 10–30% [29], except in the favorable cases of men with testicular histopathology showing hypospermatogenesis, to whom retrieval rates are approximately 80–100% [13] (Table 3.6). Nonetheless, if a previous TESA attempt had been successful in a man with NOA, its positive predictive value for a successful second attempt is 70% [30]. Based on these results, it is our opinion that TESA should be reserved for NOA individuals having a diagnostic testicular biopsy histopathology showing hypospermatogenesis or with a previous successful TESA attempt. However, if TESA fails, we neither perform a second aspiration in the same testis, at the same operative time, nor convert it to an open procedure, to avoid the risk of hematoma and testicular injury. From our clinical experience, it is very difficult to identify enlarged seminiferous tubules in such cases, even using the operating microscope, because extensive bleeding is often seen. In these occasions, we opt to perform TESA or TESE at the contralateral testis. For NOA patients without previous

Table 3.6 SRR in 176 nonobstructive azoospermic men according to the surgical method of collection stratified by histopathology results and cause of azoospermia

	Presence of testicular spermatozoa; *N* (%)
By method; *N* = 176 (100.0%)	
TESA (*N* = 90); overall SRR, *N* (%)	58/90 (64.4)
Hypospermatogenesis	26/26 (100.0)
Maturation arrest	2/6 (33.3)
Sertoli cell only	6/29 (20.7)
Not available[a]	24/29 (82.3)
Micro-TESE (*N* = 86); overall SRR, *N* (%)	45/86 (52.3)
Hypospermatogenesis	19/19 (100.0)
Maturation arrest	7/12 (58.3)
Sertoli cell only	13/39 (33.3)
Not available	6/16 (37.5)
By cause of NOA; *N* = 176 (100.0%)	
Varicocele (66)	45/66 (68.2%)
Genetic (*n* = 12)	6/12 (50.0%)
Cryptorchidism (*n* = 19)	12/19 (63.1%)
Idiopathic (63)	33/63 (52.4%)
Radiotherapy/chemotherapy (*N* = 6)	3/6 (50.0%)
Orchitis/gonadotoxin/endocrine/other (*N* = 10)	10/10 (100.0%)
Overall SRR; *N* (%)	109/176 (61.9)

Source: Androfert, Center for Male Reproduction
[a]Cases with previous successful TESA attempt

diagnostic testicular biopsy or TESA attempt, our choice is to perform sperm extraction using micro-TESE.

The use of optical magnification during TESE limits the risk of vascular injury and optimizes the chances of finding sperm [10–12]. Although no absolute predictors for sperm retrieval are available in NOA, the probability of retrieving sperm varies according to the testicular histopathology results [12, 13] (Table 3.6). Proper identification of testicular vessels under the tunica albuginea is made prior to the placement of an incision into the testis. Microsurgery also allows the preservation of intratesticular blood supply, as well as the identification of tubules more likely to harbor sperm production. Therefore, efficacy of sperm retrieval is improved while the risks of large tissue removal are minimized. Excision of large biopsy samples in conventional TESE has been shown to impair testosterone production [31]. Tissue removal in micro-TESE is often 50- to 70-fold less than standard TESE [11], and the small amount of tissue extracted facilitates sperm processing. Selection of spermatozoa from a smaller population of contaminating testicular cells allows more ease and greater speed for sperm pickup and injection process, as well as alleviates contamination and blockage of the injection needle with cells and debris. It is far less technically demanding and labor intensive to extract spermatozoa from small volume specimens than large pieces of testicular tissue that must be dissected, red blood cells lysed, and the rare spermatozoa searched for in a tedious fashion under an inverted microscope. TESE sperm processing may be incredibly labor intensive, and the searching process may miss the rare spermatozoa within a sea of seminiferous tubules and other cells. TESE/micro-TESE may be scheduled either for the day of oocyte collection and ICSI or the day before. In the latter, processed specimens are incubated in a closed HEPES-buffered culture system (microdrops under mineral oil) at room temperature, inside a laminar flow cabinet or in a clean room for a maximum of 48 h, to avoid bacterial contamination. Culture of specimens at 37°C inside the incubator should be avoided since contamination with scrotum skin-derived bacteria is often seen. From our data, optimal fertilization by ICSI using surgically retrieved sperm is obtained when the time frame from hCG administration to microinjection does not exceed 44 h [32]. Testicular tissue sperm processing, searching, and selection of viable spermatozoa for ICSI may take several hours in NOA cases. Our laboratory takes approximately 12 min to handle a single testicular spermatozoon from searching to microinjection in NOA, but only 5.5 min in OA. In other words, the average time required to perform ICSI in a standard NOA treatment cycle involving 8–12 metaphase II oocytes is approximately 2 h. Therefore, we elect to perform micro-TESE the day before oocyte collection when a busy next day IVF laboratory workload is anticipated. Additionally, we recommend that two laboratory technicians work together during the initial processing steps (one mincing the tubules and the other searching for spermatozoa) to speed up the searching process and to allow a faster feedback to the surgeon who may decide to end the procedure if sperm is found or to continue dissecting the seminiferous tubules. Our laboratory performs the processing of testicular specimens by mincing and shredding the whole tissue instead of using enzymatic digestion. The mechanical preparation has the advantage of being fast, requiring about 15–30 min, while enzymatic digestion is more time consuming, requiring at least 4 h [33]. Studies comparing both techniques show conflicting results, but large series were unable to confirm the superiority of one technique over the other for processing fresh or frozen testicular sperm [33–36].

The clinical outcomes of ICSI using testicular sperm extracted by TESA or micro-TESE from NOA individuals are significantly lower than those obtained with either ejaculated or epididymal/testicular sperm taken from men with OA [28] (Table 3.5). Our data indicate that testicular spermatozoa of men with severely impaired spermatogenesis have decreased fertility potential and may have a higher tendency to carry deficiencies such as the ones related to the centrioles and genetic material, which ultimately affect the capability of the male gamete to activate the egg and trigger the formation and development of a normal zygote and a viable embryo [28].

The concept of cryopreservation may be used in association with sperm retrieval procedures. Some centers prefer to retrieve and intentionally cryopreserve sperm for future use. This strategy offers the advantage of avoiding ovarian stimulation when no sperm is obtained from testicular specimens. If sperm is found and frozen, thawing can be done at any time, thus obviating the need to organize two operations (oocyte and sperm retrieval) at the same day. Also, cryopreservation may be an interesting tool to spare leftover specimens that would be discharged after ICSI, especially if the treatment cycle does not result in a pregnancy. Future ICSI attempts may be carried out without repeated surgical retrievals. We routinely freeze excess motile epididymal spermatozoa which are not needed for the current ICSI cycle. Most often, motile sperm will be available after thawing in such cases, and ICSI outcomes using motile fresh or frozen epididymal sperm seems not to differ [37]. Cryopreservation of testicular sperm is also advisable, especially for men with NOA who often require multiple ICSI attempts to conceive but may not have an adequate number of sperm available for repeated retrieval attempts. However, postthawed testicular sperm are often immotile or exhibit only a twitching motility, and ICSI results using immotile testicular sperm are lower than fresh ones [17, 38]. Methods for selecting immotile viable sperm for ICSI are available, but results are limited for cryopreserved specimens. HOST may not discriminate viable and nonviable frozen–thawed spermatozoa [21]. Response to motility stimulants is unpredictable, and STFT has not been validated in large series [22–27]. The application of a single laser shot to the far end of the sperm tail has been shown to cause a curling of the tail only in viable sperm, similar to the reaction observed with the HOST, but this method has not been validated in cryo-thawed specimens [39]. We currently use the STFT for discriminating viable and nonviable immotile sperm for ICSI. Using this method, normal fertilization rates obtained by our group has been fair (39.9%). In vitro incubation of fresh or frozen retrieved sperm in culture medium may aid to obtain a more viable and functionally normal sperm population that obviates the risks of using immotile unselected sperm for ICSI. Sperm culture media have the components to support normal metabolism of immotile, mature, retrieved spermatozoa that may become motile by incubation [40]. However, in vitro incubation should be limited to a maximum of 48 h since contamination by bacteria that normally come from the scrotal skin is almost a rule after a period of 36–48 h, even when strict sterile operating and laboratory conditions are used. According to each group's results, different strategies can be developed. If freezing of surgically retrieved specimens provides similar results than those obtained by using fresh sperm, then the use of freezing specimens would be preferable. If not, fresh specimens are preferable. In our hands, ICSI is performed with fresh testicular sperm whenever possible, even with the risk of submitting the female partner to unnecessary ovarian stimulation or the male to repeated retrievals. The reasons are related to the lower pregnancy rates obtained with cryo-thawed immotile testicular sperm by our group and others [18, 38, 40, 41]. To date, our technique for cryopreserve surgically-retrieved sperm is the standard liquid nitrogen vapor method using TEST-yolk buffer and glycerol as cryoprotectants [14–16]. Epididymal specimens are concentrated by washing before freezing, and testicular sperm are freed from the testicular parenchyma, i.e., testicular homogenates are frozen. Cryopreservation of few sperm into an empty zona pellucida and the use of stimulants before freezing may optimize results [15, 3, 42, 43]. Recently, it has been shown that human spermatozoa can be successfully vitrified, and this strategy may be of interest for preserving small quantities of surgically retrieved gametes [44].

Conclusions/Key Points

- PESA and TESA are simple and efficient surgical methods for epididymal and testicular sperm retrieval, respectively, in men with OA. For NOA, TESE, with or without magnification (micro-TESE), should be the preferred approach. The use of microsurgery during TESE may improve the efficacy of sperm extraction with significantly less tissue removed, which ultimately facilitates sperm processing. Sperm retrieval should be carried out either at the day of oocyte retrieval or the day before, depending on the laboratory workload.
- The primary goal of PESA/TESA/TESE sperm processing is the recovery of a clean sample containing motile sperm. Such specimens are more fragile, and often compromised in motility, as compared to the ones obtained from ejaculates. Laboratory techniques should be carried out with great caution to avoid jeopardizing the sperm fertilizing potential. The whole process starts with the surgical collection of the best quality specimen possible. During laboratory steps, minimal iatrogenic cellular damage may be achieved by strict control of centrifugation force and duration, exposure to ultraviolet light and temperature variation, laboratory air quality conditions, as well as the use of high-quality reagents, materials, and equipments.
- PESA sperm processing may be performed either by mini-gradient centrifugation or simple washing using low volumes of culture media. Testicular specimens may be processed either by mechanical mincing of seminiferous tubules or enzymatic digestion, with similar results, and homogenates are simply washed. The mechanical preparation is significantly faster than enzymatic digestion.
- The use of unselected immotile epididymal/testicular sperm for ICSI negatively impact clinical outcomes. Methods for selecting viable immotile sperm for ICSI include the HOST, STFT, and motility stimulants.
- The concept of cryopreservation may be useful for intentionally cryopreserve retrieved sperm for future use or spare leftover specimens that would be discharged after ICSI. Different strategies can be developed according to each group's results. If freezing of surgically retrieved specimens provides similar results than those obtained with the use of fresh sperm, then the use of freezing specimens would be preferable. If not, fresh specimens are preferable.

Acknowledgments The authors would like to acknowledge Christina Prudencio and Bill Seol, for their assistance in data collection and processing, and Mrs. Fabiola Bento for editorial and text revision.

References

1. Palermo G, Joris H, Devroey P, et al. Pregnancies after intracytoplasmic sperm injection of single spermatozoan into an oocyte. Lancet. 1992;340:17–8.
2. Silber S, Nagy ZP, Liu J, et al. Conventional in-vitro fertilization versus intracytoplasmic sperm injection for patients requiring microsurgical sperm aspiration. Hum Reprod. 1994;9:1705–9.

3. Devroey P, Liu J, Nagy ZP, et al. Pregnancies after testicular extraction (TESE) and intracytoplasmic sperm injection (ICSI) in non-obstructive azoospermia. Hum Reprod. 1995;10: 1457–60.
4. Esteves SC, Miyaoka R, Agarwal A. An update on the clinical assessment of the infertile male. Clinics (Sao Paulo). 2011;66:691–700.
5. Esteves SC, Glina S. Recovery of spermatogenesis after microsurgical subinguinal varicocele repair in azoospermic men based on testicular histology. Int Braz J Urol. 2005;31:541–8.
6. Craft I, Tsirigotis M, Bennett V, et al. Percutaneous epididymal sperm aspiration and intracytoplasmic sperm injection in the management of infertility due to obstructive azoospermia. Fertil Steril. 1995;63:1038–42.
7. Craft I, Tsirigotis M. Simplified recovery, preparation and cryopreservation of testicular spermatozoa. Hum Reprod. 1995;10:1623–7.
8. Raviv G, Levron J, Menashe Y, et al. Sonographic evidence of minimal and short-term testicular damage after testicular sperm aspiration procedures. Fertil Steril. 2004;82:442–4.
9. Okada H, Dobashi M, Yamazaki T, et al. Conventional versus microdissection testicular sperm extraction for nonobstructive azoospermia. J Urol. 2002;168:1063–7.
10. Tsujimura A, Matsumiya K, Miyagawa Y, et al. Conventional multiple or microdissection testicular sperm extraction: a comparative study. Hum Reprod. 2002;17:2924–9.
11. Schlegel PN. Testicular sperm extraction: microdissection improves sperm yield with minimal tissue excision. Hum Reprod. 1999;14:131–5.
12. Ramasamy R, Lin K, Gosden LV, et al. High serum FSH levels in men with nonobstructive azoospermia does not affect success of microdissection testicular sperm extraction. Fertil Steril. 2009;92:590–3.
13. Esteves SC, Verza Jr S, Prudencio C, Seol B. Sperm retrieval rates (SRR) in nonobstructive azoospermia (NOA) are related to testicular histopathology results but not to the etiology of azoospermia. Fertil Steril 2010;94:S132.
14. Esteves SC, Sharma RK, Thomas AJ, et al. Improvement in motion characteristics and acrosome status in cryopreserved spermatozoa by swim-up processing before freezing. Hum Reprod. 2000;15:2173–9.
15. Esteves SC, Spaine DM, Cedenho AP. Effects of pentoxifylline treatment before freezing on motility, viability and acrosome status of poor quality human spermatozoa cryopreserved by the liquid nitrogen vapor method. Braz J Med Biol Res. 2007;40:985–92.
16. Verza Jr S, Feijo CM, Esteves SC. Resistance of human spermatozoa to cryoinjury in repeated cycles of thaw-refreezing. Int Braz J Urol. 2009;35:581–91.
17. Nagy ZP, Liu J, Joris H, et al. The result of intracytoplasmic sperm injection is not related to any of the three basic sperm parameters. Hum Reprod. 1995;10:1123–9.
18. Dafopoulos K, Griesinger G, Schultze-Mosgau A, et al. Factors affecting outcome after ICSI with spermatozoa retrieved from cryopreserved testicular tissue in non-obstructive azoospermia. Reprod Biomed Online. 2005;10:455–60.
19. Liu J, Tsai YL, Katz E, et al. High fertilization rate obtained after intracytoplasmic sperm injection with 100% no motile spermatozoa selected by using a simple modified hypo-osmotic swelling test. Fertil Steril. 1997;68:373–5.
20. Sallam HN, Farrag A, Agameya A-F, et al. The use of the modified hypo-osmotic swelling test for the selection of immotile testicular spermatozoa in patients treated with ICSI: a randomized controlled study. Hum Reprod. 2005;20:3435–40.
21. Esteves SC, Sharma RK, Thomas Jr AJ, et al. Suitability of the hypo-osmotic swelling test for assessing the viability of cryopreserved sperm. Fertil Steril. 1996;66:798–804.
22. Soares JB, Glina S, Antunes Jr N, et al. Sperm tail flexibility test: a simple test for selecting viable spermatozoa for intracytoplasmic sperm injection from semen samples without motile spermatozoa. Rev Hosp Clin Fac Med Sao Paulo. 2003;58:250–3.
23. Oliveira NM, Sanchez RV, Fiesta SR, et al. Pregnancy with frozen-thawed and fresh testicular biopsy after motile and immotile sperm microinjection, using the mechanical touch technique to assess viability. Hum Reprod. 2004;19:262–5.

24. Esteves SC, Sharma RK, Thomas Jr AJ, et al. Cryopreservation of human spermatozoa with pentoxifylline improves the post-thaw agonist-induced acrosome reaction rate. Hum Reprod. 1998;13:3384–9.
25. Terriou P, Hans E, Giorgetti C, et al. Pentoxifylline initiates motility in spontaneously immotile epididymal and testicular spermatozoa and allows normal fertilization, pregnancy, and birth after intracytoplasmic sperm injection. J Assist Reprod Genet. 2000;17:194–9.
26. Kovacic B, Vlaisavljevic V, Reljic M. Clinical use of pentoxifylline for activation of immotile testicular sperm before ICSI in patients with azoospermia. J Androl. 2006;27:45–52.
27. Yovich JL. Pentoxifylline: actions and applications in assisted reproduction. Hum Reprod. 1993;8:1786–91.
28. Verza Jr S, Esteves SC. Sperm defect severity rather than sperm source is associated with lower fertilization rates after intracytoplasmic sperm injection. Int Braz J Urol. 2008;34:49–56.
29. Friedler S, Raziel A, Strassburger D, et al. Testicular sperm retrieval by percutaneous fine needle aspiration compared to testicular sperm extraction by open biopsy in men with non-obstructive azoospermia. Hum Reprod. 1997;12:1488–93.
30. Fasouliotis SJ, Safran A, Porat-Katz A, et al. A high predictive value of the first testicular fine needle aspiration in patients with non-obstructive azoospermia for sperm recovery at the subsequent attempt. Hum Reprod. 2002;17:139–42.
31. Schlegel PN, Su LM. Physiologic consequences of testicular sperm extraction. Hum Reprod. 1997;12:1688–92.
32. Schneider DT, Gomes AP, Verza Jr S, et al. Optimal time interval for intracytoplasmic sperm injection after administration of human chorionic gonadotrophin in severe male factor infertility. Fertil Steril. 2006;86:S155.
33. Verheyan G, De Croo I, Tournaye H, et al. Comparison of four mechanical methods to retrieve spermatozoa from testicular tissue. Hum Reprod. 1995;10:2956–9.
34. Salzbrunn A, Benson DM, Holstein AF, et al. A new concept for the extraction of testicular spermatozoa as a tool for assisted fertilization (ICSI). Hum Reprod. 1996;11:752–5.
35. Nagy ZP, Verheyen G, Tournaye H, et al. An improved treatment procedure for testicular biopsy specimens offers more efficient sperm recovery: case series. Fertil Steril. 1997;68:376–9.
36. Baukloh V. Retrospective multicentre study on mechanic and enzymatic preparation of fresh and cryopreserved testicular biopsies. Hum Reprod. 2002;17:1788–94.
37. Devroey P, Silber S, Nagy ZP, et al. Ongoing pregnancies and birth after intracytoplasmic sperm injection with frozen-thawed epididymal spermatozoa. Hum Reprod. 1995;10:903–6.
38. Fisher R, Baukloh V, Naether OGJ, et al. Pregnancy after intracytoplasmic sperm injection of spermatozoa from frozen-thawed testicular biopsy. Hum Reprod. 1996;11:2197–9.
39. Aktan TM, Montag M, Duman S, et al. Use of laser to detect viable but immotile spermatozoa. Andrologia. 2004;36:366–9.
40. Zhu J, et al. In vitro maturation of testicular spermatozoa. Hum Reprod. 1996;11:231–2.
41. Konc J, Kanya K, Cseh S. The effect of condition/state of testicular spermatozoa injected to the outcome of TESE-ICSI-ET cycles. Eur J Obstet Gynecol Reprod Biol. 2008;141:39–43.
42. Liu J, Zheng XZ, Baramki TA, et al. Cryopreservation of a small number of fresh human testicular spermatozoa and testicular spermatozoa cultured in vitro for 3 days in an empty zona pellucida. J Androl. 2000;21:409–13.
43. Levi-Setti PE, Albani E, Negri L, et al. Cryopreservation of a small number of spermatozoa in yolk-filled human zonae pellucidae. Arch Ital Urol Androl. 2003;75:195–8.
44. Isachenko E, Isachenko V, Weiss JM, et al. Acrosomal status and mitochondrial activity of human spermatozoa vitrified with sucrose. Reproduction. 2008;136:167–73.

Chapter 4
Processing Sperm Samples in HIV-Positive Patients

Thamara Viloria, Marcos Meseguer, Antonio Pellicer, José Remohí, and Nicolás Garrido

Prolonged survival of patients under HAART (highly active antiretroviral therapy) has given rise to a new demand from serodiscordant (SDC) couples who wish to have children. Unfortunately, due to the risk of transmission of viral particles through semen, the sexual intercourse in these couples should be done using protection, which eliminates any possibility to achieve pregnancies.

Thus, the only completely safe options available to these couples some years ago, to fulfill their desire for offspring, were adoption or sperm donation. Nevertheless, many couples desire genetically related offspring.

When the male partner is HIV positive, it is essential to treat the infected semen with effective laboratory techniques that not only isolate the best spermatozoa but also remove HIV-infected cells from the semen. These males need special assisted reproduction protocols in order to father children without risking transmission of their diseases to their partners and offspring [1], and these protocols mainly involve a treatment of the sperm sample and the confirmation of viral absence before any use.

For HIV, there is a low transmissibility risk, established as 1–3 infections per thousand sexual intercourses (or semen exposures) [1]. At that time, all the

T. Viloria, PhD (✉)
IVF Laboratory, Instituto Valenciano de Infertilidad (IVI), University of Valencia, Valencia, Spain
e-mail: thamara.viloria@ivi.es

M. Meseguer, PhD
In Vitro Fertilization Laboratory, IVI Valencia, Valencia, Spain
e-mail: marcos.meseguer@ivi.es

A. Pellicer, MD • J. Remohí, MD
Department of Gynecology and Obstetrics, Instituto Valenciano de Infertilidad (IVI), University of Valencia, Valencia, Spain
e-mail: antonio.pellicer@ivi.es; jose.remohi@ivi.es

N. Garrido, PhD
Andrology Laboratory and Semen Bank, Instituto Valenciano de Infertilidad (IVI), University of Valencia, Valencia, Spain
e-mail: nicolas.garrido@ivi.es

Z.P. Nagy et al. (eds.), *Clinical Embryology: A Practical Guide*,
DOI 10.1007/978-1-4614-8376-2_4,

accumulated data regarding viral transmission through semen with intrauterine insemination (IUI) is not enough to determine the real situation and must be revised. The employment of intracytoplasmic sperm injection (ICSI) on these couples is an applicable alternative to diminish this risk when using assisted reproduction technologies, because a single spermatozoon is injected directly into an oocyte, during which the pellucid zone of the oocyte is penetrated artificially.

Additionally, to prevent any accidental infection to the partner, offspring and laboratory staff during ART, we need to employ the safest methods available. To this end, we developed on SDC males, several strategies in the recent years to reduce the transmission risk to its lowest degree, maintaining reasonable and cost-effective pregnancy rates.

Our aim in this chapter is to present the reader with the information available regarding the safe employment of sperm cells for assisted reproduction in SDC couples with the male infected with HIV.

Sperm Wash and Detection of HIV-1 RNA and Proviral DNA Techniques

HIV belongs to the retroviruses family; they have the faculty to synthesize reverse transcriptase, convert the RNA form into DNA and to insert its genome in this manner into the hosts'. This issue will be very relevant for the detection methods employed [2], since we will need to demonstrate the absence of HIV in a sperm sample by analyzing both DNA and mRNA.

Several years ago, when washed sperm samples were employed for IUI treatments, immunofluorescence methods were used in the initial detection of HIV-1; at the present time, the routine detection methods for HIV-1 in sperm are based on the amplification of defined sequences of the viral nucleic acids [3, 4]. However, these methods have significant limitations, since the detection levels are 50–200 viral copies, thus not detecting viral presence below these thresholds.

Trying to improve the techniques available, we developed a protocol to reduce the detection limit to a single RNA or DNA viral copy with nested PCR (nPCR) or reverse transcription and nested PCR for RNA [5].

To this end, between August 2001 and October 2003, couples with HIV-positive males (n = 18), couples with HCV-/HIV-positive males (n = 33), and infertile couples undergoing ART where the male was HCV positive (n = 40) were studied, yielding a total number of 134 ejaculates to be washed and analyzed. All of them signed an informed consent, and the study was approved by the Institutional Review Board. The mean age of all the men included in the study was 36.6 years old (range 25–47).

The HIV-infected patients exhibit all the stages of the infection (A, B, or C) according to the Center for Disease Control (CDC) classification. The mean viral load was 48,623 copies/mL (range 78–525,000 IU/mL), with 46 patients without detectable blood viral load. The mean CD_4 cell count was 502.7 CD_4/mm^3 (range 26–1,664). Finally, the time of evolution of the disease was 11 years (range 3–20).

Semen Analysis

All the samples must be processed in a dedicated laboratory; it is necessary to employ a highly trained and experienced staff and make use of an exclusive and isolated laboratory area and set apart from work with noninfectious samples; using class II/B3 biosafety cabinet, centrifuge with safety lids, an exclusive incubator and a nitrogen tank solely for storage of these potentially infectious samples.

Samples are collected by masturbation into a sterile polypropylene container after 3–5 days of ejaculatory abstinence. After liquefaction and homogenization, semen parameters are analyzed according to the World Health Organization [6] criteria. Total count and motility before and after the wash are recorded. Sperm morphology is not analyzed for safety reasons: it is not recommended to work with cutting elements when treating HCV-/HIV-positive samples, and, as these samples are always for ICSI treatments, fresh sperm morphology is not needed.

Sperm Wash Procedure

The sperm wash consisted of three steps (Fig. 4.1):

Step 1

- An initial dilution 1:1 (vol:vol) with Sperm Medium (MediCult, Jyllinge, Denmark), of the ejaculates after liquefaction.
- Then, they were pelleted at 400 × *g* for 10 min, and the supernatants were discarded.
- An equal volume of Sperm Medium as the initial volume of was added ("first wash").

Step 2

- Prepare 3–4 conic tubes of triple density gradients of 1–1.2 mL of each layer (90, 70, and 45%, PureSperm, Nidacon, Goteborg, Sweden) and layered 1 mL approximately of "the first wash" onto each tube.
- Centrifuged 20 min at 300 × *g* and then eliminate the three upper fractions (first wash, 45 and 70% layer) of each tube.
- Each pellet was obtained and washed with 5 mL of Sperm Medium, and re-pelleted again at 400 × *g* 10 min. Supernatants were discarded.

Step 3

- After the supernatants were discarded, a swim up of 0.5–0.7 mL was done. After 45 min, the upper 0.35 mL of each tube was obtained and pooled.

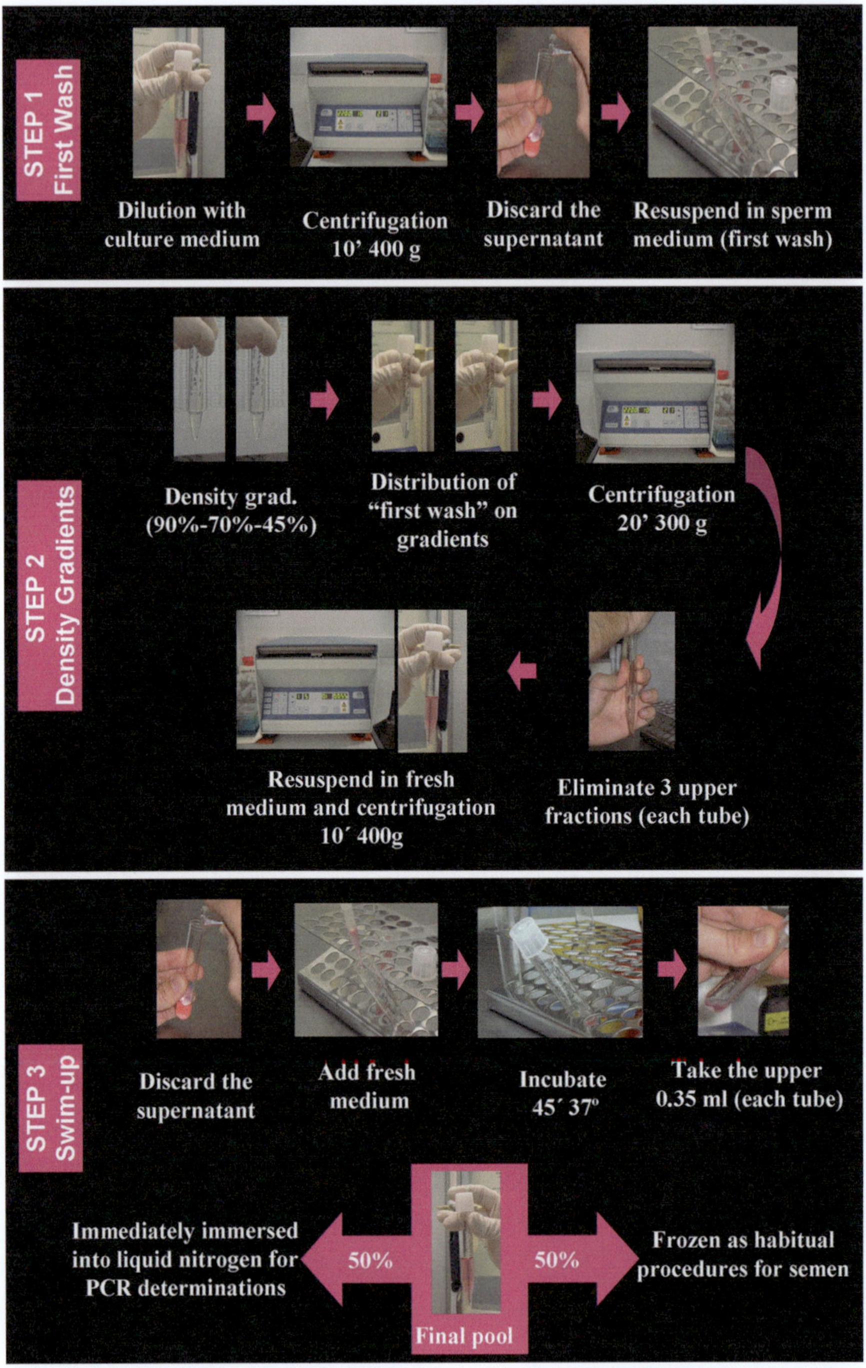

Fig. 4.1 The sperm wash procedure consists of three steps

- After evaluating the total count and motility, one half of a "pool" was immediately immersed into liquid nitrogen for PCR determinations, and the other half was frozen with Sperm Freezing Medium (MediCult, Jyllinge, Denmark), following the manufacturer's instructions, and stored until their use after a negative result of viral presence [5].

PCR Techniques for HIV Applied to Semen

Nucleic acids were extracted from the washed spermatozoa using the NucliSens (Organon-Teknika, Barcelona, Spain), following the instructions of the manufacturer. Two extractions were run in parallel, one from the spermatozoa sample and the other with the spermatozoa samples after the addition of HIV RNA obtained from HIV-infected plasma to detect the presence of transcription or amplification inhibitors after the nucleic acid extraction procedure. Both extracted samples were used for two HIV RNA transcriptions to detect genes from the *gag* and *pol* region, followed by a nested DNA amplification [7]. The same samples were used to amplify HIV proviral DNA by a nested amplification to detect both genes (*gag* and *pol*). The other extraction, run in parallel with added HIV RNA before nucleic acid extraction, was used as a positive control to detect the presence of inhibitors of the transcription or amplification. Besides negative controls to detect the presence of amplicons, contamination was carried out.

For HIV RNA transcription, we used the antisense external primers to anneal with nucleotides 1696–1676 and 3286–3265 for the *gag* and *pol* genes, respectively. Standardized conditions for transcription were followed using 100 μM DTT, 1 mM each dNTP, 0.2 μM antisense primer, 20 U RNAasin (Promega, Barcelona, Spain), and 5 U AMV transcriptase (Promega) in a final volume of 20 μL. Nested DNA amplification used the external primers to anneal with nucleotides (from ARV2/SF2 sequence) 1224–1243 and 1696–1676 and internal primers to anneal with nucleotides 1316–1335 and 1524–1504 for the gag region. External primers annealing with nucleotides 2623–2642 and 3286–3265 and internal primers annealing with nucleotides 2716–2741 and 3250–3227 for the *pol* region were used [8].

PCR standardized conditions were followed including 6 μL of reverse transcriptase (RT) or previous PCR product, 2.5 and 2 mM $MgCl_2$ for the *gag* and *pol* regions, respectively, 0.2 mM for each dNTP (Amersham Pharmacia, Madrid, Spain), 0.5 μM for each primer, and 2 U Taq polymerase (Promega) in a 50-μL final volume. β-actin (beta-actin) gene amplification was performed to confirm the presence of DNA in the extraction from spermatozoa suspension. Results were read after a 2% agarose gel electrophoresis after ethidium bromide staining [7]. In all the samples, a consistent result (either positive or negative) was obtained. The assay failure rate was zero.

The quantitative one-round PCR technique was performed according to the method of Roche Diagnostic Systems (Amplicor; Roche, Basel, Switzerland) and as described in the work by Marina and coworkers [3]. Briefly, RNA extraction was performed according to the Amplicor Specimen Preparation Kit (Roche, Barcelona, Spain).

To check for HIV RNA load, reverse transcription and amplification using SK145 and SKCC1B were carried out (amplifying a limited region of the HIV-1 *gag* gene, which translates the viral proteins p18, p24, and p55). The PCR amplified product was detected and quantified through hybridization with the use of a specific biotin-labeling probe. An ELISA was used for subsequent detection.

The results of the analysis for the detection of the presence of viral molecules after the sperm washes demonstrated that approximately 7% of sperm washes still resulted positive after the sperm wash. On those cases, the sample was reanalyzed, and the results of positive samples by nested PCR were compared with the one-round PCR protocols, finding that they resulted negative.

After 2–3 weeks, another sperm wash is programmed. We never obtained a positive result after a second wash. The assay never failed in yielding a diagnostic.

This is undoubtedly indicating that a negative sample in the protocols employing one-round PCR still had undetectable viral presence [2]. Nevertheless, different institutions employ different methodologies, with highly variable efficiency and detection limits [9, 10].

Assisted Reproduction Techniques on Serodiscordant Couples

To choose which treatment (IUI, in vitro fertilization (IVF), or ICSI) would be used, several aspects must be considered. Artificial insemination has been the alternative method for a period of time, given the low difficulty and invasiveness [3, 4]. This method may be simpler and less expensive than others, but we think that it presents some important inconveniencies, such as the need of a sperm wash result on the same day, and if a positive result is found, the cycle will be canceled; another problem is the low numbers of spermatozoa inseminated and the potential risk of viral transmission due to the exposure to thousands or even millions of "potentially infecting" spermatozoa. Also the whole sperm preparation must be inseminated within the same cycle. In this way, pregnancy rates are about 15% per cycle, with accumulative pregnancy rates of almost 60% in four consecutive treatments depending of sperm quality (considering a significant decrease of the sperm number available after sperm wash process).

We maintain a different conduct with these couples: IVF with ICSI protocols. ICSI involves a lower exposure of sperm cells compared to that in IUI (which requires millions of sperm). Despite the high cost of the ICSI process; the efficiency of this technique avoids the expensive repetitive virological semen testing and numerous cycles of ovarian stimulation. Another advantage over IUI relates to the increase in pregnancy rates per treatment cycle (two to three times higher with ICSI; nearly 50% per cycle, with cumulative pregnancy rates in three cycles of 90%) and should decrease the number of attempts needed to establish a successful pregnancy.

With ICSI, we are exposing the woman to a nearly infinitesimal risk: we just employ one single sperm for each oocyte obtained from a previously sample resulting negative by PCR.

By another way, semen samples are frozen, and nested PCR results can be confirmed as many times as needed, since that the sample is not necessarily employed the same day. Also, sperm wash can be performed before the cycle, thus not canceling any cycle due to a positive result. If sperm wash resulted negative, it can be employed several times as needed, thus avoiding the need (and expenses) of new washes.

Additionally, in men with a priori lower semen qualities, that will not be enough for optimal IUI, ICSI is the only realistic treatment option because after the extensive procedure that involves sperm wash, and in order to avoid possible positives, the sperm recovery is very low (about 5% of the initial motile sperm).

Objectively, we must keep in mind that both techniques have been employed successfully to date to help serodiscordant people succeed in their reproductive wishes safely [3, 4, 11–15].

Sperm Wash Results: Efficiency, Pregnancy, and Seroconversion Rates

Next, we are going to analyze the results of our program for SDC couples with the male infected, in terms of seroconversion and pregnancy rates when washed samples were employed. Couples with seronegative women, and HIV-positive males (n = 18), with co-infection HCV-/HIV-positive males (n = 33), and infertile couples undergoing ART where the male was HCV positive (n = 40) were included in this study, providing a total number of 134 sperm samples to be washed. The HIV infection was acquired by parenteral drug addiction in 25 of them (48.8%), plasma donation in 1 (0.2%), sexual transmission in 11 (21.6%), blood transfusion in 6 (11.7%), and 8 (15.5%) unknown. About the female population, only those with demonstrated absence of HIV and HCV antibodies were accepted in the study. They were also requested to practice sex with condoms.

Different gynecological findings were observed: 59 of them were considered as normal (64.8%), 15 of them were aged more than 36 years old (16.4%), 5 of them were low responders (5.5%), 8 of them had endometriosis (8.6%). Depending of the patient's characteristics, we treated these women with ICSI with their own oocytes or with oocytes obtained from young healthy donors. In HIV serodifferent couples, 11 procedures were made with donated eggs, while seven procedures were performed with donated eggs in HCV serodiscordant couples.

In this work, we found a global pregnancy rate of approximately 45% per cycle [1], and almost 95% of the couples finally get pregnant after four consecutive cycles. Results are shown in Table 4.1. Blood analysis after 3, 6, and 9 months confirmed no seroconversion in the women.

Table 4.1 Global cycle results depending on the infection

	HIV (total)	HIV only	HIV/HCV	HCV infected
Follicular aspirations (FA)	73	27	46	51
Oocytes obtained	920	352	568	621
Metaphase II	742	293	449	514
Zygotes	511	211	300	305
Frozen embryos	169	78	91	68
Transferred embryos	154	59	95	116
Met. II/FA	9.9 ± 2.3	10.9 ± 2.0	10.2 ± 2.0	10.5 ± 3.0
Fertilization rate/Met. II (%)	68.9 ± 6.3	72.0[a] ± 8.1	66.8 ± 6.0	59.3[a] ± 5.3
Embryos/(FA)	4.3 ± 2.0	5.1 ± 1.8	4.0 ± 2.0	3.8 ± 0.7
Cleavage rate (embryos/Met. II) (%)	57.3 ± 5.3	62.4 ± 5.6	53.4 ± 8.3	44.9 ± 10.2
Embryo transfers	64	23	41	42
Embryos/transfer	2.4	2.6	2.2	2.8
Positive pregnancy test	29	9	20	12
Negative pregnancy test	29	12	17	29
Biochemical pregnancy	5	1	4	1
Newborns	19	4	15	4
Pregnancy rate/cycle (%)	46.0	40.1	48.7	40.1
Frozen embryo (FE) transfer	10	6	4	8
FE positive pregnancy tests	2	0	2	0
FE negative pregnancy tests	8	6	2	6
FE pregnancy rates (%)	20	0	50	0

Results are expressed as total numbers, or mean ± standard error of the mean.
[a]$p < 0.05$

Influence of HIV-1 Infection on Semen Quality: The Basic Sperm Analysis and the Embryos Point of View

A posterior work was dedicated to the analysis of factors making the sperm washes fail and the sperm quality in SDC males. We evaluated male infection parameters, antiretroviral treatments received, and sperm quality to identify positive washes predictors [16].

In this study, 73 healthy seronegative males were included, as a control population, consisting in partners of women exclusively with tubaric infertility, within the same period of time. Controls and HIV males were matched by age (±2 years) and the number of days (±0.5) of sexual abstinence.

Between August 2001 and November 2003, a total of 125 males provided 136 samples to be washed. Age ranged between 21 and 54 years (median 37.1)

The viral acquisition was for the 70 HIV-infected males (45 of them also co-infected with HCV, 64.3%); 32 ex-addictions to parenteral drugs (45.7%), 2 plasma donations (3.0%), 15 heterosexual transmissions (21.4%), and finally 14 (20.0%) were from unknown origin. The length of the HIV disease was 9.6 years (range 1–20). In the CDC classification of the disease, 12 of them (17.1%) were A1, 23

Table 4.2 ROC curves analysis results for the prediction of the post-wash PCR result for infectious particles by semen parameters and HIV patient's features

Parameter (n = 73)	Area under the curve	Threshold	Sensitivity	Specificity	VPP	VPN
CD_4 (HIV)	0.59 (0.469–0.704)	≤147	37.5	92.5	37.5	92.3
Evolution (HIV)	0.53 (0.410–0.653)	≤12	85.7	30.2	12.0	95.0
Viral load (HIV)	0.49 (0.289–0.690)	≤44,000	100	36.4	22.2	100
Volume	0.49 (0.397–0.576)	>3.4	61.5	55.2	13.3	92.8
Concentration	0.65 (0.561–0.731)	≤13.6	38.5	87.9	26.3	92.7
A + B	0.55 (0.458–0.636)	>67	23.1	93.9	30.0	91.5
TMP	0.62 (0.537–0.711)	≤38.07	69.2	73.9	23.1	95.5
Volume cap.	0.55 (0.463–0.642)	≤1.1	69.2	46.5	12.9	93
Conc. post	0.57 (0.479–0.658)	>1	100	20.4	12.6	100
A + B AW	0.59 (0.507–0.685)	≤80	69.2	57.5	15.8	94.2
TMP AW	0.68 (0.600–0.769)	≤2.2	84.6	58.9	19.3	97.1
Recovery rate	0.56 (0.467–0.647)	≤0.1541	23.1	95.5	37.5	91.5

A, *B* type A and B motility, respectively (WHO statements); *TMP* total motile progressive sperm; *AW* after wash

(32.8%) A2, 5 (7.1%) A3, 3 (4.3%) B1, 7 (10%) B2, 11 (15.7%) B3, 2 (2.8%) C2, and 6 (8.5%) C3.

About antiretroviral treatments, 21 of them (30%) were treatment-free, while the remaining were receiving any combination: 2 monotherapies (2.8%), 4 bi-therapies (5.7%), 36 (51.4%) tri-therapies, tetra-therapies (8.5%), and 1 hexa-therapy (1.4%).

HIV blood load was 19,408 IU/mL (ranging from undetectable-525,000 IU/mL), while 39 patients (55.7%) showed negative viral blood load. Peripheral blood CD_4 levels median was 497.5 ranging from 26 to 1,064.

The results of this work exposed that there is no system to predict a positive result after sperm washes, as stated by the ROC curves analysis of the different factors (Table 4.2). As well, we did not found a no significant diminish in sperm quality on HIV-positive group in comparison with healthy controls, and antiretroviral treatments received are not affecting sperm quality. Another way to analyze sperm quality is by studying the embryo quality obtained from these sperm samples in comparison with healthy controls [17].

From our data, we conclude that fertilization and cleavage rates were comparable between the groups. On days 2 and 3 of embryo development, very similar embryo features were found between the groups. Additionally, there was no difference in mean number of optimal embryos on day 3; but when embryos were cultured up to 5–6 days, a significant increase on embryo blockage was found in SDC group, in comparison with control group. However, the mean number of optimal blastocysts on day 6 was comparable in both groups. Regarding number of cryopreserved and transferred embryos, implantation, pregnancy, multiple pregnancy, and miscarriage rates, difference was found between the groups.

Is Sperm Wash Possible in Oligo- or Azoospermic Samples?

To undergo these sperm wash protocols, a minimum number of motile sperm cells in the ejaculate are necessary. At least two millions are needed to perform these treatments.

Patients with Severe Oligospermia

In our institution, there are approximately 2% of the HIV- or HCV-seropositive men presenting severe oligospermia [1]. On them, the exhaustive sperm wash protocols, executed as previously described, made impossible to recover any sperm at the end of the procedure.

On males that present lower sperm count, we considered the possibility to perform modified sperm washed by serial dilutions of the sperm sample and, then, to confirm the absence of viral nucleic acids by PCR.

The first series were published in 2006, where from 7 males with severe oligospermia undergoing modified sperm washes, none resulted positive and were able to undergo assisted reproduction treatments [18]. This is, to our knowledge, the unique report from oligospermic males.

Sperm Wash Protocol on Oligozoospermic Males

Ejaculates obtained after a sexual abstinence of 3–5 days should be allowed to liquefy for 10 min at 37°C and then be diluted 1:1 (vol/vol) with human tubal fluid (HTF) medium. Then, centrifuge for 10 min at 400 × *g*, and discard the supernatants carefully. This procedure has to be repeated twice, and the resulting cells will be resuspended in a final volume of 0.5–1 mL.

One half of each sample have to be submerged immediately in liquid nitrogen for PCR determinations, and the other half be frozen as described elsewhere [2] and be stored until its usage in assisted reproduction once a negative viral presence had been confirmed.

Patients with Azoospermia

An extreme situation is presented in males without sperm in the ejaculates. Two case reports were available in the literature describing the epididymal search of motile sperm in azoospermic males presenting obstructions in the genital tract.

On these papers, only patients with epididymal sperm retrieval were presented [19, 20]. This technique could be inappropriate for some azoospermic males. For example, this method could not be applied if the obstruction is up in the genital tract, or when males presenting nonobstructive azoospermia with no spermatozoa available in the epididymal reservoir.

Furthermore, open testicular biopsies augment the chances to find motile sperm cells in azoospermic patients, although the blood and round cell presence could be increasing the risk of viral presence after wash.

Our group recently published three cases with open testicular biopsy, in azoospermia, that is also applicable to males presenting nonobstructive azoospermia [21].

Sperm Wash Protocol on Azoospermic Males

Samples were obtained from male partners by testicular sperm extraction (TESE), due to the absence of sperm in two consecutive sperm analysis, obtained and analyzed from August 2007 to November 2008. All patients had normal karyotype and no microdeletions on the Y chromosome, as expected given the causes of azoospermia.

TESE was performed as previously described [22]. Briefly, open testicular biopsies were carried out with 2% mepivacaine spermatic cord block. After opening the scrotal skin and tunica vaginalis, three small incisions were made through the tunica albuginea in different regions of each testicle, and small pieces of extruding testicular tissue were excised. Two fragments (one per testis) were embedded within Bouin's solution and were sent for histopathological examination. The remaining fragments were carried to the adjacent laboratory for sperm retrieval. Testicular tissue was placed in 2 mL of Sperm medium (MediCult, Jyllinge, Norway) and minced mechanically with sterile slides. The presence of sperm cells was checked under an inverted microscope at 3,400 magnification. If motile sperm were found, samples were immediately frozen. Before that, they were centrifuged for 10 min at 400 × *g*, and the supernatants were then carefully discarded. This procedure was repeated twice, and the resulting cells were resuspended in a final volume of 0.5–1 mL.

When this initial microscopic evaluation did not show motile spermatozoa, the sperm suspension was transferred into a Falcon tube and centrifuged at 600 × *g* for 5 min. The pellet was resuspended in 0.5 mL of Sperm Medium and incubated at 37°C and 5% CO_2 for 1 h. Then, the presence of motile sperm was checked again.

Continually, for freezing, an equal volume of Sperm Freezing Medium (MediCult) containing glycerol was added to the sperm pellet and then homogenized and placed at room temperature for 10 min. Sperm samples were frozen in small tablets using a dry ice surface for approximately 1 min and then were transferred to pre-labeled cryotubes. One half of each sample was immediately submerged in liquid nitrogen for PCR determinations, and the other half was frozen as previously described and stored into liquid nitrogen tanks until its employment in assisted reproduction once a negative viral presence had been confirmed.

For thawing, the pills were removed and transferred into 5-mL Falcon tubes, and placed in an incubator at 37°C and 5% CO_2. Then samples were washed again with Sperm Medium (MediCult) and centrifuged at 600 × *g* for 5 min. The supernatant was discarded and samples resuspended in variable amounts of medium. Thereafter, motile spermatozoa were checked again for ICSI.

After sperm washes, motile sperm were recovered to be frozen in all testicular biopsies, then guaranteeing a safe use of the spermatozoa found within the sample. Two pregnancies were achieved in five follicular aspirations, with four fresh and two frozen/thawed embryo transferences, resulting in a healthy newborn and an ongoing pregnancy.

Our results, although in a limited sequence of cases, confirm that TESE-ICSI treatments in azoospermic seropositive patients are possible, and that these males should not be rejected if these techniques, together with sperm wash and PCR confirmation of the viral absence, are available

Conclusion

The laboratory is focused on two aspects: first, we need to eliminate any viral particle, since nPCR is an extremely sensitive method, and any viral residue will be detected, thus yielding a positive result and forcing us to discard the sample. Secondly, we must optimize the sperm washing procedure to ensure that we maintain as many motile sperm as possible, to permit as many ICSI procedures as possible.

In conclusion, HIV-infected patients now have the possibility to become fathers, avoiding viral transmission to the mother and future child. Sperm parameters are not significantly different from those that the World Health Organization considers to be normal. We were unable to detect a parameter that could help us in the prediction of the sperm wash results, which remained positive in 10% of the samples.

Low CD_4 counts together with a long time of evolution of the disease are relevant for the sample, but insignificant for the whole treatment. Given these results, patients must be counseled accordingly before the initiation of a treatment.

References

1. Garrido N, Meseguer M, Bellver J, Remohi J, Simon C, Pellicer A. Report of the results of a 2 year programme of sperm wash and ICSI treatment for human immunodeficiency virus and hepatitis C virus serodiscordant couples. Hum Reprod. 2004;19:2581–6.
2. Meseguer M, Garrido N, Gimeno C, Remohi J, Simon C, Pellicer A. Comparison of polymerase chain reaction-dependent methods for determining the presence of human immunodeficiency virus and hepatitis C virus in washed sperm. Fertil Steril. 2002;78:1199–202.
3. Semprini AE, Levi-Setti P, Bozzo M, et al. Insemination of HIV-negative women with processed semen of HIV-positive partners. Lancet. 1992;340:1317–9.
4. Marina S, Marina F, Alcolea R, et al. Human immunodeficiency virus type 1—serodiscordant couples can bear healthy children after undergoing intrauterine insemination. Fertil Steril. 1998;70:35–9.
5. Meseguer M, Garrido N, Gimeno C, Remohi J, Simon C, Pellicer A. Comparison of polymerase chain reaction-dependent methods for determining the presence of human immunodeficiency virus and hepatitis C virus in washed sperm. Fertil Steril. 2002;78:1199–202.

6. World Health Organization. Laboratory manual of the WHO for the examination of human semen and sperm-cervical mucus interaction. Ann Ist Super Sanita. 2001;37:I–XII, 1–123.
7. Meseguer M, Aplin JD, Caballero-Campo P, et al. Human endometrial mucin MUC1 is up-regulated by progesterone and down-regulated in vitro by the human blastocyst. Biol Reprod. 2001;64:590–601.
8. Zazzi M, Romano L, Catucci M, et al. Low human immunodeficiency virus type 1 (HIV-1) DNA burden as a major cause for failure to detect HIV-1 DNA in clinical specimens by PCR. J Clin Microbiol. 1995;33:205–8.
9. Pasquier C, Anderson D, Andreutti-Zaugg C, et al. Multicenter quality control of the detection of HIV-1 genome in semen before medically assisted procreation. J Med Virol. 2006;78: 877–82.
10. Bujan L, Hollander L, Coudert M, et al. Safety and efficacy of sperm washing in HIV-1-serodiscordant couples where the male is infected: Results from the European CREAThE network. AIDS. 2007;21:1909–14.
11. Gilling-Smith C. HIV prevention. assisted reproduction in HIV-discordant couples. AIDS Read. 2000;10:581–7.
12. Ohl J, Partisani M, Wittemer C, et al. Assisted reproduction techniques for HIV serodiscordant couples: 18 months of experience. Hum Reprod. 2003;18:1244–9.
13. Sharma S, Gilling-Smith C, Semprini AE, Barton SE, Smith JR. View 1: assisted conception in couples with HIV infection. Sex Transm Infect. 2003;79:185–8.
14. Bujan L, Pasquier C, Labeyrie E, Lanusse-Crousse P, Morucci M, Daudin M. Insemination with isolated and virologically tested spermatozoa is a safe way for human immunodeficiency type 1 virus-serodiscordant couples with an infected male partner to have a child. Fertil Steril. 2004;82:857–62.
15. Mencaglia L, Falcone P, Lentini GM, et al. ICSI for treatment of human immunodeficiency virus and hepatitis C virus-serodiscordant couples with infected male partner. Hum Reprod. 2005;20:2242–6.
16. Garrido N, Meseguer M, Remohi J, Simon C, Pellicer A. Semen characteristics in human immunodeficiency virus (HIV)- and hepatitis C (HCV)-seropositive males: Predictors of the success of viral removal after sperm washing. Hum Reprod. 2005;20:1028–34.
17. Melo MA, Meseguer M, Bellver J, Remohi J, Pellicer A, Garrido N. Human immunodeficiency type-1 virus (HIV-1) infection in serodiscordant couples (SDCs) does not have an impact on embryo quality or intracytoplasmic sperm injection (ICSI) outcome. Fertil Steril. 2008;89: 141–50.
18. Garrido N, Remohi J, Pellicer A, Meseguer M. The effectiveness of modified sperm washes in severely oligoasthenozoospermic men infected with human immunodeficiency and hepatitis C viruses. Fertil Steril. 2006;86:1544–6.
19. Nicopoullos JD, Frodsham LC, Ramsay JW, Almeida PA, Rozis G, Gilling-Smith C. Synchronous sperm retrieval and sperm washing in an intracytoplasmic sperm injection cycle in an azoospermic man who was positive for human immunodeficiency virus. Fertil Steril. 2004;81:670–4.
20. Bujan L, Daudin M, Moinard N, Plante P, Parinaud J, Pasquier C. Azoospermic HIV-1 infected patients wishing to have children: proposed strategy to reduce HIV-1 transmission risk during sperm retrieval and intracytoplasmic sperm injection: case report. Hum Reprod. 2007;22: 2377–81.
21. Garrido N, Gil-Salom M, Martinez-Jabaloyas JM, Meseguer M. First report of the absence of viral load in testicular sperm samples obtained from men with hepatitis C and HIV after washing and their subsequent use. Fertil Steril. 2009;92:1012–5.
22. Meseguer M, Garrido N, Remohi J, et al. Testicular sperm extraction (TESE) and ICSI in patients with permanent azoospermia after chemotherapy. Hum Reprod. 2003;18:1281–5.

Part II
Embryo Culture Methods

Chapter 5
Culture Media in IVF: Decisions for the Laboratory

Jason E. Swain and Thomas B. Pool

Substantial research has been undertaken with the intent of refining and improving IVF culture media since the initial reports of human embryo culture utilizing somatic cell media, such as Ham's F10 [1, 2]. One would think that the most appropriate course of action would have been to adopt the media and culture principles being developed for animal embryos, yet clinical IVF underwent an expansive phase in the early to mid-1980s by instead using the expedient approach of borrowing simple salt solutions and complex media formulations developed for somatic cell culture [3]. Although the field is now benefiting through the clinical use of media developed systematically for mouse embryos in the laboratory of Professor John Biggers, it was through the work of pioneers like Quinn and Menezo that media designed specifically for human embryo culture in vitro initially became available [4, 5]. Modifications and refinements to these media ensued, and it is now possible to routinely grow blastocysts in vitro in defined media without the use of serum [6, 7]. This pursuit has resulted in an extensive body of literature examining various culture media formulations, culture paradigms, supplemental additives, and their impact on embryo development. Because of the breadth of these data, an exhaustive review of all media components is beyond the scope of this chapter. However, certain topics are required for embryologists to gain appreciation for the progression of the field, to understand the rationale for current media formulations, as well as to have the ability to make informed choices when it comes to selection and use of commercially available media within the laboratory. Importantly, certain aspects of IVF culture media, such as selection of media type, macromolecule supplement, and pH, are still directly controlled within the IVF laboratory and require special attention. Review of these topics is necessary to optimize laboratory efficiency and ultimately IVF outcomes.

J.E. Swain, PhD, HCLD (✉)
Department of Obstetrics and Gynecology, University of Michigan, Ann Arbor, MI, USA
e-mail: swainj@umich.edu

T.B. Pool, PhD, HCLD (ABB)
Fertility Center of Antonio, San Antonio, TX, USA

Z.P. Nagy et al. (eds.), *Clinical Embryology: A Practical Guide*,
DOI 10.1007/978-1-4614-8376-2_5,

Laboratory Choices and Culture Media

Mono vs. Sequential Culture

Commercial production and supply of various IVF culture media is one of the primary causes for dramatic improvements in the field. Utilization of ultrapure water, clean facilities, and impeccable quality control during production has helped reduce much of the variability previously encountered within the IVF laboratory. Though there is a clear consensus on the advantages of commercial media production, an ongoing debate exists with regard to the selection of optimal IVF culture media. In the last 10–15 years, there has been a dramatic shift toward the use of sequential culture media, where cleavage-stage embryos are cultured in one medium formulation for the first 1–3 days, then subsequently placed into a second medium formulation for the next 2–3 days to support morula compaction and blastocyst development. These media vary slightly in their composition, changing the levels of glucose and other energy substrates as well as altering the complement of amino acids, chelators, and other components (Fig. 5.1). The rationale behind this approach is to meet the changing needs of the embryo by attempting to emulate what is observed in vivo, where the composition of oviductal fluid differs from that of uterine fluid [8]. In addition, this approach entails replenishing embryos with

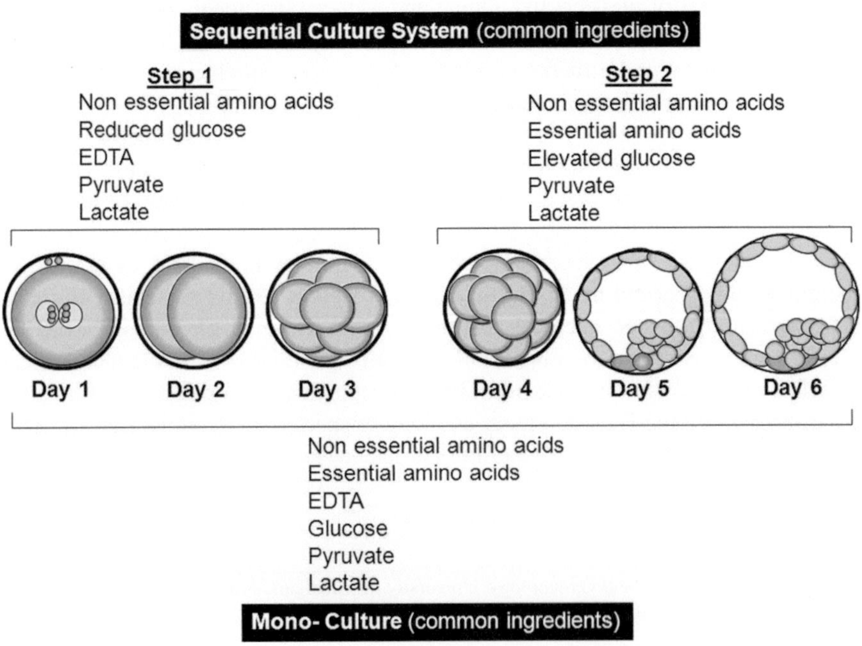

Fig. 5.1 Key energy substrate components of embryo culture media

fresh culture media, ensuring adequate supply of substrates and removal of potentially harmful by-products, such as ammonia.

In contrast, monoculture systems entail supplying a single medium formulation that is a product of exhaustive experimentation designed for "letting the embryo decide" which components it prefers [9]. The approach of replenishing media at 2–3-day intervals to supply fresh nutrients and remove waste products is also compatible with this approach. Indeed, in a number of laboratories, monoculture systems prove to be as efficient as sequential culture systems [10–12].

Extensive data on the release or depletion of nutrients by both mouse and human embryos led Leese [13] to propose the "quiet embryo hypothesis" which suggests that a reduced metabolic level is consistent with a viable phenotype. Further, environmental stresses are seen as one of the components that elevate metabolic activity resulting in heritable damage to daughter cells such as heat shock and nucleic acid damage [13, 14]. The extent to which "noisy metabolism," induced by stresses from the in vitro environment, influence embryonic responses to various metabolite challenges during medium design experiments remains unknown. But it is important to realize that all current media formulations were developed in animal models, not with human embryos, and it is not known that human zygotes respond in the same manner as those from other species to a specific environmental challenge. Medium design should therefore be considered a work in progress.

Regardless of the approach employed, the success of such a wide variety of media underscores the plasticity seen with regard to the embryo's ability to adapt to its environment. Importantly, though many media support embryo development, their efficiency needs to be evaluated in the context of their use within a particular laboratory, in conjunction with the variety of other processes that make up the complete culture system [15]. To this end, careful attention to detail and development of more sensitive endpoint assessments are needed to truly tease out minor improvements and lab-to-lab variability. Independent of which media are utilized, certain themes hold true and are important to understand in order to appreciate intricacies of embryo physiology and to assist in making informed decisions within the lab.

Energy Substrates

Glucose

Glucose has been a wide source of contention within the field of embryology and is one of the primary variables in sequential culture media. Though cleavage stage human embryos can use glucose, it is in minimal amounts compared to oxidative substrates like pyruvate [16–19]. Indeed, sequential systems utilize reduced levels of glucose (0–0.5 mM) in the first step of their system and also often include EDTA, which further suppresses glycolysis [20]. Furthermore, culture media devoid of glucose support high rates of human embryo development and pregnancy during the first 3 days of culture [21–24]. Thus, any minimal initial requirement for glucose may likely be obtained through initial exposure and carryover from handling media containing glucose, or from internal stores of glycogen. Metabolic studies indicate mammalian embryos primarily utilizing glucose during compaction and blastocyst development. Therefore, the second media employed in sequential systems raise the concentration of glucose (>2.0 mM).

Lactate/Pyruvate

Though extensive focus has been placed on glucose and its role in supporting blastocyst development, perhaps more important are the roles of energy substrates which permit the prerequisite cleavage stage embryo development. The addition of lactate to early salt solution media was instrumental in supporting development from the two-cell stage of mouse embryos [25]. Furthermore, pyruvate was discovered to be imperative for cleavage of one-cell mouse zygotes and is the primary energy substrate for cleavage stage embryos [26–28], including human, where it is used throughout development to the blastocyst stage [17, 29, 30]. Importantly, low levels of lactate can affect pyruvate metabolism [31, 32] and can also acidify internal pH [33, 34]. It has been suggested that only the metabolizable L-lactate isomer be included in culture media formations to avoid excess suppression of internal pH that may exist with use of D-/L-isomers [35].

Amino Acids

Amino acids can not only serve as energy sources to developing embryos but also serve to maintain intracellular homeostasis by acting as zwitterions to buffer pH, antioxidants, and as organic osmolytes to control cell volume [36]. As a result, amino acids are now an essential component to successful embryo culture media. Tedious sets of experiments were conducted examining effects of individual amino acids on hamster embryo development [37]. These studies demonstrated that three amino acids in particular improved development in the context of the utilized base medium: glutamine, taurine, and glycine. Additional experiments conducted by Lane and Gardner utilized commercially available mixtures of amino acids known as Eagle's "essential" and "nonessential amino acids" in a sequential culture system. These studies determined a preferential exposure sequence that improved embryo development and viability following transfer, which entailed addition of nonessential amino acids with glutamine during the first 3 days of culture, followed by inclusion of all 20 amino acids during the following 2–3 days [38]. Benefits of amino acids are also evident when included in a monoculture system, such as KSOM, yielding improved blastocyst development, cell number, and hatching rates [39–41]. Indeed, even brief exposure of mouse zygotes to media lacking amino acids can impair development [42]. Therefore, it is imperative that all media contain some source of amino acids, especially handling media utilized for oocyte retrieval and ICSI.

One potential concern with amino acids in culture, especially during cleavage stage development, is their breakdown and production of ammonia, which may impact subsequent development and health of resulting offspring [43–47]. Though debated, of particular interest is glutamine, which is the most labile of the amino acids [48]. Fortunately, dipeptide forms of glutamine, such as alanyl-glutamine [46] or glycyl-glutamine [49, 50], are stable at 37°C and help alleviate this concern. Therefore, the use of media utilizing these stabile forms of glutamine is recommended.

Osmolality

An important concept to be aware of in regard to culture media is osmolality and its resulting effect on cell volume and ultimately embryo development. High osmolality can compromise embryo development and was one of the underlying causes of the "two-cell block" observed in early embryo culture media studies (see review [51]). Osmolality of commercial culture media varies (Table 5.1). Fortunately, active mechanisms exist in oocytes and embryos to regulate cell volume, and these mechanisms depend on media ingredients. Therefore, selection of appropriate culture media is paramount. Studies demonstrate various amino acids that provide protection against high osmolality [52–54] and are thus recommended in all media to aid in this regulation [51]. Special concern exists in changing from one media to another, such as between handling media and culture media with differing ion composition. In addition, choice of culture volume can impact media osmolality due to evaporation while on heated working surfaces, as well as due to air movement over culture dishes within flow hoods. Use of larger volumes of media helps combat resulting osmolality rise, and oil overlay and use of humidified incubators are also recommended to prevent dramatic increases in osmolality.

Macromolecules

Macromolecules are an especially important consideration in IVF culture medium since their source, composition, and concentration are still largely decided within individual laboratories (Table 5.2). Therefore, as embryologists, it is our responsibility to do our due diligence and familiarize ourselves with macromolecules and their effects to help make informed decisions as to their use.

As IVF culture media advanced, the field moved toward use of a fully defined media, and the use of serum was abandoned. However, protein and other macromolecules still prove beneficial by improving embryo development, increasing cryotolerance, and also acting as surfactants and increasing colloidal osmotic pressure [55]. A common protein source utilized for in vitro culture is serum albumin, although lot-to-lot variation can be a concern [56], as well as presence of various contaminants. Therefore, recombinant albumin is also used and been found to be as

Table 5.1 Osmolality ranges of various commercial media utilized in IVF

Media	Osmolality range (MOsM)
Irvine	
P1	282–298
ECM	282–295
Single-step (SSM)	280–295
Multiblast	281–291
HTF	272–288
SAGE	
Fert media	265 ± 8
Cleavage media	265 ± 8
Blastocyst media	265 ± 8
IVM	265 ± 8
Vitrolife	
GIVF	279 ± 5
G1.5	261 ± 5
G2.5	260 ± 5
Life global	
Global	260–270 (265)
Global Fert	280–292 (285)
Blastocyst	260–270 (265)
HTF	280–292 (285)
HTFxtra	280–292 (285)
Medicult	
Universal IVF	272–288
ISM1	272–288
ISM2	272–288
EmbryoAssist	272–288
BlastAssist	272–288
Cook	
Sydney IVF cleavage	285–295
Sydney IVF blastocyst	285–295
Sydney IVF Fert	285–295

Table 5.2 Various macromolecules commercially available for inclusion in IVF culture media

Macromolecule	References
Human serum albumin (HSA)	
Recombinant albumin	[51, 52]
SSS (HSA + α (alpha) and β (beta) globulins)	[53, 54]
Dextran (DSS)	[3]
Hyaluronan	[55–57]

effective or superior to albumin in animal models [57, 58]. A growing trend in human embryo culture is the use of more complex macromolecules. Inclusion of alpha and beta globulins with human serum albumin (HSA) improved human embryo development [59] and live birth outcomes [60] and may be concentration dependent [61]. Similar products are now widely available from various commercial media companies. Additionally, macromolecules such as hyaluronan are advantageous when included in culture media [62–64]. In vivo, embryos are surrounded by various proteins and macromolecules. Thus, they likely play a physiologic role in supporting embryo growth. Potential benefit of these macromolecules may stem from nutritional roles, but may also be tied to improvement of the physical environment stemming interactions with water, as suggested by Pool and Martin [59]. These authors postulated that the more pronounced interaction of water with glycoproteins, compared to albumin, might be beneficial in the in vitro environment. As a test of this, dextran, a linear polymer of glucose and a molecule known to interact strongly with water, was added to albumin as a medium supplement [3]. This combination supported embryonic developmental rates equivalent to albumin with alpha and beta globulins and produced clinical pregnancy [3, 59]. This work led to the trial of hyaluronan as a medium supplement by others. It should also be mentioned that macromolecules might be advantageous with respect to embryo transfer media. Hyaluronan has been suggested as being advantageous for transfer and embryo implantation, though the reasoning for this is unclear as the protein cannot penetrate the zona pellucida to access the embryo and no receptors are present on the zona pellucida, though one cannot rule out direct uterine effects. Another potential rationale is that increased viscosity of transfer media may be advantageous to promote adherence of embryos to the uterine wall, and can be accomplished through use of increased protein concentrations. Macromolecules also impact cryosurvival (see review [65]). Another important factor to consider and monitor when utilizing macromolecules is their affect on media pH.

pH

While a large amount of attention in regard to IVF culture media has focused on concentrations of energy substrates or supplemental additives, the very basic principle of acid–base balance is often overlooked. Though we routinely measure this parameter indirectly during daily laboratory quality control assessments of the atmospheric content of our incubators, it is often not appreciated that we are in fact attempting to monitor medium pH (external pH, pHe). This is a very important consideration because, though commercial media companies now control many aspects of media production and quality, the laboratory itself on a day-to-day basis directly controls this aspect of culture media. Thus, greater attention to detail is given to pH in this chapter.

The pHe of culture media is simply a measure of hydrogen ion concentration, which is the result of the equilibrium between two primary components: the dissolved bicarbonate supplied in the media and the amount of CO_2 in the incubator, which dissolves in solution to yield carbonic acid. The importance of this parameter becomes more apparent when one stops to think about proper lab procedures, such as the rationale for limiting patient numbers in a single incubator, reducing incubator openings/closings, installing inner incubator doors, minimizing dish time out of the incubator, and using oil overlay. All of these practices serve to limit the amount of external stress imposed upon gametes and embryos in an attempt to optimize the in vitro culture environment by stabilizing the CO_2 environment, and ultimately pHe. The reasoning behind the need to stabilize pHe is evident from the work of Dale et al. [66]. Though mammalian embryos have various mechanisms to regulate their intracellular pH (pHi), including the Na^+/H^+ antiporter and HCO_3^-/Cl^- transporter, excursions in pHe are readily converted to variances in intracellular pH (pHi), at least initially. Additionally, oocytes have a greatly reduced ability to regulate pHi [67–69], thus reinforcing the technical need to establish a target pHe and conform to it during procedures that allow pHe to drift.

pH and Cellular Function

The need to establish a target pHe is clear when one considers pH controls several intracellular processes that can impact embryo development. Raising (~7.4) or lowering (~6.8) pHi in mouse embryos for only 3 h disrupts localization of mitochondrial and actin microfilaments compared to controls (~7.2) [70]. Even minor rises in pHi can also dramatically impact embryo metabolism through regulation of various enzymes, such as phosphofructokinase (PFK). Raising pHi ~0.1–0.15 units significantly increased embryo glycolysis and lowered oxidative metabolism [33, 71], which can dramatically impact developmental competence. Importantly, other common practices in IVF, such as vitrification, reduce the ability of these already sensitive cells to regulate pHi for about 6 h [71]. Finally, more recent evidence suggests that pHe cannot only affect embryo development, but resulting fetal development as well. Lowering the pHi of one-cell mouse embryos from 7.25 to 7.1 for 19 h resulted in significantly fewer blastocyst cell numbers, higher levels of apoptosis, and reduced fetal size/weight compared to controls [72].

Special concern for pHe exists with respect to denuded mature oocytes. These sensitive cells lack or have diminished ability to regulate pHi and are therefore heavily dependent upon pHe. Thus, in procedures such as ICSI, where the protective cumulus cells are purposefully removed, cells are created that are extremely susceptible to perturbations in pHe until several hours after fertilization occurs [73–76]. Little work has been done examining the effects of pHe on the mature oocyte. This should be concerning given the prevalence of oocyte-derived aneuploidy and the potential impact pH has on the meiotic spindle. pH is known to affect embryo actin cytoskeletal elements [70], and the oocyte cytoskeleton is responsible for positioning of the meiotic spindle [77, 78]. It is known that alkaline pH affects microtubule assembly/disassembly in bovine brain cells [79], and similar actions may be occurring with the meiotic spindle within the oocyte. Additionally, because pH can affect embryo mitochondrial localization [70], the same may hold true for oocytes. This is concerning because the distribution of oocyte mitochondria is correlated with developmental competence [80, 81]. Oocyte metabolism is also likely affected by pH, which, in turn, has been correlated with maturational status and developmental competence [82, 83]. All these factors indicate a strict regulation of pHe and avoidance of periodic deviations when dealing with oocytes.

Optimal pHe

The ability of embryos to regulate pHi is evidenced by various studies that show embryos can to develop over a pHe range of ~7.0–7.4 without any discernable effect on pHi or development [84, 85], while excursions of pHe outside this range have deleterious effects on embryo developmental competence [75, 86–89]. However, just because blastocysts can be formed over these pHe ranges does not indicate that resulting embryo quality is equivalent. Drifting too far away from the pHi of around 7.1 likely stresses the embryo, as more resources are required to maintain the proper pHi. Conventional wisdom tells us that pHe of culture media should be slightly higher than pHi to help offset the acidification that occurs as a result of intracellular metabolic processes. Thus, many laboratories culture their embryos in the range of 7.2–7.4. However, considering that pH scale is logarithmic, a range of 7.2–7.4 encompasses a >60% change in the molar [H^+], and a tighter range is likely prudent.

Unfortunately, there is no "optimum" pHe for oocytes and embryos, as this will vary from medium to medium based on specific ingredients. The amount of monocarboxylic acids, such as lactate and pyruvate, in culture media can lower pHi [33, 34]. Additionally, amino acids, particularly glycine, taurine, and glutamine, act as zwitterions and help in buffering pHi [34]. Though anecdotal observations from various laboratories suggest that perhaps culturing cleavage-stage embryos closer to pHe 7.2 may give better embryo development, the influence of media composition cannot be overlooked. Embryos grown in media with different amounts of monocarboxylic acids may have different pHi, though the pHe may be the same. Along with potential species or strain-specific requirements associated with various animal models, this likely explains variations in the literature regarding acceptable and optimal pHe [90–92]. Regardless, it would be insightful to see a properly controlled clinical trial to determine if culturing human embryos at a pH closer to 7.2 offers any benefit on embryo development, implantation, or live birth, compared to culturing embryos in the same media at a pH closer to 7.4. At the moment, there is no "ideal" pHe at which to culture embryos, and this is reflected in the wide ranges of acceptable pHe given by various commercial media companies (Table 5.3). Furthermore, despite the growing trend, it remains unknown whether early cleavage stage embryos prefer a slightly lower pHe than later stages of embryo development. However, it is known that later stages of embryos with tight junctions, like the morula and blastocysts, can regulate their pHi more rigorously than early cleavage stage embryos and can thus tolerate a wider range of pHe [33]. Interestingly, there are data to suggest that a slightly more alkaline pHe may benefit fertilization. Dale et al. [66] found higher rates of sperm binding to empty zona pellucida at pHe 7.5 compared to lower pHe. This has led to the common practice of fertilizing oocytes in a slightly higher pH, culturing day 1–3 embryos in a slightly lower pH, and culturing day 4–6 embryos in a slightly higher pH (high-low-high paradigm).

Table 5.3 Recommended pH ranges for various commercial IVF culture media

Media	Recommended pH range
Irvine	
P1	7.27–7.32
ECM	7.2–7.25
Single-step (SSM)	7.8–7.32
Multiblast	7.3–7.4
HTF	7.2–7.3
SAGE	
Fert media	7.3 ± 0.1
Cleavage media	7.2 ± 0.1
Blastocyst media	7.3 ± 01
IVM	7.2 ± 0.1
Vitrolife	
G5 Series	7.27 ± 0.07
Life global	
Global	7.2–7.4[a]
Global Fert	7.2–7.4[a]
Blastocyst	7.2–7.4[a]
HTF	7.2–7.4[a]
HTFxtra	7.2–7.4[a]
Medicult	
Universal IVF	7.3–7.4
ISM1	7.2–7.3
ISM2	7.35–7.45
EmbryoAssist	7.2–7.3
BlastAssist	7.35–7.45
Cook	
Sydney IVF cleavage	7.3–7.5
Sydney IVF blastocyst	7.3–7.5
Sydney IVF Fert	7.3–7.5

[a] Company recommends optimal of 7.3 and suggests user adjusts CO_2 readings to reach this after taking into account protein supplementation

Handling Media and Buffers

Due to the crucial nature of pH in gamete and embryo physiology, the importance of IVF handling media used for manipulations outside the incubator cannot be stressed enough. As reviewed in this chapter, the introduction of more sophisticated culture medium formulations for use within the incubator has dramatically improved our ability to produce better embryos in vitro. Altering energy substrate concentrations, use of either sequential culture or contemporary monoculture, incorporation of amino acids, and introduction of complex protein sources have all proved beneficial. However, the composition of media used for manipulations outside the laboratory incubator has been largely overlooked. These media are formulated to maintain appropriate pHe in room atmosphere, outside the elevated CO_2 concentrations of the

Table 5.4 Common zwitterionic (Good's) buffers and their p*K*a values (optimal buffering) in relation to temperature

Buffer	pH range	p*K*a 25°C	p*K*a 37°C
MOPS	6.5–7.9	7.20	7.02
TES	6.8–8.2	7.40	7.16
HEPES	6.8–8.2	7.48	7.31
DIPSO	7.0–8.2	7.60	7.35
MOBS	6.9–8.3	7.60	n/a
TAPSO	7.0–8.2	7.60	7.39

incubator. Though techniques such as oil overlay can combat this pH rise, dishes of bicarbonate-buffered culture media kept out of the incubator with oil for even brief periods can result in pH rising above 7.4 [93, 94]. Thus, for procedures such as oocyte retrieval, sperm processing, oocyte denuding, ICSI, and embryo transfer, it is often recommended that special handling media be utilized that resists changes in pHe. In the past, handling media included phosphate buffered saline (PBS) solutions, and some laboratories continue to use this medium for oocyte retrieval. However, PBS lacks essential components, such as bicarbonate and metabolic substrates. These inadequacies, coupled with elevated levels of phosphate, may compromise gamete and embryo metabolic activity, disrupt organelle distribution, and interfere with intracellular ionic homeostasis, including intracellular pH [95–97]. Indeed, even brief exposure to PBS as a handling media has been shown to compromise hamster and rabbit embryo development [98, 99] and results in aberrant gene expression in bovine embryos when compared to other buffers [100]. Therefore, a better choice, and an approach that has benefited IVF, entails adoption of handling media that contain appropriate energy substrates, bicarbonate (though at reduced levels to help maintain pHe), and synthetic organic buffers to maintain media pH within a desired range at room atmosphere. These buffers, commonly referred to as Good's buffers, are organic compounds derived from zwitterionic amino acids that provide supplemental buffering capacity over physiologic pH range of approximately 6.1–8.3 [101–103] (Table 5.4). However, different cell types display varying sensitivity to individual zwitterionic buffers [103]. Thus, determining the suitability of specific buffers for use with mammalian gametes and embryos in IVF is crucial. Two of these commonly used in commercially available handling media for ART are 4-(2-hydroxyethyl)-1-piperazineethanesulfonic acid (HEPES) and 3-(*N*-morpholino)-propanesulfonic acid (MOPS) and are selected based on their p*K*a values, an indication of their optimal buffering capacity.

Historically, HEPES at ~21 mM has been a standard for IVF handling media. More recently, at least two commercial companies also now include MOPS in their IVF handling media. Both buffers are efficient, and laboratories using media containing these buffers yield high success rates. However, though HEPES has been widely used in IVF for years, its suitability for procedures has been questioned [104, 105]. Importantly, many of the conclusions drawn concerning toxicity of HEPES are often derived from a progenitor literature that has been cited incorrectly, and the conclusions are not fully supported by the studies performed. In considering these pharmacological effects, it is essential to note that many are largely dependent on interactions with other compounds in the media, not due to toxicity of the buffers themselves. Thus, it is important to examine the use of these buffers in the context of specific base medium. Early somatic cell studies citing HEPES toxicity stemmed from light exposure and interactions with riboflavin [106, 107]. This may have also been a factor in the observations of Butler et al. [108]. Though no data were presented, authors commented that inclusion of HEPES in the medium resulted in increased oocyte degeneration; however, the medium contained riboflavin. Several studies actually indicate that HEPES is able to support oocyte maturation [109–111], fertilization [111–115], and embryo culture [104, 111, 114, 116–119]. Those studies indicating lower fertilization rates in the presence of HEPES are likely due to the simultaneous reduction in bicarbonate concentrations [115]. Embryo development is supported in the presence of HEPES when bicarbonate is present, but not when bicarbonate is absent [116]. Furthermore, when embryos are cultured at room atmosphere and compared to controls cultured in 5% CO_2, differences in development cannot be attributed to HEPES alone. Elevated CO_2 of the laboratory incubator is utilized by embryos for various biochemical processes as a carbon source [120–122] and is likely beneficial over culture at room atmosphere. It has been demonstrated that 25 mM HEPES has no adverse effect on mouse embryo development and that there are no adverse effects of up to 50 mM HEPES when cultured with 25 mM $NaHCO_3$ in ~5% CO_2 [94, 123]. Though there may be species-specific sensitivities to HEPES, or other buffer systems, data indicate that when adequately controlling for other factors such as osmolality, bicarbonate levels, gas levels, and pH, these buffers are able to successfully support mammalian embryo development.

Temperature is another variable to be aware of regarding the use of zwitterionic buffers in IVF handling media. Though it is known that temperature can affect pH probe readings and should be accounted for when measuring pH in this respect, it is often not appreciated that the p*K*a of synthetic organic buffers, as well as the actual pH of the media, changes as temperature changes [94]. As an example, MOPS was presumably selected as an alternative to HEPES for IVF media not only due to toxicity concerns but also because its p*K*a of 7.2 is the closest of the 20 zwitterionic buffers to the pHi of embryos of 7.12 [124]. Thus, MOPS would seemingly offer the best pH buffering of available options. However, the p*K*a of 7.2 for MOPS is at 25°C. Many laboratories warm their handling media to around 37°C, a temperature at which the p*K*a for MOPS is actually 7.02. This is low, considering many labs set their media pH between 7.2 and 7.4. Thus, utilization of MOPS alone, or any other single buffer for that matter, may not offer ideal pH buffering of IVF.

Future Directions

Improved Handling Media

A novel concept to address concerns with buffer toxicity in handling media, as well as the issue of temperature and optimal pH stability, is the combination of several organic buffers into a single solution [125]. Combining buffers allows for selection

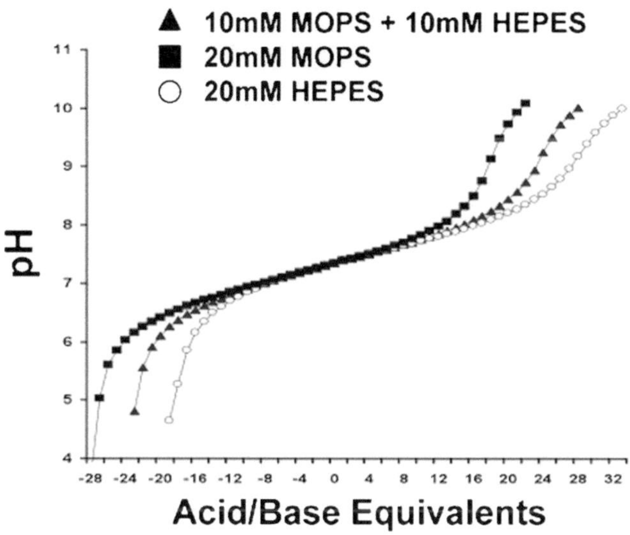

Fig. 5.2 Combining buffers allows for adjustment of p*K*a at specific temperatures

of an exact p*K*a value at a given temperature, which may be more appropriate and offer better buffering than a single buffer (Fig. 5.2). Additionally, superior buffering and combination of buffers allows for the use of lower individual buffer concentrations, thus lowering possible toxicity concerns, and may be superior to current handling media with commonly utilized 20 mM of buffer. Indeed, this approach is a valid substitute for current monobuffered handling media. Swain and Pool [94] verified that bi- and tri-buffered media with combinations of zwitterionic buffers support mouse embryo development. Preliminary data suggest that these buffers may be beneficial for ICSI over monobuffered media [94]. With further testing and verification, additional buffers could be explored and added to further refine media. In addition, specialized handling media for varying cell types may offer an avenue for further improvement. Just as sequential media have been developed to meet the differing needs of the embryos, formulating handling media to meet the differing needs of sperm, oocytes, and varying stages of embryos may be beneficial.

Media Additives-Antioxidants

Supplementation of media with various additives has proven to be a major source of IVF culture improvement. Use of the dipeptide form of glutamine has proven to be beneficial due to its increased stability in culture and resulting decrease in ammonia production [49, 50, 126]. A similar approach could be explored with other ingredients, such as pyruvate. In addition to its role as a metabolic substrate, pyruvate also acts as a powerful antioxidant [127] and can protect embryos from harmful reactive oxygen species (ROS) [128–130]. However, sodium pyruvate, the form of pyruvate added to all current embryo culture media formulations, is labile in solution [131]. By-products of pyruvate breakdown interfere with key steps in the TCA cycle, thereby compromising metabolic activity [131, 132], and are not able to scavenge ROS. Preparations of sodium pyruvate stored in media at 5°C for 1 month may produce enough by-product to inhibit embryo metabolism [132]. A potential improvement over current use of sodium pyruvate in embryo culture media entails use of esterified forms of pyruvate, such as ethyl or methyl pyruvate. These esterified forms of pyruvate have proven superior to sodium pyruvate in various experiments in somatic cells examining their protective effects against various stress paradigms [134–144]. Interestingly, both ethyl and methyl pyruvate were superior to sodium pyruvate in supporting mouse embryo development when pyruvate was the sole energy source [145]. Thus, these esterified forms of pyruvate may lend added benefit due to increased stability in solution or increased membrane permeability, factors which could have an impact on both or embryo metabolism or ability to scavenge ROS. Indeed, supplementation of IVF media with other antioxidants could provide useful in providing added protection and reduced intracellular stress to developing cells [146, 147].

Progressive Media and Microfluidics

Perhaps the most intriguing possibility for the improvement of IVF culture media lies in its use in conjunction with another technological development known as microfluidics. Through the use of automated microfluidic devices, one can potentially integrate in-line, real-time assays to monitor growth conditions. Nanosensors could theoretically detect changes in the growth environment or sense other cues from the developing cells and subsequently modify the culture environment seamlessly, without the need for removing dishes from the incubator or manually moving embryos. In essence, this would improve upon current monoculture or sequential culture systems and on practices such as splitting all cases between two media [148], by providing a customized growth environment suited to the specific needs of particular embryos, rather than expecting all embryos to adapt to a predetermined environment.

References

1. Steptoe PC, Edwards RG, et al. Human blastocysts grown in culture. Nature. 1971;229(5280):132–3.
2. Steptoe PC, Edwards RG. Reimplantation of a human embryo with subsequent tubal pregnancy. Lancet. 1976;1(7965):880–2.
3. Pool T, Atiee S, et al. Oocyte and embryo culture: basic concepts and recent advances. Infert Reprod Med Clin North Am. 1998;9(2):181–203.
4. Menezo Y, Testart J, et al. Serum is not necessary in human in vitro fertilization, early embryo culture, and transfer. Fertil Steril. 1984;42(5):750–5.

5. Quinn P, Kerin J, et al. Improved pregnancy rate in human in vitro fertilization with the use of a medium based on the composition of human tubal fluid. Fertil Steril. 1985;44:493–8.
6. Gardner DK, Pool TB, et al. Embryo nutrition and energy metabolism and its relationship to embryo growth, differentiation, and viability. Semin Reprod Med. 2000;18(2):205–18.
7. Pool TB. Recent advances in the production of viable human embryos in vitro. Reprod Biomed Online. 2002;4(3):294–302.
8. Gardner DK, Lane M, et al. Environment of the preimplantation human embryo in vivo: metabolite analysis of oviduct and uterine fluids and metabolism of cumulus cells. Fertil Steril. 1996;65(2):349–53.
9. Biggers JD, Summers MC. Choosing a culture medium: making informed choices. Fertil Steril. 2008;90(3):473–83.
10. Macklon NS, Pieters MH, et al. A prospective randomized comparison of sequential versus monoculture systems for in-vitro human blastocyst development. Hum Reprod. 2002;17(10): 2700–5.
11. Biggers JD, McGinnis LK, et al. One-step versus two-step culture of mouse preimplantation embryos: is there a difference? Hum Reprod. 2005;20(12):3376–84.
12. Reed ML, Hamic A, et al. Continuous uninterrupted single medium culture without medium renewal versus sequential media culture: a sibling embryo study. Fertil Steril. 2009;92(5): 1783–6.
13. Leese HJ. Quiet please, do not disturb: a hypothesis of embryo metabolism and viability. Bioessays. 2002;24(9):845–9.
14. Leese HJ, Baumann CG, et al. Metabolism of the viable mammalian embryo: quietness revisited. Mol Hum Reprod. 2008;14(12):667–72.
15. Gardner DK. Dissection of culture media for embryos: the most important and less important components and characteristics. Reprod Fertil Dev. 2008;20(1):9–18.
16. Hardy K, Hooper M, et al. Non-invasive measurement of glucose and pyruvate uptake by individual human oocytes and preimplantation embryos. Hum Reprod. 1989;4(2):188–91.
17. Gott A, Hardy K, et al. Non-invasive measurement of pyruvate and glucose uptake and lactate production by single human preimplantation embryos. Hum Reprod. 1990;5(1):104–8.
18. Gardner D, Lane M, et al. Uptake and metabolism of pyruvate and glucose by individual sheep preattachment embryos developed in vivo. Mol Reprod Dev. 1993;36(3):313–9.
19. Devreker F, Hardy K, et al. Noninvasive assessment of glucose and pyruvate uptake by human embryos after intracytoplasmic sperm injection and during the formation of pronuclei. Fertil Steril. 2000;73(5):947–54.
20. Lane M, Gardner DK. Inhibiting 3-phosphoglycerate kinase by EDTA stimulates the development of the cleavage stage mouse embryo. Mol Reprod Dev. 2001;60(2):233–40.
21. Conaghan J, Handyside AH, et al. Effects of pyruvate and glucose on the development of human preimplantation embryos in vitro. J Reprod Fertil. 1993;99(1):87–95.
22. Carrillo AJ, Lane B, et al. Improved clinical outcomes for in vitro fertilization with delay of embryo transfer from 48 to 72 hours after oocyte retrieval: use of glucose- and phosphate-free media. Fertil Steril. 1998;69(2):329–34.
23. Coates A, Rutherford AJ, et al. Glucose-free medium in human in vitro fertilization and embryo transfer: a large-scale, prospective, randomized clinical trial. Fertil Steril. 1999; 72(2):229–32.
24. Ben-Yosef D, Amit A, et al. Prospective randomized comparison of two embryo culture systems: P1 medium by Irvine Scientific and the Cook IVF Medium. J Assist Reprod Genet. 2004;21(8):291–5.
25. Whitten WK. Culture of tubal ova. Nature. 1957;179(4569):1081–2.
26. Brinster R. Studies on the development of mouse embryos in vitro. II. The effect of energy source. J Exp Zool. 1965;158:59–68.
27. Biggers JD, Whittingham DG, et al. The pattern of energy metabolism in the mouse oocyte and zygote. Proc Natl Acad Sci USA. 1967;58(2):560–7.
28. Gardner DK, Leese HJ. Non-invasive measurement of nutrient uptake by single cultured preimplantation mouse embryos. Hum Reprod. 1986;1(1):25–7.

29. Leese HJ, Hooper MA, et al. Uptake of pyruvate by early human embryos determined by a non-invasive technique. Hum Reprod. 1986;1(3):181–2.
30. Hardy K, Hooper MA, et al. Non-invasive measurement of glucose and pyruvate uptake by individual human oocytes and preimplantation embryos. Hum Reprod. 1989;4(2):188–91.
31. Wales RG, Whittingham DG. The metabolism of specifically labelled lactate and pyruvate by two-cell mouse embryos. J Reprod Fertil. 1973;33(2):207–22.
32. Lane M, Gardner DK. Lactate regulates pyruvate uptake and metabolism in the preimplantation mouse embryo. Biol Reprod. 2000;62(1):16–22.
33. Gibb CA, Poronnik P, et al. Control of cytosolic pH in two-cell mouse embryos: roles of H(+)-lactate cotransport and Na+/H+ exchange. Am J Physiol. 1997;273(2 Pt 1):C404–19.
34. Edwards LJ, Williams DA, et al. Intracellular pH of the preimplantation mouse embryo: effects of extracellular pH and weak acids. Mol Reprod Dev. 1998;50(4):434–42.
35. Lane M, Gardner DK. Regulation of ionic homeostasis by mammalian embryos. Semin Reprod Med. 2000;18(2):195–204.
36. Gardner DK, Lane M. Culture systems for human embryos. In: Gardner DK, Weissman A, Howles C, Zeev S, editors. Textbook of assisted reproductive technologies. Boca Raton: Informa UK Ltd; 2009. p. 219–40.
37. McKiernan SH, Clayton MK, et al. Analysis of stimulatory and inhibitory amino acids for development of hamster one-cell embryos in vitro. Mol Reprod Dev. 1995;42(2):188–99.
38. Lane M, Gardner DK. Differential regulation of mouse embryo development and viability by amino acids. J Reprod Fertil. 1997;109(1):153–64.
39. Ho Y, Wigglesworth K, et al. Preimplantation development of mouse embryos in KSOM: augmentation by amino acids and analysis of gene expression. Mol Reprod Dev. 1995;41(2): 232–8.
40. Biggers JD, McGinnis LK, et al. Amino acids and preimplantation development of the mouse in protein-free potassium simplex optimized medium. Biol Reprod. 2000;63(1):281–93.
41. Summers MC, McGinnis LK, et al. IVF of mouse ova in a simplex optimized medium supplemented with amino acids. Hum Reprod. 2000;15(8):1791–801.
42. Gardner DK, Lane M. Alleviation of the '2-cell block' and development to the blastocyst of CF1 mouse embryos: role of amino acids, EDTA and physical parameters. Hum Reprod. 1996;11(12):2703–12.
43. Gardner DK, Lane M. Amino acids and ammonium regulate mouse embryo development in culture. Biol Reprod. 1993;48(2):377–85.
44. Lane M, Gardner DK. Increase in postimplantation development of cultured mouse embryos by amino acids and induction of fetal retardation and exencephaly by ammonium ions. J Reprod Fertil. 1994;102(2):305–12.
45. Lane M, Hooper K, et al. Effect of essential amino acids on mouse embryo viability and ammonium production. J Assist Reprod Genet. 2001;18(9):519–25.
46. Lane M, Gardner DK. Ammonium induces aberrant blastocyst differentiation, metabolism, pH regulation, gene expression and subsequently alters fetal development in the mouse. Biol Reprod. 2003;69(4):1109–17.
47. Zander DL, Thompson JG, et al. Perturbations in mouse embryo development and viability caused by ammonium are more severe after exposure at the cleavage stages. Biol Reprod. 2006;74(2):288–94.
48. Biggers JD, McGinnis LK, et al. Discrepancies between the effects of glutamine in cultures of preimplantation mouse embryos. Reprod Biomed Online. 2004;9(1):70–3.
49. Biggers JD, McGinnis LK, et al. Enhanced effect of glycyl-L-glutamine on mouse preimplantation embryos in vitro. Reprod Biomed Online. 2004;9(1):59–69.
50. Summers MC, McGinnis LK, et al. Mouse embryo development following IVF in media containing either L-glutamine or glycyl-L-glutamine. Hum Reprod. 2005;20(5):1364–71.
51. Baltz JM, Tartia AP. Cell volume regulation in oocytes and early embryos: connecting physiology to successful culture media. Hum Reprod. 2010;15(2):166–76.

52. Richards T, Wang F, et al. Rescue of postcompaction stage mouse embryo development from hypertonicity by amino acid transporter substrates that may function as organic osmolytes. Biol Reprod. 2010;82(4):769–77.
53. Van Winkle LJ, Haghighat N, et al. Glycine protects preimplantation mouse conceptuses from a detrimental effect on development of the inorganic ions in oviductal fluid. J Exp Zool. 1990;253(2):215–9.
54. Lawitts JA, Biggers JD. Joint effects of sodium chloride, glutamine, and glucose in mouse preimplantation embryo culture media. Mol Reprod Dev. 1992;31(3):189–94.
55. Pool T. Blastocyst development in culture: the role of macromolecules. In: Gardner DK, Lane M, editors. ART and the human blastocyst. New York: Springer; 2001. p. 105–17.
56. McKiernan SH, Bavister BD. Different lots of bovine serum albumin inhibit or stimulate in vitro development of hamster embryos. In Vitro Cell Dev Biol. 1992;28A(3 Pt 1):154–6.
57. Bavister BD, Kinsey DL, et al. Recombinant human albumin supports hamster in-vitro fertilization. Hum Reprod. 2003;18(1):113–6.
58. Bungum M, Humaidan P, et al. Recombinant human albumin as protein source in culture media used for IVF: a prospective randomized study. Reprod Biomed Online. 2002;4(3): 233–6.
59. Pool TB, Martin JE. High continuing pregnancy rates after in vitro fertilization-embryo transfer using medium supplemented with a plasma protein fraction containing alpha- and beta-globulins. Fertil Steril. 1994;61(4):714–9.
60. Meintjes M, Chantilis SJ, et al. A randomized controlled study of human serum albumin and serum substitute supplement as protein supplements for IVF culture and the effect on live birth rates. Hum Reprod. 2009;24(4):782–9.
61. Ben-Yosef D, Yovel I, et al. Increasing synthetic serum substitute (SSS) concentrations in P1 glucose/phosphate-free medium improves implantation rate: a comparative study. J Assist Reprod Genet. 2001;18(11):588–92.
62. Lane M, Maybach JM, et al. Cryo-survival and development of bovine blastocysts are enhanced by culture with recombinant albumin and hyaluronan. Mol Reprod Dev. 2003;64(1): 70–8.
63. Gardner DK, Rodriegez-Martinez H, et al. Fetal development after transfer is increased by replacing protein with the glycosaminoglycan hyaluronan for mouse embryo culture and transfer. Hum Reprod. 1999;14(10):2575–80.
64. Palasz AT, Rodriguez-Martinez H, et al. Effects of hyaluronan, BSA, and serum on bovine embryo in vitro development, ultrastructure, and gene expression patterns. Mol Reprod Dev. 2006;73(12):1503–11.
65. Swain J, Smith G. Cryoprotectants. In: Chian R, Quinn P, editors.Cryopreservation in female fertility preservation. Cambridge:Cambridge Publishing; 2010.
66. Dale B, Menezo Y, Cohen J, et al. Intracellular pH regulation in the human oocyte. Hum Reprod 1998; 13(4): 964–970.
67. Phillips KP, Petrunewich MA, et al. The intracellular pH-regulatory HCO_3^-/Cl^- exchanger in the mouse oocyte is inactivated during first meiotic metaphase and reactivated after egg activation via the MAP kinase pathway. Mol Biol Cell. 2002;13(11):3800–10.
68. Erdogan S, FitzHarris G, et al. Mechanisms regulating intracellular pH are activated during growth of the mouse oocyte coincident with acquisition of meiotic competence. Dev Biol. 2005;286(1):352–60.
69. Fitzharris G, Baltz J. Regulation of intracellular pH during oocyte growth and maturation in mammals. Reproduction. 2009;138(4):619–27.
70. Squirrell JM, Lane M, et al. Altering intracellular pH disrupts development and cellular organization in preimplantation hamster embryos. Biol Reprod. 2001;64(6):1845–54.
71. Lane M, Lyons EA, et al. Cryopreservation reduces the ability of hamster 2-cell embryos to regulate intracellular pH. Hum Reprod. 2000;15(2):389–94.
72. Zander-Fox DL, Mitchell M, Thompson JG, Lane M. Alterations in mouse embryo intracellular pH by DMO during culture impair implantation and fetal growth. Reprod Biomed Online. 2010;21(2):219–29.

73. Fitzharris G, Baltz JM. Granulosa cells regulate intracellular pH of the murine growing oocyte via gap junctions: development of independent homeostasis during oocyte growth. Development. 2006;133(4):591–9.
74. FitzHarris G, Siyanov V, et al. Granulosa cells regulate oocyte intracellular pH against acidosis in preantral follicles by multiple mechanisms. Development. 2007;134(23):4283–95.
75. Lane M, Baltz JM, et al. Na+/H+ antiporter activity in hamster embryos is activated during fertilization. Dev Biol. 1999;208(1):244–52.
76. Phillips KP, Baltz JM. Intracellular pH regulation by HCO_3^-/Cl^- exchange is activated during early mouse zygote development. Dev Biol. 1999;208(2):392–405.
77. Zhu ZY, Chen DY, et al. Rotation of meiotic spindle is controlled by microfilaments in mouse oocytes. Biol Reprod. 2003;68(3):943–6.
78. Lenart P, Bacher CP, et al. A contractile nuclear actin network drives chromosome congression in oocytes. Nature. 2005;436(7052):812–8.
79. Regula CS, Pfeiffer JR, et al. Microtubule assembly and disassembly at alkaline pH. J Cell Biol. 1981;89(1):45–53.
80. Bavister BD, Squirrell JM. Mitochondrial distribution and function in oocytes and early embryos. Hum Reprod. 2000;15 Suppl 2:189–98.
81. Nagai S, Mabuchi T, et al. Correlation of abnormal mitochondrial distribution in mouse oocytes with reduced developmental competence. Tohoku J Exp Med. 2006;210(2):137–44.
82. Krisher RL, Bavister BD. Enhanced glycolysis after maturation of bovine oocytes in vitro is associated with increased developmental competence. Mol Reprod Dev. 1999;53(1):19–26.
83. Spindler RE, Pukazhenthi BS, et al. Oocyte metabolism predicts the development of cat embryos to blastocyst in vitro. Mol Reprod Dev. 2000;56(2):163–71.
84. John DP, Kiessling AA. Improved pronuclear mouse embryo development over an extended pH range in Ham's F-10 medium without protein. Fertil Steril. 1988;49(1):150–5.
85. Lane M, Baltz JM, et al. Regulation of intracellular pH in hamster preimplantation embryos by the sodium hydrogen (Na+/H+) antiporter. Biol Reprod. 1998;59(6):1483–90.
86. Leclerc C, Becker D, et al. Low intracellular pH is involved in the early embryonic death of DDK mouse eggs fertilized by alien sperm. Dev Dyn. 1994;200(3):257–67.
87. Zhao Y, Chauvet PJ, et al. Expression and function of bicarbonate/chloride exchangers in the preimplantation mouse embryo. J Biol Chem. 1995;270(41):24428–34.
88. Zhao Y, Baltz JM. Bicarbonate/chloride exchange and intracellular pH throughout preimplantation mouse embryo development. Am J Physiol. 1996;271(5 Pt 1):C1512–20.
89. Lane M, Bavister BD. Regulation of intracellular pH in bovine oocytes and cleavage stage embryos. Mol Reprod Dev. 1999;54(4):396–401.
90. Brinster RL. Studies on the development of mouse embryos in vitro. I. The effect of osmolarity and hydrogen ion concentration. J Exp Zool. 1965;158:49–57.
91. Hershlag A, Feng H. The effect of CO_2 concentration and pH on the in vitro development of mouse embryos. Fertil Mag. 2001;4:21–2.
92. Summers MC, Biggers JD. Chemically defined media and the culture of mammalian preimplantation embryos: historical perspective and current issues. Hum Reprod Update. 2003;9(6): 557–82.
93. Steel T, Conaghan J. pH equilibration dynamics of culture medium under oil. Fertil Steril. 2008;89 suppl 2:s27.
94. Swain JE, Pool TB. Supplementation of culture media with zwitterinoic buffers supports sperm function and embryo development within the elevated CO2 levels of the laboratory incubator. J Clinic Embryol. 2008;11(2):24.
95. Barnett DK, Bavister BD. Inhibitory effect of glucose and phosphate on the second cleavage division of hamster embryos: is it linked to metabolism? Hum Reprod. 1996;11(1):177–83.
96. Barnett DK, Clayton MK, et al. Glucose and phosphate toxicity in hamster preimplantation embryos involves disruption of cellular organization, including distribution of active mitochondria. Mol Reprod Dev. 1997;48(2):227–37.
97. Lane M, Ludwig TE, et al. Phosphate induced developmental arrest of hamster two-cell embryos is associated with disrupted ionic homeostasis. Mol Reprod Dev. 1999;54(4):410–7.

98. Farrell PS, Bavister BD. Short-term exposure of two-cell hamster embryos to collection media is detrimental to viability. Biol Reprod. 1984;31(1):109–14.
99. Escriba MJ, Silvestre MA, et al. Comparison of the effect of two different handling media on rabbit zygote developmental ability. Reprod Nutr Dev. 2001;41(2):181–6.
100. Palasz AT, Brena PB, et al. The effect of different zwitterionic buffers and PBS used for out-of-incubator procedures during standard in vitro embryo production on development, morphology and gene expression of bovine embryos. Theriogenology. 2008;70(9):1461–70.
101. Good NE, Winget GD, et al. Hydrogen ion buffers for biological research. Biochemistry. 1966;5(2):467–77.
102. Good NE, Izawa S. Hydrogen ion buffers. Methods Enzymol. 1972;24:53–68.
103. Ferguson WJ, Braunschweiger KI, et al. Hydrogen ion buffers for biological research. Anal Biochem. 1980;104(2):300–10.
104. Iwasaki T, Kimura E, et al. Studies on a chemically defined medium for in vitro culture of in vitro matured and fertilized porcine oocytes. Theriogenology. 1999;51(4):709–20.
105. Morgia F, Torti M, et al. Use of a medium buffered with N-hydroxyethylpiperazine-N-ethanesulfonate (HEPES) in intracytoplasmic sperm injection procedures is detrimental to the outcome of in vitro fertilization. Fertil Steril. 2006;85(5):1415–9.
106. Zigler Jr JS, Lepe-Zuniga JL, et al. Analysis of the cytotoxic effects of light-exposed HEPES-containing culture medium. In Vitro Cell Dev Biol. 1985;21(5):282–7.
107. Lepe-Zuniga JL, Zigler Jr JS, et al. Toxicity of light-exposed Hepes media. J Immunol Methods. 1987;103(1):145.
108. Butler JE, Lechene C, et al. Noninvasive measurement of glucose uptake by two populations of murine embryos. Biol Reprod. 1988;39(4):779–86.
109. Byrd SR, Flores-Foxworth G, et al. In vitro maturation of ovine oocytes in a portable incubator. Theriogenology. 1997;47(4):857–64.
110. Downs SM, Mastropolo AM. Culture conditions affect meiotic regulation in cumulus cell-enclosed mouse oocytes. Mol Reprod Dev. 1997;46(4):551–66.
111. Geshi M, Yonai M, et al. Improvement of in vitro co-culture systems for bovine embryos using a low concentration of carbon dioxide and medium supplemented with beta-mercaptoethanol. Theriogenology. 1999;51(3):551–8.
112. Bhattacharyya A, Yanagimachi R. Synthetic organic pH buffers can support fertilization of guinea pig eggs, but not as efficiently as bicarbonate buffer. Gamete Res. 1988;19(2):123–9.
113. Behr BR, Stratton CJ, et al. In vitro fertilization (IVF) of mouse ova in HEPES-buffered culture media. J In Vitro Fert Embryo Transf. 1990;7(1):9–15.
114. Hagen DR, Prather RS, et al. Development of one-cell porcine embryos to the blastocyst stage in simple media. J Anim Sci. 1991;69(3):1147–50.
115. Lee MA, Storey BT. Bicarbonate is essential for fertilization of mouse eggs: mouse sperm require it to undergo the acrosome reaction. Biol Reprod. 1986;34(2):349–56.
116. Mahadevan MM, Fleetham J, et al. Growth of mouse embryos in bicarbonate media buffered by carbon dioxide, hepes, or phosphate. J In Vitro Fert Embryo Transf. 1986;3(5):304–8.
117. Ali J, Whitten WK, et al. Effect of culture systems on mouse early embryo development. Hum Reprod. 1993;8(7):1110–4.
118. Ozawa M, Nagai T, et al. Successful pig embryonic development in vitro outside a CO2 gas-regulated incubator: effects of pH and osmolality. Theriogenology. 2006;65(4):860–9.
119. Liu Z, Foote RH, et al. Effect of amino acids and alpha-amanitin on the development of rabbit embryos in modified protein-free KSOM with HEPES. Mol Reprod Dev. 1996;45(2):157–62.
120. Graves CN, Biggers JD. Carbon dioxide fixation by mouse embryos prior to implantation. Science. 1970;167(924):1506–8.
121. Quinn P, Wales RG. Fixation of carbon dioxide by pre-implantation mouse embryos in vitro and the activities of enzymes involved in the process. Aust J Biol Sci. 1971;24(6):1277–90.
122. Quinn P, Wales RG. Fixation of carbon dioxide by preimplantation rabbit embryos in vitro. J Reprod Fertil. 1974;36(1):29–39.

123. Swain JE, Pool TB. New pH-buffering system for media utilized during gamete and embryo manipulations for assisted reproduction. Reprod Biomed Online. 2009;18(6):799–810.
124. Phillips KP, Leveille MC, et al. Intracellular pH regulation in human preimplantation embryos. Hum Reprod. 2000;15(4):896–904.
125. Eagle H. Buffer combinations for mammalian cell culture. Science. 1971;174(8):500–3.
126. Hashimoto S, Nishihara T, et al. Medium without ammonium accumulation supports the developmental competence of human embryos. J Reprod Dev. 2008;54(5):370–4.
127. Bunton CA. Oxidation of α-diketones and α-keto acids by hydrogen peroxide. Nature. 1949; 163:144.
128. Morales H, Tilquin P, et al. Pyruvate prevents peroxide-induced injury of in vitro preimplantation bovine embryos. Mol Reprod Dev. 1999;52(2):149–57.
129. Orsi NM, Leese HJ. Protection against reactive oxygen species during mouse preimplantation embryo development: role of EDTA, oxygen tension, catalase, superoxide dismutase and pyruvate. Mol Reprod Dev. 2001;59(1):44–53.
130. O'Fallon JV, Wright RWJ. Pyruvate revisited: a non-metabolic role for pyruvate in preimplantation embryo development. Theriogenology. 1995;43:288.
131. Montgomery CM, Webb JL. Metabolic studies on heart mitochondria. J Biol Chem. 1955; 221:359–68.
132. Montgomery CM, Webb JL. Metabolic studies on heart mitochondria. II. The inhibitory action of parapyruvate on the tricarboxylic acid cycle. J Biol Chem. 1956;221(1):359–68.
133. Wales R, Dg W. Decomposition of sodium pyruvate in culture media stored at 5°C and its effects on the development of the preimplantation mouse embryo. J Reprod Fertil. 1971; 24:126.
134. Kim JB, Yu YM, et al. Anti-inflammatory mechanism is involved in ethyl pyruvate-mediated efficacious neuroprotection in the postischemic brain. Brain Res. 2005;1060(1–2): 188–92.
135. Lin RY, Vera JC, et al. Human monocarboxylate transporter 2 (MCT2) is a high affinity pyruvate transporter. J Biol Chem. 1998;273(44):28959–65.
136. Malaisse WJ, Jijakli H, et al. Insulinotropic action of methyl pyruvate: secretory, cationic, and biosynthetic aspects. Arch Biochem Biophys. 1996;335(2):229–44.
137. Varma SD, Devamanoharan PS, et al. Prevention of intracellular oxidative stress to lens by pyruvate and its ester. Free Radic Res. 1998;28(2):131–5.
138. Sims CA, Wattanasirichaigoon S, et al. Ringer's ethyl pyruvate solution ameliorates ischemia/reperfusion-induced intestinal mucosal injury in rats. Crit Care Med. 2001;29(8): 1513–8.
139. Rocheleau JV, Head WS, et al. Quantitative NAD(P)H/flavoprotein autofluorescence imaging reveals metabolic mechanisms of pancreatic islet pyruvate response. J Biol Chem. 2004; 279(30):31780–7.
140. Zeng J, Liu J, et al. Exogenous ethyl pyruvate versus pyruvate during metabolic recovery after oxidative stress in neonatal rat cerebrocortical slices. Anesthesiology. 2007;107(4): 630–40.
141. Zeng J, Yang GY, et al. Pyruvate improves recovery after PARP-1-associated energy failure induced by oxidative stress in neonatal rat cerebrocortical slices. J Cereb Blood Flow Metab. 2007;27(2):304–15.
142. Dave SH, Tilstra JS, et al. Ethyl pyruvate decreases HMGB1 release and ameliorates murine colitis. J Leukoc Biol. 2009;86(3):633–43.
143. Di Paola R, Mazzon E, et al. Ethyl pyruvate reduces the development of zymosan-induced generalized inflammation in mice. Crit Care Med. 2009;37(1):270–82.
144. Yang R, Shaufl AL, et al. Ethyl pyruvate ameliorates liver injury secondary to severe acute pancreatitis. J Surg Res. 2009;153(2):302–9.
145. Swain JE, Pool TB. Supplementation of culture media with esterified forms of pyruvate improves mouse embryo development. In Proceedings from the ASRM Annual Meeting, San Francisco, CA; 2008.

146. Combelles CM, Gupta S, et al. Could oxidative stress influence the in-vitro maturation of oocytes? Reprod Biomed Online. 2009;18(6):864–80.
147. Wang X, Falcone T, et al. Vitamin C and vitamin E supplementation reduce oxidative stress-induced embryo toxicity and improve the blastocyst development rate. Fertil Steril. 2002;78(6):1272–7.
148. Angle M. Using two concurrent sequential culture media improves pregnancy outcomes. Clinical Embryologist. 2006;9(1):5–11.

Chapter 6
Short Culture: Day 1/Day 2/Day 3 Embryo Culture

Patrick Quinn

Louise Brown, the first successful case of human IVF, was transferred to her mother's uterus as an 8-cell embryo [1]. Normally, this early mammalian preimplantation stage resides in the fallopian tube, and when such embryos are placed in the uterus they perish or are expelled from the uterus [2, 3]. Humans appear to be the only primates in which transfer of early precompaction embryos to the uterus is successful [4]. Soon after IVF became a regular clinical procedure, successful transfer of gametes to the fallopian tube by laparoscopy (gamete intrafallopian transfer—GIFT) was reported [5], and it was suggested that the placement of these cells, and in subsequent reports, the zygote (zygote intrafallopian transfer—ZIFT) [6] and early embryo (tubal embryo transfer—TET) [7], in their correct location, the fallopian tube, was a major reason for the higher success rates of these procedures compared to IVF. However, whereas pregnancy rates of 20–25% for GIFT remained relatively constant over the decade of the 1990s, the success rates of IVF and ICSI with uterine placement of early embryos gradually improved from approximately 10% to a similar 20–25% [8]. This was proposed to be partly caused by the gradual improvement in embryo culture, primarily improvements in embryo culture media rather than any other major parameters such as better ovarian stimulation protocols or transfer of embryos at the blastocyst stage on D5 to their normal site of residence, the uterus [8]. In fact, ongoing pregnancies were also obtained by transferring the gametes directly to the uterus rather than the fallopian tube [9, 10], and although this has never become a routine clinical procedure, it does indicate the plasticity of human gametes and preimplantation embryos with respect to their successful development at various sites in the female reproductive tract albeit their replacement at the site where they would normally reside probably gives optimal results. Embryonic plasticity is also reflected, in my opinion, by embryonic development in vitro in various culture systems, and it is the purpose of this chapter to

P. Quinn, PhD, HCLD (✉)
Sage IVF, A Cooper Surgical Company, 1867 Turnstone Road, Redmond, OR 97756, USA
e-mail: Patrick.Quinn@coopersurgical.com

Z.P. Nagy et al. (eds.), *Clinical Embryology: A Practical Guide*,
DOI 10.1007/978-1-4614-8376-2_6, © Springer Science+Business Media New York 2013

focus on the factors in such culture systems that influence human embryos during Day (D)1 to D3 of development. The main focus will be on practical aspects of culture of this early developmental stage with some comments related to physiological aspects of the embryo.

Historical Perspectives of Human Embryo Culture and ET

As mentioned earlier, Louise Brown was transferred on D3 as an 8-cell embryo to her mother's uterus [1]. Trounson et al. [11] reported that embryo transfers (ETs) on D2 at the 2- to 4-cell stage produced the majority of their pregnancies, and this practice was utilized in most IVF programs worldwide in the 1980s. In some countries, D2 ET has remained a popular protocol [12, 13]. It was not until the 1990s that transfers on D3 of embryonic development became de rigueur [14, 15]. The primary reason suggested for this increased pregnancy rate with D3 ET was the ability to select better quality embryos with greater implantation potential on D3 compared to D2 and the elimination of embryos that would have arrested in development between D2 and D3 after transfer on D2 [14]. In addition, activation of the embryonic genome that occurs around D3 of development of the human embryo between the 4- and 8-cell stage [16] has been proposed as another reason for improved selection of embryos from the 8-cell stage onward [17]. Nevertheless, there have been conflicting reports concerning the superiority of ET on D2 or D3 [18, 19]. Subsequently, a similar change in ET to D5 was implemented [20]. Again, the benefits observed of later ET were based on prolonging culture, using it as a tool to select better quality embryos and cull out those that, for genetic or other physiological reasons, had a poorer prognosis for development, and the transfer of the blastocyst embryo to the uterus, the site in which it naturally resides in vivo [20]. In the initial period of D5 ET, some debate arose concerning the superiority of D5 over D3 ET [21, 22]. Some of this disputation may have been due to poor quality embryo culture medium and/or culture technique.

ET on D1 has also been used [23]. The use of this protocol was advocated in situations where adverse culture conditions were having a negative impact on success rates, and so, the early replacement of embryos into the female reproductive tract was a better environmental option for embryos than culture in vitro [24]. It has also been shown that when there is only a small number of oocytes or embryos (5 or less), higher pregnancy rates are obtained with ET on D2 rather than D3, and again, the earlier transfer of embryos to a more congenial environment in the uterus compared to that in culture has been implicated as the prime benefit of this strategy [25, 26].

All of the forgoing observations of the ability of the human oocyte and embryo to produce ongoing pregnancies and live births after transfer on various days of development to various sites in the female reproductive tract indicate the varied capacity of human embryos to fulfill their destiny to develop into a new individual. The remainder of this chapter is focused on culture techniques that participate in this process for the early human embryo.

Metabolism and Physiology of the Early Human Embryo

Energy Substrates

This has been one of the earliest subjects studied and discussed in relation to the development of preimplantation mammalian embryos. The three major substrates are pyruvate, glucose, and lactate, and the general consensus has been to supply these compounds at levels found in the fallopian tube [27]. Despite the fact that there is some debate concerning the acquisition of an accurate estimation of the concentration of these substrates [28], it has been found that low to moderate levels of all three compounds seems to work well with human embryos. The presence of pyruvate is particularly important because, as well as being an essential energy source, it also acts as a sink for removing embryotoxic level ammonium by transamination to alanine; this is one of the reasons why I have excluded alanine from my current series of media for human embryo culture [29]. Low to no levels of glucose also seems to be sufficient for the early human embryos [29]. With respect to lactate, I have combined the provision of this substrate and that of calcium in the form of calcium L-lactate, thus providing the bioactive form of lactate and avoiding excessive chemical levels of lactate by eliminating its D-isomer. The significant effect of additional D-lactate on internal pH (pHi) in the embryo that influences cellular homeostasis has led others to recommend the elimination of D-lactate from IVF media [30].

Amino Acids

Currently, nearly all media for human embryo culture contain amino acids for all stages of preimplantation development, and this is logical as these compounds are present in reproductive tract fluids [31]. Ham's F10, a medium that contains amino acids, was used in the early work of Steptoe and Edwards to culture human embryos [32]. However, in the early 1980s, the use of media such as Tyrode's T6 and my HTF medium [33] that were devoid of amino acids became popular. Subsequently, the use of amino acids became more refined by Gardner et al. [34]. when he proposed the use of nonessential amino acids in the precompaction phase from D1 to D3 of development and then the subsequent addition of essential amino acids and vitamins during the postcompaction period from D3 to D5/6. Important changes to this general theme have ensued. Studies of the consumption and production of amino acids during embryo culture have shown that alanine accumulates in the culture medium indicating its production by the embryo at all stages of preimplantation development (hence, my omission of alanine from my culture media [29]), whereas leucine is consumed by the early human preimplantation embryos, an obvious reason why this amino acid should be present during culture from D1 to D3

[35]. There has also been a call for the addition of methionine to the cleavage stage medium to lessen the frequency of monozygotic twinning [36], but this relationship needs further study.

It has been known for some time that glutamine readily deaminates, primarily by spontaneous breakdown and secondarily by embryonic metabolism to ammonium, the level of which can become toxic. The initial way to overcome this problem was to change the medium every 48 h to minimize the accumulation of ammonium. As an alternative, I substituted alanyl-glutamine, a stable form of glutamine, for both alanine and glutamine. This was done on the suggestion of Kenneth Drury and had previously been used in media for cell line culture. Subsequently, it was shown that the accumulation of ammonium in embryo culture medium was considerably reduced when using alanyl-glutamine compared to glutamine [37].

Finally, it must also be remembered that amino acids have other roles apart from being the building blocks of proteins and these include acting as energy sources after transamination and acting as internal buffers [30].

Inorganic Ions

The first successful media for preimplantation mammalian embryos were those of Whitten [38] and Brinster [39] and where based on the ionic composition of Krebs-Ringer solution. Some of the more recent changes in ionic composition that have occurred in media for preimplantation human embryos have been the reduction and/or elimination of phosphate ions [40, 41] and calcium magnesium ratios. Increased levels of exogenous magnesium ions in medium reduced the uptake of external calcium by the embryo and thus ameliorated the deleterious effects of excessive calcium within the embryo [42]. We have incorporated this change in magnesium levels in our media based on this work. In my studies with HTF medium [33], I found that excessive ratios of sodium to potassium inhibited mouse embryo development in vitro so we have been mindful of this in our human embryo media and kept the sodium to potassium ratio between 26 and 28 by adding 5 mEq/L of potassium ions. The presence of trace elements in culture media for human preimplantation embryos has not been shown to be of much importance.

pH and Temperature

One of the more important aspects of culture media, in my opinion, is the pH of the medium. Again, using the imitative principle and based on my experience when poor human embryo development was primarily associated with poor pH control [24], I have been an advocate for lower pH levels than the perceived golden role of cell culture which was 7.4 when human embryo culture first began. As far back as 1999, it was suggested that the development of early human embryos was improved using a pH in the range of 7.2 [43]. It was also reported that the internal pH (pHi) of early cleaving human embryos was about 7.12 ± 0.008 [44]. Based on these data, I have recommended a pH of 7.2 ± 0.1 for medium used to culture the early cleaving human embryo from D1 to D3 of culture. Others have recommended a similar value [30, 45]. Most laboratories that have lowered their pH to this range have anecdotally reported improvement in the development of human embryos at this stage. It is now well understood that it is more important to measure pH of the media under culture conditions rather than to just measure the CO_2 concentration in the culture atmosphere [45]. If the pH levels drift out of the recommended range for whatever reason, then CO_2 levels need adjustment to bring the pH back into range [45]. Factors affecting pH levels include altitude, temperature, and the capacity of an incubator to maintain CO_2 levels that can be affected by the frequency of opening the incubator and by leaks in the gas system from its source to within the incubator. It is also good practice to pass the gas mixture through a filter consisting of activated carbon and a HEPE filter to remove volatile organic compounds and particulate matter from the gas. Humidification of the gas is not required if all culture is done under an oil overlay.

In parallel with pH, the temperature at which gametes and embryos are handled and cultured has a critical influence on their subsequent normality and development. First, the actual optimal temperature needs to be determined for human embryos. It has been generally assumed that this is 37°C, but there is some indication that the range may be slightly lower than this, in the range of 36.5–36.9°C [46, 47]. In any event, a sustained effort is needed to keep the embryo within the required temperature limits at all times during development, and probably, the less handling of the embryo to observe the rate of the development, the better [48]. Here is where the use of time-lapse photography taken from within the incubator may play a beneficial role if indeed there are critical events that do occur in the embryo and can be observed during development without disturbing the culture system by removing it from the incubator.

Osmolality

The final aspect of culture medium to be considered is the concentration of dissolved solutes. This is referred to as osmolality. Isotonic saline, a solution of sodium chloride in water, is a fluid in which human erythrocytes neither swell nor shrink [49]. In other words, the concentration of dissolved sodium chloride in the saline solution is equal to that of dissolved solutes within the cell. Early culture media for human embryos were formulated to have an osmolarity of around 280 ± 5 mosmol/kg of water [50], but it has subsequently been shown that the human embryo can develop in media with a broader range of osmolality, for example, down to 265 ± 8 mosmol/kg. This broader range from 260 to 285 is also similar to that of mouse preimplantation embryos [51].

Formulation of Culture Media

Which Media to Use

Two general strategies, reviewed by Biggers and Summers [28], have been used in the creation of media for human embryo culture: "back to nature" and "let the embryo choose." These two strategies have subsequently come to be associated with a sequential series of media for "back to nature" and a single medium used in a nonrenewed or renewed sequence for "let the embryo choose." In the "back to nature" strategy, which I refer to as the "imitative principle" [29] media components and their concentration are chosen to mimic the chemical composition of that portion of the female reproductive tract where the embryo would be located. In humans, this would be the fallopian tube for D1–D3 and the uterine cavity for D3–D5/6. My fertilization and cleavage media used for insemination in vitro and then culture of the embryo from D1 to D3 are a very successful example of this strategy. These types of media are mainly based on the composition of human tubal fluid, but allowances are made for situations that are known to exist in other mammalian species, primarily the mouse, and studies that have shown that the presence or absence of certain substances and their concentration are of benefit. A prime example of this is the omission of alanine from my media because the embryo excretes alanine following the transamination of pyruvate, and exogenous alanine would inhibit the removal of ammonium by this reaction [29]. Media based on the "let the embryo choose" strategy have focused primarily on the amino acids in the formulation [28]. A range of amino acids that are known to be in the reproductive tract fluids are present in the medium, and it is considered that the embryo can choose which to consume or release and in what concentration [35].

It is likely that further studies, similar to a recent one that showed no difference in outcomes using a single medium for continuous culture from the zygote to the blastocyst stage compared to a sequential media series [52], are required to determine which media series used in which format (renewed vs. nonrenewed) will be the most effective in ART.

Formulation Strategies

This is a simple process providing several simple specifications are followed. It has been described in detail elsewhere [53]. All chemical components, water and vessels, pipettes, containers, etc. (glass and/or plastic) must be as pure as possible, be stored according to manufacturers' specifications, and be prescreened with a mouse embryo assay and/or sperm motility assay and tested for endotoxin levels as appropriate. Even so, there are certain procedures that need to be followed and which I have found will provide a better product. For example, it is mostly recommended that sodium pyruvate be stored at 2–8°C, but Wales and Whittingham [54] found that the stability of this compound was improved, and embryotoxicity was reduced when the solid was stored at or below −40°C. The embryotoxicity was thought to be due to the conversion of pyruvate to the metabolic inhibitor, parapyruvate. Therefore, solid sodium pyruvate should be stored at at least −20°C and not stored in the refrigerator as advised by most manufacturers.

Another practical procedure is to reduce endotoxin levels in solid sodium chloride by heating it at >200°C for at least 1 h. This depyrogenation procedure has no detrimental effect on the properties of the compound.

Amino acids are another category of components that require special attention. Because most amino acids are amphoteric, i.e., they have both acidic and basic groups, they dissolve easier at higher or lower pHs. Therefore, when making concentrated (e.g., 100×) stock solutions, one needs to add acid to get solubilization. For example, to make a 100× stock of Eagle's essential amino acids, add 30 mL of concentrated hydrochloric acid per liter of water before adding the individual components. When making the final medium solution, add components individually and stir continuously until dissolved before adding the next component. A search of the Aldrich-Sigma website (www.sigma-aldrich.com) lists the solvent used to test the solubility of various compounds, including amino acids.

To make medium, the procedure described in Tables 6.1 and 6.2 can be followed. The concentration of various components can be altered by changing the volume of the stock added and/or by changing the concentration of the component in a particular stock. As a precaution, it is advisable to test the efficacy of a particular medium with mouse embryos before using the medium with humans or other species. The method described in Tables 6.1 and 6.2 can also be used to create media to QC the various components of the medium using an appropriate bioassay such as the mouse embryo assay and/or the human sperm motility assay.

Tips and Tricks for Using ART Culture Media

Some Dos and Don'ts for Using ART Culture Media

Dos

Measure the pH of each new lot of product received. If protein is added to the medium by the end user, do so and then equilibrate the completed medium under the atmosphere it will be used at for a sufficient time (minimum of 4 h but usually overnight) and measure pH at 37°C. The most practical way is to use the Pool protocol [45]. Using a suite of media from the same manufacture (e.g., fertilization, cleavage, and blastocyst media)—only measuring the pH in the fertilization medium and then assuming that if the pH is okay in fertilization medium, then it is okay in cleavage and blastocyst media—is not a good idea. This may not be so and is not a good practice. The medium has to have pH measured with protein included. The probe can be washed in a solution containing a protease to remove protein that may have

Table 6.1 Preparation of media from stocks

Stock	Component	Source and lot #	Amount required	Actual amount
A Stability: 3 months, 2–8°C, filtered	1. NaCl 2. KCl 3. $MgSO_4.7H_2O$ 4. Gentamycin		Add appropriate amounts in grams (g) to 50 mL of water, as indicated in step 5 below 0.005 g ÷ potency, for example, 0.005 ÷ 0.63 = 0.008 g	
Other				
	5. Water		50.0 mL	
Note: Add components 1–4 to a 50-mL Falcon flask, then add the water				
B	1. $NaHCO_3$		0.752 g/50 mL	
	2. Phenol red		0.0015 g	
Add $NaHCO_3$ and phenol red to the same 50 mL of water				
C	Na pyruvate		0.036 g/10 mL[a]	
D	Ca lactate pentahydrate		0.0629 g/10 mL	
E	1a. HEPES-free acid[a] or		2.979 g/50 mL or	
	1b. HEPES Na salt[b]		3.254 g/50 mL	
	2. Phenol red		0.0015 g	
Adjust to pH 7.35 with (1a.) 1N NaOH or (1b.) 1N HCl before making up final volume to 50 mL. Add these ingredients to 40 mL H_2O. Adjust pH and make up to final volume of 50 mL				
Alternatively, mix together 1.560 g of HEPES-free acid and 1.550 g of HEPES Na salt into 50 mL of water. When 0.84 mL of this stock is added to a final volume of 10 mL of medium, as described in Table 2, it will give a 21 mM solution of HEPES with a pH of about 7.35 at 37°C				
F Stability: 3 months, −20°C	Stock solutions of amino acids		Make 100× stock in water containing 8.5 g NaCl/L; add HCl as required for dissolution	
G	EDTA Na_4 Make up several days before required; may need to hold at 37°C for several hours to get complete solution		0.004 g/10 mL[a]	
H	Glucose		0.500 g/10 mL[a]	
I	Citric acid, trisodium, dihydrate		Make solution A at 0.015 g/10 mL[a]. Make solution B by adding 1 mL of solution A + 9 mL water	
J	KH_2PO_4		0.014 g/10 mL[a]	
K	Taurine		0.013 g/10 mL[a]	
L Stability: 3 months, −20°C	Stock solutions of vitamins		Make 100 × stock in water containing 1 mL of 1 N NaOH/L	

[a]For these stocks, one can weigh out the approximate amount, divide by the concentration × 10 = volume of water to add, for example, if 0.35 g of glucose is weighed, then 0.35/0.5 × 10 = 7.0 mL water used

All stocks are stable for 3 months at 2–8°C except where noted. Frozen stocks should be thawed and used, and the remainder discarded

Table 6.2 Final preparation of media from stocks (Add the required amount of water to 0.050 g of BSA (for mouse embryos) or HSA for human embryos (see below) in a 14-mL Falcon tube)

Stock	Source (date) and/or lot #	Amount (mL)	✓ Added
H_2O		6.38	
A (salts)		1.0	
B ($NaHCO_3$)		1.0 or 0.16 for HEPES	
C (pyruvate)		0.1	
E (HEPES)		0.84	
F (amino acid stock solution)		0.1	
G (EDTA)		0.1	
H (glucose)		0.1	
I (citric acid—solution B)		0.01 (10 uL)	
J (KH_2PO_4)		0.01 (10 uL)	
Use a higher concentration in stock if a higher final concentration is required, for example, 0.050 g/10 mL			
K (taurine)		0.1	
L (vitamins)		0.1	
D (Ca lactate, pentahydrate)		1.0	
Always add this last and after thoroughly mixing all the other components. $CaCl_2.2H_2O$ and sodium lactate can also be used in place of calcium lactate			
BSA (or HSA, or another protein source; specify)		5 mg/mL, i.e., 50 mg for 10 mL	

1. Final total volume is 10 mL; adjust volume of water if different volume(s) of stock(s) is (are) being used to obtain different concentration of components
2. Mix thoroughly to dissolve all components
3. Filter sterilize
4. Add each of stocks to water, adding Ca salt stock last (otherwise, a precipitate will form). Mix thoroughly to dissolve all components. Add protein if not already done so as in step 1 above (e.g., HSA; 50 mg/10 mL = 5 mg/mL), and filter sterilize

Other specifications:
1. Osmolality: 265–280 mosmol/kg water
2. pH: 7.2–7.3, depending on concentration of $NaHCO_3$ and CO_2 used

Water: conductance 0.06 mΩ/cm; resistivity 18.0 MΩ/cm; silicate not detectable
Endotoxin: final product must be <0.1 EU/mL

stuck to the probe. An example of the protease-containing washing solution is Tergazyme [55], or buy the solution already made up [56]. When the pH of the media are known, it may then be necessary to adjust the CO_2 concentration in the incubator to obtain the desired pH in the fertilization and culture media.

Don'ts

Aliquot medium into 10-mL lots in 14-mL capped tubes and then store these in the refrigerator until the day of use. It is not good practice because handling the media like this makes them prone to microbial contamination, the pH will go up during this whole process, and when pH goes up, calcium carbonate can precipitate leading to problems as the $CaCO_3$ will not go back into solution when the pH is equilibrated down to the acceptable range.

Other practical suggestions for laboratory practice are given elsewhere [46, 48, 53].

Summary and Conclusions

To state the obvious, successful culture of human embryos, as with all other mammalian species, from the zygote stage through to D3 is an essential part of the ART process. Unless this process is optimized, further development of the embryo is doomed. The main theme that I believe I have presented is that human embryos, especially during their first 3 days of development, can be cultured in a fairly diverse range of media and give reasonable take-home baby rates. Some aspects of media composition may be more important than others. Of equal, if not more, importance is the way the media are used. In this context, pH and temperature control and the concomitant decreased observation and disturbance of the embryo during in vitro development are extremely important practical aspects of culture that are often overlooked in ART laboratories. Prospective, proactive tracking of key laboratory performance indicators is an essential feature in successful ART programs [48]. To summarize, I use the statement "a good medium used poorly produces poor outcomes."

References

1. Steptoe PC, Edwards RG. Birth after the reimplantation of a human embryo. Lancet. 1978;2:366.
2. Goto Y, Noda Y, Shiotani M, Kishi J, Nonogaki T, Mori T. The fate of embryos transferred into the uterus. J Assist Reprod Genet. 1993;10:197–201.
3. Wu JT. Development of two-cell eggs transferred into the uteri of ovariectomized rats. Biol Reprod. 1975;13:211–7.
4. Marston JH, Penn R, Sivelle PC. Successful autotransfer of tubal eggs in the rhesus monkey (*Macaca mulatta*). J Reprod Fertil. 1977;49:175–6.
5. Asch RH, Ellsworth LR, Balmaceda JP, Wong PC. Pregnancy following translaparoscopic gamete intrafallopian transfer (GIFT). Lancet. 1984;ii:1034.
6. Devroey P, Braeckmans P, Smitz J, et al. Pregnancy after translaparoscopic zygote intrafallopian transfer in a patient with sperm antibodies. Lancet. 1986;1:1329.
7. Balmaceda JP, Gastaldi C, Remohi J, et al. Tubal embryo transfer as a treatment for infertility due to male factor. Fertil Steril. 1988;50:476–9.
8. Quinn P. The development and impact of assisted reproductive technologies culture media. Fertil Steril. 2004;8:27–9.
9. Craft I, McLeod F, Green S, et al. Human pregnancy following oocyte and sperm transfer to the uterus. Lancet. 1982;319:1031–3.

10. Quinn P, Steinberg J, Schein S, Greenberg P. Direct ovum-sperm transfer (DOST) to the uterus as a mode of treatment following failed IUI but preceding IVF or GIFT. Proc 44th Annual Meeting of the Pacific Coast Fertility Society, Rancho Mirage, California; 1996. P-32:A26.
11. Trounson AO, Mohr LR, Wood C, Leeton JF. Effect of delayed insemination on IVF culture and transfer of human embryos. J Reprod Fertil. 1982;64:285–94.
12. Tremellen KP, Valbuena D, Landeras J, et al. The effects of intercourse on pregnancy rates during assisted human reproduction. Hum Reprod. 2000;15:2653–8.
13. Cooke S, Quinn P, Kime L, Ayres C, Tyler JPP, Driscoll GL. Improvement in early human embryo development using new formulation sequential stage specific culture media. Fertil Steril. 2002;78:1254–60.
14. Dawson KJ, Conaghan J, Ostera GR, Winston RM, Hardy K. Delaying transfer to the third day post insemination, to select non-arrested embryos, increases development to the fetal heart stage. Hum Reprod. 1995;10:177–82.
15. Carillo AJ, Lane B, Pridham DD, et al. Improved clinical outcomes for in vitro fertilization with delay of embryo transfer from 48 to 72 hours after oocyte retrieval: use of glucose- and phosphate-free medium. Fertil Steril. 1998;69:329–34.
16. Braude P, Bolton V, Moore S. Human gene expression first occurs between the four- and eight-cell stages of preimplantation development. Nature. 1988;332:459–61.
17. Huisman GJ, Fauser BCJM, Eijkemans MJC, Pieters MHEC. Implantation rates after in vitro fertilization and transfer of a maximum of two embryos that have undergone three to five days of culture. Fertil Steril. 2000;73:117–22.
18. Laverge H, De Sutter P, Van der Elst J, Dhont M. A prospective, randomized study comparing day 2 and day 3 embryo transfer in human IVF. Hum Reprod. 2001;16:476–80.
19. Etzeid G, Dale PO, Tanbo T, Storeng R, Kjekshus E, Abyholm T. Clinical outcome of day 2 versus day 3 embryo transfer using serum-free culture medium: a prospective randomized study. J Assist Reprod Genet. 1999;16:529–34.
20. Gardner DK, Schoolcraft WB, Wagley L, Schlenker T, Stevens J, Hesla J. A prospective randomized trial of blastocyst culture and transfer in in-vitro fertilization. Hum Reprod. 1998;13:3434–40.
21. Coskun S, Hollanders J, Al-Hassan S, Al-Sufyan H, Al-Mayman H, Jaroudi K. Day 5 versus day 3 embryo transfer: a controlled randomized trial. Hum Reprod. 2000;15:1947–52.
22. Levron J, Shulman A, Bider D, Seidman D, Levin T, Dor J. A prospective randomized study comparing day 3 with blastocyst stage embryo transfer. Fertil Steril. 2002;77:1300–1.
23. Ahuja KK, Smith W, Tucker M, Craft I. Successful pregnancies from the transfer of pronuclear embryos in an outpatient in vitro fertilization program. Fertil Steril. 1985;44:181–4.
24. Quinn P, Stone BA, Marrs RP. Suboptimal laboratory conditions can affect pregnancy outcome after embryo transfer on day 1 or day 2 after insemination in vitro. Fertil Steril. 1990;53:168–70.
25. Shen S, Rosen MP, Dobson AT, Fujimoto VY, McCulloch CE, Cedars MI. Day 2 transfer improves pregnancy outcome in in vitro fertilization cycles with few available embryos. Fertil Steril. 2006;86:44–50.
26. Bahceci M, Ulug U, Ciray N, Akman MA, Erden HF. Efficiency of changing the embryo transfer time from day 3 to day 2 among women with poor ovarian response: a prospective randomized trial. Fertil Steril. 2006;86:81–5.
27. Gardner DK, Lane M, Calderon I, Leeton J. Environment of the preimplantation human embryo in vivo: metabolite analysis of oviduct and uterine fluids and metabolism of cumulus cells. Fertil Steril. 1996;65:349–53.
28. Biggers JD, Summers MC. Choosing a culture medium: making informed choices. Fertil Steril. 2008;90:473–83.
29. Quinn P. Media used in the assisted reproductive technologies laboratories. In: Patrizio P, Tucker MJ, Guelman V, editors. A color atlas for human assisted reproduction: laboratory and clinical insights. Philadelphia: Lippincott Williams & Wilkins; 2003. p. 241–56.

30. Lane M, Gardner DK. Blastomere homeostasis. In: Gardner DK, Lane M, editors. ART and the human blastocyst. New York, NY: Springer; 2001. p. 69–90.
31. Tay JI, Rutherford AJ, Killick SR, Maguiness SD, Pertridge RJ, Leese HJ. Human tubal fluid: production, nutrient composition and response to adrenergic agents. Hum Reprod. 1997; 12:2451–6.
32. Steptoe PC, Edwards RG, Purdy JM. Human blastocysts grown in culture. Nature. 1971; 229:132–3.
33. Quinn P, Kerin JF, Warnes GM. Improved pregnancy rate in human in vitro fertilization with the use of a medium based on the composition of human tubal fluid. Fertil Steril. 1985; 44:493–8.
34. Gardner DK, Lane M. Culture and selection of viable blastocysts: a feasible proposition for human IVF? Hum Reprod Update. 1997;3:367–82.
35. Houghton FD, Hawkhead JA, Humpherson PG, et al. Non-invasive amino acid turnover predicts human embryo developmental capacity. Hum Reprod. 2002;17:999–1005.
36. Cassuto G, Chavier M, Menezo Y. Culture conditions and not prolonged culture time are responsible for monozygotic twinning in human in vitro fertilization. Fertil Steril. 2003; 80:462–3.
37. Lane M, Gardner DK. Ammonium induces aberrant blastocyst differentiation, metabolism, pH regulation, gene expression and subsequently alters fetal development in the mouse. Biol Reprod. 2003;69:1109–17.
38. Whitten WK. Culture of tubal mouse ova. Nature. 1956;177:96.
39. Brinster RL. A method for in vitro cultivation of mouse ova from two-cell to blastocyst. Exp Cell Res. 1963;32:205–8.
40. Quinn P, Moinipanah R, Steinberg JM, Weathersbee P. Successful human in vitro fertilization using a modified human tubal fluid medium lacking glucose and phosphate ions. Fertil Steril. 1995;63:922–4.
41. Pool TB, Atiee SH, Martin JE. Oocyte and embryo culture: basic concepts and recent advances. In: May JV, ed. Assisted reproduction: laboratory considerations. Infertility and Reproductive Medicine Clinics of North America. 1998;9:181–203.
42. Lane M, Bavister BD. Calcium homeostasis in early hamster preimplantation embryos. Biol Reprod. 1998;59:1000–7.
43. Ferring Pharmaceuticals. Council for the advancement of ovulation induction and assisted reproductive technology, Marrs RP, Steinkampf MP (chairpersons). The Assisted Reproductive Global Monitor, May Council Meeting, Special Meeting Reporter, Session 1. 1999.
44. Phillips KP, Leveille M-C, Claman P, Baltz JM. Intracellular pH regulation in human preimplantation embryos. Hum Reprod. 2000;15:896–904.
45. Pool TB. Optimizing pH in clinical embryology. J Clin Embryol. 2004;7:1–17.
46. Higdon HL, Blackhurst DW, Boone WR. Incubator management in an assisted reproductive technology laboratory. Fertil Steril. 2008;89:703–10.
47. Leese HJ, Baumann CG, Brison DR, McEvoy TG, Sturmey RG. Metabolism of the viable mammalian embryo: quietness revisited. Mol Hum Reprod. 2008;14:667–72.
48. Miller K. Single blastocyst transfer: the results are in the details. http://www.coopersurgical.com. Accessed September 09, 2010.
49. Saline (medicine). http://en.wikipedia.org/wiki/Saline_(medicine). Accessed September 07, 2010.
50. Quinn P, Warnes GM, Kerin JF, Kirby C. Culture factors in relation to the success of human in vitro fertilization and embryo transfer. Fertil Steril. 1984;41:202–9.
51. Dawson KM, Baltz JM. Organic osmolytes and embryos: substrates of the Gly and β transport systems protect mouse zygotes against the effects of raised osmolarity. Biol Reprod. 1997; 56:1550–8.
52. Reed ML, Hamic A, Thompson DJ, Caperton CL. Continuous uninterrupted single medium culture without medium renewal versus sequential media culture: a sibling embryo study. Fertil Steril. 2009;92:1783–6.

53. Quinn P, Pool T. Development of modern culture media. In: Fleming S, Cooke S, editors. Textbook of assisted reproduction for scientists in reproductive technology. Fremantle: Vivid; 2008. p. 65–97.
54. Wales RG, Whittingham DG. Decomposition of sodium pyruvate in culture medium stored at 5°C and its effects on the development of the preimplantation mouse embryo. J Reprod Fertil. 1971;24:126.
55. Tergazyme. http://www.alconox.com/downloads/pdf/techbull_tergazyme.pdf. Accessed September 12, 2010.
56. http://www.coleparmer.com/catalog/product_view.asp?sku=3565506. Accessed September 12, 2010.

Chapter 7
Extended Culture in IVF

David K. Gardner and Michelle Lane

Introduction

The ultimate goal of human IVF is the birth of a healthy singleton conceived through the transfer of a single embryo. The benefits that single embryo transfer (SET) brings have been well documented [1], and SET has already been proven effective in selected groups of patients [2, 3]. The relatively recent development of more effective embryo culture systems has facilitated the establishment of higher pregnancy rates, by being able to maintain the inherent viability of the gametes and subsequent embryo in vitro, and has therefore facilitated the wider introduction of SET. Furthermore, with the advent of more physiological culture media, it is possible to grow the human embryo to the blastocyst stage as a matter of routine. Thus, it is now possible to consider embryo transfer at any stage of preimplantation development. In parallel with, innovations in embryo culture has been the development of many excellent scoring systems to quantify embryo morphology [4–6], which have greatly assisted in embryo selection for transfer. Concomitantly, we are currently witnessing the application of several omic platforms (i.e., genomics, transcriptomics, proteomics, and metabolomics) in human IVF. Such technologies are generating quantifiable metrics that will assist in improving all areas of IVF, including the culture systems themselves. However, it is potentially in the area of embryo selection that omics will make their greatest impact. Clearly, human IVF has taken a huge leap forward in recent years and is entering a new exciting period. The aim of this chapter is to outline advances in embryo culture, discuss the potential benefits of blastocyst transfer and how improvements in embryo culture have also impacted on embryo selection.

D.K. Gardner, PhD (✉)
Department of Zoology, University of Melbourne, Parkville, VIC 3010, Australia
e-mail: david.gardner@unimelb.edu.au

M. Lane, BSc, PhD
Repromed, Dulwich, Adelaide, SA, Australia

Z.P. Nagy et al. (eds.), *Clinical Embryology: A Practical Guide*,
DOI 10.1007/978-1-4614-8376-2_7, © Springer Science+Business Media New York 2013

Development of Culture Systems to Support the Human Embryo

Over the past two decades, there has been a resurgence of interest in the physiology of the preimplantation embryo and in the environment within the female reproductive tract. Subsequently, culture systems for the human embryo have become more physiological, typically based on the levels of carbohydrates within the female tract, and routinely contain amino acids. The increased efficiency of these new media is reflected in an increase in implantation and pregnancy rates that the IVF community has experienced over the past decade [7]. A key aspect of the advances in culture conditions has been the ability to culture human embryos to the blastocyst stage as a matter of routine.

Some of the inherent advantages of blastocyst culture and transfer are summarized in Table 7.1. For example, not all sperm or oocytes will give rise to a viable embryo [8]. By growing the human embryo beyond the cleavage stages, i.e., past embryonic genome activation [9], one is able to consider the embryo proper, as opposed to an 8-cell embryo, which for the most part can be considered as a cleaving egg. Synchronization of embryonic stage with its relative position in the female reproductive tract is essential for the successful transfer of animal embryos. In all mammalian species studied to date, including nonhuman primates [10], the transfer of cleavage stage embryos to the uterus (i.e., prior to compaction and therefore before the generation of the first transporting epithelium) results in compromised pregnancy rates compared to the transfer of morulae or blastocysts [11]. Although the human cleavage stage embryo can develop in the uterus, in vivo the cleavage stage embryo resides in the Fallopian tube until day 4 [12]. Consequently, asynchronous transfers are being performed in the majority of IVF cases. Furthermore, it has

Table 7.1 Advantages of blastocyst transfer in human IVF

Identification of those embryos with limited, as well as those with the highest, developmental potential through morphological assessment and grading
Assessment of the embryo post genome activation
Synchronization of embryo development with the female tract to reduce cellular stress on the embryo
Minimizing exposure of the embryo to a uterine environment that has been exposed to exogenous gonadotropins
Fewer uterine contractions by day 5, thereby reducing the chance of the embryo being expelled
Demonstrated higher implantation rates, leading to a reduction in the number of embryos transferred
Ability to undertake cleavage stage embryo biopsy without the need for cryopreservation
Ability to undertake trophectoderm biopsy rather than cleavage stage biopsy, thereby increasing the number of cells analyzed (typically 6–10) and overcoming ethical/religious concerns of sampling embryonic tissue
Excellent cryosurvival
Increase in overall efficiency of IVF

been documented in animal models that the environment within the female tract following gonadotropin treatment is not as supportive to embryonic development as a nonstimulated environment [13, 14]. These data question the suitability of the uterine environment following a patient's exposure to exogenous gonadotropins. Clinical data also support the hypothesis that the uterine milieu is compromised following hyperstimulation [15]. Therefore, it may be preferable to expose embryos to such an altered uterine environment for as short a period as possible, which can be achieved through blastocyst transfer. Subsequently, the transfer of human embryos at the blastocyst stage has a sound physiological basis. Several of these advantages were perceived many years ago [16–18], but it has not been until the last 15 years that culture systems have become practical enough to use as a standard procedure in the IVF laboratory.

What Systems Can Be Used to Culture the Human Embryo?

Early culture media used in human IVF tended to either be rather basic, containing just a few salts and carbohydrates, or were tissue culture media, which contained an excess of nutrients, some of which are now known to be supraphysiological for embryos, leading to compromised development. The "simple" media, i.e., those lacking amino acids (reviewed in detail be Gardner and Lane [19]) such as those developed initially for the mouse and adapted for the human [20], were not effective in supporting human embryos past the 8-cell stage in culture. Indeed, it was not that long ago when it was considered "normal" for the majority of human embryos to arrest around the 8-cell stage in vitro (hence the adoption of cleavage stage embryo transfers). Consequently, other systems have been tried in attempts to nurture the human embryo to the blastocyst stage in culture. One such system made popular in the 1990s was co-culture, in which human embryos were cultured with monolayers of oviduct or uterine epithelial cells [17] or specific cell lines [18]. Although the development of blastocysts was facilitated by such technology, co-culture was not widely adopted, nor its efficacy ever established in randomized controlled trials. Subsequently, co-culture was replaced with the current approach of the use of more physiological culture media [21].

A major breakthrough in the formulation of embryo culture media came from the determination that amino acids have a significant role to play during embryo development [22–26] (Table 7.2). In the presence of amino acids, embryo development in culture is temporally closer to that observed in vivo: more cells are allocated to the inner cell mass (ICM) of the resultant blastocysts, energy metabolism is better supported, there is reduced apoptosis, and, most importantly, embryo viability, as assessed by implantation and fetal development, is higher [26]. However, as we are working in vitro in a system that cannot mimic many of the physical roles of the uterine epithelium, one must be mindful of in vitro artifacts, caused by working outside of the female reproductive tract. Amino acids are metabolized by embryos which subsequently release ammonium [25]. In vivo, one anticipates that this

Table 7.2 Role of amino acids during early mammalian embryo development

Role	References
Biosynthetic precursors	[96]
Energy source	[97]
Regulators of energy metabolism	[36, 98]
Osmolytes	[99]
Buffers of pHi	[100]
Antioxidants	[101]
Chelators	[102]
Signaling	[103, 104]
Regulation of differentiation	[105, 106]

ammonium is removed by the epithelial cells of the female reproductive tract, and then passes through the circulation and detoxified by the Urea cycle in the liver. However, in a static culture system, i.e., a dish in an incubator, any ammonium produced by embryonic metabolism simply builds up in the medium [25]. To add insult to injury, the amino acids themselves are labile at 37°C and spontaneously deaminate to release ammonium [25]. The significance of spontaneous ammonium build up is that it not only retards mouse and human blastocyst development in culture [27], but it has been associated with subsequent fetal retardation and neural tube defects in mice [26]. Furthermore, there appears to be a link between the concentration of ammonium in serum and the induction of fetal oversize in sheep [28, 29]. Therefore, it is advisable to renew the culture medium used at least every 48 h in order to circumvent the toxicity of ammonium. The main culprit with regard to amino acid deamination and ammonium release is glutamine. However, this amino acid can be replaced with the dipeptide alanyl-glutamine, which is stable at 37°C, and its inclusion significantly reduces ammonium release into the culture medium. However, when Gardner and colleagues measured the ammonium production by human blastocysts [30], it was found that the embryo produced significant amounts of ammonium, presumably through amino acid metabolism and transamination. The significance of these findings is that whatever culture system is employed, it is imperative to renew the medium after 48 h to ensure minimal accumulation of embryotoxic ammonium. From a practical point of view, therefore, the amount of work, cost, and embryo manipulations required is the same whether one is working with sequential media or a monophasic system (i.e., one medium formulation for the entire preimplantation period).

Of significance, the female tract provides gradients of nutrients, both carbohydrates [31] and amino acids [32, 33], which are involved in the regulation and production of energy by the developing embryo. The significance of these nutrient gradients to the embryo in culture warrants further research as existing data on the mouse indicates that such gradients in vitro impact embryo viability following transfer. For example, when the mouse zygote is cultured to the 8-cell stage and then transferred, embryo viability is highest after exposure of the embryo to a high lactate concentration (>20 mM D/L lactate), while when the embryo is cultured post compaction to the blastocyst stage, viability is highest after exposure to lower levels of lactate (<5 mM D/L lactate) [34]. These data support the hypothesis that the physiology of the developing conceptus is temporally regulated by concentration gradients of nutrients available [35].

One Medium or Two?

Sequential media were developed based on these changing environments within the female reproductive tract and to accommodate the changes in nutrient requirements and metabolism of the developing embryo [36, 37]. However, the approach of monoculture (one medium for all stages of development) is based on the principle of letting the embryo choose what it wants during development and differentiation. Clearly, such approaches have fundamental differences, and it has been questioned whether the former, more physiological approach, is really required [38]. We, therefore, decided to perform an analysis of the efficacy of such media types on the development of mouse pronucleate oocytes in vitro, and to compare their rates of development to in vivo developed embryos [39]. The media chosen were Whitten's (one of the very first mouse embryo culture media) [40], HTF (one of the first simple media developed for human embryos) [20], P1/Blastocyst (a glucose- and phosphate-free modification of HTF for 48 h after which the embryos are transferred to Ham's F10) [41], KSOM (a computer-optimized monophasic medium lacking amino acids) [42], KSOMAA (a computer-optimized monophasic medium with amino acids) [43], and G1G2 (a sequential media system based around the composition of the human female reproductive tract) [44]. All media were made with the same chemicals and water, and all embryos were transferred to fresh media after 48 h. All cultures were performed at 5% oxygen. There was no difference in cleavage time from 1- to 2-cell between any media (Fig. 7.1a). From 2- to 4-cell, embryos cultured in KSOMAA, HTF, and Whitten's media were significantly slower than those in medium G1 (Fig. 7.1b). From 4- to 8-cell, embryos cultured in all media were significantly slower than in medium G1 (Fig. 7.1c). Rates of compaction were significantly greater in embryos cultured in G1 (74.4%) compared to all other media: KSOMAA (60.2%), KSOM (65.9%), P1 (66.0%), HTF (26.4%), Whitten's (0.0%). Rates of blastocyst development were similar to in vivo developed embryos in media G1/G2 (Fig. 7.2). Blastocyst development in all other media was significantly slower to that obtained in vivo or in media G1/G2. Total blastocyst cell number was similar to in vivo blastocysts in media G1/G2, KSOMAA, and KSOM (Fig. 7.3). However, only the ICM development in G1/G2 blastocysts was equivalent to in vivo-developed blastocysts (Fig. 7.3). The data obtained demonstrate that embryos cultured in sequential media develop quicker than those in a monophasic system and that the subsequent blastocysts have the same cell number as those embryos developed in vivo. Subsequent transfers also revealed higher implantation rates of mouse embryos cultured in sequential media compared to their siblings cultured in a monophasic medium [45].

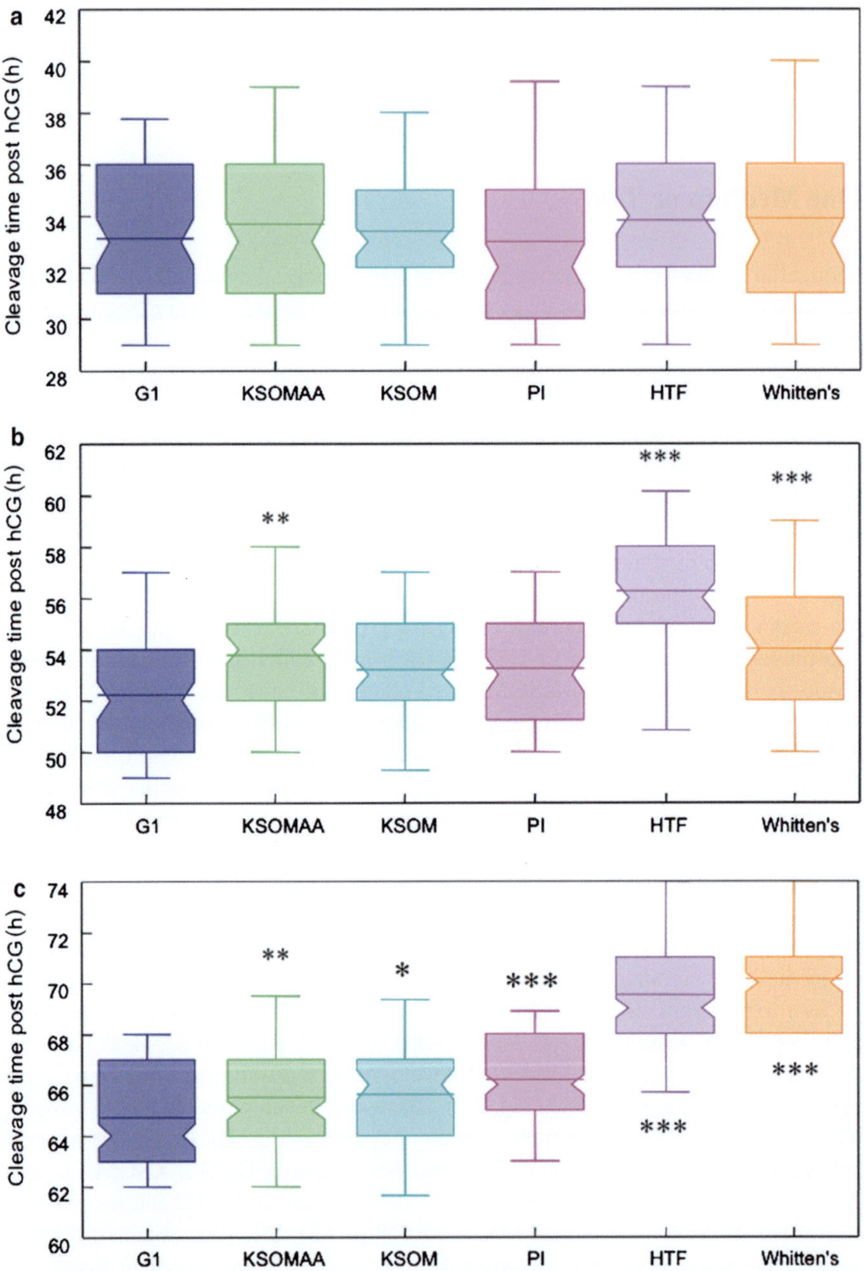

Fig. 7.1 Effect of culture media on cleavage times in hours from the zygote to the 8-cell stage. (**a**) Cleavage from the 1- to 2-cell stage. (**b**) Cleavage from the 2- to 4-cell stage. (**c**) Cleavage from the 4- to 8-cell stage. Notches represent the interquartile range (50% of the data); whiskers represent the 5 and 95% quartiles. The line across the box is the mean cleavage time. n = 100 embryos per treatment. Significantly different from G1; *$P < 0.05$; **$P < 0.01$; ***$P < 0.001$

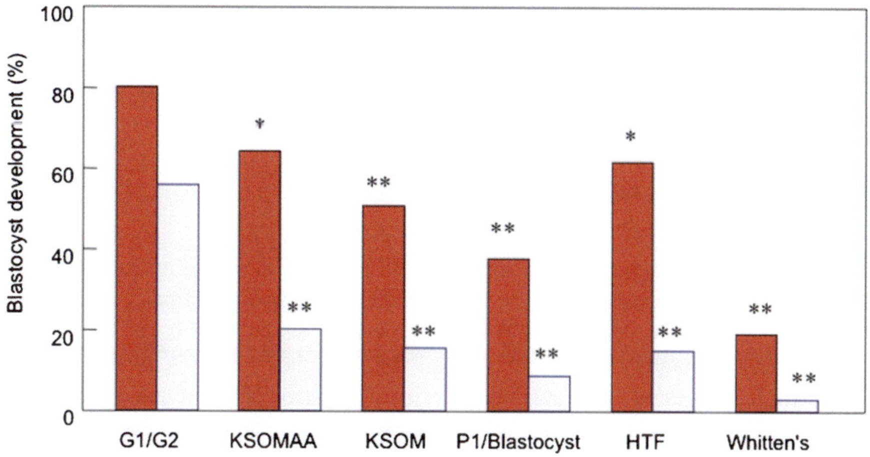

Fig. 7.2 Effect of culture conditions on blastocyst development at 94 h post-hCG. *Red bars* represent total blastocysts. *White bars* represent expanded blastocysts. Significantly different from G1/G2 embryos, $^{*}P < 0.05$, $^{**}P < 0.01$. At 94 h post-hCG, 82% of in vivo developed embryos were at the blastocyst stage

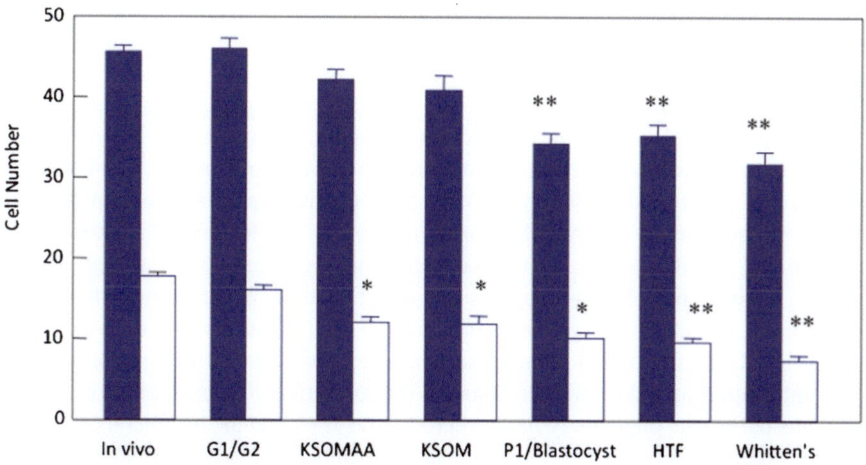

Fig. 7.3 Effect of culture conditions on blastocyst cell number and ICM development. *Blue bars* represent total cell number. *White bars* represent inner cell mass cell number. Significantly different from in vivo, $^{*}P < 0.05$, $^{**}P < 0.01$

Sequential media have now been proven to be highly effective in clinical settings. Importantly, assessment of the literature using an evidence-based Cochrane review [46] has determined that the benefit of blastocyst culture over cleavage stage culture is only evident in a sequential culture system, thereby indicating that there is a compromise in developmental competence when embryos are grown beyond the cleavage stage in a single medium. This finding for human IVF cycles mirrors the literature on animal embryos that have established developmental outcomes more similar to in vivo results after culture in sequential style culture media compared to a monophasic culture system [45].

The Holistic Approach to Embryo Culture

It is important to emphasize that the successful culture of viable human embryos entails far more than purchasing the appropriate culture media. Rather, the media is just one aspect of the overall embryo culture system, which itself is just one aspect of the overall laboratory (reviewed in detail [45]). Furthermore, it is imperative that sufficient resources be made available for quality control [47] and quality management [48], without which the lab is like a plane with no artificial horizon.

One key aspect of the laboratory that is worth reiterating, due to its significant impact on embryo development and viability, is that of oxygen concentration. The fact that both human and F1 mouse embryos can grow at atmospheric oxygen concentration (~20%) has lead to some confusion regarding the optimal concentration for embryo culture. The concentration of oxygen in the lumen of the rabbit oviduct is reported to be 2–6% [49, 50], whereas the oxygen concentration in the oviduct of hamster, and rhesus monkey is ~8% [51]. Interestingly, the oxygen concentration in the uterus is significantly lower than in the oviduct, ranging from 5% in the hamster and rabbit to 1.5% in the rhesus monkey [51].

Significantly, it has been demonstrated that optimum embryo development of several mammalian species occurs at an oxygen concentration at or below 10% [52–54]. Furthermore, it has been documented that mouse embryos cultured to the blastocyst stage in the presence of 20% oxygen have altered gene expression and a perturbed proteome compared to embryos developed in vivo [55, 56]. In contrast, culture in 5% oxygen had significantly less effect on both embryonic gene expression and proteome. Recent clinical data supports the move to the routine culture of human embryos in a reduced oxygen environment [57, 58]. Furthermore, data obtained using time-lapse incubation strongly supports the notion that at no time during the preimplantation period should the embryos be exposed to 20% oxygen [59].

Considering the physiology of the reproductive tract and the beneficial effects of using a reduced oxygen concentration as determined in controlled studies, it is advisable to culture embryos at low oxygen concentrations. This can easily be achieved with the modern tri-gas incubators or by using a premixed cylinder to purge a modular chamber/direct contact incubation system.

Implementation of Blastocyst Culture

Blastocyst transfer has now been used successfully to treat patients with poor-quality embryos [60, 61], patients with multiple IVF failures [62–64], patients with low numbers of oocytes and embryos [65], and oocyte donors [66]. Although in the examples listed above extended embryo culture has been associated with an increase in IVF success rates, there are a number of reports that question the merits of extended culture [67–69].

Parental factors also affect blastocyst formation and pregnancy-implantation rates. As maternal age increases, both the number and quality of the oocytes retrieved is reduced, thus affecting the outcome of blastocyst transfer [70, 71]. The success of blastocyst culture has also been shown to be under paternal influence [72]. Blastocyst formation is affected by the source of spermatozoa utilized for intracytoplasmic sperm injection, and in close relation to this, clinical pregnancy and implantation rates with blastocyst transfers decrease with the increase in severity of the spermatogenic disorder [73].

Gardner and Balaban [74] reviewed 16 prospective randomized trials using sequential media examining the effect of day of transfer on IVF cycle outcome [63, 68, 69, 75–87]. Of these 16 trials, seven reported a significant benefit in outcome as defined by either increased implantation rate or pregnancy rates (one study only reported pregnancy rates), when embryos were transferred at the blastocyst stage on day 5 rather than at the cleavage stage. In contrast, only one study found a significant advantage in transferring embryos at the cleavage stage [79]. The remaining eight trials reported no difference in implantation rate with respect to day of transfer.

The move to blastocyst culture has had a significant impact on reducing the number of embryos required for transfer, thereby greatly reducing the incidence of high-order multiple gestations. Although triplets can be confined to the archives of IVF, the overall multiple pregnancy rate of many programs has not decreased dramatically, as the incidence of twins is typically around 50% when two blastocysts are transferred. The only means to avoid this problem is, therefore, to consider single blastocyst transfer (SBT). In the first prospective randomized trial of single vs. two blastocyst transfers, in a population of patients with a day 3 FSH ≤10 mIU/mL and at least ten follicles >12 mm in diameter on day of hCG administration (age range 26–43 years), it was possible to establish an ongoing pregnancy rate of 60.9% without any incidence of twins [3]. Significantly, when two blastocysts were transferred, the pregnancy rate rose to 76%, but with a 47.4% incidence of twins.

Therefore, the move to SBT appears a more viable alternative to SET on day 3 in good prognosis patients. Papanikolaou and colleagues showed in a prospective randomized trial on SET that not only were higher ongoing pregnancy rates were established with blastocyst transfer, but that pregnancy loss was lower and birth rate was higher than that obtained with the transfer of cleavage stage embryos [87–89].

Blastocyst Selection for Transfer

As the embryo develops and differentiates into the blastocyst, with its distinct cell types (the ICM and trophectoderm), it becomes feasible to give a more detailed grading to the human embryo. An alphanumeric system [90] has been widely adopted and has proven valuable in assessing blastocyst viability prior to transfer [6, 91].

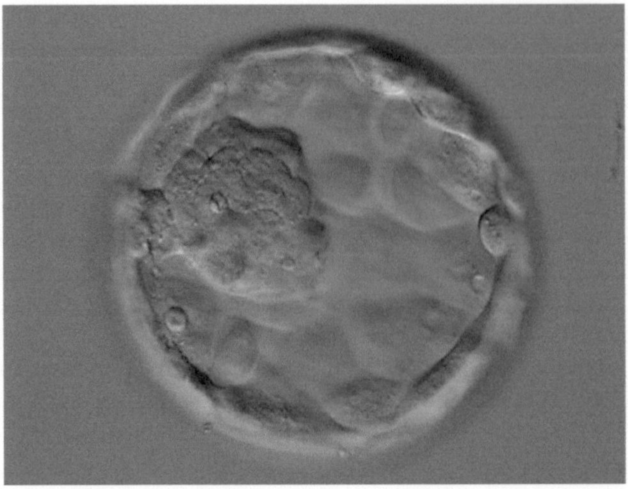

Fig. 7.4 Photomicrograph of a human blastocyst on day 5 of development. Such a blastocyst is graded as 4AA

Figure 7.4 shows a human blastocyst that has formed a well-defined ICM surrounded by a cohesive multicellular epithelium, the trophectoderm. Such an embryo from patients <38, or an oocyte donor, should ideally be transferred alone.

As discussed previously, at the blastocyst stage, one has the ability to examine the embryo proper, and using both proteomic and metabolic analysis, it is evident that even blastocysts with the same morphology have different physiologies [30, 92]. Subsequently, the analysis of embryo metabolism and its secretome will be of great value in quantitating embryonic viability prior to transfer and supporting decisions for SET. Similarly, the advent of highly sensitive molecular techniques is making karyotyping the blastocyst a reality in an IVF cycle [93]. Such molecular analyses require the cryopreservation of the embryo. The capacity to perform these analyses is supported by developments in blastocyst vitrification which have facilitated safe and effective blastocyst cryopreservation [94, 95].

Conclusions

With the advent of more physiological culture media, together with better laboratory conditions and management, it is feasible to culture the human embryo to the blastocyst as a matter of routine. The potential advantages of extended culture go beyond increases in implantation and pregnancy rates and include lower miscarriage rates, and the ability to perform comprehensive genetic and physiological analysis of the embryo proper prior to transfer. The capacity to better select a viable embryo will continue to improve the safety of IVF to the mother and child without a compromise in efficacy. The ability of blastocysts to undergo successful cryopreservation with vitrification will culminate in the transfer of genetically analyzed embryos to a naturally cycling uterus. The transfer of vitrified blastocysts in a nonstimulated cycle may ultimately be the way all future IVF is performed.

References

1. Adashi EY, Barri PN, Berkowitz R, Braude P, Bryan E, Carr J, et al. Infertility therapy-associated multiple pregnancies (births): an ongoing epidemic. Reprod Biomed Online. 2003;7(5):515–42.
2. Gerris J, De Neubourg D, Mangelschots K, Van Royen E, Vercruyssen M, Barudy-Vasquez J, et al. Elective single day 3 embryo transfer halves the twinning rate without decrease in the ongoing pregnancy rate of an IVF/ICSI programme. Hum Reprod. 2002;17(10):2626–31.
3. Gardner DK, Surrey E, Minjarez D, Leitz A, Stevens J, Schoolcraft WB. Single blastocyst transfer: a prospective randomized trial. Fertil Steril. 2004;81(3):551–5.
4. Cummins JM, Breen TM, Harrison KL, Shaw JM, Wilson LM, Hennessey JF. A formula for scoring human embryo growth rates in in vitro fertilization: its value in predicting pregnancy and in comparison with visual estimates of embryo quality. J In Vitro Fert Embryo Transf. 1986;3(5):284–95.
5. Van Royen E, Mangelschots K, De Neubourg D, Valkenburg M, Van de Meerssche M, Ryckaert G, et al. Characterization of a top quality embryo, a step towards single-embryo transfer. Hum Reprod. 1999;14(9):2345–9.
6. Gardner DK, Lane M, Stevens J, Schlenker T, Schoolcraft WB. Blastocyst score affects implantation and pregnancy outcome: towards a single blastocyst transfer. Fertil Steril. 2000;73(6):1155–8.
7. Gardner DK. Human embryonic development in vitro. In: Tan SLC, Chian R-C, Buckette WM, editors. In-vitro maturation of human oocytes. London: Informa Healthcare; 2007. p. 295–312.
8. Tesarik J. Developmental failure during the preimplanation period of human embryogenesis. In: Van Blerkom J, editor. The biological basis of early human reproductive failure. New York: Oxford University Press; 1994. p. 327–44.
9. Braude P, Bolton V, Moore S. Human gene expression first occurs between the four- and eight-cell stages of preimplantation development. Nature. 1988;332(6163):459–61.
10. Marston JH, Penn R, Sivelle PC. Successful autotransfer of tubal eggs in the rhesus monkey (*Macaca mulatta*). J Reprod Fertil. 1977;49(1):175–6.
11. Barnes FL. The effects of the early uterine environment on the subsequent development of embryo and fetus. Theriogenology. 2000;53(2):649–58.
12. Croxatto HB, Ortiz ME, Diaz S, Hess R, Balmaceda J, Croxatto HD. Studies on the duration of egg transport by the human oviduct. II. Ovum location at various intervals following luteinizing hormone peak. Am J Obstet Gynecol. 1978;132(6):629–34.
13. Van der Auwera I, Pijnenborg R, Koninckx PR. The influence of in-vitro culture versus stimulated and untreated oviductal environment on mouse embryo development and implantation. Hum Reprod. 1999;14(10):2570–4.
14. Ertzeid G, Storeng R. The impact of ovarian stimulation on implantation and fetal development in mice. Hum Reprod. 2001;16(2):221–5.
15. Pellicer A, Valbuena D, Cano F, Remohi J, Simon C. Lower implantation rates in high responders: evidence for an altered endocrine milieu during the preimplantation period. Fertil Steril. 1996;65(6):1190–5.
16. Lopata A. The neglected human blastocyst. J Assist Reprod Genet. 1992;9(6):508–12.

17. Bongso A, Fong CY, Ng SC, Ratnam S. Human embryonic behavior in a sequential human oviduct-endometrial coculture system. Fertil Steril. 1994;61(5):976–8.
18. Menezo YJ, Guerin JF, Czyba JC. Improvement of human early embryo development in vitro by coculture on monolayers of Vero cells. Biol Reprod. 1990;42(2):301–6.
19. Gardner DK, Lane M. Embryo Culture systems. In: Gardner DK, editor. In vitro fertilization a practical approach. New York: Informa Healthcare; 2007. p. 221–82.
20. Quinn P, Kerin JF, Warnes GM. Improved pregnancy rate in human in vitro fertilization with the use of a medium based on the composition of human tubal fluid. Fertil Steril. 1985;44(4): 493–8.
21. Menezo YJ, Hamamah S, Hazout A, Dale B. Time to switch from co-culture to sequential defined media for transfer at the blastocyst stage. Hum Reprod. 1998;13(8):2043–4.
22. Gwatkin RB. Amino acid requirements for attachment and outgrowth of the mouse blastocyst in vitro. J Cell Physiol. 1966;68:335–44.
23. Spindle AI, Pedersen RA. Hatching, attachment, and outgrowth of mouse blastocysts in vitro: fixed nitrogen requirements. J Exp Zool. 1973;186(3):305–18.
24. Bavister BD, Arlotto T. Influence of single amino acids on the development of hamster one-cell embryos in vitro. Mol Reprod Dev. 1990;25(1):45–51.
25. Gardner DK, Lane M. Amino acids and ammonium regulate mouse embryo development in culture. Biol Reprod. 1993;48(2):377–85.
26. Lane M, Gardner DK. Increase in postimplantation development of cultured mouse embryos by amino acids and induction of fetal retardation and exencephaly by ammonium ions. J Reprod Fertil. 1994;102(2):305–12.
27. Virant-Klun I, Tomazevic T, Vrtacnik-Bokal E, Vogler A, Krsnik M, Meden-Vrtovec H. Increased ammonium in culture medium reduces the development of human embryos to the blastocyst stage. Fertil Steril. 2006;85(2):526–8.
28. McEvoy TG, Robinson JJ, Aitken RP, Findlay PA, Robertson IS. Dietary excesses of urea influence the viability and metabolism of preimplantation sheep embryos and may affect fetal growth among survivors. Anim Reprod Sci. 1997;47(1–2):71–90.
29. Sinclair KD, McEvoy TG, Maxfield EK, Maltin CA, Young LE, Wilmut I, et al. Aberrant fetal growth and development after in vitro culture of sheep zygotes. J Reprod Fertil. 1999;116(1):177–86.
30. Gardner DK, Lane M, Stevens J, Schoolcraft WB. Noninvasive assessment of human embryo nutrient consumption as a measure of developmental potential. Fertil Steril. 2001;76(6): 1175–80.
31. Gardner DK, Lane M, Calderon I, Leeton J. Environment of the preimplantation human embryo in vivo: metabolite analysis of oviduct and uterine fluids and metabolism of cumulus cells. Fertil Steril. 1996;65(2):349–53.
32. Harris SE, Gopichandran N, Picton HM, Leese HJ, Orsi NM. Nutrient concentrations in murine follicular fluid and the female reproductive tract. Theriogenology. 2005;64(4): 992–1006.
33. Hugentobler SA, Diskin MG, Leese HJ, Humpherson PG, Watson T, Sreenan JM, et al. Amino acids in oviduct and uterine fluid and blood plasma during the estrous cycle in the bovine. Mol Reprod Dev. 2007;74(4):445–54.
34. Gardner DK, Sakkas D. Mouse embryo cleavage, metabolism and viability: role of medium composition. Hum Reprod. 1993;8(2):288–95.
35. Lane M, Gardner DK. Lactate regulates pyruvate uptake and metabolism in the preimplantation mouse embryo. Biol Reprod. 2000;62(1):16–22.
36. Gardner DK, Lane M. Culture and selection of viable blastocysts: a feasible proposition for human IVF? Hum Reprod Update. 1997;3(4):367–82.
37. Gardner DK. Changes in requirements and utilization of nutrients during mammalian preimplantation embryo development and their significance in embryo culture. Theriogenology. 1998;49(1):83–102.
38. Biggers JD, McGinnis LK, Lawitts JA. One-step versus two-step culture of mouse preimplantation embryos: is there a difference? Hum Reprod. 2005;20(12):3376–84.

39. Reed LC, Lane M, Gardner DK. In vivo rates of mouse embryo development can be attained in vitro. Theriogenology. 2003;59:349.
40. Whitten WK. Culture of tubal ova. Nature. 1957;179(4569):1081–2.
41. Behr B, Pool TB, Milki AA, Moore D, Gebhardt J, Dasig D. Preliminary clinical experience with human blastocyst development in vitro without co-culture. Hum Reprod. 1999;14(2):454–7.
42. Lawitts JA, Biggers JD. Optimization of mouse embryo culture media using simplex methods. J Reprod Fertil. 1991;91(2):543–56.
43. Ho Y, Wigglesworth K, Eppig JJ, Schultz RM. Preimplantation development of mouse embryos in KSOM: augmentation by amino acids and analysis of gene expression. Mol Reprod Dev. 1995;41(2):232–8.
44. Barnes FL, Crombie A, Gardner DK, Kausche A, Lacham-Kaplan O, Suikkari AM, et al. Blastocyst development and birth after in-vitro maturation of human primary oocytes, intracytoplasmic sperm injection and assisted hatching. Hum Reprod. 1995;10(12):3243–7.
45. Gardner D, Lane M. Towards a single embryo transfer. Reprod Biomed Online. 2003;6(4):470–81.
46. Blake DA, Farquhar CM, Johnson N, Proctor M. Cleavage stage versus blastocyst stage embryo transfer in assisted conception. Cochrane Database Syst Rev. 2007;(4):CD002118.
47. Gardner DK, Reed L, Linck D, Sheehan C, Lane M. Quality control in human in vitro fertilization. Semin Reprod Med. 2005;23(4):319–24.
48. Mortimer DM, Mortimer ST. Quality and risk management in the IVF laboratory. Cambridge: Cambridge University Press; 2005.
49. Mastroianni Jr L, Jones R. Oxygen tension within the rabbit fallopian tube. J Reprod Fertil. 1965;147:99–102.
50. Ross RN, Graves CN. O_2 levels in female rabbit reproductive tract. J Anim Sci. 1974;39:994.
51. Fischer B, Bavister BD. Oxygen tension in the oviduct and uterus of rhesus monkeys, hamsters and rabbits. J Reprod Fertil. 1993;99(2):673–9.
52. Quinn P, Harlow GM. The effect of oxygen on the development of preimplantation mouse embryos in vitro. J Exp Zool. 1978;206(1):73–80.
53. Thompson JG, Simpson AC, Pugh PA, Donnelly PE, Tervit HR. Effect of oxygen concentration on in-vitro development of preimplantation sheep and cattle embryos. J Reprod Fertil. 1990;89(2):573–8.
54. Batt PA, Gardner DK, Cameron AW. Oxygen concentration and protein source affect the development of preimplantation goat embryos in vitro. Reprod Fertil Dev. 1991;3(5):601–7.
55. Gardner DK, Lane M. Ex vivo early embryo development and effects on gene expression and imprinting. Reprod Fertil Dev. 2005;17(3):361.
56. Katz-Jaffe MG, Linck DW, Schoolcraft WB, Gardner DK. A proteomic analysis of mammalian preimplantation embryonic development. Reproduction. 2005;130(6):899–905.
57. Meintjes M, Chantilis SJ, Douglas JD, Rodriguez AJ, Guerami AR, Bookout DM, et al. A controlled randomized trial evaluating the effect of lowered incubator oxygen tension on live births in a predominantly blastocyst transfer program. Hum Reprod. 2009;24(2):300–7.
58. Nanassy L, Peterson CA, Wilcox AL, Peterson CM, Hammoud A, Carrell DT. Comparison of 5% and ambient oxygen during days 3-5 of in vitro culture of human embryos. Fertil Steril. 2010;93(2):579–85.
59. Wale PL, Gardner DK. Time-lapse analysis of mouse embryo development in oxygen gradients. Reprod Biomed Online. 2010;21(3):402–10.
60. Balaban B, Urman B, Alatas C, Mercan R, Aksoy S, Isiklar A. Blastocyst-stage transfer of poor-quality cleavage-stage embryos results in higher implantation rates. Fertil Steril. 2001;75(3):514–8.
61. Langley MT, Marek DM, Gardner DK, Doody KM, Doody KJ. Extended embryo culture in human assisted reproduction treatments. Hum Reprod. 2001;16(5):902–8.
62. Cruz JR, Dubey AK, Patel J, Peak D, Hartog B, Gindoff PR. Is blastocyst transfer useful as an alternative treatment for patients with multiple in vitro fertilization failures? Fertil Steril. 1999;72(2):218–20.

63. Levitas E, Lunenfeld E, Har-Vardi I, Albotiano S, Sonin Y, Hackmon-Ram R, et al. Blastocyst-stage embryo transfer in patients who failed to conceive in three or more day 2-3 embryo transfer cycles: a prospective, randomized study. Fertil Steril. 2004;81(3):567–71.
64. Guerif F, Bidault R, Gasnier O, Couet ML, Gervereau O, Lansac J, et al. Efficacy of blastocyst transfer after implantation failure. Reprod Biomed Online. 2004;9(6):630–6.
65. Wilson M, Hartke K, Kiehl M, Rodgers J, Brabec C, Lyles R. Integration of blastocyst transfer for all patients. Fertil Steril. 2002;77(4):693–6.
66. Schoolcraft WB, Gardner DK. Blastocyst culture and transfer increases the efficiency of oocyte donation. Fertil Steril. 2000;74(3):482–6.
67. Alikani M, Calderon G, Tomkin G, Garrisi J, Kokot M, Cohen J. Cleavage anomalies in early human embryos and survival after prolonged culture in-vitro. Hum Reprod. 2000;15(12):2634–43.
68. Coskun S, Hollanders J, Al-Hassan S, Al-Sufyan H, Al-Mayman H, Jaroudi K. Day 5 versus day 3 embryo transfer: a controlled randomized trial. Hum Reprod. 2000;15(9):1947–52.
69. Rienzi L, Ubaldi F, Iacobelli M, Ferrero S, Minasi MG, Martinez F, et al. Day 3 embryo transfer with combined evaluation at the pronuclear and cleavage stages compares favourably with day 5 blastocyst transfer. Hum Reprod. 2002;17(7):1852–5.
70. Scholtes MC, Zeilmaker GH. Blastocyst transfer in day-5 embryo transfer depends primarily on the number of oocytes retrieved and not on age. Fertil Steril. 1998;69(1):78–83.
71. Pantos K, Athanasiou V, Stefanidis K, Stavrou D, Vaxevanoglou T, Chronopoulou M. Influence of advanced age on the blastocyst development rate and pregnancy rate in assisted reproductive technology. Fertil Steril. 1999;71(6):1144–6.
72. Janny L, Menezo YJ. Evidence for a strong paternal effect on human preimplantation embryo development and blastocyst formation. Mol Reprod Dev. 1994;38(1):36–42.
73. Balaban B, Urman B, Isiklar A, Alatas C, Mercan R, Aksoy S, et al. Blastocyst transfer following intracytoplasmic injection of ejaculated, epididymal or testicular spermatozoa. Hum Reprod. 2001;16(1):125–9.
74. Gardner DK, Balaban B. Choosing between day 3 and day 5 embryo transfers. Clin Obstet Gynecol. 2006;49(1):85–92.
75. Gardner DK, Schoolcraft WB, Wagley L, Schlenker T, Stevens J, Hesla J. A prospective randomized trial of blastocyst culture and transfer in in-vitro fertilization. Hum Reprod. 1998;13(12):3434–40.
76. Utsunomiya T, Naitou T, Nagaki M. A prospective trial of blastocyst culture and transfer. Hum Reprod. 2002;17(7):1846–51.
77. Karaki RZ, Samarraie SS, Younis NA, Lahloub TM, Ibrahim MH. Blastocyst culture and transfer: a step toward improved in vitro fertilization outcome. Fertil Steril. 2002;77(1):114–8.
78. Van der Auwera I, Debrock S, Spiessens C, Afschrift H, Bakelants E, Meuleman C, et al. A prospective randomized study: day 2 versus day 5 embryo transfer. Hum Reprod. 2002;17(6):1507–12.
79. Levron J, Shulman A, Bider D, Seidman D, Levin T, Dor J. A prospective randomized study comparing day 3 with blastocyst-stage embryo transfer. Fertil Steril. 2002;77(6):1300–1.
80. Frattarelli JL, Leondires MP, McKeeby JL, Miller BT, Segars JH. Blastocyst transfer decreases multiple pregnancy rates in in vitro fertilization cycles: a randomized controlled trial. Fertil Steril. 2003;79(1):228–30.
81. Margreiter M, Weghofer A, Kogosowski A, Mahmoud KZ, Feichtinger W. A prospective randomized multicenter study to evaluate the best day for embryo transfer: does the outcome justify prolonged embryo culture? J Assist Reprod Genet. 2003;20(2):91–4.
82. Bungum M, Bungum L, Humaidan P, Andersen CY. Day 3 versus day 5 embryo transfer: a prospective randomized study. Reprod Biomed Online. 2003;7:98–104.
83. Emiliani S, Delbaere A, Vannin AS, Biramane J, Verdoodt M, Englert Y, et al. Similar delivery rates in a selected group of patients, for day 2 and day 5 embryos both cultured in sequential medium: a randomized study. Hum Reprod. 2003;18(10):2145–50.
84. Pantos K, Makrakis E, Stavrou D, Karantzis P, Vaxevanoglou T, Tzigounis V. Comparison of embryo transfer on day 2, day 3, and day 6: a prospective randomized study. Fertil Steril. 2004;81(2):454–5.

85. Kolibianakis EM, Zikopoulos K, Verpoest W, Camus M, Joris H, Van Steirteghem AC, et al. Should we advise patients undergoing IVF to start a cycle leading to a day 3 or a day 5 transfer? Hum Reprod. 2004;19(11):2550–4.
86. Hreinsson J, Rosenlund B, Fridstrom M, Ek I, Levkov L, Sjoblom P, et al. Embryo transfer is equally effective at cleavage stage and blastocyst stage: a randomized prospective study. Eur J Obstet Gynecol Reprod Biol. 2004;117(2):194–200.
87. Papanikolaou EG, D'Haeseleer E, Verheyen G, Van de Velde H, Camus M, Steirteghem AV, et al. Live birth rate is significantly higher after blastocyst transfer than after cleavage-stage embryo transfer when at least four embryos are available on day 3 of embryo culture. A randomized prospective study. Hum Reprod. 2005;29:1–6.
88. Papanikolaou V. Early pregnancy loss is significantly higher after day 3 single embryo transfer that after day 5 single blastocyst transfer in GnRH antagonist stimulated IVF cycles. Reprod Biomed Online. 2006;12(1):60–5.
89. Papanikolaou EG, Camus M, Kolibianakis EM, Van Landuyt L, Van Steirteghem A, Devroey P. In vitro fertilization with single blastocyst-stage versus single cleavage-stage embryos. N Engl J Med. 2006;354:1139–46.
90. Gardner DK, Schoolcraft WB. In vitro culture of human blastocyst. In: Jansen R, Mortimer D, editors. Towards reproductive certainty: fertility and genetics beyond. Carnforth: Parthenon; 1999. p. 378–88.
91. Balaban B, Yakin K, Urman B. Randomized comparison of two different blastocyst grading systems. Fertil Steril. 2006;85(3):559–63.
92. Katz-Jaffe MG, Gardner DK, Schoolcraft WB. Proteomic analysis of individual human embryos to identify novel biomarkers of development and viability. Fertil Steril. 2006;85(1):101–7.
93. Schoolcraft WB, Fragouli E, Stevens J, Munne S, Katz-Jaffe MG, Wells D. Clinical application of comprehensive chromosomal screening at the blastocyst stage. Fertil Steril. 2010;94(5):1700–6.
94. Lane M, Schoolcraft WB, Gardner DK. Vitrification of mouse and human blastocysts using a novel cryoloop container-less technique. Fertil Steril. 1999;72(6):1073–8.
95. Takahashi K, Mukaida T, Goto T, Oka C. Perinatal outcome of blastocyst transfer with vitrification using cryoloop: a 4-year follow-up study. Fertil Steril. 2005;84(1):88–92.
96. Crosby IM, Gandolfi F, Moor RM. Control of protein synthesis during early cleavage of sheep embryos. J Reprod Fertil. 1988;82(2):769–75.
97. Rieger D, Loskutoff NM, Betteridge KJ. Developmentally related changes in the uptake and metabolism of glucose, glutamine and pyruvate by cattle embryos produced in vitro. Reprod Fertil Dev. 1992;4(5):547–57.
98. Lane M, Gardner DK. Mitochondrial malate-aspartate shuttle regulates mouse embryo nutrient consumption. J Biol Chem. 2005;280(18):18361–7.
99. Van Winkle LJ, Haghighat N, Campione AL. Glycine protects preimplantation mouse conceptuses from a detrimental effect on development of the inorganic ions in oviductal fluid. J Exp Zool. 1990;253(2):215–9.
100. Edwards LJ, Williams DA, Gardner DK. Intracellular pH of the mouse preimplantation embryo: amino acids act as buffers of intracellular pH. Hum Reprod. 1998;13(12):3441–8.
101. Liu Z, Foote RH. Development of bovine embryos in KSOM with added superoxide dismutase and taurine and with five and twenty percent O_2. Biol Reprod. 1995;53(4):786–90.
102. Lindenbaum A. A survey of naturally occurring chelating ligands. Adv Exp Med Biol. 1973;40:67–77.
103. Wu G, Morris Jr SM. Arginine metabolism: nitric oxide and beyond. Biochem J. 1998;336(Pt 1):1–17.
104. Martin PM, Sutherland AE, Van Winkle LJ. Amino acid transport regulates blastocyst implantation. Biol Reprod. 2003;69(4):1101–8.
105. Lane M, Gardner DK. Differential regulation of mouse embryo development and viability by amino acids. J Reprod Fertil. 1997;109(1):153–64.
106. Martin PM, Sutherland AE. Exogenous amino acids regulate trophectoderm differentiation in the mouse blastocyst through an mTOR-dependent pathway. Dev Biol. 2001;240(1):182–93.

Chapter 8
In Vitro Maturation of Human Oocytes

Baris Ata, Jack Huang, and Ri-Cheng Chian

Today, pregnancy rates achieved with in vitro fertilization (IVF) treatment have exceeded that achieved in natural cycles [1–3]. These figures are achieved with simultaneous transfer of multiple embryos in a given treatment cycle. Traditionally, production of multiple embryos has been only possible after development of controlled ovarian stimulation (COS) protocols.

In a natural menstrual cycle, several antral follicles are present in the human ovary. The interactions between the growing follicles, the pituitary gland, and the hypothalamus prevent multifollicular growth and allow only one follicle complete maturation and reach ovulation in the majority of cycles. COS with exogenous gonadotropins and gonadotropin releasing hormone analogs enables overriding this natural selection process and collection of multiple mature oocytes which are amenable to fertilization. COS has been an integral part of conventional IVF treatment for over 20 years.

COS requires multiple daily injections and frequent monitoring scans creating direct and indirect costs, loss of working time, and inconvenience. Unfortunately, the cost of drugs used for COS poses a substantial financial burden and at times prevents a couple's access to treatment. The most important medical problem associated with COS is the risk of ovarian hyperstimulation syndrome (OHSS). OHSS is a potentially lethal condition, most commonly occurring as an iatrogenic complication of COS [4]. It is characterized by ovarian enlargement and increased

B. Ata, MD
Assisted Reproduction Unit, Department of Obstetrics and Gynecology,
Uludag University, Bursa, Turkey

J. Huang, MD, PhD
Center for Reproductive Medicine, Weill Cornell Medical College,
New York Presbyterian Hospital, New York, NY, USA

R.-C. Chian, PhD (✉)
Department of Obstetrics and Gynecology, Royal Victoria Hospital,
Women's Pavilion F, 687 Pine Avenue West, Montreal, QC, Canada H3A 1A1
e-mail: Ri-cheng.chian@muhc.mcgill.ca

Z.P. Nagy et al. (eds.), *Clinical Embryology: A Practical Guide*,
DOI 10.1007/978-1-4614-8376-2_8,

capillary permeability, causing fluid shift to the third space. This results in ascites formation, hypovolemia, hemoconcentration, and hypercoagulability. OHSS may be further complicated by acute renal failure, hypovolemic shock, thromboembolic episodes, and adult respiratory distress syndrome (ARDS), and in extreme cases, it can be fatal. The risk of OHSS can be as high as 6% in young women with polycystic ovarian syndrome (PCOS) [5]. More recently, the altered hormonal milieu during COS has been suggested to have detrimental effects on developing oocytes, embryos derived from these oocytes, and/or endometrial receptivity [6, 7].

Collection and in vitro maturation (IVM) of the already existing immature oocytes in the smaller antral follicles can provide multiple mature oocytes that can be fertilized or cryopreserved for future use. The technique has been named IVM. Using immature oocytes collected in a nonstimulated cycle to produce multiple embryos avoids the costs, inconvenience, and risks associated with conventional IVF.

Research on immature oocytes dates as far back as the 1930s [8]. These oocytes are shown to resume meiosis upon removal from the follicle, have the capacity to complete meiotic division, and can be fertilized in vitro. More than 80% of oocytes were reported to resume meiosis independent of the menstrual cycle day and gonadotropin support in IVM medium [9]. The first pregnancy and live birth from in vitro-matured oocytes in humans was only reported by Veeck and colleagues in 1983 in the context of a stimulated IVF cycle [10]. They reported two pregnancies resulting from IVM of immature oocytes collected alongside mature oocytes in gonadotropin-stimulated IVF cycles. However, IVF with COS had already become the norm, and it was not until 1991 when Cha and colleagues first reported intentional collection of immature oocytes from women undergoing gynecological surgery that IVM began to gain momentum [11]. The immature oocytes donated by these women were matured in vitro, and the resulting embryos were transferred to a recipient with premature ovarian failure [11]. The recipient delivered healthy triplet girls.

Three years later, Trounson and colleagues reported the collection of immature oocytes from women with PCOS for their own use [12]. The immature oocytes collected were matured in vitro with gonadotropin-enriched medium, then fertilized, and a healthy live birth following transfer of resultant embryos was reported. Unfortunately, the initial pregnancy rates were low, and it took another 5 years to allow success rates to exceed 35% per cycle in appropriately selected patient groups [13–24].

Indications for IVM Treatment

Infertility with PCO or PCOS

Young women with high antral-follicle counts achieve the highest pregnancy rates with IVM [25]. IVM has become an established treatment option for women with PCO or PCOS who need ART. However, the clinical application of IVM technology can be expanded to benefit other patient populations.

High Responders to Gonadotropin Stimulation

IVM combined with IVF can be a valid option for patients who demonstrate an overresponse to COS and are considered to be at risk of OHSS during an already started IVF cycle. The only method proven to prevent OHSS completely is to avoid the injection of human chorionic gonadotropin (HCG) for final oocyte maturation [4]. However, this strategy requires cancelation of the treatment cycle, leading to frustration in both the patient and the physician. Giving the HCG injection when the leading follicle size is 12–14 mm, before the conventional HCG criteria for IVF is met, followed by oocyte collection 36–38 h later may prove to be an effective strategy. Lim et al. reported a 36.6% clinical pregnancy rate using a similar strategy in 123 women who had ≥20 follicles with a mean diameter ≥10 mm after ≥5 days of gonadotropin stimulation [26]. None of the women in this cohort developed OHSS. As a further note, 18.9% of 1,554 oocytes collected were in vivo matured.

Poor Responders to Gonadotropin Stimulation

Unfortunately, all women do not respond similarly to COS, and some fail to develop a reasonable number of mature follicles in stimulated IVF cycles. The most common cause of poor response seems to be the age-related decline in ovarian reserve, but it also occurs in some younger women.

For women in whom poor ovarian response does not seem to be due to a rectifiable cause inherent to the particular treatment cycle; i.e., inappropriate choice of stimulation protocol, skipped medication, etc., trying further stimulated cycles can prove useless. IVM may provide a viable option in such cases. In two studies involving women with a history of poor ovarian response in a stimulated IVF cycle, pregnancy rates of 31.6 and 40.4% were achieved with IVM [27, 28]. In eight women with a poor response, defined as ≤4 follicles growing or oocytes collected in a previous stimulated IVF cycle, we achieved a similar number of embryos available for transfer in the subsequent IVM cycle [29]. Six women reached embryo transfer (75%), and one achieved a live birth, yielding a 16.7% live birth rate per transfer in this small sample.

Oocyte Donation

Young women who have high ovarian reserve are preferred as oocyte donors. Unfortunately, such women comprise a high risk population for early OHSS in stimulated IVF cycles. Besides the risk of OHSS, the inconvenience of the numerous injections required and the theoretical risk of cancer associated with repeated use of ovulation induction drugs cause reluctance on the part of some potential oocyte donors. IVM can be an appropriate method for oocyte donation cycles as young women with high antral-follicle counts comprise the best candidates for IVM and yield good pregnancy rates.

We reported collection of an average of 12.8 immature oocytes from 12 oocyte donors with a mean age of 29 years. Sixty-eight percent of the oocytes matured in vitro and 62 embryos were available for transfer to 12 recipients with a mean age of 37.7 years [30]. On average, four embryos were transferred (range 2–6) and a clinical pregnancy rate of 50% was achieved. Two women had first-trimester miscarriages while four had healthy live births, yielding a live birth rate of 33%.

Fertility Preservation

The American Society of Clinical Oncology and American Society of Reproductive Medicine have endorsed IVF and embryo cryopreservation (EC) as the only method of female fertility preservation [31, 32]. IVM expands the fertility preservation options for women who are not candidates for IVF–EC for various medical and social reasons. Women with hormone-sensitive tumors may undergo immature oocyte collection and cryopreserve resultant embryos. The advantages of IVM are not limited to eliminating the need for expensive drugs as well as their administration and avoiding hormone-sensitive tumors: IVM enables oocyte retrieval at any phase of the menstrual cycle and completion of the fertility preservation procedure in 2–10 days, preventing a delay in treatment of the primary disease [33, 34]. We reported three women without male partners seeking fertility preservation prior to chemotherapy, who presented for the first time in the luteal phase of their menstrual cycle and were to undergo gonadotoxic treatment immediately [34]. Five to seven immature oocytes were recovered with luteal-phase oocyte retrieval from these patients. Three to five M-II oocytes were vitrified following IVM. Two of these three women later underwent one and two more collections, respectively, in the follicular phase of the next cycle(s), and additional immature oocytes were vitrified following IVM.

Immature oocytes can also be harvested from ovarian biopsy specimens and can be vitrified following IVM [35]. This combination of ovarian-tissue cryobanking and IVM represents a new strategy for fertility preservation. We retrieved 11 immature oocytes from a wedge resection specimen in a 16-year-old patient with mosaic Turner syndrome. Eight of these oocytes were vitrified following IVM [36]. In four women with cancer, we harvested 11 immature and eight mature oocytes from wedge biopsy specimens. Eight of the 11 immature oocytes reached M-II stage following IVM and were vitrified [35].

Step-by-Step Protocol for IVM Treatment

Monitoring and Management of an IVM Cycle

Monitoring starts with a baseline scan performed in the early follicular phase of the menstrual cycle, preferably between days 2 and 5 of a natural menstrual cycle or a withdrawal bleed, induced with progesterone administration in amenorrheic women.

The number and size of the antral follicles and endometrial texture and thickness are recorded. The uterus and ovaries are examined for any abnormalities. A second scan is performed about a week later when it is anticipated that the largest follicle has reached 10–12 mm in diameter and the endometrial thickness is at least 6 mm. The presence of a dominant follicle does not require cancelation of the treatment cycle because smaller follicles are found to contain viable oocytes, even in the presence of a dominant follicle [37, 38].

The role of gonadotropin administration before oocyte collection is still controversial. Randomized controlled trials comparing the outcome of gonadotropin-primed IVM cycles with that of IVM cycles without any priming have yielded conflicting results [20, 22, 39, 40]. When data from these studies are combined, there is a trend toward higher clinical pregnancy rates with FSH/HMG administration or HCG priming in women with polycystic ovaries (PCO)/PCOS; however, the difference is not statistically significant. Differences in patient characteristics, gonadotropin administration protocols, and the limited total number of patients included in these studies prevent a definitive conclusion, and further research is needed. Based on our own experience and the favorable trend observed in trials of HCG priming, the current routine IVM protocol at the McGill Reproductive Centre (MRC) involves HCG administration priming regardless of cycle regularity.

Our preferred HCG dose is 10,000 IU i.m. 36–38 h before oocyte collection. The decision on dosage is based on failure to observe any improvement in laboratory or clinical outcomes with a higher HCG dose of 20,000 IU in a randomized controlled trial conducted in our unit [41]. On the other hand, in a retrospective analysis, we found an increase in the number of in vivo-matured oocytes collected, the rate of oocyte maturation in the first 24 h after collection, and the embryo implantation and clinical pregnancy rates when the interval between HCG administration and oocyte collection was extended to 38 h rather than the traditional 35 h [42]. The relevance of the latter findings is supported by the following studies. Our results suggest that the presence of in vivo-matured oocytes can be associated with higher pregnancy rates in HCG-primed IVM cycles [43]. A significantly higher proportion of embryos derived from in vivo-matured oocytes attained good morphological characteristics compared with those derived from in vitro-matured oocytes in these cycles. Moreover, oocytes that complete IVM in the first 24 h after collection seem to have a higher rate of cleavage, and embryos derived from such oocytes have a higher rate of blastocyst formation compared with their counterparts that complete maturation later [44].

Both the size of the leading follicle and endometrial thickness are taken into consideration regarding timing of oocyte retrieval. We prefer the size of the dominant follicle to range between 7 and 12 mm at the day of HCG administration, i.e., 36–38 h before oocyte collection, because embryo implantation and clinical pregnancy rates were found to be significantly lower in cycles where the mean diameter of the dominant follicle measured >14 mm compared with cycles that produced smaller dominant follicles with a mean diameter of 10–14 mm or ≤10 mm at the time of oocyte collection [37]. The highest implantation (14.3%) and pregnancy rates (40.3% per transfer) were achieved in cycles with a 10–14-mm-sized dominant follicle.

In a retrospective analysis of 155 unstimulated IVM cycles, we have found mean endometrial thickness to be significantly higher in conception cycles, though the absolute difference was only 0.8 mm (10.2 vs. 9.4 mm in conception and nonconception cycles respectively, $p = 0.04$). More interestingly, a trend analysis demonstrated a significant increase in pregnancy rates in parallel with endometrial thickness (clinical pregnancy rates were 9.4, 15.9, 27.6, and 28% for endometrial thickness of <8, 8–9.9, 10–11.9, and ≥12 mm, respectively; chi square test for trend, $p = 0.036$) [45]. Interestingly, endometrial texture, categorized as "triple line" or "non-triple line," was not found to be predictive for treatment outcome in the same study.

If the endometrial thickness is <6 mm on the day of the second scan, HCG administration can be delayed if the size of the largest follicle is less than 12 mm. Sometimes, if the largest follicle is close to 10–12 mm but the endometrium is very thin, we would use estradiol alone in a dose of 12 mg/day. This increases the endometrial thickness and delays follicle growth.

For women whose endometrial thickness was less than 6 mm on the day of the second scan, we later adopted an additional strategy of administering HMG in a dose of 150 IU/day and/or starting estradiol earlier. The rationale is increasing endogenous estrogen levels with limited support to the continuing growth of the follicles in the cohort. A retrospective comparison of the two strategies in 48 cycles demonstrated a similar increase in mean endometrial thickness with both methods, from 4.5 to 7.7 mm and from 4.7 to 7.3 mm in HMG and estradiol cycles, respectively [46]. However, compared with oral administration of 17β estradiol, HMG injections were associated with an increase in the number of in vivo-matured oocytes collected (cycles with more than one in vivo-matured oocyte, 54.5 vs. 34.6%), implantation (15 vs. 8.2%), and pregnancy rates (36.4 vs. 23.1%). The differences were not statistically significant, arguably due to the limited sample size of the study. Currently, we prefer HMG over estradiol for women with a thin endometrium. HMG injections are continued until endometrial thickness reaches 8 mm or the leading follicle reaches a mean diameter of 12 mm.

Oocyte Collection Procedure

The principles of transvaginal ultrasound-guided oocyte retrieval for IVM are the same as those for IVF oocyte collection. There are a few modifications in both the technique and equipment. Most patients easily tolerate the procedure under conscious sedation and with paracervical block achieved with 1% bupivacaine injection. A smaller-gauge needle (19–20G) with a shorter bevel is used. The aspiration pressure is set at 75–80 mmHg, approximately half the conventional IVF aspiration pressure, in order to minimize the risk of oocyte denudation during aspiration. This precaution is carried out because immature oocytes need the presence of surrounding granulosa cells during the nuclear maturation process. The fine-bore needle may be blocked frequently with bloodstained aspirate and ovarian stroma.

Therefore, multiple punctures are often needed, and flushing the needle lumen with heparinized saline between punctures is required. Sometimes external abdominal pressure may be required to fix the mobile ovaries during collection. Patients with difficult-to-reach ovaries or poor pain control may do better under limited general anesthesia with propofol.

Laboratory Procedure

Similar to IVF, the follicular aspirate is first examined under a stereomicroscope to identify cumulus-oocyte complexes (COC). Since identification of small immature oocytes surrounded by scarce granulosa cells which are not widely dispersed is more difficult with the conventional technique as they can be overlooked, follicular aspirate is filtered through a nylon mesh strainer (Fig. 8.1) with 70 μm pores after removal of initially identified COCs. The filtered aspirate can be reexamined after washing with HEPES-buffered human serum albumin (HSA)-containing medium.

In order to determine whether the oocyte is mature or not, a special observation technique called "sliding method" can be employed without denuding cumulus cells from oocyte. Briefly, COC is allowed to slide slowly from one side to the other on the bottom of the Petri dish, while being observed under the stereomicroscope (Fig. 8.2). During COC sliding, it is possible to observe clearly whether or not the oocyte cytoplasm contains a germinal vesicle (GV) or if the oocyte has extruded a first polar body (1PB) into perivitelline space (PVS) (Fig. 8.3). If neither GV is seen in the oocyte cytoplasm nor 1PB found in PVS, the oocyte is defined as germinal vesicle breakdown (GVBD) or metaphase-I (M-I) stage.

The immature COCs (maximum of ten) are incubated in an Organ Tissue Culture Dish (Falcon, 60 × 15 mm) (Fig. 8.4) containing 1 mL oocytc maturation medium supplemented with a final concentration of 75 mIU/mL FSH and 75 mIU/mL LH at 37°C in an incubator with an atmosphere of 5% CO_2 and 95% air with high humidity (prefer with triple gas mixture, 90% N_2, 5% CO_2, and 5% O_2 with 100% humidity). Oocyte maturation medium should be prepared for equilibration at least 2 h before immature oocyte retrieval (particularly, it can be made 1 day before). Some commercial available oocyte maturation medium does not contain protein source. In that case, the oocyte maturation medium needs to be supplemented with some protein source, such as HSA or maternal serum. If maternal serum is going to be used, it is better prepared in advance and inactivated (56°C 30 min) before using.

Oocytes reaching metaphase-II (M-II) stage on the day of collection are denuded and fertilized together with any in vivo-matured oocytes, while immature oocytes are cultured in IVM medium for 24–48 h. Twenty-four hours after maturation in culture (Fig. 8.5), all COCs are stripped for identification of oocyte maturity. COCs are denuded using a finely drawn glass pipette following 1 min of exposure to a commercially available hyaluronidase solution. The mature oocytes are then subjected to insemination by either IVF or intracytoplasmic sperm injection (ICSI) after stripping. The remaining immature oocytes (GV and M-I) will remain in

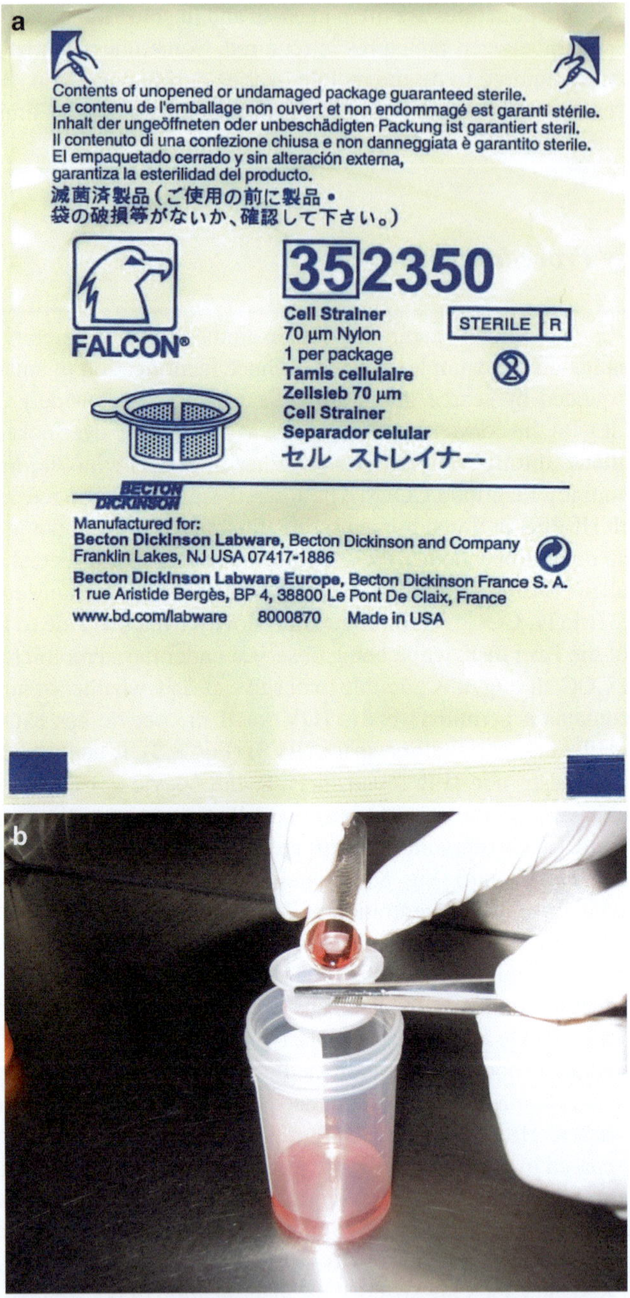

Fig. 8.1 (**a**) Labeling on Cell Strainer (Falcon, Becton Dickinson and Company, USA); (**b**) follicular aspirates are filtered with a Cell Strainer

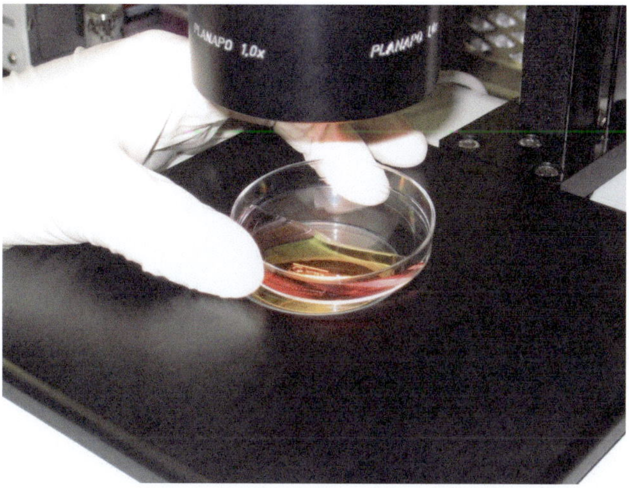

Fig. 8.2 Sliding technique for observation of oocyte maturity. COCs are allowed to slide slowly from one side to the other on the bottom of the Petri dish, while being observed under the stereomicroscope

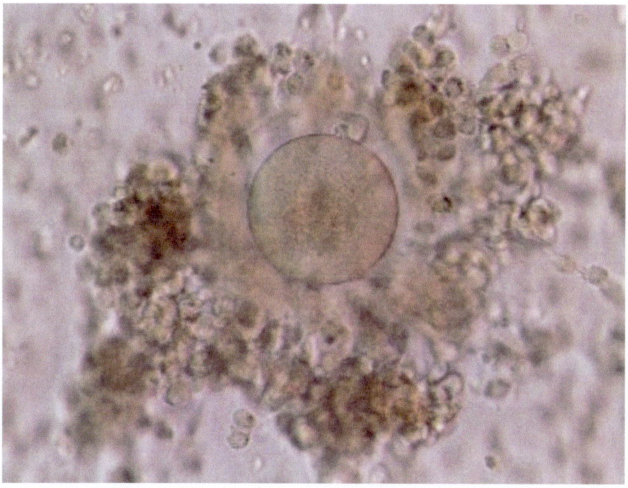

Fig. 8.3 During COC sliding, it is possible to observe clearly whether or not the oocyte has extruded a first polar body (1PB) into perivitelline space (PVS)

culture for another 24 h. Forty-eight hours after oocyte retrieval, the remaining stripped oocytes are reexamined, and if any have matured at this point, they will be inseminated by either IVF or ICSI.

Since in vivo-matured oocytes can be retrieved after HCG priming from leading or dominant follicles, it has been argued that such "IVM treatment" is not genuine.

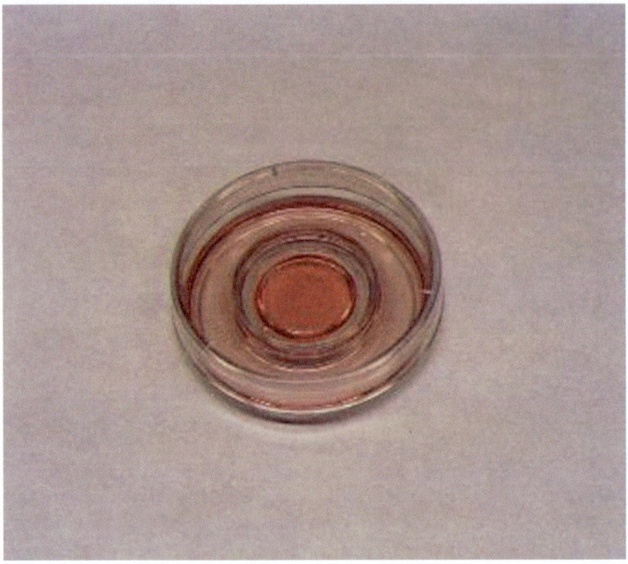

Fig. 8.4 Organ Tissue Culture Dish (Falcon, 60 × 15 mm) containing 1 mL oocyte maturation medium in the inner well and 2 mL of oocyte maturation medium in the outer well

Accordingly, the treatment has been reworded as "natural-cycle IVF combined with IVM," simply referred to as natural-cycle IVF/M [38, 47–49].

Although similar implantation and pregnancy rates have been reported following fertilization of in vitro-matured oocytes with ICSI or IVF, ICSI has been commonly practiced in IVM cycles due to a theoretical risk of zonal hardening during the in vitro culture period [50, 51]. In fact, fertilization rates with ICSI were shown to be higher than with IVF in the same study (84.1 vs. 56.3%) [51]. Another reason for preferring ICSI over IVF in IVM cycles is some immature oocytes being denuded for assessment of polar-body extrusion. Oocytes devoid of cumulus cells may have decreased chemotactic potential for sperm in the medium [52]. ICSI is the fertilization method routinely used in the McGill IVM program. The preferred time for ICSI is 2–4 h after polar-body extrusion [52].

Culture conditions for fertilized oocytes and cleavage-stage embryos derived from in vitro-matured oocytes are the same as those in IVF cycles. Embryo development and quality are similarly assessed, based on the number of blastomeres and the amount of nuclear fragments.

Embryo Transfer

The timing of embryo transfer and the number of embryos to be transferred are dictated by the number and quality of available embryos. Embryo transfer is

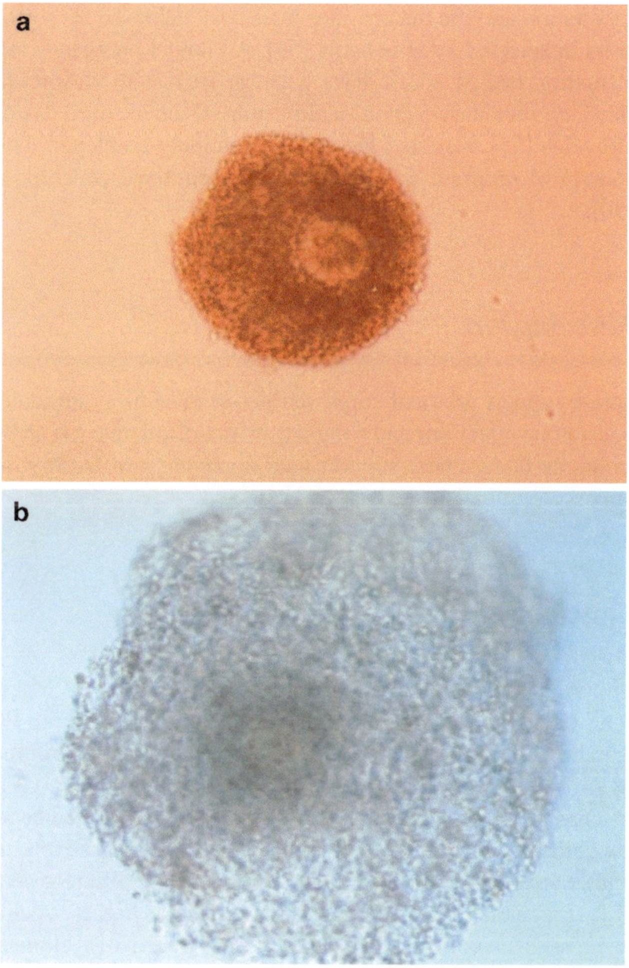

Fig. 8.5 Morphological changes of immature COC before and after culture in the oocyte maturation medium. (**a**) Immature COC immediately after retrieval from the ovary; (**b**) the same COC after 24 h of culture in the oocyte maturation medium. Note that the cumulus mass has almost doubled in size compared with its mass before culture (two photos with the same magnification)

commonly performed on the third day after oocyte collection. Growth and quality of available embryos are evaluated with regard to fertilization time of each embryo. A group of best embryos for days is transferred using essentially the same technique as that employed in IVF cycles. In general, embryo implantation rates in IVM cycles are lower than in IVF cycles. Therefore, on average, more embryos are transferred in order to maintain similar pregnancy rates. However, as expected, this fact does not seem to increase multiple pregnancy rates after IVM [53, 54].

High implantation and pregnancy rates have been achieved by performing blastocyst transfers in selected IVM patients [55]. A clinical pregnancy rate of 51.9% and an implantation rate of 26.8% have been reported with blastocyst transfer in patients with >7 zygotes and >3 good-quality embryos on the third day postfertilization in IVM cycles [55]. Assisted hatching is routinely employed before embryo transfer in our IVM program due to the above-mentioned concerns about zonal hardening [50].

Luteal-Phase Support

The luteal-phase support protocol employed in our IVM program includes 50 mg/day i.m. progesterone injections and 6 mg/day estradiol valerate p.o. in three divided doses. We continue luteal-phase support until completion of the first trimester for pregnant patients.

Clinical Outcome of IVM Treatment

The most important determinants of pregnancy following an IVM cycle are the female age and the number of oocytes collected. Young women with PCO seem to be the best candidates for IVM treatment. In 2007, we achieved an embryo implantation rate of 15% and a clinical pregnancy rate per embryo transfer (CPR) of 36.7% in women younger than 35 years of age. However, for women aged between 35 and 40 years, implantation and CPR were 10.1 and 29.3%, respectively, in the same period. Similarly successful results have been reported by different centers around the world [14]. Pregnancy rates seem to be significantly higher when an in vivo-matured oocyte has been collected. Recently, we reported a 40% clinical pregnancy rate in such cycles in young women with PCO [43].

Pregnancy Loss

Biochemical pregnancy loss rates were similar among 1,581 women who had a positive pregnancy test following assisted reproduction treatment (ART) with IVM, IVF, or ICSI in our unit during a 5-year period (17.5% for IVM pregnancies, 17% for IVF, and 18% for ICSI pregnancies, $p = 0.08$). However, the clinical miscarriage rate was significantly higher in IVM pregnancies (25.3%) than in IVF (15.7%) and ICSI (12.6%) pregnancies ($p < 0.01$) [56]. However, the incidence of PCOS in the IVM group was 80%, whereas only 8% and <1% of women in the IVF and ICSI groups had PCOS, respectively. Miscarriage rates reaching 25% after ovulation induction, and ranging from 25 to 37% following IVF, have been reported in women with PCOS [57–59]. Arguably, the higher incidence of PCOS in IVM patients in this series can be the reason of the higher miscarriage rate observed in the IVM group. Critically, miscarriage rates were not different between IVM and IVF pregnancies among women with PCOS, 24.5 vs. 22.8%, respectively.

Obstetric Outcome

IVM pregnancies comprised 15.9% of 344 ART pregnancies in a retrospective analysis of all pregnancies delivered at the McGill University Health Centre during a 5-year period from Jan 1, 1998, to Dec 31, 2003 [54]. The incidence of multiple or high-order multiple pregnancies was not different among IVM (21 and 5%), IVF (20 and 3%), and ICSI (17 and 3%) pregnancies. Although cesarean delivery rates of ART pregnancies were higher than spontaneous conceptions, the incidence of cesarean delivery was similar among singleton pregnancies conceived with different treatments (IVM 39%, IVF 36%, and ICSI 36%). Likewise, the mean birth weights of all infants conceived with ART were similar among all ART groups, but lower than those of spontaneous conceptions.

Congenital Abnormalities and Physical and Neuromotor Development

In the above-mentioned study, the odds ratios (ORs) for any congenital abnormality, calculated with spontaneous conceptions serving as the reference, were 1.42 (95% confidence interval (CI) 0.52–3.91) for IVM, 1.21 (95% CI 0.63–2.32) for IVF, and 1.69 (95% CI 0.88–3.26) for ICSI, respectively [54]. None of these were statistically significant. Interestingly, the odds ratio was lower for IVM than for ICSI, even though ICSI was used for all IVM cases. This suggests that the reported high congenital abnormality rate with ICSI is more likely to be due to poor sperm per se because ICSI with normal sperm used in IVM cycles did not increase the odds of congenital abnormality to the same extent.

Shu-Chi et al. analyzed the chromosomal constitution and mental development of 21 children born after IVM and compared with 21 spontaneously conceived children. All of the IVM children were found to have normal karyotype and mean developmental index score, similar to controls in this small-sized study [60]. Another study of 46 IVM babies born to 40 women reported similar findings [61]. The neuropsychological development of children was assessed until 24 months and was found to be within population standards. The physical growth of IVM children seems to be similar to that of spontaneously conceived children [60, 61]. Currently available data seem reassuring and do not suggest an increased risk of congenital malformations and physical or neurological developmental delay in IVM children.

Summary

IVM is a relatively new technology compared to conventional IVF. IVM should be regarded as a complementary assisted reproductive technology that provides unique opportunities rather than merely a competitor of IVF. Patients who are at high risk of OHSS, those with unexpectedly hyper- or poor responses during controlled ovarian hyperstimulation, those with recurrent unexplained IVF failures, as well as those who are facing imminent gonadotoxic chemotherapy and are in need of fertility preservation can benefit from advantages of IVM.

Essentially, all ART laboratory procedures can be performed with in vitro-matured oocytes if the need arises. The first successful IVM cycles combined with preimplantation genetic screening and percutaneous testicular sperm aspiration have already been reported by our team [62, 63]. IVM has enabled successful treatment of patients with empty follicle syndrome in previous stimulated IVF cycles [64]. Patients can undergo several IVM cycles, and we previously reported a series of patients who achieved repeated live births with IVM treatment [65].

References

1. Tan SL, Royston P, Campbell S, et al. Cumulative conception and livebirth rates after in-vitro fertilisation. Lancet. 1992;339:1390–4.
2. Nyboe Andersen A, Goossens V, Bhattacharya S, et al. Assisted reproductive technology and intrauterine inseminations in Europe, 2005: results generated from European registers by ESHRE: ESHRE. The European IVF Monitoring Programme (EIM), for the European Society of Human Reproduction and Embryology (ESHRE). Hum Reprod. 2009;24:1267–87.
3. The Society for Assisted Reproductive Technology. National data summary. 2007. wwwsartorg. Accessed 15 December 2009.
4. Ata B, Tulandi T. Pathophysiology of ovarian hyperstimulation syndrome and strategies for its prevention and treatment. Expert Rev Obstet Gynecol. 2009;4:299–311.
5. MacDougall MJ, Tan SL, Balen A, Jacobs HS. A controlled study comparing patients with and without polycystic ovaries undergoing in-vitro fertilization. Hum Reprod. 1993;8:233–7.
6. Baart EB, Martini E, Eijkemans MJ, et al. Milder ovarian stimulation for in-vitro fertilization reduces aneuploidy in the human preimplantation embryo: a randomized controlled trial. Hum Reprod. 2007;22:980–8.
7. Martinez-Conejero JA, Simon C, Pellicer A, Horcajadas JA. Is ovarian stimulation detrimental to the endometrium? Reprod Biomed Online. 2007;15:45–50.
8. Pincus G, Enzmann E. The comparative behaviour of mammalian eggs in vivo and in vitro. I J Exp Med. 1935;62:665–75.
9. Edwards RG. Maturation in vitro of human ovarian oocytes. Lancet. 1965;2:926–9.
10. Veeck LL, Wortham Jr JW, Witmyer J, et al. Maturation and fertilization of morphologically immature human oocytes in a program of in vitro fertilization. Fertil Steril. 1983;39:594.
11. Cha KY, Koo JJ, Ko JJ, Choi DH, Han SY, Yoon TK. Pregnancy after in vitro fertilization of human follicular oocytes collected from nonstimulated cycles, their culture in vitro and their transfer in a donor oocyte program. Fertil Steril. 1991;55:109–13.
12. Trounson A, Wood C, Kausche A. In vitro maturation and the fertilization and developmental competence of oocytes recovered from untreated polycystic ovarian patients. Fertil Steril. 1994;62:353–62.

13. Cha KY, Chian RC. Maturation in vitro of immature human oocytes for clinical use. Hum Reprod Update. 1998;4:103–20.
14. Chian RC, Buckett WM, Tan SL. In-vitro maturation of human oocytes. Reprod Biomed Online. 2004;8:148–66.
15. Barnes FL, Crombie A, Gardner DK, et al. Blastocyst development and birth after in-vitro maturation of human primary oocytes, intracytoplasmic sperm injection and assisted hatching. Hum Reprod. 1995;10:3243–7.
16. Barnes FL, Kausche A, Tiglias J, Wood C, Wilton L, Trounson A. Production of embryos from in vitro-matured primary human oocytes. Fertil Steril. 1996;65:1151–6.
17. Chian RC, Buckett WM, Too LL, Tan SL. Pregnancies resulting from in vitro matured oocytes retrieved from patients with polycystic ovary syndrome after priming with human chorionic gonadotropin. Fertil Steril. 1999;72:639–42.
18. Chian RC, Buckett WM, Tulandi T, Tan SL. Prospective randomized study of human chorionic gonadotrophin priming before immature oocyte retrieval from unstimulated women with polycystic ovarian syndrome. Hum Reprod. 2000;15:165–70.
19. Chian RC, Gulekli B, Buckett WM, Tan SL. Priming with human chorionic gonadotropin before retrieval of immature oocytes in women with infertility due to the polycystic ovary syndrome. N Engl J Med 1999;341:1624, 6.
20. Mikkelsen AL, Smith SD, Lindenberg S. In-vitro maturation of human oocytes from regularly menstruating women may be successful without follicle stimulating hormone priming. Hum Reprod. 1999;14:1847–51.
21. Suikkari AM, Tulppala M, Tuuri T, Hovatta O, Barnes F. Luteal phase start of low-dose FSH priming of follicles results in an efficient recovery, maturation and fertilization of immature human oocytes. Hum Reprod. 2000;15:747–51.
22. Mikkelsen AL, Lindenberg S. Benefit of FSH priming of women with PCOS to the in vitro maturation procedure and the outcome: a randomized prospective study. Reproduction. 2001;122:587–92.
23. Mikkelsen AL, Host E, Blaabjerg J, Lindenberg S. Time interval between FSH priming and aspiration of immature human oocytes for in-vitro maturation: a prospective randomized study. Reprod Biomed Online. 2003;6:416–20.
24. Lin YH, Hwang JL, Huang LW, et al. Combination of FSH priming and hCG priming for in-vitro maturation of human oocytes. Hum Reprod. 2003;18:1632–6.
25. Tan SL, Child TJ, Gulekli B. In vitro maturation and fertilization of oocytes from unstimulated ovaries: predicting the number of immature oocytes retrieved by early follicular phase ultrasonography. Am J Obstet Gynecol. 2002;186:684–9.
26. Lim KS, Yoon SH, Lim JH. IVM as an alternative for over-responders. In: Tan SL, Chian RC, Buckett W, editors. In-vitro maturation of human oocytes. London: Informa Healthcare; 2007.
27. Liu J, Lu G, Qian Y, Mao Y, Ding W. Pregnancies and births achieved from in vitro matured oocytes retrieved from poor responders undergoing stimulation in in vitro fertilization cycles. Fertil Steril. 2003;80:447–9.
28. Liu J, Lim JH, Chian RC. IVM as an alternative for poor responders. In: Tan SL, Chian RC, Buckett W, editors. In-vitro maturation of human oocytes. Basic science to clinical applications. London: Informa Healthcare; 2007. p. 333–44.
29. Child TJ, Gulekli B, Chian RC, Abdul-Jalil AK, Tan SL. In-vitro maturation (IVM) of oocytes from unstimulated normal ovaries of women with a previous poor response to IVF. Fertil Steril. 2000;74:S45.
30. Holzer H, Scharf E, Chian RC, Demirtas E, Buckett W, Tan SL. In vitro maturation of oocytes collected from unstimulated ovaries for oocyte donation. Fertil Steril. 2007;88:62–7.
31. The American Society for Reproductive Medicine. Fertility preservation and reproduction in cancer patients. Fertil Steril. 2005;83:1622–8.
32. Lee SJ, Schover LR, Partridge AH, et al. American Society of Clinical Oncology recommendations on fertility preservation in cancer patients. J Clin Oncol. 2006;24:2917–31.
33. Rao GD, Chian RC, Son WS, Gilbert L, Tan SL. Fertility preservation in women undergoing cancer treatment. Lancet. 2004;363:1829–30.

34. Demirtas E, Elizur SE, Holzer H, et al. Immature oocyte retrieval in the luteal phase to preserve fertility in cancer patients. Reprod Biomed Online. 2008;17:520–3.
35. Huang JY, Tulandi T, Holzer H, Tan SL, Chian RC. Combining ovarian tissue cryobanking with retrieval of immature oocytes followed by in vitro maturation and vitrification: an additional strategy of fertility preservation. Fertil Steril. 2008;89:567–72.
36. Huang JY, Tulandi T, Holzer H, et al. Cryopreservation of ovarian tissue and in vitro matured oocytes in a female with mosaic Turner syndrome: case report. Hum Reprod. 2008;23:336–9.
37. Son WY, Chung JT, Herrero B, et al. Selection of the optimal day for oocyte retrieval based on the diameter of the dominant follicle in hCG-primed in vitro maturation cycles. Hum Reprod. 2008;23:2680–5.
38. Chian RC, Buckett WM, Abdul-Jalil AK, et al. Natural-cycle in vitro fertilization combined with in vitro maturation of immature oocytes is a potential approach in infertility treatment. Fertil Steril. 2004;82:1675–8.
39. Son WY, Yoon SH, Lim JH. Effect of gonadotrophin priming on in-vitro maturation of oocytes collected from women at risk of OHSS. Reprod Biomed Online. 2006;13:340–8.
40. Fadini R, Dal Canto MB, Mignini Renzini M, et al. Effect of different gonadotrophin priming on IVM of oocytes from women with normal ovaries: a prospective randomized study. Reprod Biomed Online. 2009;19:343–51.
41. Gulekli B, Buckett WM, Chian RC, Child TJ, Abdul-Jalil AK, Tan SL. Randomized, controlled trial of priming with 10,000 IU versus 20,000 IU of human chorionic gonadotropin in women with polycystic ovary syndrome who are undergoing in vitro maturation. Fertil Steril. 2004;82:1458–9.
42. Son WY, Chung JT, Chian RC, et al. A 38 h interval between hCG priming and oocyte retrieval increases in vivo and in vitro oocyte maturation rate in programmed IVM cycles. Hum Reprod. 2008;23:2010–6.
43. Son WY, Chung JT, Demirtas E, et al. Comparison of in-vitro maturation cycles with and without in-vivo matured oocytes retrieved. Reprod Biomed Online. 2008;17:59–67.
44. Son WY, Lee SY, Lim JH. Fertilization, cleavage and blastocyst development according to the maturation timing of oocytes in in vitro maturation cycles. Hum Reprod. 2005;20:3204–7.
45. Child TJ, Gulekli B, Sylvestre C, Tan SL. Ultrasonographic assessment of endometrial receptivity at embryo transfer in an in vitro maturation of oocyte program. Fertil Steril. 2003; 79:656–8.
46. Elizur SE, Son WY, Yap R, et al. Comparison of low-dose human menopausal gonadotropin and micronized 17beta-estradiol supplementation in in vitro maturation cycles with thin endometrial lining. Fertil Steril. 2009;92:907–12.
47. Lim JH, Park SY, Yoon SH, Yang SH, Chian RC. Combination of natural cycle IVF with IVM as infertility treatment. In: Tan SL, Chian RC, Buckett W, editors. In-vitro maturation of human oocytes. Basic science to clinical application. London: Informa Healthcare; 2007. p. 353–60.
48. Lim JH, Yang SH, Chian RC. New alternative to infertility treatment for women without ovarian stimulation. Reprod Biomed Online. 2007;14:547–9.
49. Lim JH, Yang SH, Xu Y, Yoon SH, Chian RC. Selection of patients for natural cycle in vitro fertilization combined with in vitro maturation of immature oocytes. Fertil Steril. 2009;91: 1050–5.
50. Nagy ZP, Cecile J, Liu J, Loccufier A, Devroey P, Van Steirteghem A. Pregnancy and birth after intracytoplasmic sperm injection of in vitro matured germinal-vesicle stage oocytes: case report. Fertil Steril. 1996;65:1047–50.
51. Soderstrom-Anttila V, Makinen S, Tuuri T, Suikkari AM. Favourable pregnancy results with insemination of in vitro matured oocytes from unstimulated patients. Hum Reprod. 2005;20: 1534–40.
52. Oren-Benaroya R, Orvieto R, Gakamsky A, Pinchasov M, Eisenbach M. The sperm chemoattractant secreted from human cumulus cells is progesterone. Hum Reprod. 2008;23:2339–45.
53. Holzer H. World status of babies born through IVM. Proceedings of the 1st European congress on in vitro maturation of human oocytes in assisted reproduction. 2008.

54. Buckett WM, Chian RC, Holzer H, Dean N, Usher R, Tan SL. Obstetric outcomes and congenital abnormalities after in vitro maturation, in vitro fertilization, and intracytoplasmic sperm injection. Obstet Gynecol. 2007;110:885–91.
55. Son WY, Lee SY, Yoon SH, Lim JH. Pregnancies and deliveries after transfer of human blastocysts derived from in vitro matured oocytes in in vitro maturation cycles. Fertil Steril. 2007;87:1491–3.
56. Buckett WM, Chian RC, Dean NL, Sylvestre C, Holzer HE, Tan SL. Pregnancy loss in pregnancies conceived after in vitro oocyte maturation, conventional in vitro fertilization, and intracytoplasmic sperm injection. Fertil Steril. 2008;90:546–50.
57. Balen AH, Tan SL, MacDougall J, Jacobs HS. Miscarriage rates following in-vitro fertilization are increased in women with polycystic ovaries and reduced by pituitary desensitization with buserelin. Hum Reprod. 1993;8:959–64.
58. Kousta E, White DM, Franks S. Modern use of clomiphene citrate in induction of ovulation. Hum Reprod Update. 1997;3:359–65.
59. Homburg R. Pregnancy complications in PCOS. Best Pract Res Clin Endocrinol Metab. 2006;20:281–92.
60. Shu-Chi M, Jiann-Loung H, Yu-Hung L, Tseng-Chen S, Ming IL, Tsu-Fuh Y. Growth and development of children conceived by in-vitro maturation of human oocytes. Early Hum Dev. 2006;82:677–82.
61. Soderstrom-Anttila V, Salokorpi T, Pihlaja M, Serenius-Sirve S, Suikkari AM. Obstetric and perinatal outcome and preliminary results of development of children born after in vitro maturation of oocytes. Hum Reprod. 2006;21:1508–13.
62. Ao A, Jin S, Rao D, Son WY, Chian RC, Tan SL. First successful pregnancy outcome after preimplantation genetic diagnosis for aneuploidy screening in embryos generated from natural-cycle in vitro fertilization combined with an in vitro maturation procedure. Fertil Steril. 2006;85:1510.e9–11.
63. Abdul-Jalil AK, Child TJ, Phillips S, Dean N, Carrier S, Tan SL. Ongoing twin pregnancy after ICSI of PESA-retrieved spermatozoa into in-vitro matured oocytes: case report. Hum Reprod. 2001;16:1424–6.
64. Hourvitz A, Maman E, Brengauz M, Machtinger R, Dor J. In vitro maturation for patients with repeated in vitro fertilization failure due to "oocyte maturation abnormalities". Fertil Steril. 2009;94(2):496–501.
65. Al-Sunaidi M, Tulandi T, Holzer H, Sylvestre C, Chian RC, Tan SL. Repeated pregnancies and live births after in vitro maturation treatment. Fertil Steril. 2007;87:1212.e9–12.

Chapter 9
In Vivo Embryo Culture Device

Claude Ranoux

The intravaginal culture (IVC) called the INVO procedure is a unique option for patients seeking treatment in infertility. The INVO procedure was created to simplify the process of in vitro fertilization (IVF) and early embryo development and reduce the sophisticated laboratory instrumentation required. Mild ovarian stimulation or natural cycle combined with the INVO procedure makes possible the treatment to infertile couples in a medical office setting such as the office of an infertile specialist [1], a satellite unit of a reproductive center, or in some areas an ob-gyn's office. The INVO procedure using the INVOcell device substitutes the CO_2 incubator used in conventional IVF with the vaginal cavity of the patient.

History of the Intravaginal Culture Also Called INVO

Since the birth of Louise Brown, the first baby born by IVF in 1978, several scientific milestones have been accomplished in assisted reproductive technologies (ART). Most of these scientific advances such as controlled ovarian hyperstimulation, embryo cryopreservation, and intracytoplasmic sperm injection (ICSI) have not only increased the embryo implantation rates but also created clinical, ethical, and legal issues and dramatically complicated the IVF procedure. These complicated technical advances have contributed to increased costs of IVF. The high cost of IVF has resulted in rejection of reimbursement by the insurance companies thus restricting IVF access to infertile couples who can afford to pay out of pocket. These technical advances have also contributed to the creation of governmental regulations for ART in many countries. All these factors have slowed the expansion of IVF technologies—a major factor that explains why, after more than 30 years

C. Ranoux, MD, MS (✉)
INVO Bioscience, 100 Cummings Center, Suite 207P, Beverly, MA 01915, USA
e-mail: clauderanoux@invobioscience.com

Z.P. Nagy et al. (eds.), *Clinical Embryology: A Practical Guide*,
DOI 10.1007/978-1-4614-8376-2_9, © Springer Science+Business Media New York 2013

of existence, so many infertile couples cannot and do not receive IVF treatment. The INVO procedure performed by a trained physician and embryologist in an office or satellite unit becomes accessible to many more insured and noninsured infertile couples.

Principle

The INVO procedure consists of utilizing the vaginal cavity environment for the oocyte fertilization and early embryo development [2]. The INVOcell device is specially designed for the INVO procedure [3]. The vaginal cavity provides the pCO_2, pO_2, and temperature for the culture of the gametes and the embryos [4]. The INVOcell device is permeable to gas and allows the equilibrium between the pCO_2 of the vagina and the pCO_2 of the culture medium. This system maintains the pH of the culture medium between 7.2 and 7.4 during the entire period of vaginal incubation. This in vivo fertilization and early embryo development involves the participation of the patient giving a more natural approach to the assisted conception.

Discovery of the Intravaginal Culture

The INVO technique was discovered around 1985. The laboratory IVF incubators at the time had CO_2 distribution controlled by a bead system. The rate of CO_2 mixed with the air was very imprecise and had peaks of low and high CO_2 concentrations that resulted in major variations in the pH of the culture medium. When cells or mouse gametes were placed in the same incubator in plastic tubes filled with culture medium and hermetically closed, the passage of CO_2 through the wall of the sealed plastic tubes altered the peaks of CO_2 and dramatically reduced the variations of pH in the culture medium. To simplify the process, the natural vaginal cavity providing CO_2 and O_2 was used. There was originally a concern of potential lesions of the uterine cervix from the prototype device during incubation that could interfere with the quality of the embryo transfer. This was eliminated by tests that demonstrated no lesions or interference. This was later confirmed by the results of the first INVO procedures showing comparable embryo implantations to conventional IVF.

Prototype and Initial Results with the Prototype

Prototype

During the initial cases and publications utilizing the INVO procedure, a prototype which was a simple plastic tube was used [2]. The tube chosen showed the best

Table 9.1 Initial results of INVO using the prototype device

Number of publications	Countries	Number of INVO cycles	Clinical pregnancy rate/cycle (%)
9	Austria, France, Germany, Japan, Netherland, UK, USA	815	19.6

sealed closure among several prototypes that were initially tested. The prototype device was filled with culture medium first to avoid air bubbles. Air bubbles could be caught by the viscous cumulus of the mature oocytes causing them to float up and decreasing the chances of fertilization. These air bubbles could modify the pH of the culture medium. With the prototype tube, oocytes could also be lost in the overflow during the closing of the prototype.

Initial Results with the Prototype

Several publications in international medical journals [1, 2, 4–10] were issued at this time reporting the results obtained by INVO using this prototype device (Table 9.1).

Some of these publications clearly indicated equivalent pregnancy rates between INVO using the prototype device and conventional IVF [2, 5, 9].

From the Prototype to the Improved INVOcell Device

The first practitioners using the INVO prototype device had many difficulties. The device could only be opened and closed once. There were observations of variations in pH of the culture medium, bacterial contamination, accidental openings of the prototype in the vaginal cavity, loss of embryos, and increased risk of vaginal bacteriosis. A new device, the INVOcell made of three parts, was designed to address all these identified technical problems [3].

The Inner Chamber

The inner chamber houses the culture medium and the gametes. A rotating valve allows several openings and closings of the inner chamber without introduction of air or contamination of the culture medium. The rotating valve has a small orifice at a bottom of a small well which prevents major variations in pH of the culture medium and loss of gametes due to possible overflow while filling. The volume of the chamber has been reduced to 1.08 mL from the initial 3 mL. At the bottom of the main chamber, a microchamber collects the embryos after incubation. This

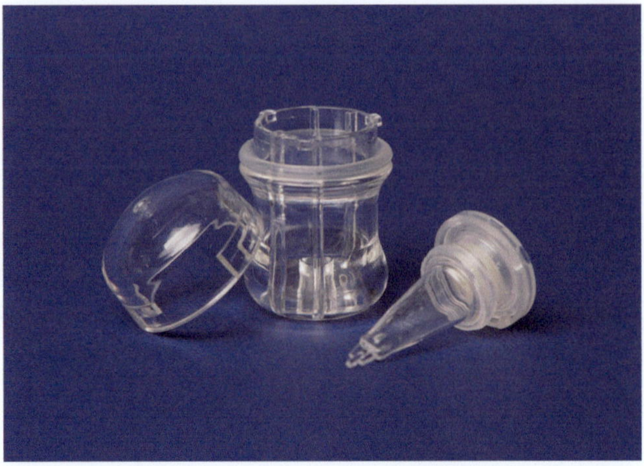

Fig. 9.1 Inner chamber and open outer rigid shell of the INVOcell device

microchamber allows direct observation and selection of the embryos without transfer to a culture dish. Loading of the embryos can be done directly from the microchamber with the embryo transfer catheter.

The Outer Rigid Shell

The outer rigid shell protects the inner chamber from vaginal contaminations and keeps the inner chamber sterile (Fig. 9.1). It has a smooth external surface to prevent any lesions or irritations of the vagina and cervix during the 3 days of vaginal incubation. The wall is permeable to CO_2 and O_2. The rigid shell could be grasped if necessary with a forceps to remove it from the vagina. A locking position prevents any unexpected device opening during vaginal incubation.

The Retention System

The retention system has also been improved. Holes have been perforated in the membrane of the diaphragm for the elimination of the vaginal secretions during incubation (Fig. 9.2). Tests of comfort and retention, requested by regulatory agencies for approval of the device, were performed using the INVOcell and its retention system. The INVOcell device does not cause any discomfort or irritation of the vaginal cavity and does not increase incidence of bacterial vaginosis from the 3 days of incubation. No device expulsion was observed when the retention system was used. These results were confirmed by the first INVO procedures using the INVOcell.

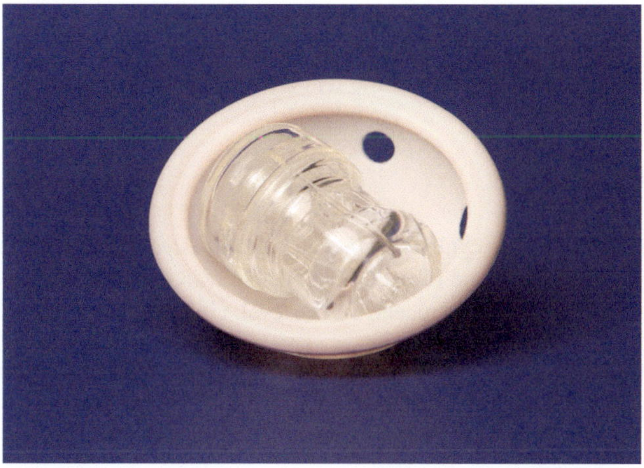

Fig. 9.2 Fully assembled INVOcell placed in the retention system and ready to be positioned in the vagina

The INVO Cycle

INVO Cycle

The indications for using an INVO cycle are similar to the indications using conventional IVF. INVO is not recommended in severe oligoasthenoteratozoospermia. All other indications can be treated by INVO.

Natural Cycle or Mild Ovarian Stimulation Protocols

Current stimulation protocols use the association of gonadotropin-releasing hormone (GnRH) agonist and high doses of human menopausal gonadotropin (hGM) or follicle-stimulating hormone (FSH). These protocols recruit a lot of follicles and show complications such as severe ovarian hyperstimulation syndromes (OHSS) as well as multiple pregnancies with premature deliveries, birth defects, and maternal complications. The use of these protocols and their complications represent a very costly burden for society. The governments of several countries and specialized associations such as the American Society for Reproductive Medicine (ASRM) have developed regulations and guidance concerning the numbers of embryos to transfer. This has contributed to a returned interest in natural cycle and mild stimulation protocols that produce less embryos and are safer for the female. The introduction of GnRH antagonists [11, 12] or indomethacin [13, 14] in preventing premature LH surges and ovulations has also contributed to the reintroduction of the natural cycle and mild ovarian stimulation protocols. Mild stimulations and natural cycle protocols with the INVO procedure contribute equally to the simplicity, low complication rates, and low cost of the INVO cycle.

Modified Natural Cycle

The monitoring of natural cycle is simple and inexpensive. Generally, an average of four rapid immunoenzymatic blood assays, when available, and two or three ultrasound exams starting at day 8 precede the retrieval. GnRH antagonist (0.25 mg daily) or indomethacin (50 mg 3× per day, as used in Dr. Lucina's study and discussed later) is started at day 8 or when the leading follicle reached 15 mm and is used to prevent premature ovulation. Triggering of ovulation is performed by the injection of 5,000 IU of human chorionic gonadotropin (hCG) when the size of the follicle reaches 18 mm and the estradiol 180 pg (pictogram)/mL, when dosage is available.

Clomiphene Citrate Protocol

The monitoring of the stimulation and the control of the premature ovulation are identical to the modified natural cycle. Induction of the ovulation is based on the same follicular size (18 mm) of the dominant follicle and is done using 10,000 IU of hCG. Clomiphene citrate (CC) is generally used at a dose of 100 mg/day from day 3 to day 7. In developing countries, an aromatase inhibitor, letrozole (2.5–7.5 mg/day), is used from day 3 to day 7 and is preferred to CC due to its lower antiestrogenic action and better embryo implantation, and it requires less exogenous gonadotropins [15] (letrozole is not allowed in the USA and Europe). Gonadotropin, hMG, or FSH, 75 units, may be added every day starting on day 3 or day 5 of the cycle depending of the number of follicles to recruit. Generally, two to seven oocytes are retrieved.

Luteal Phase Support

Luteal phase is usually supported by progesterone (200–600 mg a day) started after the follicle retrieval and continued until the 10th week of pregnancy when the placenta takes over the progesterone secretion. Estradiol support (4 mg a day) is also used in association with progesterone.

Follicle Retrieval

Transvaginal follicle aspiration using ultrasound vaginal probe is performed 36 h after hCG injection to get the best oocyte maturity from the dominant follicle(s).

Mild ovarian stimulation protocols recruit few follicles, allowing a short retrieval time. The use of conscious sedation makes the retrieval procedure well tolerated by the patient without the need for general anesthesia [1, 2]. A pump with control of vacuum pressure (120 mm hg) is recommended for the follicle aspiration; if not available, a follicular aspiration using 10-mL syringes can be done [2].

INVO Procedure

In INVO, the vagina provides the proper incubation temperature and the correct CO_2 supplementation required for embryo development. The INVOcell device has been designed to maximize the transfer of CO_2 present in the vaginal cavity to the culture medium, maintain the pH of the culture medium during the period of incubation, and reduce the quantity of O_2 transfer to the medium. The INVOcell eliminates the need for a complex laboratory and simplifies all the steps of the assisted fertilization and early embryo development.

Sperm Preparation

In the INVO procedure, the sperm preparation takes place before oocyte retrieval, so the oocytes can be inseminated immediately after the retrieval procedure without major exposure to a detrimental environment.

Sperm collection: Collection is generally performed by masturbation; if the collection is done by intercourse, a nontoxic condom should be provided.

Sperm washing and selection: Currently, the “swim-up” and the density gradient separation are the techniques used for sperm preparation. These two different techniques have the same principles wash the sperm to eliminate the seminal fluid and components which may interfere on fertilization and select the most motile spermatozoa. Density gradients have demonstrated a better selection of motile spermatozoa in oligoasthenozoospermia.

Insemination Using the INVOcell

Insemination using the INVOcell is performed immediately after oocyte retrieval. This point is very important, especially when the facility performing the INVO procedure does not have a CO_2 incubator or any CO_2 supplementation. It minimizes the exposure of the oocytes to the ambient atmosphere that is low in CO_2 and rich in oxygen (O_2). To maintain the proper pH of the culture medium during the short exposures to the ambient atmosphere, it is recommended to use HEPES media.

INVOcell preparation: The INVOcell parts, the inner chamber, the rigid outer shell, and the retention system are prewarmed before use. The inner chamber is rinsed with culture medium and then filled with 1.08 mL of fresh culture medium. The inner chamber is closed and replaced in the incubator until the placement of the gametes. Several culture media have been used successfully with the INVOcell; they have to be bicarbonate-buffered. The media have to support 3 days of culture. Media with the addition of small amounts of phenol red are recommended especially when no CO_2 incubator is available as the phenol red is a very sensitive pH indicator.

Placement of the gametes: The fraction of motile spermatozoa is introduced first into the inner chamber. A total number of *30,000 motile spermatozoa* are used for insemination regardless of the number of eggs placed in the device. In case of oligoasthenoteratozoospermia, the sperm number may be increased to 50,000 motile spermatozoa. The oocytes, immediately after retrieval, are placed in warmed culture medium with HEPES. When all the oocytes have been collected, they are rinsed in one drop of buffered bicarbonate culture medium to eliminate the HEPES and then are transferred in the inner chamber. The rotating valve is then closed. The inner chamber is placed into the bottom of the outer rigid shell. The outer rigid shell top is then closed in a locked position. The device is now ready for placement in the vagina (Fig. 9.2). If for any reason the patient is not ready for the placement of the device, put the device back into the incubator until it can be placed in the vaginal cavity. It is essential to transfer the device into the vaginal cavity as soon as possible after insemination; the vaginal cavity provides the correct gas environment.

In Vivo Embryo Culture

The fully assembled INVOcell device should be inserted into the vagina manually by the physician. The use of a speculum makes the process more difficult for the physician and very uncomfortable for the patient.

Vaginal incubation: The device is designed to be held in the fornix or in front of the cervix during the 2 or 3 days of incubation and maintained in place using the retention system. It is recommended that the couple have no intercourse during the period of incubation. Female patients can shower, but no bath, swimming, or vaginal douche is allowed due to the potential changes in vaginal temperature that could affect incubation. Normal daily activities can be performed during the 3 days of incubation. Instructions including recommendations are provided to the patient.

Embryo(s) Transfer

The embryo transfer is generally performed 3 days after the insemination at the reproductive unit.

Device removal: The device and retention system are removed manually by grasping the ring of the retention system and pulling them out. The device is rinsed with prewarmed saline solution to clean off the vaginal secretions.

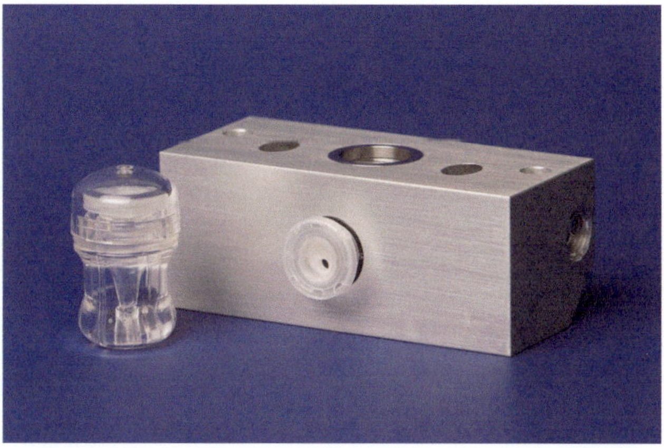

Fig. 9.3 Fully assembled INVOcell in vertical position and inner chamber positioned in the holding block for observation

Embryo Settling

The laboratory has a CO_2 incubator: The outer rigid shell is opened and discarded. The inner chamber is placed in a vertical position in the holding block in the CO_2 incubator for 15 min. During this time, the embryo(s) settle at the bottom into the microchamber.

The laboratory has no CO_2 incubator: If no CO_2 gas is available, keep the inner chamber in the outer rigid shell. The layer of gas captured between the inner chamber and the outer rigid shell will help to maintain the pH and temperature of the medium during embryo sedimentation. Place the cleaned device in a plastic sterile container in a vertical position in the incubator for 15 min. Just before the embryo observation, discard the rigid shell and place the inner chamber in the holding block (Fig. 9.3).

Embryo(s) observation and selection: The holding block containing the inner chamber is removed from the incubator and put on the microscope stage. The holding block has been designed not only to maintain the correct temperature and pH of the culture medium in the inner chamber but also to allow microscopic observation of the gametes and embryos directly through the wall of the inner chamber. In the holding block, the inner chamber is immersed in mineral oil which will eliminate irregularities of the device allowing clear viewing of the embryos directly from the microchamber. With the block in the vertical position, the oil is located internally in a reservoir (6.5 mL). During the microscopic observation, the block is flipped in a horizontal position. The microchamber is centered in the observation window and covered by the mineral oil coming from the reservoir of the block. When the embryo(s) have been located, the magnification is increased to grade and evaluate the stage of their development (two to eight cells). It is recommended that no more

Table 9.2 Results of the prelaunch clinical trial using the INVOcell

		Clinical pregnancy	
Groups	Cleavage rate (%)	Rate per cycle	Rate per transfer
Group 1 ≤10 Oocytes retrieved	52.20	31.80% (7/22)	38.90% (7/18)
Group 2 >10 Oocytes retrieved	49.30	11.70% (7/60)	13.50% (7/52)
Total	49.90	17.10% (14/82)	17.10% (14/82)

than two quality embryos be transferred to minimize the risk of multiple pregnancies. However, in some special circumstances, this number may be increased to three after discussing with the couple and after obtaining their agreement.

Embryo Transfer Catheter Loading

Embryo(s) can be loaded directly from the inner chamber: The embryo transfer catheter filled with culture medium is placed through the orifice of the open valve of the inner chamber positioned in the holding block. The embryo(s) can be visually selected and withdrawn from the microchamber into the transfer catheter by moving the syringe plunger attached to the transfer catheter up and down.

Embryo(s) loaded from a culture dish: A volume of 100 μL is aspirated from the microchamber under microscopic observation using a long pipette tip. This volume is transferred into a culture dish containing HEPES culture medium for observation and selection of the embryos for transfer. The selected embryos are then rinsed in fresh medium and loaded as classically into the embryo transfer catheter.

Embryo transfer into the uterus: The embryo transfer is performed using ultrasound guidance and an abdominal transducer to visualize the correct position of the catheter in the uterus. Any bleeding should be carefully avoided during the embryo transfer as it negatively impacts the prognosis of the procedure.

Preliminary Results

Prelaunch Trial

During the development of the new INVOcell device and its clearance by regulatory agencies, a lot of tests have been performed including a clinical trial. Results of this trial are shown in Table 9.2. A high number of oocytes, over ten per retrieval, were obtained in almost three-fourths of the cases (group 2) as all the stimulation protocols used GnRH agonist with high doses of gonadotropins. By agency request, no more than ten eggs could be placed in the INVOcell. Therefore, the embryologist

Table 9.3 Results of the first postlaunch INVO procedures using INVOcell

Countries	Number of cycles	Clinical pregnancies (rate)
Austria, Bolivia, Brazil, Ecuador, India, Mexico, Nicarragua, Pakistan, Panama, Peru, Spain, Turkey, Venezuela	457	128 (28%)

Table 9.4 Results of the clinical trial performed at CECOLFES

Number of cycles	125
Number of embryos per transfer	2.4
Number of single pregnancies	40
Number of multiple pregnancies	10
Total number of pregnancies	50
Clinical pregnancy rate/cycle	40%
Clinical pregnancy rate/transfer	43.9%[a]

[a] Eleven embryo transfers were not performed, nine due to poor or no fertilization. In the two last cases, the husbands were not available at the embryo transfer, and embryos were cryopreserved by vitrification

had to select ten oocytes with the best maturity among the 20–30 retrieved oocytes. This factor certainly explains the low pregnancy rate obtained in group 2. In group 1, patients received the same regimen of drugs but developed only ten or less than ten oocytes. In this group of low responders with the highest pregnancy rate, all the oocytes were placed in INVOcell without preselection by the embryologist.

Only the two best embryos were transferred, resulting in 14 clinical pregnancies with 12 births of normal babies and only one set of twin.

Postlaunch INVO Cycles

Since the launch of the product at the end of 2008, several hundred procedures have been done with the INVO procedure using the INVOcell. Only results of one fraction of these procedures are reported in Table 9.3, the ones for which data have been obtained and confirmed. These procedures were performed in different countries in reproductive centers as well as in newly created INVO units.

Clinical Trial at CECOLFES (Colombia)

In addition to these INVO procedures, a clinical trial has been performed by one of the first users of INVO, the Dr. Elkin Lucena at CECOLFES in Colombia. Dr. Lucena gave us the permission to report the results of the first 125 INVO procedures that he will published in a peer review journal (Table 9.4) [16]. These procedures were done in female population including 40 years old patients and older with an average age of 33.8. These 120 infertile couples should have been treated with a conventional IVF. Severe male factors needing ICSI were excluded. Mild ovarian stimulation was only used with indomethacin started at day 8 to block the ovulation. An average number of 6.5 oocytes were obtained per punction of which an average of 4.2 was inseminated in INVO. The excess oocytes (2.3 per punction) if matures were cryopreserved for future use.

Potential Disadvantages/Advantages

Potential Disadvantages

Products of degradation from dead cells and metabolism of the live cells are known to be detrimental to fertilization and embryo development. In the INVO procedure, the concentration of motile sperm has been deliberately reduced to 30,000–35,000 motile sperm per milliliter. This concentration represents less than a third of the sperm concentration generally used in conventional IVF. It has been demonstrated that this sperm concentration gives the best fertilization rates, with the lowest production of degradation products and rate of polyspermic embryos (unpublished study). The absence of embryo checking at 16–20 h postinsemination could fail to identify polyspermic embryos. Polyspermic embryos were frequently observed at the beginning of IVF due to an immaturity of the retrieved oocytes and a very high motile sperm concentration used for insemination. The formation of pronuclei is a dynamic process; it seems irrational to try eliminating polyspermic embryos by a few seconds of observation. Eliminate the main causes for polyspermic embryo formation by a better oocyte maturity and by decreasing the sperm concentration has seemed to us a more logical approach.

Advantages

1. INVO dramatically reduces and simplifies gametes and embryos handling and manipulations.
2. An embryologist with little experiences in reproductive technologies can be trained quickly and obtain excellent results.
3. The fixed laboratory equipment is low cost and not complex allowing creation of INVO units requiring little equipment maintenance and quality controls.
4. The frequent electric breakdowns observed in developing countries that affect the results of IVF/ICSI, even when battery backup or generators are available, did not impact the result of INVO.
5. The gametes and embryos are not stored in the laboratory during the 3 days of incubation. Therefore, gas supplementation, battery backup, positive pressure and air filtration, alarm system, and embryologist on call are not necessary. All these factors have contributed to the decreased cost of INVO.
6. The risk of mixing up gametes or embryos has been reduced, and INVO gives the patient a new sense of participation with in vivo conception.

Table 9.5 Preliminary results using the INVOcell for oocyte maturation and embryo development after ICSI

Procedure	Countries	Number of cycles	Number of clinical pregnancies (rate)
ICSI	Austria, Brazil, Colombia, Peru, Turkey	190	66
IVM, ICSI	Colombia, Venezuela	7	2
Total		197	68 (34.5%)

Other Applications of the INVOcell

Gamete and embryo transportation in INVOcell have been reported [9] and are still performed by users of INVO. Reproductive centers have incubators overloaded with eggs and embryos requiring frequent openings of the doors and creating major variations in CO_2 and temperature. The INVOcell has been used successfully to vaginally incubate embryos inseminated through ICSI. The INVOcell has also been used to mature immature oocytes intravaginally and later to incubate the embryos inseminated by ICSI as shown in Table 9.5.

What Did We Learn from INVO?

Oocyte In Vitro Maturation After Retrieval Is Not Required

From the beginning, the oocytes that have being retrieved after hCG induction were immediately inseminated. This was possible by using 36 h between the hCG injection and the oocyte retrieval.

Low Sperm Concentrations Are Used Successfully for Insemination

INVO has always been used with very low sperm concentrations for oocyte insemination. A concentration of 30,000 motile spermatozoa/mL is generally used and gives comparable fertilization rate and pregnancy rates to the conventional IVF. Concentrations as low as 5,000 motile spermatozoa/mL were also used but abandoned due to inconsistency in fertilization (nonpublished).

Embryo Development in Low Oxygen Concentration ($\approx$ 5%)

The INVOcell device is permeable to gas and equilibrates the pCO_2 and pO_2 of the culture medium of the inner chamber with the pCO_2 and pO_2 of the vagina. In this system, the vagina works as a CO_2 generator and an O_2 reducer. The INVO process was the first fertilization system using low oxygen concentration in air.

Cumulus Cells Perform as a Homologous Coculture System

The INVO procedure was the first coculture system using cumulus cells. This coculture system is simple, non-labor intensive, and safest for the patient [17, 18]. These cumulus cells filter and absorb the toxins and nitrogenous residues produced by the dead cells and the metabolism of the live.

Embryo Cumulus Cells Are Removed Naturally During Incubation

Spontaneous removal of embryo cumulus and corona cells has always been observed after 2 or 3 days of incubation in the INVO device. This natural and complete denudation, a sign of quality culture conditions, is the result of the enzymatic action of the spermatozoa as well as a mechanical action related to the patient mobility during the period of incubation. In the INVO procedure, culture media change is not performed so the presence of infection or toxins cannot be tolerated. The oocytes are trapped in a cumulus mass dense and viscous when any toxicity is present during the 2 or 3 days of incubation.

Positioning of INVO Among the Current Reproductive Techniques

The INVO procedure is a new infertility treatment positioned between intrauterine insemination (IUI)—simple, inexpensive, but not very successful (less than 10% of birth per cycle) [19]—and conventional IVF—complex, very expensive, but very successful (28–32% birth per cycle have been reported by several international registries for patient under 40 years old). INVO when associated with mild stimulation is a simple and successful procedure. INVO presents the advantage to treat more indications of infertility than IUI (85 vs. 50%) and to offer a diagnostic value (fertilization or not) that IUI does not.

Potential Role of INVO in Developed Countries

Governmental regulations are in place in many of the developed countries restricting the use of infertility treatments to reproductive centers. These centers have already invested in complex equipment reducing the cost saving of the INVO cycle. However, the simplicity of INVO allows performing three to four INVO cycles for one cycle of IVF or ICSI. Reproductive centers can treat a lot more patient without overloading incubators or investing in new equipment and increasing the number of embryologists. INVO may also be used in satellite units to extend the geographic influence of the reproductive center.

Role of INVO in Developing Countries

It seems irrational to treat infertility in developing countries that are frequently overpopulated, have difficulties in feeding their existing population, and have other medical priorities than to treat their infertile population. However, infertility has major socioeconomical consequences in developing countries [20, 21]. Couples who do not have children are rejected socially and do not provide offspring that economically support the elderly population. It is estimated that by 2050 most of the developing countries will not be able to renew their population [21]. The main cause of infertility is blocked tubes due to infectious diseases. Unfortunately, IVF or ICSI, the most effective treatments, is not available due to the cost to build a reproductive center and the cost of a treatment cycle. The low cost of equipment used in an INVO unit, the low maintenance of this equipment, and the rapid training of an embryologist with little experience are factors which will contribute to the expansion of the role of INVO in the treatment in infertility in developing countries.

Future Implications and Developments of the INVO Technology

Only a low percentage of infertile couples in the world can benefit from the treatment of assisted reproduction techniques due to their cost and availability.

If the cost per pregnancy using INVO confirms to be lower than the cost per pregnancy using IUI, INVO should replace IUI as the first treatment option for infertility. The diagnostic value of INVO and its ability to treat a larger percentage of the infertile population than IUI are other contributing factors for using INVO as the first-line treatment of an infertile couple.

In developing countries or regions of the world where IVF/ICSI is not available or is not affordable for a large majority of infertile couples, INVO combined with natural cycle or mild stimulation and performed in INVO satellite units represents an attractive infertility treatment option. These INVO units can be built very rapidly and do not need a large financial investment in fixed equipment. The maintenance does not require a lot of expenses and need little quality controls. The units can work even when gas supplies and electric power are erratic. The trainings of the clinician and the embryologist can be completed rapidly. The INVO procedure is so simple that the results are highly reproducible even with an embryologist with little experience. INVO involves the participation of the patient in the process of fertilization and early embryo development. INVO is an in vivo conception with a high level of acceptance among the patients who benefited from the procedure especially patients with religious convictions and ethical concerns for conventional IVF.

References

1. Taymor M, Ranoux C, Gross G. Natural oocyte retrieval with intravaginal fertilization: a simplified approach to in vitro fertilization. Obstet Gynecol. 1992;80:888–91.
2. Ranoux C, Foulot H, Aubriot FX, Poirot C, Dubuisson JB, Chevallier O, Cardone V. A new in vitro fertilization technique: intravaginal culture. Fertil Steril. 1988;49:654–7.
3. Frydman R, Ranoux C. INVO: a simple, low cost effective assisted reproductive technology. ESHRE Monographs, Special task force on 'Developing countries and infertility'. Hum Reprod. 2008;163:85–9.
4. Fukuda M, Fukuda K, Ranoux C. Unexpected low oxygen tension of intravaginal culture. Hum Reprod. 1996;11:1293–5.
5. Sterzik K, Rosenbusch B, Sasse V, Wolf A, Beier HM, Lauritzen C. A new variation of in vitro fertilization: intravaginal culture of human oocytes and cleavage stages. Hum Reprod Suppl. 1989;4(8 Suppl):83–6.
6. Ranoux C, Seibel MM. New techniques in fertilization: intravaginal culture and microvolume straw. J In Vitro Fert Embryo Transf. 1990;7:6–8.
7. Freude G, Artner B, Leodolter S. Intravaginal culture—simplification of IVF. Wien Med Wochenschr. 1990;140:498–501.
8. Wiegerinck MAHM, Moret E, Van Dop PA, Wijnberg M, Beerendonk CDMB. Intra vaginal culture (IVC), the Eindhoven experience. In: Evers JHL, Heineman MJ, editors. Ovulation to implantation. Elsevier Science: BV; 1990. p. 349–51.
9. Sharma S, Hewitt J. Intravaginal culture for IVF. Bombay Hosp J. 1993;35:155–60.
10. Batres F, Mahadevan M, Maris M, Miller M, Moutos D. Stimulated cycle and intravaginal culture fertilization in an office setting: a preliminary study. Poster presentation (P-196) at the annual meeting of ASRM, Cincinnati, OH; 1997.
11. Rongieres-Bertrand C, Olivennes F, Righini C, Fanchin R, et al. Revival of the natural cycles in in-vitro fertilization with the use of a new gonadotropin-releasing hormone antagonist (Cetrorelix): a pilot study with minimal stimulation. Hum Reprod. 1999;14:683–8.
12. Lee TH, Lin YH, Seow KM, et al. Effectiveness of cetrorelix for the prevention of premature luteinizing hormone surge during controlled ovarian stimulation using letrozole and gonadotropins: a randomized trial. Fertil Steril. 2008;90:113–20.
13. De Silva M, Reeves JJ. Indomethacin inhibition of ovulation in the cow. J Reprod Fertil. 1985;75:547–9.
14. Nargund G, Waterstone J, Bland J. Cumulative conception and live birth rate in natural (unstimulated) IVF cycles. Hum Reprod. 2001;16:259–62.
15. Requina A, Herrero J, Landeras J, Navarro E, et al. Use of letrozole in assisted reproduction: a systematic review and meta-analysis. Hum Reprod Update. 2008;14:571–82.
16. Lucena E, Saa AM, Navarro DE, Lombana C, Moran A. Invo Procedure: minimally invasive IVF as an alternative treatment option for infertile couples. The Scientific World Journal. 2012; (in press).
17. Quinn P. Use of coculture with cumulus cells in insemination medium in human in vitro fertilization (IVF). J Assist Reprod Genet. 1994;11:270–7.
18. Carrel DT, Peterson CM, Jones KP, Hatasaka HH, et al. A simplified coculture system using homologous, attached cumulus tissue results in improved human embryo morphology and pregnancy rates during in vitro fertilization. J Assist Reprod Genet. 1999;16:344–9.

19. Ombelet W, Campo R, Bosmans E, Nijs M. Intrauterine insemination (IUI) as a first-line treatment in developing countries and methodological aspects that might influence IUI success. ESHRE Monographs, Special task force on 'Developing countries and infertility'. Hum Reprod. 2008;2008(1):64–72. doi:10.1093/den,165:64-72.
20. Ombelet W, Nargund G. The patient from the developing world. In: Macklon NS, Greer IA, Steegers EAP, editors. Textbook of periconceptional medicine. London.: Informa Healthcare; 2009. p. 261–71.
21. Ombelet W. False perceptions and common misunderstandings surrounding the subject of infertility in developing countries. Hum Reprod. ESHRE Monographs, Special task force on 'Developing countries and infertility'. Hum Reprod. 2008;204:8–11.

Chapter 10
Microfluidics for Gamete Manipulation and Embryo Culture

Gary D. Smith, Charles Bormann, and Shuichi Takayama

Assisted reproductive technologies (ART) have evolved over the last 3 decades with the development of new technologies that have resulted in refinement of in vitro production of mammalian embryos which is central to several other areas of biotechnology. In vitro production of mammalian embryos is utilized for treatment of human infertility [1], derivation of genetically modified animals for biomedical research and enhanced food production [2], cryopreservation of gametes, and nuclear transfer [3]. Continuous refinements of ARTs have been achieved through modification of medium components, their concentrations, and supplementation of new components at specific time points. While there have been many advances in IVP in regard to efficiency and embryo quality, these embryos are still suboptimal compared to their in vivo counterparts. Differences in the quality of embryos produced in vitro vs. in vivo are believed to result from stresses imposed on oocytes/embryos during the in vitro production procedure. These stresses begin as early as oocyte retrieval, as even a small variations in handling temperature affects ability of oocytes to continue through the in vitro production procedure [4]. Additionally, ART procedures entail as numerous washes and transfers to different culture drops that potentially impose stress (change in pH, osmolarity, and temperature) on

G.D. Smith, PhD (✉)
Departments of OB/GYN, Physiology, and Urology, University of Michigan, Ann Arbor, MI, USA

Reproductive Sciences Program, A Taubman Consortium for Stem Cell Therapies, University of Michigan, Ann Arbor, MI, USA
e-mail: smithgd@med.umich.edu

C. Bormann, PhD
Reproductive Endocrinology, Wisconsin Oncofertility Clinic, UW Hospital and Clinics, Madison, WI, USA

S. Takayama, PhD
Department of Biomedical Engineering, Macromolecular Science and Engineering Program, University of Michigan, Ann Arbor, MI, USA

Z.P. Nagy et al. (eds.), *Clinical Embryology: A Practical Guide*,
DOI 10.1007/978-1-4614-8376-2_10,

gametes and embryos [5]. Finally, human factors associated with ARTs have potential to introduce oocyte/embryo loss at each handling step. In treatment of human infertility, where costs of embryos are high, loss of an oocyte or embryo at any stage could be problematic. Historically, scientists have worked to develop tools that would allow gamete/embryo manipulation under more in vivo-like conditions, with the idea that this would reduce stress imposed during in vitro production and potential human error. Today, significant developments in fabrication of micro-/nanotechnology devices are positioned to impact biology and medicine and have the potential to significantly improve laboratory ARTs for humans infertility treatment, domestic animals food production, rodents biomedical research, and stem cell research and the search for treatments and cures for human health diseases.

Integration of microdevices into biological research and medical treatments has progressed rapidly [6–9]. Developments of micro-/nanodevices have enabled the study of cells at single-cell and subcellular levels in ways not previously possible. These devices may allow us the ability to track protein production, metabolism, as well as additional viability markers in living cells vs. current fixed cell systems. These types of tools become especially important when the availability of cells is limited, such as when dealing with gametes and embryos in treating human infertility. In addition, microfluidic devices could allow development of more in vivo-like systems for cell culture [10] and embryo development [11] by precise environmental control at the microscale.

Microdevice and Microfluidic Technologies

Advancements in nanotechnology and miniaturization of bioanalytical procedures have allowed scientists a powerful platform to study biological systems. Deoxyribonucleic acid (DNA) sequencing, PCR, electrophoresis, DNA separation, and cell counting and sorting are just a small list of biological systems that have begun transformation from the macro- to microscale [9]. Microfluidics is one area of advancement with great promise. Microfluidics deals with the behavior, specific control, and manipulation of microliter and nanoliter volumes of fluid. This technology first emerged in the 1990s and has enabled molecular biology procedures and single cell-based bioassays. One example of how this technology has been applied was in development of a polydimethylsiloxane (PDMS)-based microfluidic device for the analysis of a single rat pheochromocytoma (PC12) cell. This system maintained cell viability and could be utilized to transport a single PC12 cell into a microchamber where nicotine was introduced and microelectrodes were used to effectively monitor release of dopamine from the cell [12].

Microfluidic systems have been designed for a unidirectional flow of oocytes, embryos, sperm, medium, and medium components [6, 13–16]. In some instances, microscale design of these microfluidic devices permits laminar flow, characterized as parallel streams flowing without disruption between currents. When laminar flow is present, mixing between streams occurs predominately by diffusion [9] with a slight meniscus between the laminar flowing streams. Similar methodology could be used to spatially and temporally expose gametes, embryos, and embryonic stem cells to different molecules with subcellular precision. In addition, one could develop molecular gradients to investigate migratory events of gametes, embryos, and stem cells. The unique physical, spatial, and temporal environment obtained with microdevices opens countless avenues to increase knowledge of basic gamete/embryo physiology that were not previously possible.

Assisted Reproductive Technologies

Currently, in vitro production of mammalian embryos is relatively inefficient due to suboptimal starting materials and artificial stresses imposed on gametes and embryos in their in vitro environment. During the laboratory ART process, oocytes/embryos are moved numerous times between media, requiring removal from their incubator environment. These manipulations introduce stresses such as changes in temperature, pH, osmolarity, and mechanical stress. Past efforts to reduce biochemical stress to gametes and embryos have involved manipulation of media and its composition. Relatively little attention has been paid to improving the mechanical platform on which gamete/embryo manipulation occurs.

In Vitro Oocyte Maturation

Oocyte maturation in vitro is the first step of in vitro production of domestic animal embryos. While human oocytes are usually obtained at mature state following in vivo maturation, there are groups working on human oocyte in vitro maturation (IVM) [17–20]. Oocyte maturation can be divided into two independent events: nuclear maturation (progression to metaphase II [MII]) and cytoplasmic maturation (preparation of the cytoplasm to support development to MII, subsequent fertilization, and embryo development). Given that embryo viability closely reflects oocyte quality, it is clear that optimal oocyte maturation is essential for successful preimplantation development.

Oocyte IVM is an emerging technology that holds great potential for treatment of human infertility (see reviews [17–20]). This technology, once efficient, will reduce the need for ovarian hormone stimulation, limiting the risk of ovarian hyperstimulation (OHSS) and reducing the cost associated with in vitro fertilization (IVF) [21]. Additionally, oocyte IVM may provide an alternative to cancelation of treatment cycles for patients with a poor response to ovarian stimulation [22, 23]. Finally, IVM may be a useful tool coupled with oocyte, follicle, or ovarian tissue cryopreservation for preserving fertility in women undergoing gonadotoxic chemo- or radiation therapy for cancers and/or autoimmune diseases. Today, human IVM is relatively inefficient with many questions regarding safety of this technique

[24–26]. Thus, it is imperative to develop a culture system that adequately supports nuclear and cytoplasmic maturation of oocytes.

It can be hypothesized that oocyte IVM in a microfluidic environment more closely resembles oocyte maturation conditions in vivo and thus may benefit oocyte maturation and subsequent embryo development. This is especially important as it has been shown that events during oocyte maturation affect subsequent embryonic development [27–29]. Walters and colleagues reported that, despite inferior cumulus expansion, PDMS microchannels did not inhibit porcine oocyte nuclear maturation (71% compared to control cultured oocytes 61%) [30]. Hester and coworkers subsequently demonstrated a significant increase ($P < 0.05$) in embryos cleaved from total oocytes matured in PDMS/borosilicate microchannels (67%) compared to controls (49%) [31]. This improvement in embryo development was speculated to result from improved cytoplasmic maturation. These initial experiments on oocyte maturation using microfluidics are promising and may provide a more supportive in vivo-like culture environment for maturing human oocytes in the future.

Sperm Selection and Isolation

Nearly 40% of human infertility is male factor-related [32]. IVF was originally developed as a treatment for tubal infertility; however, high rates of males with poor semen quality have led to development of several methods to isolate motile sperm. Under in vivo conditions, potentially fertile spermatozoa are separated from immotile spermatozoa, debris, and seminal plasma in the female genital tract [33]. The three most commonly used techniques to artificially isolate motile sperm from an ejaculate include density gradient centrifugation, sperm migration or "swim-up," and simple dilution and washing [34]. Both sperm migration and gradient centrifugation result in recovery of motile sperm; yet, several investigators have raised concern as to whether these methods of sperm isolation damage sperm DNA or impair motile sperm by exposing them to reactive oxygen species [35–37]. It has been shown that increased levels of sperm DNA damage during IVF correlate with reduction in embryo morphology at early cleavage stages [38], failure to advance to the blastocyst stage in vitro [39, 40], decreased pregnancy rates [41–43], and result in an increase in spontaneous abortions [44]. Furthermore, these separation techniques are suboptimal for patients with severe oligozoospermia, as samples from many of these patients have large amounts of debris, and recovery rates from initial sperm samples have been reported to be as low as 0.8% for direct sperm migration [45, 46].

Reduced spermatozoa quality or quantity during IVF results in poor and sometimes failed fertilization. In these cases, fertilization by injecting a single spermatozoon into the ooplasm of a mature oocyte is possible and referred to as intracytoplasmic sperm injection (ICSI) [47]. Although only a single healthy sperm is required for ICSI, processing, isolating, and selecting the most viable sperm can be challenging with current sperm separation techniques. Importantly, one can recognize that ICSI is an invasive technique and circumvents processes of natural

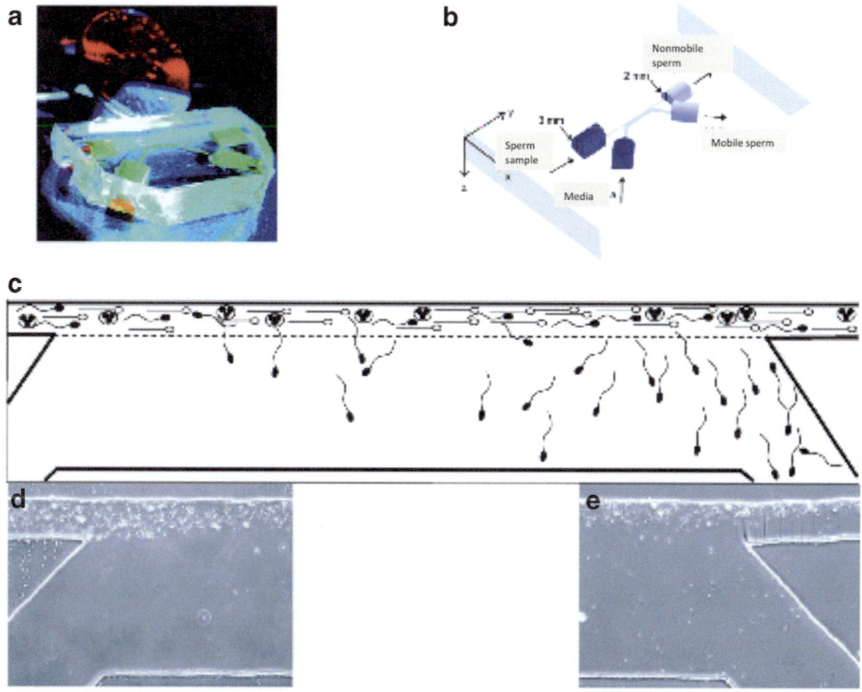

Fig. 10.1 (**a**) Picture of microfluidic sperm sorter next to a penny for size reference. (**b**) Three-dimensional view of microfluidic sperm sorter. (**c**) Theoretical vision for microfluidic sperm sorter. Media and semen flows from left to right. Semen sample is loaded into the upper stream inlet, and fresh media is placed in the lower stream inlet. (**d**, **e**) Motile sperm deviate from the initial streamline and cross the interface of the laminar flow streams, exiting into the lower stream outlet for recovery. Debris, nonmotile sperm, and seminal plasma exit the device in the upper stream outlet. From Cho et al. [13]. Used with permission

fertilization [48]. Because of its invasiveness, even in fully competent hands, this technique can result in lysis and death of 5–7% of injected oocytes [49, 50]. Considering that ICSI bypasses all normal sperm selection processes, it is imperative to have an efficient artificial selection process that minimizes stress and damage to sperm and maximizes the probability of successful pregnancy, birth, and healthy offspring [48]. Therefore, separation of sperm using microfluidics has been investigated as a possible alternative to traditional sperm isolation techniques.

Advances in microfabrication have made it possible to easily construct any desired [51, 52] microstructures. Using soft lithography, Cho and colleagues developed a novel gravity-driven pumping system to sort sperm samples [13]. The device, termed a microscale integrated sperm sorter (MISS), contained inlet/outlet ports, fluid reservoirs, gravity-driven power sources, and converging microchannels with laminar flow; all integrated components working together to facilitate sperm sorting (Fig. 10.1) [13]. The premise for this design was based on a natural phenomenon of parallel laminar flow, characteristic of fluid movement at the microscale [16]. The orientation, geometry, and size of the MISS reservoirs were designed to balance gravitational forces and surface tension forces and provide a pumping system, free of external energy, that generates steady flow rates over extended periods of time [13]. This device was designed so that converging stream of semen and media would flow in parallel, in a laminar fashion within a microchannel. The two parallel streams only mix by diffusion at the interface between streams, but motile sperm are able to swim across the contacting streamline and into the media for collection. Nonmotile sperm, cellular debris, and seminal plasma do not cross this barrier and flow uninterrupted into a waste reservoir.

For unprocessed semen, the device consistently produced a sorted fraction with increased motility (mean 98% motile) and improved strict sperm morphology (mean 22% normal forms) vs. the initial specimen (mean 44 and 10%, respectively) [16]. For debris-filled samples, the device not only concentrated motile sperm (mean 98% motile) within the collected fraction but also produced a round cell: sperm ratio of 1:33 compared with a 10:1 ratio in the starting specimen [16]. This device provides a simple, safe method of obtaining motile sperm of enriched normal morphology from both unprocessed normal semen and poor-quality specimens containing significant debris.

A limitation of the current microfluidic device is that it is not capable of processing an entire sample due to its small capacity, yet such limitations can be circumvented by parallel processing. Additionally, it does not isolate every motile sperm, but this again can be elevated, if need be, by integrating a semen recirculatory system to current chip designs. Nevertheless, isolation of motile sperm is fast and easy and can be readily used for isolating sperm for ICSI, for insemination in microdrops under oil, or for insemination in a microfluidic environment. Because no centrifugation is employed in MISS-sperm isolation, there is reduced opportunity to cause sublethal structural or DNA damage to sperm that may be used for insemination. Additional modifications of the current system are underway, which may allow for large-scale processing of semen.

In Vitro Fertilization

Species differences exist in the relative difficulty in achieving IVF. This is especially apparent in animal systems, such as the pig, where polyspermy occurs at a high frequency and lab-to-lab variations are seen in the blastocyst formation (25–30%). In general, IVF involves coincubation of oocytes with an appropriate concentration of motile and morphologically normal sperm. Media volumes may range from 20 μL microdrops to 1 mL in dishes at a minimum concentration of 500,000 sperm/mL [34]. The volume of media in which insemination occurs varies between laboratories and between total numbers of motile sperm collected from an individual. Because traditional insemination in a microdrop requires such a high number of sperm which then deplete metabolic substrates and produce potentially harmful waste products in the IVF media [53, 54], there is an emphasis to develop new technologies for in vitro insemination to reduce numbers of sperm needed to achieve successful IVF.

Several systems have been developed for insemination, including the climbing-over-a-wall (COW) method used by Funahashi and Nagai and straw IVF [55, 56]. The COW method has been performed with frozen-thawed boar sperm placed into an outer chamber filled with tris-buffered medium for fertilization of porcine oocytes positioned in the inner well of the COW chamber. This system was designed to select high-quality sperm in terms of progressive motility and viability and potentially mimics the in vivo system of the reproductive tract. The COW-IVF method resulted in high penetration rates at increased sperm concentrations of 0.5, 1.0, and 5.0×10^5 cells/mL while still maintaining monospermic penetration rates comparable to the traditional IVF microdrop system [55]. Similarly, the straw IVF method was developed to reduce the incidence of polyspermy and maintain penetration rates [56] and utilizes a 0.25-mL straws with oocytes in medium (~5 cm length) at one end of the straw and an adjacent 1-cm section of medium containing spermatozoa. Thus, sperm must swim to the oocytes in order to initiate fertilization, and this method reduced the number of sperm at the site of fertilization by selecting the highest quality sperm [56]. Both the COW and straw IVF methods limit the total number of sperm reaching the egg, enriching the population for those with the best motility. Similar methodologies have also been applied to human IVF with some success [57–59]. However, these techniques have not gained widespread acceptance.

Advancements in microfluidics and soft lithography have made it possible to more closely mimic the oviductal (site of in vivo fertilization) environment in vitro. Research by Clark and colleagues studied porcine fertilization in a microchannel designed to recapitulate function and structure of the oviduct [60]. In this study, oocytes in microchannels had a significantly higher incidence of monospermic penetration ($P < 0.05$) as compared to oocytes fertilized in a traditional microdrop system, with comparable penetration and male pronuclear formation rates [60]. These results demonstrate that the biomimetic microchannel IVF system can reduce polyspermy and thereby increase number of potentially viable embryos without reducing overall in vitro production efficiency.

It has been well demonstrated that only a few hundred sperm eventually reach the ampulla of the oviduct for fertilization in humans [61, 62]. Advancements in microchannel design and microfluidics may ultimately provide an alternative method of in vivo-like insemination by decreasing volume of media and numbers of sperm needed, while increasing oocyte-sperm interaction in a dynamic environment. Suh and colleagues demonstrated that mouse IVF can be conducted quickly and successfully within microfluidic channels [63]. In this experiment, a PDMS-based microfluidic insemination channel was fabricated consisting of a single microchannel separated by a barrier grate manufactured in three dimensions (Fig. 10.2). This grate permits unimpeded flow of sperm and media through the microchannel but prevents migration of the oocyte [63]. Fertilization rates were significantly increased in microchannels, compared to conventional means of insemination, when the concentration of sperm used for insemination was limited [63]. Not only were less sperm required for fertilization because of the small

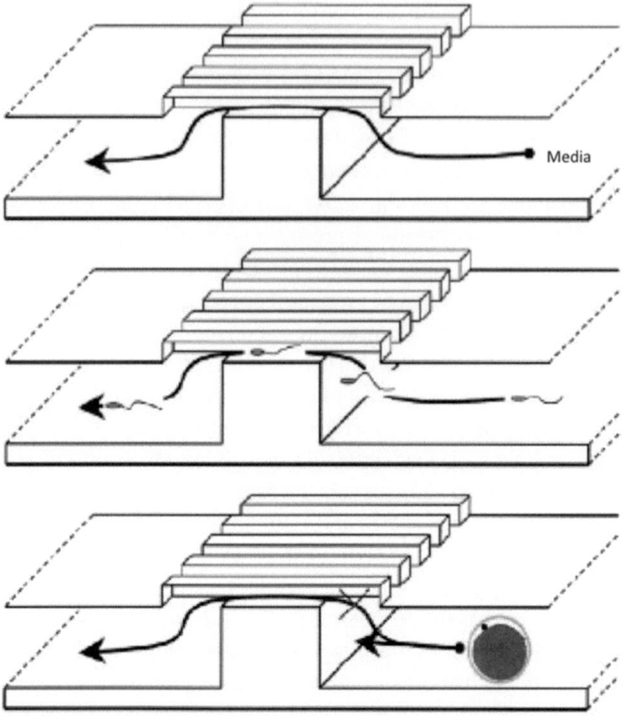

Fig. 10.2 Schematic of a microfluidic device composed of a microchannel for coincubation of sperm and oocytes for IVF. The three-dimensional construct of the channel prevents movement of the oocyte beyond the grate but allows for flow of medium and sperm through the channel. The potential to recirculate media and sperm exists. From Suh et al. [63]. Used with permission

amounts of media needed for microfluidic culture, but also a lower concentration of sperm was required because of constrained space and direct delivery of sperm to the oocyte, further reducing the number of sperm needed for successful fertilization [63]. The use of microfluidics and flow results in a predictable delivery of sperm to oocytes and may reduce the randomness of sperm and oocyte interaction that takes place in larger volumes during standard IVF [63]. Finally, this method may be useful when inseminating with sexed semen and/or [47] samples with compromised sperm numbers due to cryopreservation and thawing.

Embryo Culture

In vivo preimplantation mammalian embryos develop in the absence of direct cell contact with the reproductive tract for approximately 5–7 days before implanting in the uterus. These embryos are free floating, lack a blood supply, and move continuously within the female reproductive tract through a changing fluid environment.

During this time, the embryo is undergoing mitotic divisions and differentiation. Preimplantation embryo's nutrition is derived from internal stores or maternal-derived products obtained from luminal secretions of the oviduct and uterus. Its cellular activities, including division, gene expression, and metabolism, are influenced by the environment and factors contained within the embryo, produced by the embryo itself, and produced by cells of the reproductive tract.

Success of IVF may be compromised by limitations of current embryo culture methods, resulting in impaired embryo development and decreased viability [34]. Improvements in embryo culture methods have been based on simulating in vivo conditions and meeting the ever-changing needs of the embryo. Research into sequential media methods of embryo culture takes this hypothesis one step further [64]. Conventional embryo culture systems, however, mostly employ a single medium, or double media system, from the time of insemination until embryo transfer. In vivo, the embryo is bathed in a constantly changing environment as it moves through the oviduct to the uterus. Conditions required by the embryo at one point of development may be detrimental at later stages.

Current embryo culture technologies are not ideal for sequential media embryo culture systems. Embryos must be handled during media changes, and environments are voluminous compared to in vivo conditions which may temper the presence of embryotrophic factors. Microfluidics is well suited to meet the needs of embryo culture. Changing of media is straightforward, and no manipulation of the embryo is necessary. The media can be gradually changed around the embryo, rather than subjecting it to sudden changes in microenvironment. In theory, microenvironment that exists within microfluidic devices might simulate physiological conditions and therefore also may benefit embryo development [6].

Thus far, there have been encouraging outcomes with microfluidic embryo culture technology. Glasgow and coworkers first established that manipulation and movement of an embryo in a microfluidic environment are possible at low flow rates. In this experiment, microchannels were tested and designed with constriction areas that prevented movement of the embryo down the channel while allowing for flow of media around and past the embryo. No deformation or injury to the embryo was noted at the low flow rates used [65]. Once the feasibility of embryo handling and media flow within a microchannel was established, mouse embryos were cultured and development rates compared [6]. A significantly higher percentage of embryos within the microfluidic channels reached the morula, blastocyst, and hatched blastocyst stage compared with controls. In addition, early embryonic development was investigated to determine if PDMS/borosilicate microchannels under static conditions could support development of in vivo-derived four-cell porcine embryos to blastocysts. There was no difference ($P > 0.05$) in the blastocyst formation in microchannels (79%) compared to control drops (84%) [66]. In addition, some microchannel-produced blastocysts were transferred to a recipient and produced five live piglets with normal birth and weaning weights and subsequently went on to reproduce normally [66].

In 2004, experiments were conducted to determine if microchannel culture could support development of two-cell mouse embryos. Using PDMS/borosilicate glass microchannels, it was reported that there were significantly more ($P > 0.01$) blastocysts in the microchannels than in controls following 72 h of culture (73, 43%, respectively) [67]. Using another prototype (silicon wafer, borosilicate sandwich), it was demonstrated that percentage of blastocysts were also increased compared to control and the kinetics of development was more in vivo-like. Birth of live offspring was achieved following culture in microchannels [66].

Similarly, Heo and coworkers demonstrated an advantage of culturing mouse embryos on a microfluidic platform with dynamic media flow [68]. These experiments utilized a computer-controlled, integrated microfluidic system with on-chip pumps and valves, powered by individually actuated Braille pins to pump fresh media through a series of elastomeric capillaries [69]. This system takes advantage of the resilient yet elastic nature of PDMS microchannels fabricated with soft lithography, together with the movement of Braille pins to "squeeze" fluid through channels. When synchronized to various valving patterns, each stroke of a Braille pin generates forward or backward flow of media through microchannels. Results from these experiments showed embryos cultured under dynamic conditions had significantly more cells than those cultured under static conditions. Furthermore, blastocyst cell counts following microfluidic dynamic embryo culture more closely mirrored results obtained from their in vivo counterparts [68]. These results suggest that development of embryos in a dynamic microenvironment may closely mimic in vivo embryo growth conditions. In addition, these improved embryo development rates obtained in microfluidic dynamic culture experimentally translated into improved implantation and ongoing pregnancy rates. Most importantly, these preimplantation embryo developmental kinetics, implantation, and ongoing pregnancy rates more closely resembled those observed when embryos developed in utero in comparison to embryos grown under conventional static conditions. Live offspring were also produced. Collectively, results from these comparative controlled studies suggest that the microenvironment obtained by combining microfluidics, dynamic pulsatile fluid flow, and microfunnel embryo detainment supports enhanced embryo development compared to conventional culture conditions. One could question whether this improved embryo development was a consequence of suboptimal development of control embryos. It is impossible to compare results from different laboratories, strains of mice, initial stage of embryo development, soluble culture components, gaseous environments, timing of end-point measures, and specifics of end-point measures. However, our advanced blastocyst development rates, total blastocyst cell count, implantation rates, and ongoing pregnancy rates for controls are representative of contemporary reports [70–75]. Using the same culture device design, Bormann and coworkers (unpublished data) showed a significant improvement in percentage of IVF bovine embryos reaching the blastocyst stage compared to static controls. These results further demonstrate the importance of physical and mechanical environment on embryo development as well as the potential wide application of this technology in gamete/embryo culture.

To begin elucidation of mechanisms imparting improved embryonic developmental competence in pulsatile dynamic microfluidic culture, we ask the question of whether fluid flow influenced embryo development in a temporal- or developmental-stage-specific manner. We found that developmental impact of pulsatile media flow is not developmental stage specific [68]. This is especially important when one considers that mouse zygotic genome activation occurs at the one- to two-cell transition [76] during the first 48 h of culture, in conjunction with global chromatin remodeling, altered histone acetylation, and release from a transcriptionally repressive state [77]. The lack of differential benefit of pulsatile media flow between the first and last 48 h of culture would also suggest that the developmental benefit is not specific toward latter preimplantation developmental events such as compaction at the eight-cell stage [78], initiation of cellular polarity at the eight-cell to morula stage [79], or blastocoel formation at the transition form morula to blastocyst [80]. These results would suggest that benefits of microfluidic-generated pulsatile fluid flow on embryonic developmental competence may be due to subtle changes in the culture microenvironment that produces embryo development that is more in vivo-like and significantly advanced compared to static culture. This leads one to consider dynamic culture, embryo development, and microenvironment in relation to retention of autocrine factors, removal of waste products, and disruption of concentration gradients that may form at cell surfaces.

Embryos may develop better in small volumes or in the presence of multiple embryos, presumably due to beneficial autocrine effects [81, 82]. Some identified autocrine factors include leukemia inhibitory factor [83], interleukin-1 [84], insulin-like growth factor [85], platelet-derived growth factor [86], epidermal growth factor [87], and transforming growth factor [88]. Utilization of embryo-secreted autocrine factors is advantageous over exogenous delivery of mitogens because (i) embryos produce a complex mixture of biochemicals which are difficult to completely mimic with exogenous biomolecules and (ii) addition of exogenous growth factors has inherent limitations in spatial and temporal exposure and can sometimes lead to developmental abnormalities such as large offspring syndrome (LOS) [89, 90]. Heo and coworkers employed a computational modeling system (Fig. 10.3) to simulate fluid flow and biomolecular transport within the microfunnel culture systems. The results show that the microfunnel culture systems retain greater amounts of biomolecules compared to microchannels with flow, which had suboptimal embryo development [91]. However, retention of beneficial autocrine factors cannot fully explain the benefits of microfunnel pulsatile culture since this occurs to a greater extent in microdrops, which displayed reduced embryo developmental competence compared to the microfunnel dynamic system.

Embryos culture in small droplets may allow accumulation of toxic substances such as ammonia- [92] and oxygen-derived radicals [93], which may harm embryos [75]. Periodic media changes could prevent toxin accumulation, but it needs to be balanced with elimination of positive-acting auto- and paracrine factors [94]. The microfunnel pulsatile embryo culture system provided periodic media refresh, moderate retention of biomolecules, agitation of fluid surrounding the embryo, and removal of media. This combination appears to be advantageous.

Another concept to acknowledge within a microfluidic/microfunnel/dynamic culture system is the inherent fluid movement and mechanical agitation of embryos during culture that can disrupt concentration gradients of substrates, secretory

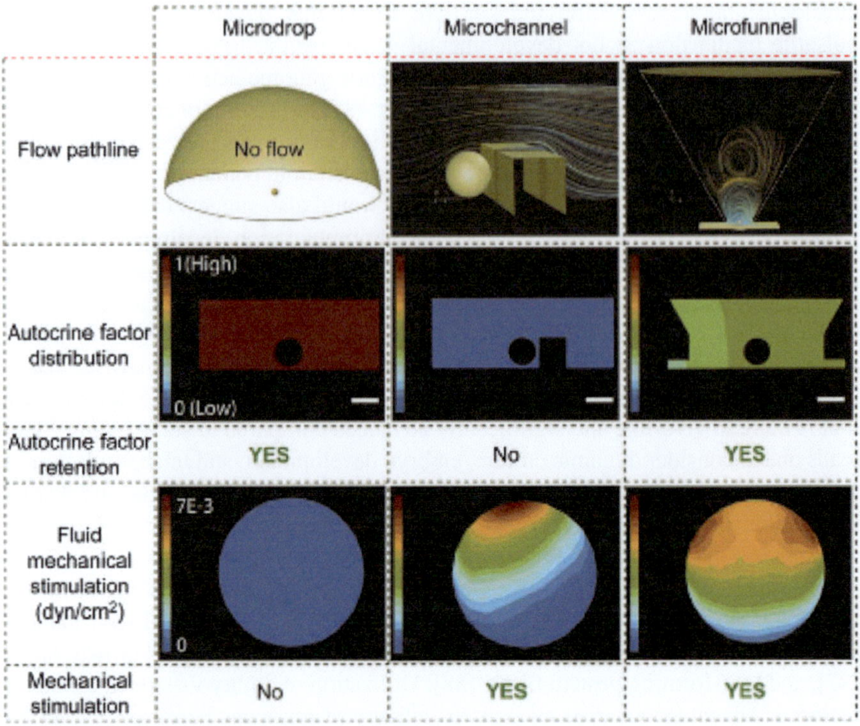

Fig. 10.3 Dynamic microfunnel culture provides fluid mechanical stimulation with retention of autocrine factors. Summary of flow path lines, mechanical stimulation, and autocrine factor distribution/retention provided by different embryo culture methods as simulated using Fluent. Microdrops retain autocrine factors but do not provide mechanical stimulation. Microchannels provide mechanical stimulation but do not retain autocrine factors. Dynamic microfunnel cultures provide both. From Heo et al. [68]. Used with permission

molecules, dissolved gases, and waste products. Movement ensures that unstirred layers do not form around the embryo and likely facilitate exchange of gases and/or metabolites. While such point-of-contact concentrations of gases, substrates, or metabolites are difficult to measure, one can envision that such disruptions of gradients could occur with media flow and embryo agitation. In conclusion, a portable computerized microfluidic system has been designed for embryo culture. Its user-friendly architecture, flexibility in microchannel and chip design, and programmability of fluid actuation system allow convenient and practical manipulation of chemical and mechanical microenvironments for in vitro embryo production. Improved pregnancy outcomes may alleviate current inefficiencies in embryo production for biomedical research, genetic gain in domestic species, and fertility treatment in humans. Combining physiological mechanical stimulation with retention of beneficial autocrine factors may also benefit a broad range of cell culture technologies beyond the dynamic microfunnel embryo culture systems described here.

Integrated ART Microfluidic Device

A significant advantage of using microfluidics is in the ability to integrate various aspects of ART and cell monitoring systems on a single chip. Clark and colleagues reported the integration of two different techniques of ART (maturation and fertilization) in a single microchannel with porcine oocytes [95]. Additional research is needed in design and development of a platform that can meet all the needs of ARTs on a single chip. This will not only mirror more closely the maternal microenvironment but will also eliminate technician-dependent variability and error.

Integration of detection devices with somatic cell culture has already been achieved using microfluidics. Cheng and colleagues demonstrated the ability to monitor Ca^{2+} transients, extracellular pH, and relative amounts of intra- and extracellular lactate production from a single cardiomyocyte [96]. Furthermore, Shackman and colleagues developed a novel system for high-resolution monitoring of insulin secretion from single islets of Langerhans [97], and Mehta and colleagues developed a method to measure oxygen content in real time in microfluidic perfusion systems [98]. Such assays, if applied to a microfluidic platform for gamete/embryo culture and analysis, could function as a monitoring system for culture condition optimization and real-time selection of embryos with the greatest implantation potential.

Embryo Bioanalysis

An unmet need in the infertility laboratory is selecting the most viable embryo for transfer from a pool of visually similar embryos. Accepted practice in most human clinics is to transfer embryos either on day 3 (approximately the eight-cell stage) or on days 5 and 6 (blastocyst stages). It is difficult to predict which day 3 embryos will continue to develop to the blastocyst stage, and importantly, this developmental stage coincides with the maternal to embryonic genomic transition in which a high percentage of embryos undergo developmental arrest. Therefore, many programs transfer multiple embryos to obtain acceptable pregnancy rates. Appropriate efforts currently focus on reducing the number of multiple pregnancies by move toward single blastocyst transfer [99], making embryo selection even more critical. In the past and present, embryo selection was/is based primarily on morphological characteristics such as cleavage rate, cell number, blastomere size, and degree of fragmentation. These methods of selection are subjective and lack predictive power.

One of the most reliable indicators of embryo viability is the rate at which an embryo consumes glucose or pyruvate from the culture medium and produces lactate and other metabolic waste products. Lane and Gardner showed embryos with glycolytic activity similar to their in vivo counterparts have a fourfold increase in pregnancy rate compared to embryos selected and transferred at random [100]. Recently, Bormann and colleagues (unpublished data) developed a metabolic assay that can be readily integrated into a microfluidic platform. This will allow noninvasive quantification of metabolism by individual preimplantation embryo

[101]. This assay along with others currently being developed may soon be used to assess embryo quality and viability.

Advancements in proteomics have made it possible to identify minute quantities of secreted peptides from preimplantation stage embryos. Using microliquid chromatography electrospray ionization mass spectrometry and matrix-assisted laser desorption ionization time-of-flight mass spectrometry, Katz-Jaffe and coworkers analyzed the proteome of individual human embryos and related protein expression profiles to morphology [102, 103]. Protein profiling has many benefits and potential applications in assisted reproduction. By measuring an embryo's secretome, it may be possible in the future to identify certain markers for male and female embryos and determine the sex of the developing embryo without using invasive approaches. This may be an important diagnostic tool in circumventing X-linked congenital disorders. Furthermore, another benefit to this noninvasive approach to profiling developing embryos would be to detect embryos with chromosome abnormalities or other health issues. Further advances in protein profiling would not just enable selection of the best quality embryo but may also allow identification of abnormal embryos without having to perform invasive procedures such as embryo biopsy and preimplantation genetic screening.

Conclusions and Future Directions

Upon recent developments of microscaled systems similar in size to mammalian gametes and preimplantation embryos, the birth of a new era has begun for assisted reproduction. Important functions necessary for carrying out basic ART laboratory procedures, including oocyte maturation, insemination, and embryo culture, can be performed in microfluidic devices. The idea of integration of numerous techniques into an "ART lab on a chip" is now possible and will allow for automation and chemical and mechanical manipulation. Microfluidic platforms may provide insight as to why ART-produced embryos are suboptimal compared to those derived in vivo. Such platforms also will provide general information to improve our knowledge of basic gamete/embryo physiology and developmental biology. Lastly, new prototypes of microfluidic devices for ARTs will be developed that enable real-time live oocyte/embryo metabolic and secretome analysis, without human manipulation-introduced error. Such live-cell assays will enhance our understanding of cellular physiological processes and provide additional parameters to measure oocyte/embryo health and viability.

Acknowledgments The authors would like to thank Dr. Carrie Smith for critically reviewing this manuscript. We recognize and appreciate financial support from National Institutes of Health (NIH; HD 049607–01—S.T & G.D.S), United States Department of Agriculture (USDA; 2005–35203-16148—G.D.S & S.T), the Michigan Economic Development Corporation (MEDC; GR 696—S.T & G.D.S) Support for C.B. was provided by NIH Training Grant in Reproductive Sciences T32-HD07048 (G.D.S). We apologize to those whose work we have not cited owing to space limitation.

References

1. Hagmann M. Fertility therapy may aid gene transfer. Science. 1999;284:1097–8.
2. Velander WH, Lubon H, Drohan WN. Transgenic livestock as drug factories. Sci Am. 1997;276:70–4.
3. Polejaeva IA, Chen SH, Vaught TD, et al. Cloned pigs produced by nuclear transfer from adult somatic cells. Nature. 2000;407:86–90.
4. Ravindranatha BM, Nandi S, Raghu HM, Reddy SM. In vitro maturation and fertilization of buffalo oocytes: effects of storage of ovaries, IVM temperatures, storage of processed sperm and fertilization media. Reprod Domest Anim. 2003;38:21–6.
5. Xie Y, Wang F, Zhong W, et al. Shear stress induces preimplantation embryo death that is delayed by the zona pellucida and associated with stress-activated protein kinase-mediated apoptosis. Biol Reprod. 2006;75:45–55.
6. Beebe D, Wheeler M, Zeringue H, Walters E, Raty S. Microfluidic technology for assisted reproduction. Theriogenology. 2002;57: 125–35.
7. Beebe DJ, Mensing GA, Walker GM. Physics and applications of microfluidics in biology. Annu Rev Biomed Eng. 2002;4:261–86.
8. Quake SR, Scherer A. From micro- to nanofabrication with soft materials. Science. 2000;290: 1536–40.
9. Sia SK, Whitesides GM. Microfluidic devices fabricated in poly(dimethylsiloxane) for biological studies. Electrophoresis. 2003;24:3563–76.
10. Walker G, Ozers M, Beebe DJ. Insect cell culture in microfluidic channels. Biomed Microdevices. 2002;4:161–6.
11. Raty S, Beebe DJ, Rodriguez-Zas SL, Wheeler MB. Culture in microchannels enhances in vitro embryonic development of preimplantation mouse embryos. Theriogenology. 2001;55:241.
12. Huang WH, Cheng W, Zhang Z, et al. Transport, location, and quantal release monitoring of single cells on a microfluidic device. Anal Chem. 2004;76:483–8.
13. Cho BS, Schuster TG, Zhu X, et al. Passively driven integrated microfluidic system for separation of motile sperm. Anal Chem. 2003;75:1671–5.
14. Davis JA, Raty S, Eddington DT, Glasgow IK, Zeringue HC, Wheeler MB, et al. Development of microfluidic channels for the culture of mammalian embryos. In: First annual international IEEE-EMBS special topic conference on microtechnologies in medicine & biology proceedings; 2000. p. 307–10.
15. Glasgow IK, Zeringue HC, Beebe DJ, Choi SJ, Lyman J, Wheeler MB. Individual embryo transport on a chip for a total analysis system. In: Third international symposium on micro-total analysis system; 1998. p. 13–16.
16. Schuster TG, Cho B, Keller LM, Takayama S, Smith GD. Isolation of motile spermatozoa from semen samples using microfluidics. Reprod Biomed Online. 2003;7:75–81.
17. Jurema MW, Nogueira D. In vitro maturation of human oocytes for assisted reproduction. Fertil Steril. 2006;86:1277–91.
18. Mikkelsen AL. Strategies in human in-vitro maturation and their clinical outcome. Reprod Biomed Online. 2005;10:593–9.
19. Papanikolaou EG, Platteau P, Albano C, et al. Immature oocyte in-vitro maturation: clinical aspects. Reprod Biomed Online. 2005;10:587–92.
20. Piquette GN. The in vitro maturation (IVM) of human oocytes for in vitro fertilization (IVF): is it time yet to switch to IVM-IVF? Fertil Steril. 2006;85:833–5; discussion 841.
21. Brinsden PR, Wada I, Tan SL, Balen A, Jacobs HS. Diagnosis, prevention and management of ovarian hyperstimulation syndrome. Br J Obstet Gynaecol. 1995;102:767–72.
22. Check ML, Brittingham D, Check JH, Choe JK. Pregnancy following transfer of cryopreserved-thawed embryos that had been a result of fertilization of all in vitro matured metaphase or germinal stage oocytes. Case report. Clin Exp Obstet Gynecol. 2001;28: 69–70.

23. Liu J, Lu G, Qian Y, Mao Y, Ding W. Pregnancies and births achieved from in vitro matured oocytes retrieved from poor responders undergoing stimulation in in vitro fertilization cycles. Fertil Steril. 2003;80:447–9.
24. Albertini DF, Sanfins A, Combelles CM. Origins and manifestations of oocyte maturation competencies. Reprod Biomed Online. 2003;6:410–5.
25. Fauser BC, Bouchard P, Coelingh Bennink HJ, et al. Alternative approaches in IVF. Hum Reprod Update. 2002;8:1–9.
26. Hardy K, Wright CS, Franks S, Winston RM. In vitro maturation of oocytes. Br Med Bull. 2000;56:588–602.
27. Hendriksen PJ, Vos PL, Steenweg WN, Bevers MM, Dieleman SJ. Bovine follicular development and its effect on the in vitro competence of oocytes. Theriogenology. 2000;53:11–20.
28. Krisher RL, Lane M, Bavister BD. Developmental competence and metabolism of bovine embryos cultured in semi-defined and defined culture media. Biol Reprod. 1999;60: 1345–52.
29. Spindler RE, Pukazhenthi BS, Wildt DE. Oocyte metabolism predicts the development of cat embryos to blastocyst in vitro. Mol Reprod Dev. 2000;56:163–71.
30. Walters EM, Beebe DJ, Wheeler MB. In vitro maturation of pig oocytes in polydimethylsiloxane (PDMS) and silicon microfluidic devices. Theriogenology. 2001;55:497.
31. Hester PN, Roseman HM, Clark SG, Walters EM, Beebe DJ, Wheeler MB. Enhanced cleavage rates following in vitro maturation of pig oocytes within polydimethylsiloxane-borosilicate microchannels. Theriogenology. 2002;57:723.
32. Mosher WD, Pratt WF. Fecundity and infertility in the United States: incidence and trends. Fertil Steril. 1991;56:192–3.
33. Mortimer D. Sperm transfer in the human female reproductive tract. Oxford: Oxford University Press; 1989.
34. Trounson A, Gardner DK. Handbook of in vitro fertilization. Boca Raton: CRC Press LLC; 2000.
35. Aitken RJ, Clarkson JS. Significance of reactive oxygen species and antioxidants in defining the efficacy of sperm preparation techniques. J Androl. 1988;9:367–76.
36. Zini A, Finelli A, Phang D, Jarvi K. Influence of semen processing technique on human sperm DNA integrity. Urology. 2000;56:1081–4.
37. Zini A, Mak V, Phang D, Jarvi K. Potential adverse effect of semen processing on human sperm deoxyribonucleic acid integrity. Fertil Steril. 1999;72:496–9.
38. Virant-Klun I, Tomazevic T, Meden-Vrtovec H. Sperm single-stranded DNA, detected by acridine orange staining, reduces fertilization and quality of ICSI-derived embryos. J Assist Reprod Genet. 2002;19:319–28.
39. Benchaib M, Braun V, Lornage J, et al. Sperm DNA fragmentation decreases the pregnancy rate in an assisted reproductive technique. Hum Reprod. 2003;18:1023–8.
40. Seli E, Gardner DK, Schoolcraft WB, Moffatt O, Sakkas D. Extent of nuclear DNA damage in ejaculated spermatozoa impacts on blastocyst development after in vitro fertilization. Fertil Steril. 2004;82:378–83.
41. Bungum M, Humaidan P, Spano M, et al. The predictive value of sperm chromatin structure assay (SCSA) parameters for the outcome of intrauterine insemination, IVF and ICSI. Hum Reprod. 2004;19:1401–8.
42. Henkel R, Hajimohammad M, Stalf T, et al. Influence of deoxyribonucleic acid damage on fertilization and pregnancy. Fertil Steril. 2004;81:965–72.
43. Tesarik J, Greco E, Mendoza C. Late, but not early, paternal effect on human embryo development is related to sperm DNA fragmentation. Hum Reprod. 2004;19:611–5.
44. Carrell DT, Liu L, Peterson CM, et al. Sperm DNA fragmentation is increased in couples with unexplained recurrent pregnancy loss. Arch Androl. 2003;49:49–55.
45. Englert Y, Van den Bergh M, Rodesch C, et al. Comparative auto-controlled study between swim-up and Percoll preparation of fresh semen samples for in-vitro fertilization. Hum Reprod. 1992;7:399–402.

46. Smith S, Hosid S, Scott L. Use of postseparation sperm parameters to determine the method of choice for sperm preparation for assisted reproductive technology. Fertil Steril. 1995;63: 591–7.
47. Palermo G, Joris H, Devroey P, Van Steirteghem AC. Pregnancies after intracytoplasmic injection of single spermatozoon into an oocyte. Lancet. 1992;340:17–8.
48. Schultz RM, Williams CJ. The science of ART. Science. 2002;296:2188–90.
49. Palermo GD, Alikani M, Bertoli M, et al. Oolemma characteristics in relation to survival and fertilization patterns of oocytes treated by intracytoplasmic sperm injection. Hum Reprod. 1996;11:172–6.
50. Nagy ZP, Liu J, Joris H, et al. The influence of the site of sperm deposition and mode of oolemma breakage at intracytoplasmic sperm injection on fertilization and embryo development rates. Hum Reprod. 1995;10:3171–7.
51. Anderson JR, Chiu DT, Jackman RJ, et al. Fabrication of topologically complex three-dimensional microfluidic systems in PDMS by rapid prototyping. Anal Chem. 2000;72: 3158–64.
52. Unger MA, Chou HP, Thorsen T, Scherer A, Quake SR. Monolithic microfabricated valves and pumps by multilayer soft lithography. Science. 2000;288:113–6.
53. Dietl JA, Rauth G. Molecular aspects of mammalian fertilization. Hum Reprod. 1989;4: 869–75.
54. Hickman DL, Beebe DJ, Rodriguez-Zas SL, Wheeler MB. Comparison of static and dynamic medium environments for culturing of pre-implantation mouse embryos. Comp Med. 2002; 52:122–6.
55. Funahashi H, Fujiwara T, Nagai T. Modulation of the function of boar spermatozoa via adenosine and fertilization promoting peptide receptors reduce the incidence of polyspermic penetration into porcine oocytes. Biol Reprod. 2000;63:1157–63.
56. Li YH, Ma W, Li M, et al. Reduced polyspermic penetration in porcine oocytes inseminated in a new in vitro fertilization (IVF) system: straw IVF. Biol Reprod. 2003;69:1580–5.
57. Ranoux C, Poirot C, Foulot H, et al. Human egg fertilization in capillary tubes. J In Vitro Fert Embryo Transf. 1988;5:49–50.
58. Ranoux C, Seibel MM. New techniques in fertilization: intravaginal culture and microvolume straw. J In Vitro Fert Embryo Transf. 1990;7:6–8.
59. van der Ven HH, Hoebbel K, al-Hasani S, Diedrich K, Krebs D. Fertilization of human oocytes in capillary tubes with very small numbers of spermatozoa. Hum Reprod. 1989;4:72–6.
60. Clark SG, Haubert K, Beebe DJ, Ferguson CE, Wheeler MB. Reduction of polyspermic penetration using biomimetic microfluidic technology during in vitro fertilization. Lab Chip. 2005;5:1229–32.
61. Ahlgren M. Sperm transport to and survival in the human fallopian tube. Gynecol Invest. 1975;6:206–14.
62. Settlage DS, Motoshima M, Tredway DR. Sperm transport from the external cervical os to the fallopian tubes in women: a time and quantitation study. Fertil Steril. 1973;24:655–61.
63. Suh RS, Zhu X, Phadke N, et al. IVF within microfluidic channels requires lower total numbers and lower concentrations of sperm. Hum Reprod. 2006;21:477–83.
64. Gardner DK, Lane M. Culture of viable human blastocysts in defined sequential serum-free media. Hum Reprod. 1998;13(Suppl 3):148–59; discussion 160.
65. Glasgow IK, Zeringue HC, Beebe DJ, et al. Handling individual mammalian embryos using microfluidics. IEEE Trans Biomed Eng. 2001;48:570–8.
66. Walters EM, Clark S, Roseman HM, Beebe DJ, Wheeler MB. Production of live piglets following in vitro embryo culture in a microfluidic environment. Theriogenology. 2003;59:353.
67. Raty S, Walters EM, Davis J, et al. Embryonic development in the mouse is enhanced via microchannel culture. Lab Chip. 2004;4:186–90.
68. Heo Y, Cabrera L, Bormann C, et al. Dynamic microfunnel culture enhances mouse embryo development and pregnancy rates. Hum Reprod. 2010;25:613–22.
69. Gu W, Zhu X, Futai N, Cho BS, Takayama S. Computerized microfluidic cell culture using elastomeric channels and Braille displays. Proc Natl Acad Sci USA. 2004;101:15861–6.

70. Manser R, Leese H, Houghton F. Effect of inhibiting nitric oxide production on mouse preimplantation embryo development and metabolism. Biol Reprod. 2004;71:528–33.
71. Biggers J. History of KSOM, a single medium for embryo culture. Fertil World. 2005;3: 4–5.
72. Summers MC, McGinnis LK, Lawitts JA, Biggers JD. Mouse embryo development following IVF in media containing either L-glutamine or glycyl-L-glutamine. Hum Reprod. 2005;20:1364–71.
73. Feil D, Lane M, Roberts CT, et al. Effect of culturing mouse embryos under different oxygen concentrations on subsequent fetal and placental development. J Physiol Lond. 2006;572: 87–96.
74. Mitchell M, Cashman K, Gardner D, Thompson J, Lane M. Disruption of mitochondrial malate-aspartate shuttle activity in mouse blastocysts impairs viability and fetal growth. Biol Reprod. 2009;80:295–301.
75. Lane M, Gardner DK. Ammonium induces aberrant blastocyst differentiation, metabolism, pH regulation, gene expression and subsequently alters fetal development in the mouse. Biol Reprod. 2003;69:1109–17.
76. Schultz R. Regulation of zygotic gene activation in the mouse. Bioessays. 1993;15:531–8.
77. Ma J, Svoboda P, Schultz R, Stein P. Regulation of zygotic gene activation in the preimplantation mouse embryo: global activation and repression of gene expression. Biol Reprod. 2001;64:1713–21.
78. Johnson M, Ziomek C. Induction of polarity in mouse 8-cell blastomeres: specificity, geometry, and stability. J Cell Biol. 1981;91:303–8.
79. Johnson M, Maro B, Takeichi M. The role of cell adhesion in the synchronisation and orientation of polarisation in 8-cell mouse blastomeres. J Embryol Exp Morphol. 1986;93:239–55.
80. Borland R, Biggers J, LeChene C. Studies on the composition and formation of mouse blastocoele fluid using electron probe microanalysis. Dev Biol. 1977;55:1–8.
81. Hardy K, Spanos S. Growth factor expression and function in the human and mouse preimplantation embryo. J Endocrinol. 2002;172:221–36.
82. Diaz-Cueto L, Gerton GL. The influence of growth factors on the development of preimplantation mammalian embryos. Arch Med Res. 2001;32:619–26.
83. Lavranos TC, Rathjen PD, Seamark RF. Trophic effects of myeloid leukaemia inhibitory factor (LIF) on mouse embryos. J Reprod Fertil. 1995;105:331–8.
84. Zolti M, Bider D, Benrafael Z, et al. Cytokine involvement in oocytes and early embryos. Fertil Steril. 1991;56:265–72.
85. Rappolee DA, Sturm KS, Behrendtsen O, et al. Insulin-like growth factor-II acts through an endogenous growth pathway regulated by imprinting in early mouse embryos. Genes Dev. 1992;6:939–52.
86. Osterlund C, Wramsby H, Pousette A. Temporal expression of platelet-derived growth factor (PDGF)-A and its receptor in human preimplantation embryos. Mol Hum Reprod. 1996;2: 507–12.
87. Brice EC, Wu JX, Muraro R, Adamson ED, Wiley LM. Modulation of mouse preimplantation development by epidermal growth-factor receptor antibodies, antisense RNA, and deoxyoligonucleotides. Dev Genet. 1993;14:174–84.
88. Babalola GO, Schultz RM. Modulation of gene-expression in the preimplantation mouse embryo by TGF-alpha and TGF-beta. Mol Reprod Dev. 1995;41:133–9.
89. Young LE, Sinclair KD, Wilmut I. Large offspring syndrome in cattle and sheep. Rev Reprod. 1998;3:155–63.
90. Young LE, Fernandes K, McEvoy TG, et al. Epigenetic change in IGF2R is associated with fetal overgrowth after sheep embryo culture. Nat Genet. 2001;27:153–4.
91. Hickman DL, Beebe DJ, Rodriguez-Zas SL, Wheeler MB. Comparison of static and dynamic medium environments for culturing of pre-implantation mouse embryos. Comp Med. 2002;52:122–6.
92. Gardner DK, Lane M. Amino-acids and ammonium regulate mouse embryo development in culture. Biol Reprod. 1993;48:377–85.

93. Johnson MH, Nasresfahani MH. Radical solutions and cultural-problems—could free oxygen radicals be responsible for the impaired development of preimplantation mammalian embryos in-vitro. Bioessays. 1994;16:31–8.
94. Fukui Y, Lee ES, Araki N. Effect of medium renewal during culture in two different culture systems on development to blastocysts from in vitro produced early bovine embryos. J Anim Sci. 1996;74:2752–8.
95. Clark SG, Walters EM, Beebe DJ, Wheeler MB. A novel integrated in vitro maturation and in vitro fertilization system for swine. Theriogenology. 2003;59:441.
96. Cheng W, Klauke N, Sedgwick H, Smith GL, Cooper JM. Metabolic monitoring of the electrically stimulated single heart cell within a microfluidic platform. Lab Chip. 2006;6: 1424–31.
97. Shackman JG, Dahlgren GM, Peters JL, Kennedy RT. Perfusion and chemical monitoring of living cells on a microfluidic chip. Lab Chip. 2005;5:56–63.
98. Mehta G, Mehta K, Sud D, et al. Quantitative measurement and control of oxygen levels in microfluidic poly(dimethylsiloxane) bioreactors during cell culture. Biomed Microdevices. 2007;9:123–34.
99. Papanikolaou EG, Camus M, Fatemi HM, et al. Early pregnancy loss is significantly higher after day 3 single embryo transfer than after day 5 single blastocyst transfer in GnRH antagonist stimulated IVF cycles. Reprod Biomed Online. 2006;12:60–5.
100. Lane M, Gardner DK. Selection of viable mouse blastocysts prior to transfer using a metabolic criterion. Hum Reprod. 1996;11:1975–8.
101. Bormann CL, Chisolm CN, Heo YS, Takayama S, Smith GD. Development of a sensitive assay to measure lactate production of preimplantation embryos. Fertil Steril. 2006;86:S115.
102. Katz-Jaffe MG, Gardner DK, Schoolcraft WB. Proteomic analysis of individual human embryos to identify novel biomarkers of development and viability. Fertil Steril. 2006;85: 101–7.
103. Katz-Jaffe MG, Schoolcraft WB, Gardner DK. Analysis of protein expression (secretome) by human and mouse preimplantation embryos. Fertil Steril. 2006;86:678–85.

Part III
Insemination Procedures

Chapter 11
Intrauterine Insemination

Gautam N. Allahbadia and Rubina Merchant

Introduction

Despite revolutionary advances in the field of assisted reproduction, such as in vitro fertilization (IVF), intracytoplasmic sperm injection (ICSI), and subzonal insemination (SUZI), intrauterine insemination (IUI) remains an inexpensive, noninvasive, and effective first-line therapy for selected patients with cervical factor, moderate male factor, unexplained infertility, immunological infertility, and infertility due to ejaculatory disorders and is now also proposed as a therapy for endometriosis, ovarian dysfunction, and even for tubal factor. Though the technique of IUI has essentially remained the same, several advances in the type of stimulation protocols, gonadotropins, sperm preparation techniques, and ultrasound monitoring have led to promising success rates with IUI. IUI involves a preprocedure evaluation including a thorough physical, clinical, and laboratory evaluation to determine the duration and etiology of infertility, semen quality, functional tubal status, and the follicular and uterine status. Controlled ovarian hyperstimulation with close monitoring of folliculogenesis and ovulation to avoid adverse complications, such as ovarian hyperstimulation syndrome (OHSS) and multiple pregnancies, may be used to obtain the adequate number of follicles. Following induction of ovulation with human chorionic gonadotropin (hCG), the processed semen sample is then inseminated in the uterine cavity. The objective in terms of preovulatory follicle number must be determined prior to stimulation in order to optimize the cycle outcome with a singleton birth [1]. IUI is the preferred conception-enhancing technique for women <35 years, functional tubes, short period of infertility, and moderate male infertility, particularly in technology-limited settings, and four to six IUI cycles may

G.N. Allahbadia, MD, DNB, FNAMS (✉) • R. Merchant, PhD
Rotunda - The Center for Human Reproduction, Bandra, Rotunda Blue Fertility Clinic and Keyhole Surgery Center, Shivaji Park, Rotunda Fertility Clinic and Keyhole Surgery Center, Andheri, Mumbai, India
e-mail: drallah@gmail.com; rubinamm@gmail.com

Z.P. Nagy et al. (eds.), *Clinical Embryology: A Practical Guide*,
DOI 10.1007/978-1-4614-8376-2_11,

be performed before considering alternate therapy such as IVF [2, 3]. It is the method of choice vs. timed intercourse or natural cycle IUI [1]. The following sections will deal with the indications for IUI, technique, stimulation protocols, alternative insemination techniques, and prognostic factors that determine the outcome.

Indications for IUI

Cervical Factor Infertility

In couples with a cervical factor, diagnosed by a well-timed, nonprogressive postcoital test with normal semen parameters [4], higher pregnancy rates (PRs) have been reported following IUI compared to expectant management (51% vs. 33%, respectively) [5] with acceptable pregnancy rates even without COH (9.7%) and without an increased risk for multiple pregnancy compared to COH (12.7%) [4]. Cumulative pregnancy rates of 19.7%, 36.8%, and 36.8% have been reported for a maximum of three IUI cycles in patients with a cervical factor without superovulation [6].

Male Factor Infertility

A male factor may be diagnosed if the semen analysis at an initial microscopic examination demonstrates low sperm count, motility, morphology, antisperm antibodies, or any combination of these, or advanced testing indicates subnormal sperm function. While IUI is considered the best first-line treatment and most cost-effective procedure for moderate male factor subfertility [7], severe male factor infertility with a significant deterioration in sperm parameters or function may necessitate a direct referral to IVF or ICSI in that order, depending on the degree of severity [8]. Pregnancy rates of 12.8%, 29.3%, and 38.3% for a maximum of three cycles have been reported in couples with a male factor without superovulation [6], 7% per cycle following COH-IUI with clomiphene citrate (CC), and 12% per cycle with follicle-stimulating hormone (FSH) with multiple birth rates averaging 13% [9].

Unexplained Infertility

Despite the belief that IVF may be a more cost-effective primary treatment option compared to IUI in lieu of the low success rates with IUI and the subsequent requirement for IVF in the event of failure [10], the results of randomized controlled trials (RCTs) using live birth rates rather than pregnancy rates, and taking into account efficacy, complications, especially multiple pregnancy rates, patient compliance and cost-efficiency, suggest that the initial treatment for idiopathic infertility should be IUI as opposed to IVF [11]. Although the pregnancy rate per cycle was higher in the IVF group than in the IUI groups [12.2% vs 7.4% (spontaneous cycle) and 8.7% (COH-IUI), respectively; $p = 0.09$], the cumulative pregnancy rate for IVF was not significantly better than that for IUI. Moreover, the drop-out rates before a maximum of six attempts were higher in the IVF group compared to the IUI groups (42% vs. 15% and 16%, respectively; $p < 0.01$) [12].

Tubal Factor

Lower cumulative PRs have been reported in couples with isolated unilateral tubal occlusion compared to unexplained infertility after three cycles of COH-IUI (30.9% vs. 42.6%); cumulative PRs were lower in to women with mid-distal or distal tubal occlusion compared to women with proximal tubal occlusion (19% vs. 38.2%) and significantly lower than in women with unexplained infertility (19% vs. 42.6%, respectively). Hence, though, COH-IUI can be suggested as the initial treatment of choice in patients with unilateral proximal tubal occlusion, patients with mid-distal or distal tubal occlusion on hysterosalpingography (HSG) should be referred for laparoscopic assessment or IVF [13].

Endometriosis

An estrogen-dependent disorder, defined as the presence of endometrial tissue outside of the uterine cavity, endometriosis is a leading cause of infertility with a prevalence of 0.5–5% in the fertile and 25–40% in infertile women [14]. Controlled ovarian hyperstimulation with IUI is recommended in early-stage and surgically corrected endometriosis when the pelvic anatomy is normal, while combined surgery with gonadotropin-releasing hormone (GnRH) analogue treatment has been proposed to be a first-line therapy followed by IVF as second-line therapy in advanced cases [15]. Comparable clinical PRs per cycle have been reported in women with minimal, mild endometriosis and unexplained infertility (21% vs. 18.9% vs. 20.5%) following COH-IUI with comparative cumulative live birth rates within four cycles of COH and IUI (70.2%, 68.2%, 66.5%, respectively); CPR/cycle with or without COH-IUI was lower in women with surgically untreated minimal to mild endometriosis than in women with unexplained infertility [16]. However, in patients with minimal or mild endometriosis with pathological utero-tubal transport documented by hysterosalpingoscintigraphy (HSSG), IUI yields poor pregnancy rates despite normal semen parameters and patent Fallopian tubes, necessitating recourse to IVF/ICSI [17]. Though IVF reduces time to pregnancy in early-stage disease compared to controls, it does not increase the chance of pregnancy after three years [18].

In patients with stage IV endometriosis and in women >38 years of age, significantly higher PR, fecundity, and cumulative fecundity have been reported following IVF-ET compared to COH-IUI. Hence, IVF-ET should be the first-line approach in the management of infertility in such patients, and if COH-IUI is attempted, it should not exceed 3–4 cycles [19].

Contraindications

IUI may be contraindicated in women with sperm-immobilizing antibodies owing to antibodies secreted in the female reproductive tract that might impair sperm passage, inhibit fertilization, and prevent normal postfertilization processes [20]. Couples with severe male factor infertility, abnormal pelvic anatomy, not amenable to microsurgical repair, Fallopian tube disease with an impaired ampullary mucosal architecture, advanced stage endometriosis (stages III and IV), or minimal/mild endometriosis (stages I and II) with documented failure in tubal transport may directly benefit from IVF/ICSI with or without surgical interventions. The total antral follicle number is reported to decrease with age ($P < 0.0001$). In women >35 years with antral follicle counts (AFCs) <5, the application of COH/IUI may not be indicated [21].

Workup Before IUI

Major causes of infertility include male factors, ovarian dysfunction, tubal disease, endometriosis, and uterine or cervical factors. A careful history and physical examination of each partner can reveal the underlying etiology and guide further management of infertility.

Investigations that must be carried out in the female partner include:

- Evaluation of folliculogenesis and documentation of ovulation by transvaginal sonography (TVS) or with a home urinary luteinizing hormone kit.
- Evaluation of the functional tubal status by HSG, confirmed by a laparohysteroscopy in case of an abnormality, which has diagnostic and therapeutic power and may guide future management.

Further, a HSSG in patients with minimal or mild endometriosis may help document pathological uterotubal transport characteristic of the disease, necessitating IVF/ICSI despite normal semen parameters [17].

- A complete hormone evaluation including FSH, luteinizing hormone (LH), thyroid hormone profile.
- Ovarian reserve testing of FSH and estradiol (E2) levels on day 3 of the menstrual cycle, the clomiphene citrate challenge test, or pelvic ultrasonography for

AFC in women >35 years to determine treatment options and the likelihood of success [22].
- Testing for antisperm antibodies (ASAB) in the serum and cervical mucus.
- Infections such as chlamydial salpingitis, genital tract tuberculosis trachomatis, *Chlamydia trachomatis, and Neisseria gonorrhea.*
- Testing for HIV/hepatitis.

Male Partner

- A thorough semen analysis. Abnormal seminograms of infertile men may be classified as azoospermia-no sperm in the ejaculate, oligozoospermia (sperm count <15 million/mL), cryptozoospermia (spermatozoa absent from fresh preparations but observed in a centrifuged pellet), teratozoospermia (normal sperm morphology <4%), asthenozoospermia (progressive motility <32%), necrozoospermia (>58% dead sperm), or a combination of any of these conditions.
- Sperm function tests to evaluate sperm survival, viability, acrosome reaction, sperm fertilizing ability.
- Testing for antisperm antibodies.
- Semen culture and sensitivity to evaluate infection.
- Testing for HIV/hepatitis.

Natural Cycles or Controlled Ovarian Hyperstimulation?

IUI may be performed with or without controlled ovarian hyperstimulation depending on the patient characteristics.

Natural Cycles

A majority of studies have reported better IUI outcomes in terms of the number of preovulatory follicles, clinical and ongoing pregnancy rates (OPRs), and live birth rates following ovulation induction (OI) compared with the natural cycle [23–28]. Significantly higher pregnancy rates have been reported following ovulation induction with CC/CC + gonadotropins/gonadotropins alone compared to natural cycles in husband (AIH) inseminations [26, 27] (Table 11.1), while no significant differences were observed between natural cycles and donor insemination cycles [27]. The overall pregnancy rates for AIH and DI cycles were 8.6% and 20.2%, respectively [27] Pittrof et al. [23] reported a significantly higher number of preovulatory follicles (43.6%, 59.9%, 12.6%, $P < 0.0001$) and significantly higher pregnancy rates ($P = 0.038$) in CC/tamoxifen + gonadotropin – stimulated cycles

Table 11.1 Comparison in the clinical pregnancy rates following stimulation with various regimens and IUI

		Stimulation regimens								
	Natural		CC + gonadotropins			Aromatase inhibitors		Gonadotropins		
Study	cycles	CC	hMG	rFSH	Tx + G	Letrozole	L + rFSH	hMG	rFSH	*P* value
Baysoy et al. [41]						18.4		15.7[a]		
Tehrani Nejad et al. [40]			14.3			32.8				<0.01
Gregoriou et al. [45]						8.9			14.0	
Barroso et al. [38]				20			23.8[b]			
Mitwally and Casper [43]							26.5		18.5	
Bedaiwy et al. [42]							15.77		18.07	
Mahani and Afnan [25]	2.0 (12.0)	4.0 (7.0)	7.0 (16.0)					9.0 (23.0)		
Pittrof et al. [23]	20.1		23.6		29.9					0.038
Chen and Liu [26]	11.35		19.61							<0.01
Custers et al. [27]	6.3	12.5	16.4					11.2		

CC was administered at a dose of 100 mg/day from day 3 to 7 of the menstrual cycle. Letrozole was administered at a dose of 5 mg/day from day 3 to 7 of the menstrual cycle unless otherwise specified. Gonadotropins were administered at a dose of 75 IU from day 6 to 7 of the menstrual cycle until hCG administration

Values in brackets represent CPR/patient

Tx + G tamoxifen + gonadotropins

[a]hMG was administered on day 3 at a dose of 75 IU for women <30 years old and 150 IU for women >30 years old

[b]Letrozole was administered at a dose of 2.5 mg/day from day 3 to 7 of the menstrual cycle

compared to natural cycles [23]. However, Chen and Liu [26] concluded that though stimulated IUI is superior to natural cycle IUI cycles in patients <35 years, natural cycle is preferable for patients ≥35 years. There were no significant differences in the abortion and delivery rates between the OI and the natural cycle insemination ($P > 0.05$) [26]. IUI in the spontaneous cycle carries fewer health risks than does IUI after mild hormonal stimulation and therefore, should be the first-choice treatment [12].

Controlled Ovarian Hyperstimulation

Controlled ovarian hyperstimulation (COH) can be used in conjunction with IUI in couples with infertility factors not involving the Fallopian tubes to increase the number of available oocytes at the site of fertilization [29, 30]. Ovarian stimulation is initiated after the selection of the dominant follicle, mostly on the fifth day of the cycle. Several drugs, including clomiphene citrate (CC), tamoxifen, aromatase inhibitors, and gonadotropins alone or in conjunction with GnRH agonist/antagonist, have been used for ovulation induction in various protocols that may be individually tailored according to the patient. These regimens and protocols and clinical evidence of their benefits are discussed in the following sections.

Clomiphene Citrate

Ovarian stimulation by clomiphene citrate (CC) and IUI remains the first-choice treatment for ovulatory dysfunction, unexplained infertility, endometriosis, or male subfertility [27] with pregnancy rates averaging 7% per cycle [8]. Clomiphene citrate, an antiestrogenic agent is often administered for 5 days from day 3 to 7 of the menstrual cycle in doses of 50 mg once/twice a day. However, pelvic abnormalities, especially ovarian cysts, must be excluded prior to CC administration. Owing to the negative influence of CC on endometrial thickness, the medication should be reduced to 3 days in patients with retarded endometrial growth confirmed by ultrasonography [31]. Though no consensus exists about the drug of first choice to be used as hyperstimulation and there are no significant differences in clinical pregnancy (38% vs. 34.3%) and live birth rates (28.2% vs. 26.9%) between CC and rFSH, a randomized multicenter parallel trial concluded that being less expensive, CC seems the more cost-effective drug and therefore, can be offered as drug of first choice [32].

Gonadotropins

Gonadotropins, such as FSH and human menopausal gonadotropin (hMG), alone or in conjunction with GnRH agonist/antagonist, are often used for ovulation induction. The dose and mode of administration of gonadotropins are adjusted according to the individual patient and may be varied depending on the response. The response of the patient to gonadotropins is monitored regularly by TVS.

A meta-analysis of 43 trials involving 3,957 women concluded that gonadotropins might be the most effective drugs when IUI is combined with ovarian hyperstimulation, yielding higher pregnancy rates compared to antiestrogens, comparable PRs with different types of gonadotropins, no improvement with GnRH agonist or antagonist but increased multiple pregnancy rates and OHSS rates with increased doses of gonadotropins, and significantly higher multiple pregnancy rates with the agonist. When gonadotropins are used for ovarian stimulation, low-dose protocols are advised since pregnancy rates do not differ from those obtained with high-dose regimens, whereas the chances to encounter negative effects from ovarian stimulation such as multiple pregnancies and OHSS are limited with low-dose gonadotropins. Further research is needed for each comparison made [33]. No significant differences have been reported among low-dose gonadotropin protocols that differed in gonadotropin dosage (4/6/8/ampoules of 75 IU FSH) or the mode of administration in terms of cycle parameters, suggesting that an individualized and more intensive approach to ovarian stimulation is necessary for many women with unexplained infertility [34]. Lyophilized urinary hMG (HP-hMG) and rFSH are equally suitable in mild ovarian stimulation for IUI in patients with unexplained infertility. However, data derived from a larger study population are needed to determine whether higher amounts of two gonadotropins in this subgroup might produce any benefits or unfavorable effects [35].

With regard to the mode of administration, daily recombinant FSH (follitropin-beta) stimulation has been associated with higher CPRs (42% vs. 19%, respectively), higher total recombinant FSH dose (825 IU vs. 625 IU), and endometrial thickness (10.1 mm vs. 9.3 mm) compared to alternate-day FSH stimulation in women with anovulatory or unexplained infertility for over 12 months who had not responded to or not conceived with CC treatment though the duration of stimulation and the median number of follicles over 14 mm, AFC, and day-3 serum FSH were comparable between the groups. However, prospective randomized trials would be needed to determine whether this is indeed the case [36]. Mahani and Afnan [25] reported the highest CPRs/cycle and CPR/patient following IUI in patients stimulated with hMG compared with CC, CC + hMG, or natural cycle.

Combination Protocols

Clomiphene citrate may be used in conjunction with gonadotropins/dexamethasone for stimulation. Combination protocols are less costly and equally effective, with potentially fewer multiple births than with gonadotropins alone with fewer days of injections and fewer ampoules used. The advantages of a combination protocol in terms of pregnancy rates are depicted in Table 11.1. Although tamoxifen (40 mg/day from day 3 to 9) may not be a first-line treatment in patients with adequate endometrium, it may be a promising alternative for patients with a thin endometrium, yielding increased endometrial thickness ($P < 0.001$), CPR ($P = 0.015$), decreased early miscarriage rate ($P = 0.001$), and thus, improved ongoing pregnancy ($P < 0.001$) rate compared to CC (100 mg/day for 5 days) and despite a higher gonadotropin dose and stimulation duration and fewer follicles larger than 14 mm than clomiphene-treated patients [37].

Aromatase Inhibitors

Studies have reported a beneficial effect of the use of the aromatase inhibitor Letrozole (2.5–5 mg/day from day 3 to 7 of the IUI cycle) alone/coadministered with gonadotropins compared to CC, CC + gonadotropins, or gonadotropins alone in terms of comparable if not higher CPR/cycle and take home baby rates. Significantly higher serum levels of LH, endometrial thickness, and progesterone at the time of hCG administration have been observed despite a significantly lower serum E2 level [37–39] with significantly lower costs, risks, and patient inconvenience in patients with unexplained infertility [37, 38, 40, 41] endometriosis, and combined indications [42], and lower FSH dose requirement and IUI cancelation rates in patients with ovulatory infertility [43] and older infertile women [39]. Letrozole may be more effective than clomiphene and tamoxifen in a combination protocol [44] and beneficial in patients who fail to respond to CC [45] (Table 11.1). The improved follicular response to aromatase inhibitors has been attributed to aromatase inhibition, a release in the estrogenic negative feedback, increased endogenous FSH secretion, and increased follicular sensitivity to FSH [43].

Stimulation Protocols

Various gonadotropin stimulation protocols have been employed depending on the patient characteristics. Stimulation may be initiated on the first day of a cycle (the short protocol), or in the cycle preceding the "proper" stimulation cycle (the long protocol).

The Short GnRH Analogue Protocol

GnRH analogue (0.1 mg Decapeptyl/triptorelin) is administered daily from the first day of a cycle until hCG administration resulting in a gonadotropin flare-up effect. Gonadotropin administration (hMG/FSH) is initiated from the third day of the cycle in a step-up/step-down protocol, doses being adjusted individually according to patient requirements.

Step-Up Protocol

Generally, hMG is administered in a daily dose of 150 IU that may be stepped up to 225 IU when one or more follicles are ≥14 mm and the dose maintained until hCG administration. Low-dose step-up FSH treatment has been associated with a significant reduction in the incidence of OHSS compared to the conventional dose (8.3% vs. 27.1%, $P < 0.05$) and a significant decrease in the incidence of moderate OHSS requiring hospitalization (0% vs. 16.7%, $P < 0.01$) in patients with unexplained infertility despite comparable pregnancy rates. However, multiple pregnancies cannot be completely prevented with the low-dose protocol [46].

Step-Down Protocol

Gonadotropins (hMG) are administered in a daily dose of 225 IU that may be stepped down to 150 IU if an excessive reaction to stimulation is expected.

The Short GnRH Antagonist Protocol

Fixed Dose Protocol

Following the initiation of gonadotropins on day 3 of the menstrual cycle, antagonists, such as cetrorelix/ganirelix, are administered in a fixed dose (0.25–0.5 mg/day) when one or more follicles are ≥14 mm until hCG administration.

Incremental Dose Protocol

Following the initiation of gonadotropins on day 3 of the menstrual cycle, antagonists, cetrorelix/ganirelix, are administered in an incremental dose (0.25 mg/day when the leading follicles are 14 mm and increased to 0.5 mg when the leading follicles are 16 mm) until hCG administration.

The Long GnRH Analogue Protocol

The long agonist protocol involves the subcutaneous (s.c.) administration of 0.1 mg Decapeptyl from the midluteal phase (the 21st day of the cycle preceding the proper stimulation cycle) and until hCG administration. Optimally, gonadotropin stimulation is initiated following pituitary downregulation, identified by estradiol (E2) levels <50 pg/mL and no ovarian follicle larger than 14 mm. However, stimulation may be started if there is a follicle >14 mm with E2 levels <50 pg/mL. Gonadotropins may be administered in a step-up or step-down protocol [32].

Ultralong Agonist Protocol

The ultralong agonist protocol (ULP) involves the subcutaneous (s.c.) administration of a single injection of 3.75 mg Decapeptyl followed by daily s.c. Decapeptyl (0.1 mg) administration 4 weeks later and until hCG administration. Gonadotropin stimulation is initiated once pituitary desensitization is achieved as assessed by serum E2 levels ≤100 MIU/mL. hCG, 10,000 IU, is administered when one or more leading follicles are ≥18 mm followed by IUI on evidence of follicular rupture on TVS or 34–36 h after hCG administration.

A protocol of recombinant FSH (50 IU daily) and ganirelix (0.25 mg) fixed dose protocol is reported to represent an effective and safe regimen for ovulation induction, associated with a lower rate of mono-ovulation (53.3% vs. 78.8%, $P = 0.06$), and higher CPR per initiated cycle (34.4% vs. 5.9%, $P = 0.005$) compared to alternate-day FSH treatment in couples with unexplained infertility or moderate male subfertility [47]. However, the efficacy of the antagonist in preventing premature luteinization is disputed with some studies reporting in favor [48] and others against [49, 50].

Expectant Management

Some randomized trials report that COH-IUI and unstimulated IUI do not offer substantial benefit in couples with unexplained subfertility in terms of CPRs, OPRs, or live birth rates compared with expectant management, and expectant management for a period of 6 months therefore appears justified in these couples [51, 52].

Semen Parameters and Processing

Semen Parameters to Consider

Semen parameters that must be considered in an IUI program include the semen processing time, processed total motile sperm count, rapid progressive motility after processing, sperm morphology before and after processing, inseminating motile sperm count (IMSC), IUI insemination time, and 24-h sperm survival.

Delaying semen processing from 30 min up to 1 h and/or delaying IUI from 90 min up to 2 h after collection compromises the pregnancy outcome in gonadotropin-IUI cycles [53]. A universal threshold level above which IUI can be performed with acceptable pregnancy rates has not been determined yet [7]. However, IUI success may be impaired in couples with processed total motile sperm (PTMS) <10 million [54] sperm survival <70% [55], <5% normal spermatozoa, inseminating motile count (IMC) $<1 \times 10^6$ [7], and prewash IUI-semen pregnancy score (IUI-SPS) <150 [56], necessitating alternative therapy. The PTMS count has been independently associated with fertility after IUI (P = 0.0014) [54]. PTMS $\geq 10 \times 10^6$, their 24-h sperm survival threshold of ≥70% [55], normal morphology before sperm separation ≥15.5% [odds ratio (OR) = 2.2, (P = 0.02)], rapid, progressive motility ≥25.5% after sperm separation (P = 0.029), and curvilinear velocity (VCL) after sperm separation ≥102.65 μm/s (P = 0.002) independently predict pregnancy outcome in patients with male factor infertility [57]. These variables would be helpful in counseling patients for future management [57].

Semen Preparation Techniques

The rationale behind semen preparation techniques for assisted reproduction is the separation of motile morphologically normal spermatozoa from leucocytes, bacteria, and dead spermatozoa that produce oxygen radicals that negatively influence the ability of sperm to fertilize the egg [58].

There are several sperm separation techniques, and these are based on different principles like migration, filtration, or density gradient centrifugation (DGC). However, the kind of technique employed entirely depends on the quality of the semen ejaculate (i.e., count, motility, morphology, sperm survival, vitality) at an initial evaluation, prior to processing the sample. An ideal preparation technique would be rapid and inexpensive, would isolate all the motile sperms without damaging their fertilizing capacity, and would ensure that the adequate number of motile, functionally normal spermatozoa is present at the site of fertilization following IUI.

The double DGC with different media (IxaPrep, Nycodenz, SilSelect, PureSperm, or Isolate) and the swim-up technique are the standard techniques in use and have been detailed in other chapters in the book. The swim-up technique (with or without centrifugation) depends entirely on the initial sperm count and percentage of progressive motility. Though swim-up yields a high number of progressively motile sperm and effectively separates sperm from bacteria and cell debris, it is of limited use in cases of low sperm count. DGC involves the use of different density gradients to separate cells by the density during centrifugation. It may be used to obtain a high yield of motile spermatozoa from poor quality samples with borderline to moderate oligozoospermia/asthenozoospermia. Discretion at this point is very essential. It must be remembered that while a single sperm defect, i.e., a poor count may be rescued with DGC, a combination of defects will yield poor postprocess results. The glass wool filtration technique may also be used for a high yield of motile spermatozoa. Owing to concerns that centrifugation increases reactive oxygen species (ROS) formation in semen and that high levels of ROS are associated with sperm membrane injury through spontaneous lipid peroxidation, which may alter sperm function, ejaculates with ROS production should not be centrifuged. The time of centrifugation is more important than the *g*-force for inducing ROS formation in semen, and a shorter centrifugation period in the preparation of sperm for assisted reproductive techniques may be beneficial [28].

Swim-down, refrigeration/heparin techniques, and filtration methods, such as the SpermPrep method and membrane-based electrophoretic filtration system [Cell

Sorter-10 (CS-10)], are some of the other techniques that have been in use. The SpermPrep method is a Sephadex preparation with a different bead size that offers quicker, improved semen manipulation for patients with oligozoospermia and/or asthenozoospermia [59] while the Cell Sorter-10 (CS-10) preferentially isolates spermatozoa with very low levels of DNA damage. Noncentrifugation methods include a novel Zech device that is a dual-chamber capillary dish that obviates the potential harmful effects of centrifugation on sperm.

Advanced Sperm Preparation Methods

The advanced methods for semen preparation include molecular sperm selection strategies such as hyaluronic acid-mediated sperm selection, annexin V magnetic-activated cell separation (MACS) that utilizes colloidal superparamagnetic micro-beads (approximately 50 nm in diameter) conjugated with annexin V to separate apoptotic and nonapoptotic spermatozoa, and annexin V molecular glass wool filtration [60].

Density Gradient Centrifugation versus Swim-Up/Sperm Wash

DGC techniques, utilizing PureSperm, yield significantly higher median total motile sperm counts (TMSC) [32.2×10^6 vs. 17.6×10^6], higher recovery rates of mature motile sperm (69.2% vs. 50.0%), longevity at 4 h (83.0% vs. 55.0%), postthaw recovery, and better preserve semen quality in fresh and cryopreserved semen compared to swim-up [61]. They yield higher pregnancy rates compared to sperm wash (14.3% vs. 11.6%, respectively; 18% vs. 4%, respectively for samples with <22 million motile sperm in the inseminate) [62] and significant sperm enrichment compared to Isolate (50% and 90%) [sperm recovery rates (30.0% vs. 19.7%, respectively)] [61]. Swim-up yields a significantly higher mean percentage of viable sperm but significantly lower recovery rates of total motile, progressively motile, and viable sperm compared with DGC despite similar low rates of apoptotic sperm [63]. Hence, while samples with an acceptable number of motile sperm can be processed efficiently by wash only, poor quality semen samples should be processed using DGC. The percentage of sperm in the original semen sample with a velocity of ≥80 μm/s for the wash method influences the pregnancy outcome [62]. However, a meta-analysis of five parallel RCTs failed to demonstrate a significant benefit of one technique over the other and concluded insufficient evidence to recommend any specific preparation technique. Further, large high-quality randomized trials are warranted [58].

The combination of DGC and MACS is reported to be superior to all other sperm preparation methods, providing motile, viable, and nonapoptotic spermatozoa [64], improved cryosurvival rates [65], significant improvement in induced acrosome reaction test (IART) ($P < 0.001$) [66] with an improved ability to fertilize eggs using the hamster oocyte penetration assay [60], and significantly reduced levels of apoptotic markers versus DGC alone ($P < 0.001$) [66]. Because of a wide variety of ejaculate qualities, which influence the functions of spermatozoa to a great extent, the efficacy of different preparation methods will vary; hence, the technique to be used must be individually tailored.

IUI in Practice: Description of the Procedure

Timing of Insemination

IUI may be timed 34–36 h after the administration of 10,000 IU hCG intramuscularly, which may be timed following evidence of one or more follicles ≥18 mm during ultrasound monitoring of folliculogenesis and an endometrial thickness >7 mm (with triple-line development). Alternatively, IUI may be timed following sonographic evidence of follicular rupture and free fluid in the pouch of Douglas, or following biochemical evidence of an LH surge. A meta-analysis of seven controlled trials (2,623 patients), examining the effectiveness of hCG administration before IUI on CPRs in comparison with LH detection, failed to demonstrate a consistent, clinically important benefit of hCG-induced ovulation compared with LH monitoring of spontaneous ovulation for IUI timing [67]. Despite comparable pregnancy rates between hCG-induced ovulation and LH surge (an increase in LH level ≥200% over a mean of preceding 2 days) timed IUI, a significantly longer time to IUI, significantly higher cancelation rates (31% vs. 11%) attributed mainly to failure to detect an LH surge [68], and favorable outcomes limited only to CC-induced cycles [69] have been reported suggesting that the decision to use hCG for IUI timing should be influenced by factors other than pregnancy rates [68]. Postponing IUI until the observation of follicle rupture at transvaginal ultrasonography may yield a higher pregnancy rate (23.5% vs. 8.8%, respectively; $p < 0.001$) in couples with unexplained infertility and male factor subfertility [70].

With regard to the ovulation inducing agent, a subcutaneous injection of a relatively low dose of GnRHa [triptorelin (Decapeptyl), 0.1 mg] can be as effective as hCG (10,000 IU) after follicular maturation in producing pregnancy in COH-IUI treatment cycles in patients presenting with amenorrhea, oligomenorrhea, or unexplained infertility with comparative conception rates (15.3% vs. 26.5%), abortion rates (18.2% vs. 33.3%), and term pregnancy rates (13.6% vs. 19.0%), respectively [71].

Insemination Procedure

IUI is performed with the patient in the dorsal lithotomy position on an empty bladder. The Cusco speculum is inserted, the cervical os is identified, and the cervix is cleaned with a swab of sterile saline. The os may be held in place with a volsellum, if necessary. Meanwhile, in the laboratory, an atraumatic Wallace ET catheter is loaded with 0.5 mL of processed sperm. The catheter is inserted into the uterine cavity without touching the fundus and the sperm suspension is gradually released. The patient is advised to rest in the same position for 15–20 min prior to discharge. Immobilization for 15 min after insemination yields significantly higher OPR per couple (27% vs. 18%) and live birth rates (27% vs. 17%) compared to the control group [72].

Luteal Phase Support

Following IUI, luteal phase support may be achieved with transvaginal administration of micronized progesterone (200 mg/day) or vaginal progesterone gel (Crinone 8% gel) for 2 weeks. A clinical pregnancy may be documented following sonographic evidence of a gestational sac with heart beats at 6 weeks of amenorrhea, and an ongoing pregnancy by >12 weeks of amenorrhea. Luteal phase support with vaginal progesterone gel (Crinone 8% gel) significantly affects the success of ovarian stimulation and IUI cycles in patients with unexplained infertility, yielding significantly higher CPR/cycle and per patient (21.1% and 39.4%, respectively) compared to patients who received no luteal phase support (12.7% and 23.8%, respectively) [73]. Alternatively, intranasal administration of a GnRH agonist (buserelin) could be effective in providing luteal support with good pregnancy rates (28%) [74].

Postprocedure Care

Patients can pursue their routine activity following IUI but must take care to avoid excess physical exertion. Signs of spotting or bleeding must be reported immediately.

Single vs. Double Insemination

Studies have reported significantly better pregnancy outcomes following double insemination (12 and 34 h after hCG administration) versus single insemination (34–36 h after hCG administration) in couples with ovulatory dysfunction, endometriosis, male factor, unexplained infertility, tubal factor, and combined diagnoses, particularly within gonadotropin protocols and ovulatory dysfunction and male factor diagnostic categories, and despite a significantly lower female age in the single IUI group [75] and slightly higher cost of double IUI [76]. However, a recent meta-analysis of six RCTs, involving 829 women, failed to demonstrate a clear benefit of double IUI versus single IUI in the overall CPR in couples with unexplained infertility [77]. Despite the 36th h being the preferred timing for IUI, no statistical difference regarding pregnancy rates has been reported between single 24th h and double 12th- and 36th-h inseminations in patients with unexplained infertility, male factor, and ovulatory dysfunction following COH with gonadotropin + IUI, suggesting that that the 24th-h IUI might be preferred in demanding situations [78].

IUI vs. Timed Intercourse (TI)

Despite evidence of a significant benefit of IUI over TI in two large meta-analyses in terms of the probability of conception, both in natural cycles and in COH cycles, with COH (gonadotropins)-IUI offering the best chance of conception in couples with male subfertility [29] and ovulatory infertility [79], a recent meta-analysis [80] failed to demonstrate a significant clinical benefit in terms of pregnancy rates between stimulated and natural cycle IUI, natural cycle TI/IUI, or stimulated IUI/TI. It concluded insufficient data to perform a statistical analysis or to recommend or advise against IUI with or without COH above TI, or vice versa, or to document adverse outcomes such as OHSS, multiple pregnancy, miscarriage rate, and ectopic pregnancy [80]. Timed intercourse following IUI with a low number of motile sperm is an alternative treatment that appears to be a practical, simple, and an inexpensive addition that significantly increases the pregnancy rates over IUI alone (27.7% vs. 10.5%, $P = 0.023$) in infertile couples with a normal sperminogram [81].

Number of Cycles

There is general agreement in the literature that 4–6 IUI cycles may be performed with acceptable pregnancy rates before resorting to alternative therapy [62, 82] though studies have reported acceptable OPR in high-order IUI cycles up to nine [27]. More than four cycles of CC-IUI can compensate for low pregnancy rates due to age, semen quality, or follicle number in patients with ovulation dysfunction. Significantly lower mean PRs have been reported in patients ≥43 years with poor semen quality, single preovulatory follicles, and diagnoses other than ovulatory dysfunction compared to those after four (CPRs 46% for ovulatory dysfunction; 38% for cervical factor, male factor, and unexplained infertility; 34% for endometriosis; and 26% for tubal factor) or six (CPRs 65% for ovulation dysfunction, 35% for endometriosis, and unchanged for other diagnoses) cycles [82]. Morshedi et al. [62] reported 88% of pregnancies in the first three cycles of IUI and 95.5% within the first four cycles with an overall CPR/cycle of 13.0% and CPR/patient of 28.3% per with a miscarriage rate of 34.0% [62]. Aboulghar et al. [83] reported significantly higher cycle fecundity in the first three trials of COH-IUI than in cycles 4–6 (16.4% vs. 5.6%, $P < 0.001$, $n = 594$, 1,112 cycles) suggesting that COH-IUI for the treatment of unexplained infertility should be limited to a maximum of three trials and patients should be offered IVF or ICSI if they fail to conceive after three trials of COH and IUI [83]. Moreover Qublan et al. [84] reported an increased incidence and recurrence rate of luteinized unruptured follicle (LUF) among patients with preexisting LUF undergoing multiple IUI cycles. The incidence of LUF was 56.5% in the second cycle of IUI treatment with recurrence rate of 78.6%, and 58.9% among patients who underwent three consecutive IUI cycles with a recurrence rate of 90%. In these patients, other options of infertility treatment might be justified [84]. The use of clomiphene citrate for unexplained fertility for more than 12 cycles of IUI has been associated with a threefold increase in risk of ovarian cancer [85].

Intrauterine versus Other Forms of Artificial Insemination

Intracervical Insemination

Sperm may be deposited in or around the endocervical canal (cervical insemination—CI) or in the uterine cavity itself (IUI). IUI has been considered potentially more effective than CI as the sperm bypass the cervical mucus and are deposited closer to the Fallopian tubes. The cost and risks of IUI, on the other hand, may be higher because of the need for sperm preparation, the introduction of foreign material into the uterus [86] and the consequent risk of infection and anaphylaxis [87]. Significantly improved pregnancy rates and live birth rates without a statistically significant evidence of an effect on multiple pregnancies or miscarriages have been reported following six cycles of stimulated IUI with CC/gonadotropins using cryopreserved sperm in comparison to cervical insemination [86].

Fallopian Tube Sperm Perfusion

Fallopian tube sperm perfusion (FSP) is based on the pressure injection of 4 mL of sperm suspension with the attempt of sealing of the cervix to prevent semen reflux [34] and ensures the presence of higher sperm densities in the Fallopian tubes at the time of ovulation than does standard IUI [88]. The IUI technique on the other hand is based on intrauterine injection of 0.5 mL of sperm suspension without flushing the tubes [30]. Despite previous reports of the advantages of FSP in terms of higher CPR and OPR/patient, reduced cost and complications in couples with unexplained infertility compared to IUI [89, 90], a recent meta-analysis of eight randomized controlled studies involving 595 couples with nontubal subfertility including a subgroup analysis in couples with unexplained subfertility reported no clear benefit for FSP over IUI [88]. In couples with long-standing infertility, intraperitoneal insemination (IPI), FSP, and IUI have similar efficacy in the achievement of a clinical pregnancy [91].

Intrauterine tuboperitoneal insemination (IUTPI) with 10 mL of inseminate has been proposed as a useful technique in the treatment of unexplained infertility, mild or moderate male infertility, and mild or moderate endometriosis compared to FSP (CPR/cycle 29.4% vs. 17.6%), and three attempts of IUTPI may be beneficial before moving on to more invasive and expensive methods of assisted reproduction [92].

Risks and Complications of IUI

Early Complications: Risks of the Procedure

Though complications after IUI are rare, studies have reported slight cervical contact bleeding and mild abdominal discomfort and/or cramps [93]. Vaginal administration of misoprostol at the time of IUI is associated with a significant increase in vaginal bleeding and abdominal cramping rates and does not seem to enhance the outcome [94]. Spontaneous abortions, blighted ovum, and ectopic pregnancies have been reported in 7.8%, 2.6%, and 1.3% of the pregnancies, respectively in COH-IUI cycles [95]. Infectious complications associated with IUI are frequently cited, though rarely reported. According to Sacks and Simon [96], most reported cases of infection fail to show evidence for the actual presence of infection, and the prevalence is unaltered by the administration of prophylactic antibiotics or washing the semen sample with antibiotics. *Escherichia coli* septicemia has been reported subsequent to IUI [97]. *Chlamydia trachomatis* infection, acquired as an intrauterine infection, as well as during transit through the birth channel, may result in a number of adverse pregnancy outcomes, including ectopic pregnancy, early and late abortion, intrauterine infections of the fetus, stillbirth, prematurity, premature rupture of the membranes (PROM), and postpartum endometritis [97].

Late Complications

Although IUI itself is less invasive and expensive than other techniques of assisted reproduction, the adverse effects of COH, such as OHSS and multiple pregnancies, are a concern [22, 24, 80]. Miscarriage rates ranging from 11.8% [6] to 34.0% [4] have been reported following COH-IUI.

Multiple Births

Multiple pregnancy rates following IUI are significantly influenced by age and etiology of the patient. Multiple pregnancy rates of 6.0% in unexplained and male subfertility [33], 13.2% in anovulatory infertility [98], and 23.5% in couples with exclusive female factors, such as anovulation, cervical factors, or unexplained infertility and a maximum of three IUI cycles, have been reported [99]. Multifollicular growth is associated with increased pregnancy rates following COH-IUI. Surpassing the recruitment of two follicles would lead to a dramatic increase in the risk of OHSS and multiple pregnancies without a substantial gain in overall pregnancy rate [100, 101]. According to van Rumste et al. [100], one stimulated follicle should be the goal if safety is the primary concern, whereas two follicles may be accepted after careful patient counseling. They reported an absolute pregnancy rate of 8.4% for monofollicular and 15% for multifollicular growth. Compared with monofollicular growth, pregnancy rates increased by 5% and 8%, while the risk of multiple pregnancies increased by 6%, 14%, and 10% when stimulating two, three, and four follicles. The absolute rate of multiple pregnancies was 0.3% after monofollicular and 2.8% after multifollicular growth [100]. In patients <35 years old, the incidence of multiple pregnancies, particularly ≥3 implantations tripled when ≥6 follicles were ≥12 mm in CC, hMG, and CC + hMG cycles, and when E2 levels were >1,000 pg mL in hMG and CC + hMG cycles. In patients ≥35 years, pregnancy rates in hMG and CC + hMG cycles doubled when six or more follicles were ≥12 mm, or E2 levels were >1,000 pg mL, whereas three or more implantations were not significantly increased [101].

Treatment strategies to reduce the incidence of multiple pregnancies in ovulation induction programs can be targeted to reduce multiple follicular development and subsequent ovulation by a more aggressive cancelation policy, follicle reduction by fine needle aspiration, conversion to IVF or dealing with the problem of multiple gestation after it has occurred (i.e., multifetal pregnancy reduction) [102]. Specifically, tailoring the rate of multifollicular development according to the duration and type of infertility (etiology, primary or secondary, female age) would prove to be a safer approach for achieving pregnancy as well as avoiding adverse effects such as the risk of OHSS and multiple pregnancies [103]. Withholding hCG or IUI in CC, hMG, and CC + hMG cycles when six or more follicles are ≥12 mm may reduce triplet and higher-order implantations by 67% without significantly reducing pregnancy rates for patients under 35 years of age [101]. According to Ragni et al. [104] in COH-IUI cycles, daily administration of 50 IU recombinant FSH with the use of GnRH antagonists and a policy of strict cancelation (if three or more follicles ≥16 mm and/or five or more follicles ≥11 mm) based on echographic criteria are associated with a satisfactory pregnancy rate per initiated cycle and a low risk of high-order multiple pregnancies. The CPR per initiated cycle was 9.2% with a 9.5% and 0% incidence of twins and high-order multiple pregnancies, respectively [104].

Success Rates with IUI

Factors Affecting Outcome

Overall CPRs/cycle ranging from 9.2% to 22% have been reported in the literature following stimulated IUI [4, 6, 7, 79, 96, 120] with live birth rates of 10% for CC-stimulated and 8.7% for rFSH-stimulated cycles [37]. Guven et al. [105] reported a PR of 7.9% in the primary infertility group and 21.4% in the secondary infertility group. However, these results are largely determined by the patient selection criteria, the sperm and follicular characteristics, and the stimulation protocol in the various studies.

Characterization of prognostic factors for pregnancy is essential, particularly those for women at risk of multiple pregnancies after IUI [106].

Favorable Predictors of IUI Outcome

The following factors have been reported as significant predictors of the pregnancy outcome following IUI.

- Patient's age ≤35 years, irrespective of the method of sperm preparation used [62]. A higher birth rate (25.8%) has been reported in women <35 years undergoing COH-IUI compared to women ≥35 years (14.0%) when four or more follicles were greater than or equal to 12 mm [107].
- Infertility etiology. Pregnancy rates/cycle may vary among women with different etiologies, being highest in anovulatory infertility (19.2%) and lowest in endometriosis-based infertility (11.9%). The cumulative pregnancy rates varied greatly by diagnosis from 16% for patients with male factor infertility to 60% for patients with ovulatory disorder [108]. Cervical factor yields a favorable outcome [109].
- Sperm parameters
  - Total motile sperm count (TMSC) before sperm preparation ($P > 0.05$) [105].
  - Sperm motility. Patients with original sperm motility ≥30% had a higher cumulative pregnancy rate (74%) than patients with motility <30% ($P < 0.005$) with a four times increase in PR with an increase in motility of ≥30% [110].
  - Progressive motility [99].
  - Normal sperm morphology [105, 106]. Significantly higher PRs have been reported with samples with normal sperm morphology of >4% (according to Kruger's criteria) compared to ≤4% (22.2% vs. 6.7%, respectively; $p = 0.003$) [105].
  - Processed total motile sperm count (PTMS) count $\geq 10 \times 10^6$ and 24-h survival of ≥70% can predict the IUI outcome with a 94% sensitivity and an 86% specificity [2]. An average TMSC of ten million may be a useful threshold value for decisions about treating a couple with IUI or IVF [111].
- Mild controlled ovarian hyperstimulation [107, 109, 112]. A significantly higher incidence of follicles (81% vs. 53%; $P < 0.05$) as well as cycles (63% vs. 49%; $P < 0.05$) with uniformly high-grade vascularity has been observed by transvaginal power Doppler ultrasonography on the day of insemination (32–36 h post-hCG administration) in COH-IUI cycles compared with unstimulated or clomiphene-induced donor cycles [112].

- Follicular dynamics.
  - Increase in the number of preovulatory follicles (1–4) at the time of hCG administration [2, 99, 109, 113].
  - Increase in AFC and, hence, increase in the dominant follicle number and E2 level on the day of hCG [7].
  - Serum E2 levels. Birth rate increased from 3.6% when E2 was <500 pg/mL to 19.6% when E2 was ≥2,500 pg/mL [109].
  - High-grade follicular vascularity. Higher pregnancy and lower early pregnancy loss rates have been observed in cycles with uniformly high-grade follicular vascularity, possibly attributed to COH, compared with other vascularity grades [112]. However, a recent study by Ragni et al. [114] reported that follicular vascularity (follicles with a mean diameter ≥16 mm) does not predict the chance of pregnancy in women undergoing mild COH and IUI [114].
- Endometrial thickness [99].
- Shorter duration of infertility [99].
- Cervical mucus aspiration before IUI [60].

The etiology of infertility and the stimulation protocol used may have a significant effect on the pregnancy outcome. Pregnancy rates of 36%, 25.0%, and 30% have been reported following stimulation with sequential CC and hMG and three follicles in patients with anovulatory infertility, male infertility, and combined infertility, respectively, 21.1% following CC stimulation in endometriosis-based infertility, and 24.3% with an IMC >30 × 10^6. Ovarian stimulation in unexplained infertility resulted in PRs of 24.2% and 19.8% with three follicles and an IMC >30 × 10^6, respectively [98].

Factors Predicting a Poor Prognosis

A significant negative correlation of the following factors with the IUI pregnancy outcome has been reported:

- Increasing maternal age ≥35 [107–109]. A 0.0% cumulative probability of ongoing pregnancy following three cycles of IUI in women ≥40 years has been reported compared to women <40 years (28.2%) irrespective of the infertility history, use of ovarian stimulation, or baseline semen parameters, suggesting that the treatment of male and/or cervical factor by IUI is ineffective for women ≥40 years [115]. Treatment with CC is ineffective, and delivery rates following COH with gonadotropins and IUI are <5%. Therefore, it is recommended that after a short trial of gonadotropins and IUI, women aged 40–41 years should be quickly referred to IVF. At an older age, IVF is the primary treatment option [116].
- Decreased basal AFC. In women >35 years with AFCs <5, the application of COH-IUI may not be indicated [21]. Low basal AFC is associated with lower clinical pregnancy and live birth rates in unexplained subfertile couples treated with COH-IUI [117].

- Male factor infertility with initial sperm motility <30% ($P < 0.002$), initial sperm count $<5 \times 10^6$ per mL ($P < 0.01$) [114], and normal sperm morphology <14% [112].
- Postwash TMSC ≤20 million/mL [108].
- Endometriosis and tubal factor-associated infertility [106–109].
- Uterine anomalies [109].
- Increasing number of cycles with more than four treatment cycles [107, 109].
- Longer duration of subfertility [109].
- Low midluteal progesterone (P4) level ≤25 nmol/L [118].

A recent study by Merviel et al. [119] concluded that the couple with the best chance of pregnancy following COH (gonadotropin)-IUI can be described as a woman <30 years with cervical or anovulatory infertility and a man with a TMS ≥5 million spermatozoa. The "ideal" stimulation cycle enables the recruitment of two follicles measuring >16 mm with an E2 concentration >500 pg/mL on the day of hCG administration. The best results are obtained when IUI is performed using a soft catheter [119]. Though male and female factors contribute to pregnancy outcome, the clinician can influence prognosis by increasing the number of follicles, especially in severe male factor cases [106].

Recent Advances

The transcriptome of spermatozoa used in homologous IUI reveals profound differences between expression profiles of sperm samples that impregnate successfully and those that do not. These differences might improve the predictive power of sperm evaluation to estimate IUI success by complementing the basic sperm analysis [120]. Three-dimensional (3D) and 3D power Doppler (PD) when used with 2D ultrasound and color Doppler for pre-hCG follicular assessment improve pregnancy rates in IUI cycles by enabling an assessment of the follicular volume, perifollicular resistance index, and perifollicular vascularity index, all of which may influence the conception rates [121].

Conclusion

IUI is a simple, cost-effective, noninvasive first-line therapy for cervical factor, anovulatory infertility, moderate male factor, unexplained infertility, and immunological infertility with CPRs ranging from 10% to 20%. Optimal pregnancy rates following COH with a low-dose gonadotropin protocol and IUI may be obtained in couples with a short duration of infertility where the woman's age is ≤35 years with a PTMS count $\geq 10 \times 10^6$ and a 24-h survival of ≥70%, normal sperm morphology of >4% (according to Kruger's criteria), 2–3 follicles ≥16 mm with uniformly high-grade vascularity and E2 levels >500 pg/mL on the day of hCG, adequate endometrium with a trilaminar pattern during insemination, and appropriately timed insemination using a soft atraumatic catheter. Strict patient selection criteria and individualized stimulation protocols tailored according to the age and etiology of the patient with a strict cycle cancelation policy will help to reduce the associated complications, such as multiple pregnancies and OHSS, while maximizing the overall pregnancy outcome. Three to six IUI cycles may be offered before considering alternate therapy. However, patients with advanced maternal age, severe male factor infertility, tubal pathology, or severe endometriosis will benefit from a direct referral to IVF/ICSI. Couples should be fully informed about the risks of IUI and COH as well as alternative treatment options. Larger randomized prospective controlled trials, investigating the important outcomes including live births, multiple pregnancies, miscarriage rates, and risk of ovarian hyperstimulation following IUI, are warranted.

References

1. De Sutter P. Rational diagnosis and treatment in infertility. Best Pract Res Clin Obstet Gynaecol. 2006;20(5):647–64.
2. Abdelkader AM, Yeh J. The potential use of intrauterine insemination as a basic option for infertility: a review for technology-limited medical settings. Obstet Gynecol Int. 2009; 2009:584837.
3. Katzorke T, Kolodziej FB. [Significance of insemination in the era of IVF and ICSI] (Article in German). Urologe A. 2010;49:842–6.
4. Steures P, van der Steeg JW, Verhoeve HR, van Dop PA, Hompes PG, Bossuyt PM, van der Veen F, Habbema JD, Eijkemans MJ, Mol BW. Does ovarian hyperstimulation in intrauterine insemination for cervical factor subfertility improve pregnancy rates? Hum Reprod. 2004;19(10):2263–6.
5. Steures P, van der Steeg JW, Hompes PG, Bossuyt PM, Habbema JD, Eijkemans MJ, Schöls WA, Burggraaff JM, van der Veen F, Mol BW, CECERM (Collaborative Effort for Clinical Evaluation in Reproductive Medicine). Effectiveness of intrauterine insemination in subfertile couples with an isolated cervical factor: a randomized clinical trial. Fertil Steril. 2007; 88(6):1692–6.
6. Check JH, Bollendorf A, Zaccardo M, Lurie D, Vetter B. Intrauterine insemination for cervical and male factor without superovulation. Arch Androl. 1995;35(2):135–41.
7. Ombelet W, Deblaere K, Bosmans E, Cox A, Jacobs P, Janssen M, Nijs M. Semen quality and intrauterine insemination. Reprod Biomed Online. 2003;7(4):485–92.
8. Aboulghar M, Baird DT, Collins J, Evers JL, Fauser BC, Lambalk CB, Somigliana E, Sunde A, Crosignani PG, Devroey P, Diczfalusy E, Diedrich K, Fraser L, Geraedts JP, Gianaroli L, Glasier A, Van Steirteghem A, Collins J, Crosignani PG, ESHRE Capri Workshop Group. Intrauterine insemination. Hum Reprod Update. 2009; 15(3):265–77.
9. ESHRE Capri Workshop Group, Aboulghar M, Baird DT, Collins J, Evers JL, Fauser BC, Lambalk CB, Somigliana E, Sunde A, Crosignani PG, Devroey P, Diczfalusy E, Diedrich K, Fraser L, Geraedts JP, Gianaroli L, Glasier A, Van Steirteghem A, Collins J, Crosignani PG. Intrauterine insemination. Hum Reprod Update. 2009;15(3):265–77.
10. Pashayan N, Lyratzopoulos G, Mathur R. Cost-effectiveness of primary offer of IVF vs. primary offer of IUI followed by IVF (for IUI failures) in couples with unexplained or mild male factor subfertility. BMC Health Serv Res. 2006;6:80.

11. Homburg R. The case for initial treatment with intrauterine insemination as opposed to in vitro fertilization for idiopathic infertility. Hum Fertil (Camb). 2003;6(3):122–4.
12. Goverde AJ, McDonnell J, Vermeiden JP, Schats R, Rutten FF, Schoemaker J. Intrauterine insemination or in-vitro fertilisation in idiopathic subfertility and male subfertility: a randomised trial and cost-effectiveness analysis. Lancet. 2000;355(9197):13–8.
13. Farhi J, Ben-Haroush A, Lande Y, Fisch B. Role of treatment with ovarian stimulation and intrauterine insemination in women with unilateral tubal occlusion diagnosed by hysterosalpingography. Fertil Steril. 2007;88(2):396–400.
14. Ozkan S, Murk W, Arici A. Endometriosis and infertility: epidemiology and evidence-based treatments. Ann N Y Acad Sci. 2008;1127:92–100.
15. Ozkan S, Arici A. Advances in treatment options of endometriosis. Gynecol Obstet Invest. 2009;67(2):81–91.
16. Werbrouck E, Spiessens C, Meuleman C, D'Hooghe T. No difference in cycle pregnancy rate and in cumulative live-birth rate between women with surgically treated minimal to mild endometriosis and women with unexplained infertility after controlled ovarian hyperstimulation and intrauterine insemination. Fertil Steril. 2006;86(3):566–71.
17. Kissler S, Hamscho N, Zangos S, Gätje R, Müller A, Rody A, Döbert N, Menzel C, Grünwald F, Siebzehnrübl E, Kaufmann M. Diminished pregnancy rates in endometriosis due to impaired uterotubal transport assessed by hysterosalpingoscintigraphy. BJOG. 2005;112(10):1391–6.
18. Hansen KA, Eyster KM. A review of current management of endometriosis in 2006: an evidence-based approach. S D Med. 2006;59(4):153–9.
19. Dmowski WP, Pry M, Ding J, Rana N. Cycle-specific and cumulative fecundity in patients with endometriosis who are undergoing controlled ovarian hyperstimulation-intrauterine insemination or in vitro fertilization-embryo transfer. Fertil Steril. 2002;78(4):750–6.
20. Shibahara H, Koriyama J, Shiraishi Y, Hirano Y, Suzuki M, Koyama K. Diagnosis and treatment of immunologically infertile women with sperm-immobilizing antibodies in their sera. J Reprod Immunol. 2009;83(1–2):139–44.
21. Chang MY, Chiang CH, Chiu TH, Hsieh TT, Soong YK. The antral follicle count predicts the outcome of pregnancy in a controlled ovarian hyperstimulation/intrauterine insemination program. J Assist Reprod Genet. 1998;15(1):12–7.
22. Massin N, Cédrin-Durnerin I, Hugues JN. [Intrauterine insemination: spontaneous or medically-assisted ovulation?] (Article in French). Gynecol Obstet Fertil. 2004;32(10):898–903.
23. Pittrof RU, Shaker A, Dean N, Bekir JS, Campbell S, Tan SL. Success of intrauterine insemination using cryopreserved donor sperm is related to the age of the woman and the number of preovulatory follicles. J Assist Reprod Genet. 1996;13(4):310–4.
24. Verhulst SM, Cohlen BJ, Hughes E, Te Velde E, Heineman MJ. Intra-uterine insemination for unexplained subfertility. Cochrane Database Syst Rev. 2006;(4):CD001838.
25. Mahani IM, Afnan M. The pregnancy rates with intrauterine insemination (IUI) in superovulated cycles employing different protocols (clomiphene citrate (CC), human menopausal gonadotropin (HMG) and HMG + CC) and in natural ovulatory cycle. J Pak Med Assoc. 2004;54(10):503–5.
26. Chen L, Liu Q. [Natural cycle versus ovulation induction cycle in intrauterine insemination] (Article in Chinese). Zhonghua Nan Ke Xue. 2009;15(12):1112–5.
27. Custers IM, Steures P, Hompes P, Flierman P, van Kasteren Y, van Dop PA, van der Veen F, Mol BW. Intrauterine insemination: how many cycles should we perform? Hum Reprod. 2008;23(4):885–8.
28. Shekarriz M, DeWire DM, Thomas Jr AJ, Agarwal A. A method of human semen centrifugation to minimize the iatrogenic sperm injuries caused by reactive oxygen species. Eur Urol. 1995;28(1):31–5.
29. Cohlen BJ, Vandekerckhove P, te Velde ER, Habbema JD. Timed intercourse versus intrauterine insemination with or without ovarian hyperstimulation for subfertility in men. Cochrane Database Syst Rev. 2000;(2):CD000360.

30. Cantineau AE, Cohlen BJ, Al-Inany H, Heineman MJ. Intrauterine insemination versus fallopian tube sperm perfusion for non tubal infertility. Cochrane Database Syst Rev. 2004;(3):CD001502.
31. Krzysztof L. Optimizing stimulation protocols. In: Allahbadia GN, Merchant R, editors. Contemporary perspectives in assisted reproductive technology. India: Reed Elsevier; 2005. p. 10–7.
32. Dankert T, Kremer JA, Cohlen BJ, Hamilton CJ, Pasker-de Jong PC, Straatman H, van Dop PA. A randomized clinical trial of clomiphene citrate versus low dose recombinant FSH for ovarian hyperstimulation in intrauterine insemination cycles for unexplained and male subfertility. Hum Reprod. 2007;22(3):792–7.
33. Cantineau AE, Cohlen BJ, Heineman MJ. Ovarian stimulation protocols (anti-oestrogens, gonadotrophins with and without GnRH agonists/antagonists) for intrauterine insemination (IUI) in women with subfertility. Cochrane Database Syst Rev. 2007;(2):CD005356.
34. Hughes EG, Collins JA, Gunby J. A randomized controlled trial of three low-dose gonadotrophin protocols for unexplained infertility. Hum Reprod. 1998;13(6):1527–31.
35. Kocak M, Dilbaz B, Demır B, Taşci Y, Tarcan A, Dede S, Haberal A. Lyophilised hMG versus rFSH in women with unexplained infertility undergoing a controlled ovarian stimulation with intrauterine insemination: a prospective, randomised study. Gynecol Endocrinol. 2010;26:429–34.
36. Kabli N, Sylvestre C, Tulandi T, Buckett W. Comparison of daily and alternate day recombinant follicle-stimulating hormone stimulation protocols for intrauterine insemination. Fertil Steril. 2009;91(4):1141–4.
37. Wang CW, Horng SG, Chen CK, Wang HS, Huang HY, Lee CL, Soong YK. Ovulation induction with tamoxifen and alternate-day gonadotrophin in patients with thin endometrium. Reprod Biomed Online. 2008;17(1):20–6.
38. Barroso G, Menocal G, Felix H, Rojas-Ruiz JC, Arslan M, Oehninger S. Comparison of the efficacy of the aromatase inhibitor letrozole and clomiphene citrate as adjuvants to recombinant follicle-stimulating hormone in controlled ovarian hyperstimulation: a prospective, randomized, blinded clinical trial. Fertil Steril. 2006;86(5):1428–31.
39. Bedaiwy MA, Shokry M, Mousa N, Claessens A, Esfandiari N, Gotleib L, Casper R. Letrozole co-treatment in infertile women 40 years old and older receiving controlled ovarian stimulation and intrauterine insemination. Fertil Steril. 2009;91(6):2501–7.
40. Tehrani Nejad ESh, Abediasl Z, Rashidi BH, Azimi Nekoo E, Shariat M, Amirchaghmaghi E. Comparison of the efficacy of the aromatase inhibitor letrozole and clomiphene citrate gonadotropins in controlled ovarian hyperstimulation: a prospective, simply randomized, clinical trial. J Assist Reprod Genet. 2008;25(5):187–90.
41. Baysoy A, Serdaroglu H, Jamal H, Karatekeli E, Ozornek H, Attar E. Letrozole versus human menopausal gonadotrophin in women undergoing intrauterine insemination. Reprod Biomed Online. 2006;13(2):208–12.
42. Bedaiwy MA, Forman R, Mousa NA, Al Inany HG, Casper RF. Cost-effectiveness of aromatase inhibitor co-treatment for controlled ovarian stimulation. Hum Reprod. 2006;21(11): 2838–44.
43. Mitwally MF, Casper RF. Aromatase inhibition reduces the dose of gonadotropin required for controlled ovarian hyperstimulation. J Soc Gynecol Investig. 2004;11(6):406–15.
44. Ryan GL, Moss V, Davis WA, Sparks AE, Dokras A, Van Voorhis BJ. Oral ovulation induction agents combined with low-dose gonadotropin injections and intrauterine insemination: cost- and clinical effectiveness. J Reprod Med. 2005;50(12):943–50.
45. Gregoriou O, Vlahos NF, Konidaris S, Papadias K, Botsis D, Creatsas GK. Randomized controlled trial comparing superovulation with letrozole versus recombinant follicle-stimulating hormone combined with intrauterine insemination for couples with unexplained infertility who had failed clomiphene citrate stimulation and intrauterine insemination. Fertil Steril. 2008;90(3):678–83.
46. Sengoku K, Tamate K, Takaoka Y, Horikawa M, Goishi K, Komori H, Okada R, Tsuchiya K, Ishikawa M. The clinical efficacy of low-dose step-up follicle stimulating hormone administration for treatment of unexplained infertility. Hum Reprod. 1999;14(2):349–53.

47. Ragni G, Alagna F, Brigante C, Riccaboni A, Colombo M, Somigliana E, Crosignani PG. GnRH antagonists and mild ovarian stimulation for intrauterine insemination: a randomized study comparing different gonadotrophin dosages. Hum Reprod. 2004;19(1):54–8.
48. Lambalk CB, Leader A, Olivennes F, Fluker MR, Andersen AN, Ingerslev J, Khalaf Y, Avril C, Belaisch-Allart J, Roulier R, Mannaerts B. Treatment with the GnRH antagonist ganirelix prevents premature LH rises and luteinization in stimulated intrauterine insemination: results of a double-blind, placebo-controlled, multicentre trial. Hum Reprod. 2006;21(3):632–9.
49. Lin YH, Seow KM, Chen HJ, Hsieh BC, Huang LW, Tzeng CR, Hwang JL. Effect of cetrorelix dose on premature LH surge during ovarian stimulation. Reprod Biomed Online. 2008;16(6):772–7.
50. Crosignani PG, Somigliana E, Intrauterine Insemination Study Group. Effect of GnRH antagonists in FSH mildly stimulated intrauterine insemination cycles: a multicentre randomized trial. Hum Reprod. 2007;22(2):500–5.
51. Steures P, van der Steeg JW, Hompes PG, Bossuyt PM, van der Veen F, Habbema JD, Eijkemans MJ, Broekmans FJ, Verhoeve HR, Mol BW. [Intra-uterine insemination with controlled ovarian hyperstimulation compared to an expectant management in couples with unexplained subfertility and an intermediate prognosis: a randomised study] (Article in Dutch). Ned Tijdschr Geneeskd. 2008;152(27):1525–31.
52. Bhattacharya S, Harrild K, Mollison J, Wordsworth S, Tay C, Harrold A, McQueen D, Lyall H, Johnston L, Burrage J, Grossett S, Walton H, Lynch J, Johnstone A, Kini S, Raja A, Templeton A. Clomifene citrate or unstimulated intrauterine insemination compared with expectant management for unexplained infertility: pragmatic randomised controlled trial. BMJ. 2008;337:a716.
53. Yavas Y, Selub MR. Intrauterine insemination (IUI) pregnancy outcome is enhanced by shorter intervals from semen collection to sperm wash, from sperm wash to IUI time, and from semen collection to IUI time. Fertil Steril. 2004;82(6):1638–47.
54. Miller DC, Hollenbeck BK, Smith GD, Randolph JF, Christman GM, Smith YR, Lebovic DI, Ohl DA. Processed total motile sperm count correlates with pregnancy outcome after intrauterine insemination. Urology. 2002;60(3):497–501.
55. Branigan EF, Estes MA, Muller CH. Advanced semen analysis: a simple screening test to predict intrauterine insemination success. Fertil Steril. 1999;71(3):547–51.
56. Bedaiwy MA, Sharma RK, Alhussaini TK, Mohamed MS, Abdel-Aleem AM, Nelson DR, Thomas Jr AJ, Agarwal A. The use of novel semen quality scores to predict pregnancy in couples with male-factor infertility undergoing intrauterine insemination. J Androl. 2003; 24(3):353–60.
57. Shibahara H, Obara H, Ayustawati, Hirano Y, Suzuki T, Ohno A, Takamizawa S, Suzuki M. Prediction of pregnancy by intrauterine insemination using CASA estimates and strict criteria in patients with male factor infertility. Int J Androl. 2004;27(2):63–8.
58. Boomsma CM, Heineman MJ, Cohlen BJ, Farquhar C. Semen preparation techniques for intrauterine insemination. Cochrane Database Syst Rev. 2007;(4):CD004507.
59. Ohashi K, Saji F, Wakimoto A, Kato M, Tsutsui T, Tanizawa O. Preparation of oligozoospermic and/or asthenozoospermic semen for intrauterine insemination using the SpermPrep semen filtration column. Fertil Steril. 1992;57(4):866–70.
60. Paasch U, Grunewald S, Glander HJ. Sperm selection in assisted reproductive techniques. Soc Reprod Fertil Suppl. 2007;65: 515–25.
61. Allamaneni SS, Agarwal A, Rama S, Ranganathan P, Sharma RK. Comparative study on density gradients and swim-up preparation techniques utilizing neat and cryopreserved spermatozoa. Asian J Androl. 2005;7(1):86–92.
62. Morshedi M, Duran HE, Taylor S, Oehninger S. Efficacy and pregnancy outcome of two methods of semen preparation for intrauterine insemination: a prospective randomized study. Fertil Steril. 2003;79 Suppl 3:1625–32.
63. Ricci G, Perticarari S, Boscolo R, Montico M, Guaschino S, Presani G. Semen preparation methods and sperm apoptosis: swim-up versus gradient-density centrifugation technique. Fertil Steril. 2009;91(2):632–8.

64. Zhang Y, Qian Y, Feng T, Cai L, Liu J. [Separation of high-quality sperm by PureSperm centrifugation applied to intrauterine insemination cycles] (Article in Chinese). Zhonghua Nan Ke Xue. 2004;10(5):348–50.
65. Said TM, Agarwal A, Zborowski M, Grunewald S, Glander HJ, Paasch U. Utility of magnetic cell separation as a molecular sperm preparation technique. Andrology. 2008;29(2):134–42.
66. Lee TH, Liu CH, Shih YT, Tsao HM, Huang CC, Chen HH, Lee MS. Magnetic-activated cell sorting for sperm preparation reduces spermatozoa with apoptotic markers and improves the acrosome reaction in couples with unexplained infertility{dagger}. Hum Reprod. 2010;25(4):839–46.
67. Kosmas IP, Tatsioni A, Fatemi HM, Kolibianakis EM, Tournaye H, Devroey P. Human chorionic gonadotropin administration vs. luteinizing monitoring for intrauterine insemination timing, after administration of clomiphene citrate: a meta-analysis. Fertil Steril. 2007;87(3): 607–12.
68. Lewis V, Queenan Jr J, Hoeger K, Stevens J, Guzick DS. Clomiphene citrate monitoring for intrauterine insemination timing: a randomized trial. Fertil Steril. 2006;85(2):401–6.
69. Mitwally MF, Abdel-Razeq S, Casper RF. Human chorionic gonadotropin administration is associated with high pregnancy rates during ovarian stimulation and timed intercourse or intrauterine insemination. Reprod Biol Endocrinol. 2004;2:55.
70. Kucuk T. Intrauterine insemination: is the timing correct? J Assist Reprod Genet. 2008;25(8): 427–30.
71. Shalev E, Geslevich Y, Matilsky M, Ben-Ami M. Induction of pre-ovulatory gonadotrophin surge with gonadotrophin-releasing hormone agonist compared to pre-ovulatory injection of human chorionic gonadotrophins for ovulation induction in intrauterine insemination treatment cycles. Hum Reprod. 1995;10(9):2244–7.
72. Custers IM, Flierman PA, Maas P, Cox T, Van Dessel TJ, Gerards MH, Mochtar MH, Janssen CA, van der Veen F, Mol BW. Immobilisation versus immediate mobilisation after intrauterine insemination: randomised controlled trial. BMJ. 2009;339:b4080. doi:10.1136/bmj.b4080.
73. Erdem A, Erdem M, Atmaca S, Guler I. Impact of luteal phase support on pregnancy rates in intrauterine insemination cycles: a prospective randomized study. Fertil Steril. 2009;91(6):2508–13.
74. Pirard C, Donnez J, Loumaye E. GnRH agonist as novel luteal support: results of a randomized, parallel group, feasibility study using intranasal administration of buserelin. Hum Reprod. 2005;20(7):1798–804.
75. Randall GW, Gantt PA. Double vs. single intrauterine insemination per cycle: use in gonadotropin cycles and in diagnostic categories of ovulatory dysfunction and male factor infertility. J Reprod Med. 2008;53(3):196–202.
76. Ragni G, Maggioni P, Guermandi E, Testa A, Baroni E, Colombo M, Crosignani PG. Efficacy of double intrauterine insemination in controlled ovarian hyperstimulation cycles. Fertil Steril. 1999; 72(4):619–22.
77. Polyzos NP, Tzioras S, Mauri D, Tatsioni A. Double versus single intrauterine insemination for unexplained infertility: a meta-analysis of randomized trials. Fertil Steril. 2009;94: 1261–6.
78. Tonguc E, Var T, Onalan G, Altinbas S, Tokmak A, Karakaş N, Gulerman C. Comparison of the effectiveness of single versus double intrauterine insemination with three different timing regimens. Fertil Steril. 2010;94:1267–70.
79. Costello MF. Systematic review of the treatment of ovulatory infertility with clomiphene citrate and intrauterine insemination. Aust N Z J Obstet Gynaecol. 2004;44(2):93–102.
80. Bensdorp AJ, Cohlen BJ, Heineman MJ, Vandekerckhove P. Intra-uterine insemination for male subfertility. Cochrane Database Syst Rev. 2007;(4):CD000360.
81. Huang FJ, Chang SY, Chang JC, Kung FT, Wu JF, Tsai MY. Timed intercourse after intrauterine insemination for treatment of infertility. Eur J Obstet Gynecol Reprod Biol. 1998;80(2): 257–61.

82. Dickey RP, Taylor SN, Lu PY, Sartor BM, Rye PH, Pyrzak R. Effect of diagnosis, age, sperm quality, and number of preovulatory follicles on the outcome of multiple cycles of clomiphene citrate-intrauterine insemination. Fertil Steril. 2002;78(5):1088–95.
83. Aboulghar M, Mansour R, Serour G, Abdrazek A, Amin Y, Rhodes C. Controlled ovarian hyperstimulation and intrauterine insemination for treatment of unexplained infertility should be limited to a maximum of three trials. Fertil Steril. 2001;75(1):88–91.
84. Qublan H, Amarin Z, Nawasreh M, Diab F, Malkawi S, Al-Ahmad N, Balawneh M. Luteinized unruptured follicle syndrome: incidence and recurrence rate in infertile women with unexplained infertility undergoing intrauterine insemination. Hum Reprod. 2006;21(8):2110–3.
85. Hughes E, Brown J, Collins JJ, Vanderkerchove P. Clomiphene citrate for unexplained subfertility in women. Cochrane Database Syst Rev. 2010;(1):CD000057.
86. Besselink DE, Farquhar C, Kremer JA, Marjoribanks J, O'Brien P. Cervical insemination versus intra-uterine insemination of donor sperm for subfertility. Cochrane Database Syst Rev. 2008;(2): CD000317.
87. O'Brien P, Vandekerckhove P. Intra-uterine versus cervical insemination of donor sperm for subfertility. Cochrane Database Syst Rev. 2000;(2):CD000317.
88. Cantineau AE, Cohlen BJ, Heineman MJ. Intra-uterine insemination versus fallopian tube sperm perfusion for non-tubal infertility. Cochrane Database Syst Rev. 2009;(2):CD001502.
89. Fanchin R, Olivennes F, Righini C, Hazout A, Schwab B, Frydman R. A new system for fallopian tube sperm perfusion leads to pregnancy rates twice as high as standard intrauterine insemination. Fertil Steril. 1995;64(3):505–10.
90. Ricci G, Nucera G, Pozzobon C, Boscolo R, Giolo E, Guaschino S. A simple method for fallopian tube sperm perfusion using a blocking device in the treatment of unexplained infertility. Fertil Steril. 2001;76(6):1242–8.
91. Noci I, Dabizzi S, Evangelisti P, Cozzi C, Cameron Smith M, Criscuoli L, Fuzzi B, Branconi F. Evaluation of clinical efficacy of three different insemination techniques in couple infertility. A randomized study. Minerva Ginecol. 2007;59(1):11–8.
92. Mamas L. Comparison of fallopian tube sperm perfusion and intrauterine tuboperitoneal insemination: a prospective randomized study. Fertil Steril. 2006;85(3):735–40.
93. Aribarg A, Sukcharoen N. Intrauterine insemination of washed spermatozoa for treatment of oligozoospermia. Int J Androl. 1995;18 Suppl 1:62–6.
94. Billiet K, Dhont M, Vervaet C, Vermeire A, Gerris J, De Neubourg D, Delbeke L, Ombelet W, De Sutter P. A multi-center prospective, randomized, double-blind trial studying the effect of misoprostol on the outcome of intrauterine insemination. Gynecol Obstet Invest. 2008;66(3):145–51.
95. Zadehmodarres S, Oladi B, Saeedi S, Jahed F, Ashraf H. Intrauterine insemination with husband semen: an evaluation of pregnancy rate and factors affecting outcome. J Assist Reprod Genet. 2009;26(1):7–11.
96. Sacks PC, Simon JA. Infectious complications of intrauterine insemination: a case report and literature review. Int J Fertil. 1991;36(6):331–9.
97. Mårdh PA. Influence of infection with Chlamydia trachomatis on pregnancy outcome, infant health and life-long sequelae in infected offspring. Best Pract Res Clin Obstet Gynaecol. 2002;16(6):847–64.
98. Ahinko-Hakamaa K, Huhtala H, Tinkanen H. Success in intrauterine insemination: the role of etiology. Acta Obstet Gynecol Scand. 2007;86(7):855–60.
99. Tomlinson MJ, Amissah-Arthur JB, Thompson KA, Kasraie JL, Bentick B. Prognostic indicators for intrauterine insemination (IUI): statistical model for IUI success. Hum Reprod. 1996;11(9): 1892–6.
100. van Rumste MM, Custers IM, van der Veen F, van Wely M, Evers JL, Mol BW. The influence of the number of follicles on pregnancy rates in intrauterine insemination with ovarian stimulation: a meta-analysis. Hum Reprod Update. 2008;14(6):563–70.
101. Dickey RP, Taylor SN, Lu PY, Sartor BM, Rye PH, Pyrzak R. Relationship of follicle numbers and estradiol levels to multiple implantation in 3,608 intrauterine insemination cycles. Fertil Steril. 2001;75(1):69–78.

102. Hale L. Prevention of multiple pregnancy during ovulation induction. Twin Res. 2003;6(6): 540–2.
103. Bry-Gauillard H, Coulondre S, Cédrin-Durnerin I, Hugues JN. [Benefits and risks of ovarian stimulation before intrauterine insemination] (Article in French). Gynecol Obstet Fertil. 2000; 28(11):820–31.
104. Ragni G, Caliari I, Nicolosi AE, Arnoldi M, Somigliana E, Crosignani PG. Preventing high-order multiple pregnancies during controlled ovarian hyperstimulation and intrauterine insemination: 3 years' experience using low-dose recombinant follicle-stimulating hormone and gonadotropin-releasing hormone antagonists. Fertil Steril. 2006;85(3):619–24.
105. Guven S, Gunalp GS, Tekin Y. Factors influencing pregnancy rates in intrauterine insemination cycles. J Reprod Med. 2008;53(4):257–65.
106. Montanaro Gauci M, Kruger TF, Coetzee K, Smith K, Van Der Merwe JP, Lombard CJ. Stepwise regression analysis to study male and female factors impacting on pregnancy rate in an intrauterine insemination programme. Andrologia. 2001;33(3):135–41.
107. Dickey RP, Olar TT, Taylor SN, Curole DN, Rye PH, Matulich EM. Relationship of follicle number, serum estradiol, and other factors to birth rate and multiparity in human menopausal gonadotropin-induced intrauterine insemination cycles. Fertil Steril. 1991;56(1):89–92.
108. Tay PY, Raj VR, Kulenthran A, Sitizawiah O. Prognostic factors influencing pregnancy rate after stimulated intrauterine insemination. Med J Malaysia. 2007;62(4):286–9.
109. Steures P, van der Steeg JW, Mol BW, Eijkemans MJ, van der Veen F, Habbema JD, Hompes PG, Bossuyt PM, Verhoeve HR, van Kasteren YM, van Dop PA, CECERM (Collaborative Effort in Clinical Evaluation in Reproductive Medicine). Prediction of an ongoing pregnancy after intrauterine insemination. Fertil Steril. 2004;82(1):45–51.
110. Yalti S, Gürbüz B, Sezer H, Celik S. Effects of semen characteristics on IUI combined with mild ovarian stimulation. Arch Androl. 2004;50(4):239–46.
111. Van Voorhis BJ, Barnett M, Sparks AE, Syrop CH, Rosenthal G, Dawson J. Effect of the total motile sperm count on the efficacy and cost-effectiveness of intrauterine insemination and in vitro fertilization. Fertil Steril. 2001;75(4):661–8.
112. Bhal PS, Pugh ND, Gregory L, Goacher L, Wells C, Shaw RW. The potential effect of controlled ovarian hyperstimulation on follicular vascular perfusion: a study applying power Doppler ultrasonography within a treatment programme using donor sperm. J Obstet Gynaecol. 2001;21(5):507–12.
113. Marchetti C, Dewailly D. [Intrauterine insemination: indications and methods] (Article in French). Rev Prat. 2006;56(5):500–6.
114. Ragni G, Anselmino M, Nicolosi AE, Brambilla ME, Calanna G, Somigliana E. Follicular vascularity is not predictive of pregnancy outcome in mild controlled ovarian stimulation and IUI cycles. Hum Reprod. 2007;22(1):210–4.
115. Check JH, Lurie D, Peymer M, Katsoff D, Long R. Efficacy of intrauterine insemination without ovarian hyperstimulation for male or cervical factor in women aged 40 or over. Arch Androl. 2000;44(3):193–6.
116. Tsafrir A, Simon A, Margalioth EJ, Laufer N. What should be the first-line treatment for unexplained infertility in women over 40 years of age—ovulation induction and IUI, or IVF? Reprod Biomed Online. 2009;19 Suppl 4:4334.
117. Erdem M, Erdem A, Guler I, Atmaca S. Role of antral follicle count in controlled ovarian hyperstimulation and intrauterine insemination cycles in patients with unexplained subfertility. Fertil Steril. 2008;90(2):360–6.
118. Costello MF, Emerson S, Lukic J, Sjoblom P, Garrett D, Hughes G, Steigrad S. Predictive value of mid luteal progesterone concentration before luteal support in controlled ovarian hyperstimulation with intrauterine insemination. Aust N Z J Obstet Gynaecol. 2004; 44(1):51–6.
119. Merviel P, Heraud MH, Grenier N, Lourdel E, Sanguinet P, Copin H. Predictive factors for pregnancy after intrauterine insemination (IUI): an analysis of 1038 cycles and a review of the literature. Fertil Steril. 2010;93(1):79–88.

120. García-Herrero S, Meseguer M, Martínez-Conejero JA, Remohí J, Pellicer A, Garrido N. The transcriptome of spermatozoa used in homologous intrauterine insemination varies considerably between samples that achieve pregnancy and those that do not. Fertil Steril. 2009; 94:1360–73.
121. Panchal S, Nagori CB. Pre-hCG 3D and 3D power Doppler assessment of the follicle for improving pregnancy rates in intrauterine insemination cycles. J Hum Reprod Sci. 2009; 2(2):62–7.

Chapter 12
Conventional IVF Insemination

Liesl Nel-Themaat, Thomas Elliott, Ching-Chien Chang, Graham Wright, and Zsolt Peter Nagy

As with most other medical practices, infertility specialists customize patient treatment plans according to the need and characteristics of each individual case. This is especially true for ovarian stimulation and synchronization of the patient's cycle prior to oocyte retrieval, where the physician makes decisions based on several different variables along the course of the treatment. Once oocytes have been obtained, this decision-making process continues in the laboratory.

Often, the first of such choices that embryologists are faced with is which method of insemination to use. Conventional in vitro fertilization (IVF) and intracytoplasmic sperm injection (ICSI) are distinct in methodology, and deciding which of these routes to follow can be quite complex. Numerous factors play a role in the appropriateness and outcome of each method. Furthermore, embryologists may choose to split the oocytes into two different groups and perform ICSI on one group and IVF on the other group. In such cases, the treatment is referred to as split IVF/ICSI.

This section is aimed at describing the method and some important elements of conventional IVF (from here on, IVF refers to conventional IVF). We will also compare the advantages and disadvantages of the three options and discuss the different factors that should be taken into consideration when deciding which insemination method to use. Figure 12.1 was compiled in attempt to aid the decision-making process. We hope this will help embryologists, physicians, and patients to make the most appropriate and informed choices.

L. Nel-Themaat, PhD • T. Elliott, BSc • C.-C. Chang, PhD • G. Wright, BSc
Z.P. Nagy, MD, PhD, HCLD (ABB), EMB (ACE) (✉)
Scientific and Laboratory, Reproductive Biology Associates, 1100 Johnson Ferry Rd.
Suite 200, Atlanta, GA 30342, USA
e-mail: zsolt.peter.nagy@gmail.com

Z.P. Nagy et al. (eds.), *Clinical Embryology: A Practical Guide*,
DOI 10.1007/978-1-4614-8376-2_12, © Springer Science+Business Media New York 2013

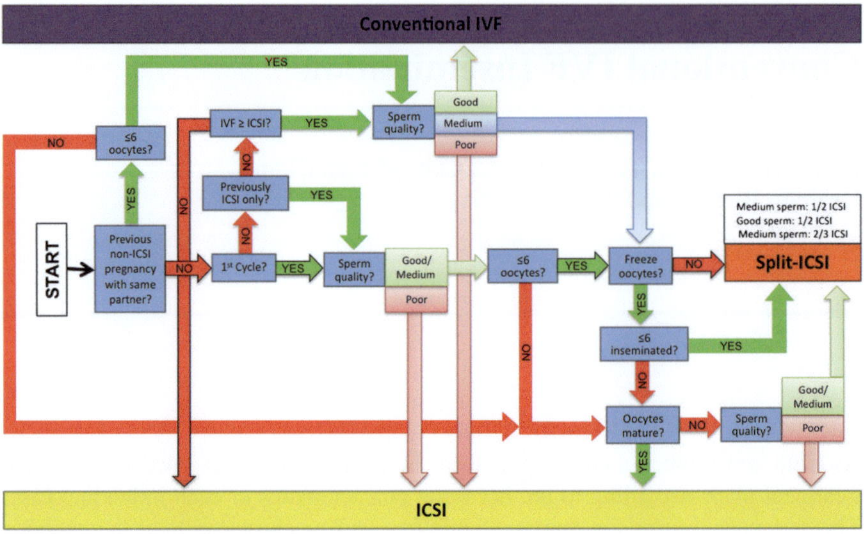

Fig. 12.1 Flow chart for decision-making in insemination choices

History of In Vitro Fertilization

The first report of IVF came from Spallanzani in the 1700s, when he demonstrated the fertilization of frog oocytes by mixing them with semen (for review, see ref. [1]). Although he had previously seen spermatozoa using his various microscopes, at the time, it was believed that spermatozoa were parasites instead of the fertilizing agent. Only in the next century, with much opposition, were Prevost and Dumas able to demonstrate that spermatozoa are *secreted* by the testes and responsible for the fertilizing capability of semen [1]. This was followed by von Baer's discovery of the mammalian oocyte in 1827 and eventually successful IVF and births in the rabbit by Chang [2]. Realizing the clinical value of this discovery, several groups in Europe, Australia, and the USA competed to achieve successful IVF in humans. On 25 July 1978, Louise Brown, the first human birth resulting from IVF, came from Steptoe and Edwards in the UK [3]. More live births followed shortly in Australia (1980), the USA (1981), and Sweden, France, and Austria (1982), with a subsequent worldwide explosion of ART clinics and research programs (for review, see refs. [1, 4–6]). One debated topic was the use of stimulated vs. natural cycles, as Louise Brown was a result of a natural cycle after hormonal stimulation was abandoned by Steptoe and Edwards due to repeated failure [3]. Eventually, successful stimulation protocols that allowed multiple oocyte collection were developed [7]. This allowed production of multiple embryos from a single cycle, embryo selection, and the ability to cryopreserve the extras. Furthermore, having numerous oocytes opened up the possibility to use more than one method of insemination in a single cycle. We will elaborate on this topic in subsequent sections.

Initially, IVF was the only available option for creating *test-tube babies*. This meant that for successful fertilization, spermatozoa that were placed in large numbers in the same tube (dish) as oocytes had to find an oocyte, infiltrate the cumulus, bind to and penetrate the zona pellucida, attach to the oolemma, and finally deposit its nuclear material in the ooplasma, all under in vitro conditions [3, 8]. It also meant that during IVF, many of the natural selection processes were still in place. For example, to successfully fertilize the oocyte, the spermatozoan had to, among other factors, be progressively motile to enter the cumulus mass and be able to undergo the acrosome reaction to penetrate the zona [8]. It was soon realized that for certain cases, some of these events had to be circumvented in order to obtain fertilization. This was particularly true for patients with male-factor infertility that would not normally qualify for IVF due to abnormal morphology, low motility, and low sperm concentration [910]. Therefore, experimentation for alternative modes of fertilization was underway. Initially, studies focused on assisting spermatozoa microsurgically to get through the zona pellucida. Methods included making an opening for sperm to enter through the zona either mechanically (i.e., partial zona dissection) or chemically (zona drilling) [11], or by injecting the sperm into the perivitelline space (subzonal sperm injection) [12]. Although these techniques increased fertilization rates, they had drawbacks, such as increased rates of polyspermy and the fact that the sperm still needed the capacity to bind to the oolemma [13]. Eventually, a procedure known to be successful in rabbits [14] and cattle [15], in which the spermatozoa were injected directly into the ooplasma, led to the first human pregnancies and subsequent birth from ICSI [16].

Development of ICSI gave embryologist the *luxury* of a choice between two different approaches, IVF or ICSI, each with unique advantages and disadvantages, which will be discussed below. The ability to choose, however, is only beneficial if factors that determine success rates for each method are carefully considered and understood.

Elements of Conventional IVF

In one sentence, conventional IVF can be described as follows: Obtain oocytes from a natural or stimulated cycle, obtain sperm either surgically or from ejaculate, mix the gametes in a dish with appropriate culture medium, and culture overnight. The next day, fertilization is accessed by the presence of male and female pronuclei. Although this may sound pretty straight forward, there are dozens of elements throughout the procedure that have been fine-tuned over more than 30 years to obtain the success we see today. The most basic ones include factors involving gamete collection, processing, and subsequent embryo culture. Previous chapters have described these techniques in detail. Therefore, this section will only give a brief overview of the insemination procedure and then focus on some aspects that have not been discussed.

The In Vitro Insemination Procedure

Different programs use different protocols for IVF. This brief description corresponds to the methods that are utilized at our practice, but are not necessarily superior to differing protocols.

Gametes are collected and processed as previously described. Oocyte maturity is assessed at time of retrieval, based on cumulus maturation [17, 18]. Although oocytes that appear immature can still be inseminated, the embryologist should keep record of the number of immature oocytes. This will help with more accurately evaluating fertilization outcomes.

Prior to insemination, it is of utmost importance to cross-check patient sample identification numbers to make sure that the correct oocytes are inseminated with the correct sperm. Needless to say, error at this step can have dire consequences. A carefully labeled Petri dish with drops of fertilization medium under mineral oil can be prepared the night before to ensure thorough equilibration in the incubator overnight.

Insemination normally takes place roughly 5 h after oocyte retrieval and 40–41 h after hCG administration. Processed sperm is added to the insemination drop to obtain a final concentration of approximately 1×10^5 cells per mL. For a cell suspension of 10×10^6 per mL, the addition of 10 μL sperm preparation to an insemination drop of 90 μL should provide the appropriate concentration. Oocyte-cumulus complexes (OCCs) are then added to the fertilization drops. We typically add no more than 4 OCCs to a drop of roughly 100 μL (~25 μL of medium per OCC). Gametes are cultured overnight in a humidified incubator, usually at 5% CO_2 (depending on medium formulation) in *fertilization medium*.

The next day, oocytes are washed, manually stripped of cumulus (the details of the stripping procedure is described in Chap. 12), and transferred to fresh drops of *cleavage medium*. Fertilization is assessed by the presence of two pronuclei, and subsequent embryo evaluation is performed as described.

Timing of Insemination

To achieve successful fertilization, oocytes need to be fully matured in preparation for interaction with sperm upon fertilization. This includes nuclear and cytoplasmic maturation of the oocyte, expansion of the cumulus and corona, preparation of the zona pellucida and oolemma for sperm binding, and extrusion of the first polar body. The result is a fully matured oocyte arrested in metaphase II, ready for the complex cascade of sperm-oocyte interactions that will follow (for recent reviews, see refs. [8, 19, 20]). In a natural cycle, these events are timed by the gonadotropins synthesized in the anterior pituitary. They are controlled by gonadotropin-releasing hormone (GnRH) from the hypothalamus and ensure completion of oocyte maturation prior to sperm exposure and fertilization. Follicle-stimulating hormone (FSH) initiates follicular recruitment of FSH receptor-bearing, recruitable follicles, which leads to growth of the cohort and eventually maturation of the dominant follicle. At the end of the follicular phase, due to a positive feedback by estrogen on the pituitary, the LH surge occurs and triggers ovulation. A delicate relationship is maintained between the oocyte and follicular cells so that maturation of both is carefully synchronized, leading to ovulation only once the oocyte has fully matured [21]. The oocyte is released into the peritoneal cavity, captured by the fimbria, and transported to the oviductal ampulla, where fertilization typically occurs [8, 22]. Therefore, after ovulation, an unspecified window (minutes to hours) of time elapses between ovulation and fertilization, during which final oocyte maturation processes can be completed.

In a stimulated cycle, the woman is treated with high doses of gonadotropins to ensure that numerous follicles will mature while ovulation is suppressed (for review, see ref. [23, 24]). Maturation and ovulation is then initiated by hCG treatment, followed by oocyte aspiration (instead of ovulation) 35–36 h later, mimicking the in vivo LH-to-ovulation time frame, but not necessarily allowing completion of maturation. It should also be noted that should insemination be performed immediately following oocyte retrieval, the time of capture and transport to the ampulla is essentially lost, implying that a significant percentage of oocytes may not have had the opportunity to fully mature.

There appears to be asynchrony between the somatic cells and the oocyte in stimulated cycles, which leads to lower fertilization rates when insemination is performed immediately after oocyte retrieval [25]. In fact, Trounson et al. [26] reported the highest fertilization and pregnancy rates after a 5–6-h delay of insemination following oocyte retrieval 34–37-h post-hCG. They also found that fertilization rates dramatically decreased as the timing of insemination after oocyte retrievals decreased. Considering these results and the mentioned asynchrony in the OCC, it is not surprising that Cohen et al. found that after hCG stimulation, the percentage of visible meiotic spindles increased with time elapsed after hCG injection, even in oocytes that already extruded the first polar body [27]. As a result, the authors suggested postponing ICSI to 38–42 h after hCG administration, which apparently compensates for some of the asynchrony and lost migration time.

These and other reports indicate that timing of insemination in relation to hCG administration is imperative to achieve oocyte maturation and successful fertilization. It also appears that the timing of insemination after oocyte collection is less critical since the last phases of the maturation process is initiated by hCG administration and not by removal of the oocyte from the follicles. Needless to say, follicles should have reached a minimum level of maturity (usually 1.4 cm in diameter) before hCG and aspiration is attempted to make sure the OCC is receptive for stimulation.

Nuclear maturation can occur outside of the follicle, providing that the minimum threshold of maturation has been reached (i.e., fully grown germinal vesicle stage). However, cytoplasmic maturation is also essential for fertilization, which is supported by the somatic cells [21]. The OCCs therefore has the ability to continue the maturation process in vitro and may potentially be fertilized hours after their sibling oocytes, as long as they are given enough time and have the support of the maturation-promoting cumulus [28]. We will discuss handling of these immature OCCs in subsequent sections, but in general, recommend that oocytes should be inseminating no less than 38 h after hCG.

Concentration of Spermatozoa During Insemination

The main objective of IVF is to achieve fertilization outside of the body. As the procedure became more common, so did the challenges that embryologists faced. The first measure of success that is evaluated in the laboratory is fertilization, as indicated by the presence of two pronuclei and the second polar body the day after insemination (following mechanical removal of the cumulus, the procedure that is described in detail in Chap. 12). Failed fertilization was one such a problem that had to be faced early on. Researchers started trying different procedures in attempt to increase the chances of fertilization, which led to development of several new techniques, including ICSI. One such method that received significant attention in the late 1980s and 1990s was to increase the sperm concentration for patients with sperm morphology abnormalities or those that previously had failed IVF cycles [29, 30]. This was called the high oocyte insemination concentration (HIC) procedure. The idea was that even if there is just a small percentage of motile, morphologically normal spermatozoa in the ejaculate, increasing the insemination concentration would lead to a sufficient number of sperm to fertilize the oocyte.

Literature on the topic is very contradictory. While some groups reported higher fertilization rates with HIC-IVF [29, 31], others found that in couples with total fertilization failure, increased sperm concentration did not rescue fertilization [30]. In patients with severe teratozoospermia, Oehninger et al. [32] obtained higher fertilization rates in oocytes inseminated by HIC than for those on which ICSI was performed. The ICSI group, however, produced embryos with higher morphology scores, and there was no difference in implantation rates between the two treatment groups. The mentioned studies used inconsistent procedures. For example, some denuded oocytes prior to insemination, while others left the OCCs intact. These variations in protocols make results from different publications hard to compare.

At the moment, most research shows superiority of ICSI over conventional IVF to overcome failed fertilization, even when compared with HIC. Therefore, most groups abandoned HIC-IVF in favor of ICSI for couples with a history of failed fertilization following conventional IVF.

Advantages and Disadvantages for Conventional IVF and ICSI

In order to make an informed decision of when to use which procedure, it is important to understand the major advantages and disadvantages of one method over the other.

Conventional IVF is a less invasive, more natural procedure that provides a longer window of opportunity for sperm to fertilize the oocytes, rather than insemination at a specific time point. It maintains several natural selection criteria for sperm as well as oocytes, which may allow for some unknown mechanism to reduce developmental defects. Reports exist of developmental delays in children conceived by ICSI when compared to those from IVF or natural conception [33–36], but whether the lack of such mechanisms in ICSI offspring is responsible for these findings remains to be confirmed.

It is much less labor intensive and cheaper to perform than ICSI, and a large wealth of information is available on the subject since it has been intensively studied in humans for over 30 years. One of the biggest drawbacks of IVF over ICSI is a higher occurrence of failed fertilization [37, 38]. This can be attributed to various causes, such as poor sperm quality, or oocyte defects such as an abnormal zona pellucida or oolemma that renders sperm incapable of fertilizing the oocyte (for recent reviews, see refs. [8, 20]). Therefore, semen quality has to be higher when used for IVF vs. ICSI.

Another disadvantage of IVF is that embryologists generally do not know the maturation status of oocytes, since they are not denuded before insemination. This may skew success rates when comparing the techniques. To minimize this problem, the cumulus maturation aspect can be used as an indication of oocyte maturity [17, 39]. It is also possible to individually examine each OCC in a small volume of media by pulling away the thickest parts of the cumulus to look for the presence of a polar body [18]. This technique, coined *cumulus spreading*, is of course a very time-consuming and tedious procedure.

The most value of the ICSI procedure is that the sperm does not have to bind to or penetrate cumulus and corona, the zona pellucida or the oolemma, as it is injected directly into the ooplasm. Thus, morphologically abnormal or low-motility sperm that may be unable to fertilize oocytes during IVF can be used for injection. It also provides the opportunity to examine each oocyte closely prior to injection, which results in more accurate portrayal of success rates. While denuding adds some advantages, it may affect the oocytes negatively, as hyaluronidase treatment and manual stripping can damage the oocytes. ICSI requires a very high level of skill and precision, which increases the workload of the laboratory exponentially.

As this brief discussion indicated, there are definite advantages and disadvantages to both techniques, and ideally, clinics should find a way to combine their use to reap the benefit of both techniques.

Deciding on IVF, ICSI, or Split-ICSI

Although conventional IVF was the original method of insemination outside of the body, many laboratories have completely switched to ICSI as their preferred method of insemination, regardless of oocyte and semen qualities. There are good arguments for doing strictly ICSI, such as a single, standardized protocol to maintain and less emphasis placed on semen evaluation. However, there are advantages in the ability to perform both techniques, depending on specific case parameters. In doing so, a more customized treatment plan is followed for each patient. Several important factors should be considered when deciding which method, IVF, ICSI, or split-ICSI, to perform. The latter is taking advantages of both methods and thereby essentially *covering all the bases* [38, 40].

It would be very challenging to discuss each issue that determines the most appropriate method of insemination individually. Instead of a simple formula, the decision-making process is very complex, as each aspect is influenced by the others. Furthermore, there are external issues that may alter the preferred route (discussed later). We therefore generated a flow chart that includes the most important factors to consider (Fig. 12.1). These are represented as questions, and the philosophies behind them for the decision-making process are discussed below. Importantly, the chart is by no means all inclusive, but is meant as a guide for physicians and embryologists. There are numerous additional factors that may influence the method of choice, and endless unique situations that may arise and are not on the chart. Such issues were omitted from the flow chart and discussed separately in attempt to simplify it.

Previous Non-ICSI Pregnancy with Same Partner

It is of utmost importance to look at a patient's fertility record if one is to understand the full scope of the treatment options. The question of whether or not a patient previously had a non-ICSI pregnancy gives an indication of former sperm-oocyte interaction. If the answer is yes, it is likely that the sperm has (or at least at some point had) the ability to fertilize the oocytes without injection. The time since the last successful pregnancy (or fertilization using IVF) should be noted, as quality parameters of either gametes may have changed over time. Nonetheless, this history indicates that they are (or at least once were) compatible. If a patient has never conceived without ICSI with her current partner, but both partners previously had proven fertility with different partners, there may be compatibility issues between their gametes regardless of the quality. This may especially affect younger couples with seemingly good-quality semen and oocytes. In such a case, although IVF could be successful, ICSI nevertheless may be necessary to obtain fertilization.

First Cycle

Much information about a patient and the expected outcomes can be gathered from previous cycles. By looking at former cycles, the embryologists should/can get idea of the fertilization capacity of the oocytes and sperm. This is especially true for patients that previously had all IVF or split-ICSI cycles. For example, if a patient responded poorly to IVF but well to ICSI, IVF should not be considered for the next cycle. However, if a patient had better fertilization rates with IVF than ICSI, the lab may opt to do all IVF or split-ICSI, depending on sperm quality and the number of oocytes available on the day. Therefore, it is essential to thoroughly examine previous cycles and use what was learned from them in subsequent cycles.

In a patient's first cycle, it is especially valuable to do split-ICSI as a means to gather such information for subsequent cycles. The first cycle may even be treated as a test cycle specifically for this purpose and in essence serve as a diagnostic tool. For example, in couples that had fertility with different partners, failure to get pregnant may arise from incompatibility between the sperm and oocytes of that particular couple (see discussion section "Previous Non-ICSI Pregnancy with Same Partner"). In such a case, we would expect high fertilization rates with ICSI and low rates with IVF. To benefit most from such a diagnostic cycle, it should still conform to downstream requirements, as depicted in Fig. 12.1. If the semen quality is poor, doing an ICSI split may not yield accurate information to use in subsequent cycles, and it may be better to treat the cycle as a regular cycle with maximum fertilization the main objective. In that case, according to the flow diagram, only ICSI should be performed.

Sperm Quality

For successful IVF, the sperm needs to have the ability to fertilize the oocyte without assistance. This means that there should be minimum number of morphologically normal, motile sperm in the insemination drop to achieve fertilization (discussed above). If sperm quality is poor and cannot be improved by processing, ICSI should be performed. Good, medium, and poor sperm refer to relative standards, and each sample should be evaluated for specific criteria [41] to estimate whether there would be enough normal, motile sperm from the ejaculate to perform IVF.

Generally, the concentration of sperm in the fertilization drop should be about 100,000–150,000/mL motile, morphologically normal cells. If raw semen quality is too low to meet these criteria, quality should be classified as poor, and all ICSI should be performed to maximize fertilization rates. If the above criteria can be reached but it appears borderline or still have low progressive motility (<40%) or some morphological abnormality, at least 50% of the oocytes should be allocated to ICSI in case IVF fails. Good sperm quality, with sufficient concentration, motility, and morphology, may be used for all IVF or up to 50% IVF in split-ICSI cases. Sperm quality is the final determinant of whether all IVF or split-ICSI will be performed for patient that are known to respond better to IVF than ICSI.

Oocyte Number Recovered from the Patient: If <6 Oocytes

The number of oocytes for this question should be internally standardized for each lab. In general, patients with six or more oocytes should be considered for split-ICSI. More conservative groups may choose a larger number as their cutoff.

During an in vitro cycle, the most critical aim of the lab is to achieve fertilization, since embryos and pregnancies cannot be obtained without it. Therefore, if there is a limited number of oocytes, it becomes more important to focus on the method that will result in higher fertilization rates, which is ICSI [37, 42]. As discussed, conventional IVF has some advantages over ICSI. Therefore, if a patient has more than the specified number of good-quality mature oocytes, a percentage of them can be assigned to IVF. We recommend that split-ICSI should be performed if a patient has a minimum of six mature, morphologically normal oocytes. Each lab, however, should decide their standard cutoff oocyte number for split-ICSI. Typically, oocytes will be divided evenly between the two treatment methods. In some cases, the lab may decide to adjust this ratio based on other parameters, for example, allocate two thirds to ICSI and one third to IVF if sperm quality is medium or below (see Fig. 12.1).

Should We Freeze Excess Oocytes?

Patients with large numbers of oocytes may opt for (partial) oocyte freezing. This will reduce the number of oocytes to inseminate. The number of remaining oocytes left for insemination should thus be considered when determining which method to use. If more than the lab standard remains (typically six or more), split-ICSI should be performed. However, if fewer are left for insemination, the maturity of the cumulus should be considered as described below (also see section "Ethical Concerns").

Should We Inseminate Fewer Than Six Oocytes, When There Is Choice?

In cases where a patient decided to freeze a portion of her oocytes, the number remaining for insemination will determine whether IVF or split-ICSI should be performed (see section "Oocyte Number Recovered from the Patient: If <6 Oocytes"). It should also be taken into account that oocyte cryopreservation requires decumulation of oocytes, which will necessitate ICSI for subsequent fertilization cycles.

Oocytes Maturity

Upon oocyte retrieval, embryologists mostly have to rely on the status of the cumulus to estimate the maturity status of the oocytes [39]. However, when a patient has fewer than 6 oocytes, the preferred protocol of many labs and as recommended by our criteria is to do all ICSI. When a significant percentage of those oocytes are immature ($\geq$50%), this decision may prove complicated. Many laboratories by default denude all the oocytes in a small cohort, while standard practice for IVF requires an intact OCC, since inseminating denuded oocytes typically result in low fertilization rates (personal communication). However, Taylor et al. [43] found that IVF resulted in higher fertilization rates in sibling oocytes with increased immaturity. This is most likely because IVF gives the oocyte time to mature and be fertilized by the already-present sperm once it has matured, as conventional IVF insemination is typically performed overnight and provides a longer time window during which immature oocytes can mature, resulting in optimization of sperm-oocyte interaction and fertilization. With a smaller number of oocytes, each should be examined individually based on cumulus appearance and possibly for the presence of a polar body (see above). For those that are immature, IVF may yield better fertilization. Should these immature oocytes be denuded prior to determining maturation, they are typically cultured overnight to perform day 1 ICSI. However, this means that the oocyte may mature several hours before ICSI will be performed, possibly missing the window in which it can be successfully fertilized, emphasizing the importance of cumulus evaluation prior to denuding.

Should the oocytes be denuded and then it is discovered that a high percentage are immature, IVF can still be attempted, as some groups achieved good fertilization rates after inseminating denuded oocytes [44–46].

When Previous Insemination Was Only ICSI

This question is asked subsequent to whether it is the patient's first cycle. If it is not the first cycle and previously only ICSI was performed, there are no data available on IVF for those patients. There should thus not be a preference toward either technique without considering the factors downstream in Fig. 12.1. Essentially, neither ICSI nor IVF will be penalized on previous cycles. If the patient previously had both ICSI and IVF, the outcome of each technique in those cycles should be compared, as discussed in the next section.

How to Divide Oocytes for Insemination: IVF ≥ ICSI?

This question is to find out if the previous outcome of IVF was equal to or better than that of ICSI when considering fertilization, development, and the number and quality of resulting embryos. In patients that had cycles where IVF and ICSI were performed, embryologists have a considerable advantage in knowing the outcome of both techniques for the specific couple. Generally, the technique that previously proved more successful should be repeated, providing oocyte and sperm parameters are sufficient. This should be determined not only by fertilization rates but also by embryo quality, as the end goal is to obtain the largest number of good-quality embryos. If these outcomes were equal, the decision should lean more in favor of IVF, as it is a less invasive technique that is easier to perform and generally a more natural process (see above).

Other Factors

Apart from considerations outlined in previous sections, there are other factors that may influence the decision-making process that is external to the laboratory. These include issues that can be very patient specific and may essentially override the decision that the lab would typically make based on the flow chart (Fig. 12.1). Some programs may choose not to treat patients with criteria that negatively affect pregnancy rates. This is where science, ethics, and human emotions become merged to create very complicated situations for the clinics as well as the patients. These factors are discussed below:

Costs

As with most labor-intensive medical care, infertility treatment is not cheap. While most essential procedures are covered, at least partially, by medical insurance, this is not the case with most nonessential issues, such as infertility. Whether or not insurance will cover in vitro treatment is dependent on state and the specific insurance company and plan at hand. The cost schedule also varies greatly between different laboratories. Therefore, regardless of the diagnosis and recommended treatment, it should be confirmed that the patient has sufficient funds for the chosen procedure. Unfortunately, some patients will not be able to afford certain treatment plans. In general, ICSI is more expensive than IVF, whereas labs may charge for both procedures should split-ICSI be performed. Therefore, the choice of insemination method may sometimes be made purely on the financial capabilities of the patient. This information should be discussed with the patient prior to start of treatment.

Ethical Concerns

IVF has always been, and will continue to be, a very controversial subject. This is especially true when religious beliefs are considered. Some patients are against the ICSI procedure since it is essentially in the hands of another human being to choose which sperm fertilizes the oocyte. These patients often request IVF only, regardless of oocyte numbers and sperm quality. The laboratory should always respect these requests, even if they may lower success rates. Other patients may not want to have too many embryos produced, since they do not feel comfortable with discarding or donating extra embryos and do not want the burden of having to deal with a large number of frozen embryos. In such cases, patients may want to freeze all oocytes except for a small number for insemination. Again, this will affect the choice of which procedure to use.

Technical Competence of Staff

Individual laboratories have staff with different skill levels. Each group should calculate their own fertilization and embryo development rates for ICSI and IVF.

This is especially important for new, less-experienced groups. If there is a big difference in competence for the two procedures, the embryologists may want to adjust the ratio in favor of the one in which they are more proficient until they become more experienced and increase success rates with the other procedure. Well-trained, competent embryologists are key to obtaining desired results. It should also be considered that ICSI is labor intensive and therefore increases the workload on the lab. Incorporating IVF may relieve some of this stress in growing programs and give technicians extra time to improve other techniques. Naturally, decreasing workload should never be the sole motivation for choosing IVF, especially if it could lower the patient's chance of pregnancy.

Literature of IVF and ICSI Outcomes

Although often preliminary in nature, literature exists that indicates differences in the developmental potential of children conceived by ICSI and IVF [33–36]. There are also studies that suggest differences in the sex ratio obtained from the two procedures [47]. Furthermore, a wealth of often-inaccurate information is available on the Internet. Patients tend to research such topics and may approach the clinic with strong opinions about the different aspects of their treatment.

Influence of Friends and Family Members

Patients going through infertility treatment tend to share their experiences with family members and friends to get opinions from people they trust. Sometimes, these confidants may have gone through treatments themselves, or know people who have. In such cases, their opinions may carry a significant weight in the patient's decision of treatment. This can have an enormous implication of the preferred treatment choice. For example, a patient's sister may have had IVF and became pregnant on her first cycle. Thus, the patient wants the exact same treatment, although her oocyte and semen qualities are far inferior or superior to those of her younger sister. Despite the effort of the doctor and embryologist to better educate and advise the patient, she may not change her mind, which means that she will receive IVF or ICSI while she would probably have better chances of conceiving with ICSI (or it would not be necessary to perform ICSI).

Conclusions

Our objective with this chapter was to give a brief overview of the conventional IVF procedure and some of the factors that determine success. The decision-making process of whether to do conventional IVF, ICSI, or split-ICSI is, as discussed above, very complex. We presented the influencing factors in a manner that allows thorough evaluation of every case, resulting in an educated, well thought through decision of which insemination method to use. Subsequently (mostly to help us wrap our heads around the subject in preparation for writing this chapter), we developed a flow chart to indicate step by step how a decision is reached (Fig. 12.1). We believe it will assist embryologists in deciding which method of fertilization to use in their labs. The flow chart should be especially valuable for new, less-experienced groups that are considering both ICSI and IVF, but are unsure of how to implement both techniques into their treatment plans. We also hope that it will stimulate laboratories that are doing strictly ICSI to consider IVF and split-ICSI, as it may benefit both the patient and the lab by improving success rates, reducing costs, and minimizing workload.

Acknowledgments The authors would like to thank the members of Reproductive Biology Associates for valuable intellection contributions during composition of this chapter.

References

1. Clarke GN. A.R.T. and history, 1678–1978. Hum Reprod. 2006;21:1645–50.
2. Chang MC. Fertilization of rabbit ova in vitro. Nature. 1959;184 Suppl 7:466–7.
3. Steptoe PC, Edwards RG. Birth after the reimplantation of a human embryo. Lancet. 1978;2:366.
4. Cohen J, Trounson A, Dawson K, Jones H, Hazekamp J, Nygren KG, Hamberger L. The early days of IVF outside the UK. Hum Reprod Update. 2005;11:439–59.
5. Edwards RG. An astonishing journey into reproductive genetics since the 1950's. Reprod Nutr Dev. 2005;45:299–306.
6. Fauser BC, Edwards RG. The early days of IVF. Hum Reprod Update. 2005;11:437–8.
7. Trounson AO, Leeton JF, Wood C, Webb J, Wood J. Pregnancies in humans by fertilization in vitro and embryo transfer in the controlled ovulatory cycle. Science. 1981;212:681–2.
8. Ikawa M, Inoue N, Benham AM, Okabe M. Fertilization: a sperm's journey to and interaction with the oocyte. J Clin Invest. 2010;120:984–94.
9. Hall J, Fishel S. In vitro fertilization for male infertility: when and how? Baillieres Clin Obstet Gynaecol. 1997;11:711–24.
10. Cohen J, Alikani M, Adler A, Berkeley A, Davis O, Ferrara TA, Graf M, Grifo J, Liu HC, Malter HE, et al. Microsurgical fertilization procedures: the absence of stringent criteria for patient selection. J Assist Reprod Genet. 1992;9:197–206.
11. Malter HE, Cohen J. Partial zona dissection of the human oocyte: a nontraumatic method using micromanipulation to assist zona pellucida penetration. Fertil Steril. 1989;51:139–48.
12. Ng SC, Bongso A, Ratnam SS, Sathananthan H, Chan CL, Wong PC, Hagglund L, Anandakumar C, Wong YC, Goh VH. Pregnancy after transfer of sperm under zona. Lancet. 1988;2:790.
13. Garrisi GJ, Talansky BE, Grunfeld L, Sapira V, Navot D, Gordon JW. Clinical evaluation of three approaches to micromanipulation-assisted fertilization. Fertil Steril. 1990;54:671–7.
14. Hosoi Y, Miyake M, Utsumi K, Iritani A. Development of rabbit oocytes after microinjection of spermatozoon. Proc 11th Congr Anim. Reprod Artif Insem 1988;331–3.
15. Goto K, Kinoshita A, Takuma Y, Ogawa K. Fertilisation of bovine oocytes by the injection of immobilised, killed spermatozoa. Vet Rec. 1990;127:517–20.
16. Palermo G, Joris H, Devroey P, Van Steirteghem AC. Pregnancies after intracytoplasmic injection of single spermatozoon into an oocyte. Lancet. 1992;340:17–8.

17. Coticchio G, Sereni E, Serrao L, Mazzone S, Iadarola I, Borini A. What criteria for the definition of oocyte quality? Ann N Y Acad Sci. 2004;1034:132–44.
18. Veeck LL. Oocyte assessment and biological performance. Ann N Y Acad Sci. 1988;541: 259–74.
19. Marteil G, Richard-Parpaillon L, Kubiak JZ. Role of oocyte quality in meiotic maturation and embryonic development. Reprod Biol. 2009;9:203–24.
20. Nixon B, Aitken RJ, McLaughlin EA. New insights into the molecular mechanisms of sperm-egg interaction. Cell Mol Life Sci. 2007;64:1805–23.
21. Russell DL, Robker RL. Molecular mechanisms of ovulation: co-ordination through the cumulus complex. Hum Reprod Update. 2007;13:289–312.
22. Croxatto HB. Physiology of gamete and embryo transport through the fallopian tube. Reprod Biomed Online. 2002;4:160–9.
23. Balasch J. The role of FSH and LH in ovulation induction: current concepts. In: Gardner DK, Weissman A, Howles CM, Shoham Z, editors. Textbook of assisted reproductive technologies. Laboratory and clinical perspectives. 3rd ed. London: Informa Healthcare; 2009.
24. Hugues JN, Cedrin-Durnerin I. Endocrine characteristics of the ART cycle. In: Gardner DK, Weissman A, Howles CM, Shoham Z, editors. Textbook of assisted reproductive technologies. Laboratory and clinical perspectives. 3rd ed. London: Informa Healthcare; 2009.
25. Sundstrom P, Nilsson BO. Meiotic and cytoplasmic maturation of oocytes collected in stimulated cycles is asynchronous. Hum Reprod. 1988;3:613–9.
26. Trounson AO, Mohr LR, et al. "Effect of delayed insemination on in-vitro fertilization, culture and transfer of human embryos." J Reprod Fertil. 1982;64(2):285–94.
27. Cohen Y, Malcov M, Schwartz T, Mey-Raz N, Carmon A, Cohen T, Lessing JB, Amit A, Azem F. Spindle imaging: a new marker for optimal timing of ICSI? Hum Reprod. 2004;19: 649–54.
28. Yokoo M, Sato E. Cumulus-oocyte complex interactions during oocyte maturation. Int Rev Cytol. 2004;235:251–91.
29. Oehninger S, Acosta AA, Morshedi M, Veeck L, Swanson RJ, Simmons K, Rosenwaks Z. Corrective measures and pregnancy outcome in in vitro fertilization in patients with severe sperm morphology abnormalities. Fertil Steril. 1988;50:283–7.
30. Kastrop PM, Weima SM, Van Kooij RJ, Te Velde ER. Comparison between intracytoplasmic sperm injection and in-vitro fertilization (IVF) with high insemination concentration after total fertilization failure in a previous IVF attempt. Hum Reprod. 1999;14:65–9.
31. Baker HW, Liu DY, Bourne H, Lopata A. Diagnosis of sperm defects in selecting patients for assisted fertilization. Hum Reprod. 1993;8:1779–80.
32. Oehninger S, Kruger TF, Simon T, Jones D, Mayer J, Lanzendorf S, Toner JP, Muasher SJ. A comparative analysis of embryo implantation potential in patients with severe teratozoospermia undergoing in-vitro fertilization with a high insemination concentration or intracytoplasmic sperm injection. Hum Reprod. 1996;11:1086–9.
33. Bowen JR, Gibson FL, Leslie GI, Saunders DM. Medical and developmental outcome at 1 year for children conceived by intracytoplasmic sperm injection. Lancet. 1998;351:1529–34.
34. Knoester M, Helmerhorst FM, Vandenbroucke JP, van der Westerlaken LA, Walther FJ, Veen S. Perinatal outcome, health, growth, and medical care utilization of 5- to 8-year-old intracytoplasmic sperm injection singletons. Fertil Steril. 2008;89:1133–46.
35. Knoester M, Helmerhorst FM, Vandenbroucke JP, van der Westerlaken LA, Walther FJ, Veen S. Cognitive development of singletons born after intracytoplasmic sperm injection compared with in vitro fertilization and natural conception. Fertil Steril. 2008;90:289–96.
36. Papaligoura Z, Panopoulou-Maratou O, Solman M, Arvaniti K, Sarafidou J. Cognitive development of 12 month old Greek infants conceived after ICSI and the effects of the method on their parents. Hum Reprod. 2004;19:1488–93.
37. van der Westerlaken L, Helmerhorst F, Dieben S, Naaktgeboren N. Intracytoplasmic sperm injection as a treatment for unexplained total fertilization failure or low fertilization after conventional in vitro fertilization. Fertil Steril. 2005;83:612–7.

38. van der Westerlaken L, Naaktgeboren N, Verburg H, Dieben S, Helmerhorst FM. Conventional in vitro fertilization versus intracytoplasmic sperm injection in patients with borderline semen: a randomized study using sibling oocytes. Fertil Steril. 2006;85:395–400.
39. Veeck LL. The morphological assessment of human oocytes and early conception. In: Keel BA, Webster BW, editors. Handbook of the laboratory diagnosis and treatment of infertility. Boca Raton: CRC Press; 1990. p. 353.
40. Hershlag A, Paine T, Kvapil G, Feng H, Napolitano B. In vitro fertilization-intracytoplasmic sperm injection split: an insemination method to prevent fertilization failure. Fertil Steril. 2002;77:229–32.
41. WHO laboratory manual for the examination and processing of human semen. 5th ed. Geneva, Switzerland: WHO Press; 2010.
42. Tournaye H, Verheyen G, Albano C, Camus M, Van Landuyt L, Devroey P, Van Steirteghem A. Intracytoplasmic sperm injection versus in vitro fertilization: a randomized controlled trial and a meta-analysis of the literature. Fertil Steril. 2002;78:1030–7.
43. Taylor TH, Wright G, Jones-Colon S, Mitchell-Leef D, Kort HI, Nagy ZP. Comparison of ICSI and conventional IVF in patients with increased oocyte immaturity. Reprod Biomed Online. 2008;17:46–52.
44. Lavy G, Boyers SP, DeCherney AH. Hyaluronidase removal of the cumulus oophorus increases in vitro fertilization. J In Vitro Fert Embryo Transf. 1988;5:257–60.
45. Magier S, van der Ven HH, Diedrich K, Krebs D. Significance of cumulus oophorus in in-vitro fertilization and oocyte viability and fertility. Hum Reprod. 1990;5:847–52.
46. Mahadevan MM, Trounson AO. Removal of the cumulus oophorus from the human oocyte for in vitro fertilization. Fertil Steril. 1985;43:263–7.
47. Hentemann MA, Briskemyr S, Bertheussen K. Blastocyst transfer and gender: IVF versus ICSI. J Assist Reprod Genet. 2009;26:433–6.

Chapter 13
Oocyte Denuding

Roberta Maggiulli, Filippo Ubaldi, and Laura Rienzi

Overview of the Technique

The term *oocyte denuding* refers to the removal of the somatic cell layers that surround the oocytes. During the preovulatory growth, within the follicle, the oocyte is surrounded by two different cell layers: *granulosa and thecal cells* that sustain oocyte nutrition and maturation providing essential metabolites, hormones, and growth factors [1–4]. However, the oocentric perspective of folliculogenesis highlights the central role of the oocyte itself in directing its own development as well as the follicle differentiation [5–9]. In this regard, the oocyte is deemed capable of modulating the follicular environment in order to guarantee correct preantral, antral, and preovulatory development.

During folliculogenesis, granulosa cells differentiate in two different specialized subpopulations: the cumulus oophorus, whose innermost layer, immediately adjacent to the zona pellucida, is called corona radiata, and the parietal granulosa cells. Cells of the corona radiata extend their cytoplasm toward the oocyte through the zona pellucida, creating gap junctions with oocytes microvilli. Communications (either paracrine interaction or gap junction) occur between the oocyte and the cumulus–corona cells, allowing oocyte nutrition and maturation from the diplotene to the MII stage [10, 11]. During ovulation and resumption of meiosis (induced by the preovulatory peak of LH in natural cycles), a definitive retraction of corona cell process and changes in the organization of corona radiata are observed. In parallel, a considerable active secretion of hyaluronic acid occurs, causing further expansion of cumulus–corona mass that appears finally as an expanded and mucified layer. The hyaluronic acid is a glycosaminoglycan that interposes among cells and separates them, conferring to the cumulus–corona mass a fluffy appearance. Whereas in

R. Maggiulli, PhD (✉) • F. Ubaldi, MD, MSc • L. Rienzi, MSc
GENERA Centre for Reproductive Medicine, Clinica Valle Giulia, Rome, Italy
e-mail: maggiulli@generaroma.it

Z.P. Nagy et al. (eds.), *Clinical Embryology: A Practical Guide*,
DOI 10.1007/978-1-4614-8376-2_13,

natural cycles the stage of oocyte nuclear maturation is coupled to an increased expansion and mucification of the cumulus layer [12], in stimulated cycles, it may be observed as asynchrony of these two processes [13]. This may be caused by a different sensitivity of the oocyte and the cumulus–corona mass to the stimulants [13, 14].

Besides their well-established role in supporting oocyte maturation, cumulus–corona cells might also be involved later on in embryonic development. These cells are supposed to be involved in embryonic metabolism, either stimulating gene expression [15] or reducing oxidative stress [16].

When oocyte denuding is thus performed, the oocyte is exposed for a variable amount of time to culture conditions without the protection of these layers and prior to its activation induced by the sperm entry at fertilization. The effect of this is unknown and still unexplored.

Ovum Pickup and Cumulus–Corona–Oocyte Complex Harvesting

In stimulated cycles, oocyte retrieval is usually performed at 36 h after hCG administration by ultrasound-guided transvaginal aspiration. The harvesting is carried out using an aspiration unit composed by a vacuum pump, a collection tube connected to a 17-gauge needle, and a collecting test tube. Today, several sophisticated vacuum pumps with adjustable aspiration pressure are available commercially. Since during the collection, oocytes are exposed to an increasing pressure that may affect their integrity, a maximum pressure of about 120 mmHg is recommended to avoid the risk to damage the oocytes [17]. Moreover, to minimize changes in temperature, the collection tubes should be kept in a tube warmer before being connected to the collection system.

Once the ovaries are visualized, ovarian follicles are aspirated in a systematic fashion. Immediately after the collection, the adjoining laboratory examines the follicular fluid. Cumulus–corona–oocyte complexes (CCOC) are identified in sterile plastic dishes, rinsed, transferred in preequilibrated IVF medium tube, and incubated at 37°C in an adequate atmosphere. During the entire procedure, efforts should be made to minimize the oocyte exposure to even transient temperature and pH fluctuations that may have a detrimental effect to the oocyte competence.

Indications

The evaluation of oocyte morphology prior to standard IVF is tricky because of the presence of the somatic cells. The quality and the degree of expansion of these cells do not always represent a reliable index of oocyte maturity and are mostly dependent on the type of ovarian stimulation protocol used [12, 13, 18–20].

With the introduction of assisted-fertilization techniques such as PZD (partial zona dissection), SUZI (subzonal insemination), and finally ICSI (intracytoplasmic

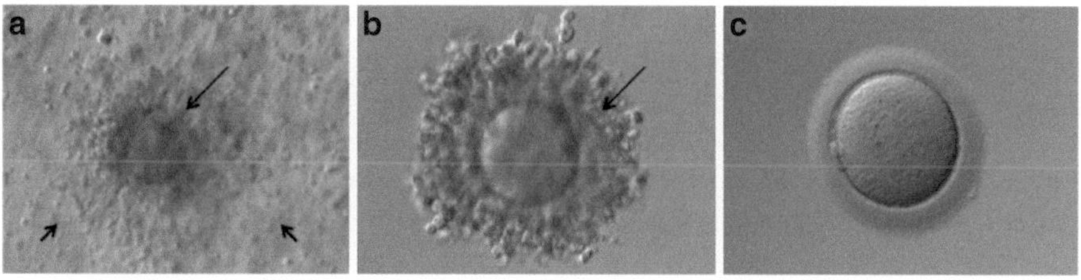

Fig. 13.1 Oocyte denudation steps. (**a**) Oocyte surrounded by corona radiata (*short arrow*) and cumulus cells (*long arrow*); (**b**) oocyte after the enzymatic-induced dispersion of cumulus cells; (**c**) MII denuded oocyte

sperm injection) [21], the removal of cumulus cells became a crucial step before fertilization since it allowed an unequivocal evaluation of oocyte nuclear maturity and easier handling of the oocytes during the micromanipulation procedure. Moreover, direct observation of oocyte morphology, including the extracytoplasmic components, is feasible only after denudation of its cumulus and corona layers.

In order to avoid sperm contamination, ICSI has been indicated as the preferred insemination method when preimplantation genetic diagnosis is required. To this end, complete and meticulous removal of somatic cells is of crucial importance, since extraneous DNA from maternal cumulus cells may also represent a potential source of contamination if a PCR-based technology is used [22].

Equipment and Procedure

The cumulus and corona cells are removed prior to any micromanipulation procedure by using a combined enzymatic and mechanical treatment [23]. Since hyaluronic acid is a major component of the mucified cumulus mass that surrounds the mature oocyte, hyaluronidase is employed for enzymatic removal of these cells. The type and concentration of this enzyme will be discussed later.

The procedure is usually performed under a stereomicroscope in different wells or microdrops containing buffered medium, normally covered by oil, on a warming plate.

A limited number of COCCs are normally placed into the first well/droplet containing the enzyme to disperse the cumulus cells (Fig. 13.1a). To enhance enzymatic removal of the cumulus and corona cells, the stripping of cumulus cells is performed by pipetting repeatedly the oocytes through a glass/plastic pipette with an inner diameter of approximately 250 μm for up to 30–40 s.

Once initial cell dissociation is observed (Fig. 13.1b), oocytes are moved to the second well/droplet containing clean buffered medium, taking care to carry over a minimum amount of enzyme. Then, further denudation is carried out by glass or plastic denuding pipettes with decreasing inner diameters (170–130 μm) to remove the corona cells (Fig. 13.1c). An accurate washing of denuded oocytes is then required to wash out completely the enzyme.

It has been proposed that a two-step denuding procedure involving an incubation period after oocytes exposure to the enzyme and before the mechanical step [24] may expedite the removal of cumulus cells while minimizing mechanical-induced oocyte damage. After partial removal of the cumulus cells by a short exposition to buffered medium containing the enzyme, the oocytes are rinsed in preequilibrated culture medium and place back into the incubator for 30 min. This further step leads to a weakening of the hyaluronan matrix, allowing an easier cumulus cell removal by gently pipetting oocytes with 150-μm inner diameter stripper. After denudation, the oocytes can be examined under an inverted microscope to assess integrity and the stage of maturation.

Timing

The oocyte denudation is usually performed between 37 and 40 h post-hCG administration and immediately before the insemination. Already in 1982, Trounson et al. [25] postulated that preincubation of cumulus–corona–oocyte complexes before conventional insemination was beneficial for the accomplishment of complete oocyte maturation and assured high rates of fertilization and embryo development in vitro.

However, no differences between the effect of early (1–2 h after retrieval) and late (5–6 h after retrieval) denudation and injection on early embryo development was reported by Van de Velde [26]. The authors assumed that the stimulation protocol involved in the study allowed a well-synchronized nuclear–cytoplasmic maturation hiding the potential contribution of cumulus–corona complex preincubation.

To evaluate whether the timing of ICSI has an effect on ICSI outcome, we analyzed the possible effects of preincubation of CCOC on fertilization and embryo development rates after ICSI [27]. In agreement with Ho and coauthors [28], we observed that a preincubation period of at least 3 h between oocyte retrieval and ICSI could improve the fertilization rate and embryo quality. This time might be necessary for some oocytes to reach full cytoplasmic maturity, leading to a higher activation rate upon microinjection.

Our observations have been challenged by Yanagida et al. [29] who showed that oocytes retained sufficient potential for fertilization between 1 and 9 h after oocyte collection. On the other hand, they observed that extended preincubation time might be responsible of reduced embryo quality.

Oocyte Evaluation

Cumulus–Corona–Oocyte Complex Assessment

Several scoring systems for cumulus–corona–oocyte complex evaluation have been introduced aiming to predict the nuclear maturity of the overshadowed oocytes and identify the proper timing for insemination [19, 30–36]. Early studies from

Table 13.1 Cumulus–corona–oocyte complex evaluation

Groups	CCOC morphology
Mature	Expanded cumulus Radiant corona Distinct zona pellucida, clear ooplasm Expanded well-aggregated membrana granulosa cells
Approximately mature	Expanded cumulus mass Slightly compact corona radiata Expanded well-aggregated membrana granulosa cells
Immature	Dense compact cumulus if present Adherent compact layer of corona cells Ooplasm if visible with the presence of germinal vesicle Compact and nonaggregated membrane granulosa cells
Postmature	Expanded cumulus with clumps Radiant corona radiata, yet often clumped, irregular, or incomplete Visible zona, slightly granular or dark ooplasm Small and relatively nonaggregated membrana granulosa cells
Atretic	Rarely with associated cumulus mass Clumped and very irregular corona radiata if present Visible zona, dark and frequently misshapen ooplasm Membrana granulosa cells with very small clumps of cells

Adapted from Lin et al. [35], with permission

Rattanachaiyanont et al. [19], performed on oocytes scheduled for denudation and insemination by ICSI, reported no correlation between oocyte–corona–cumulus complex morphology and nuclear maturity, fertilization rate, and embryo cleavage. On the other hand, other authors reported that CCOC scoring related to fertilization and pregnancy rates [34] as well as to blastocyst quality and development [35]. Recently, Lin and colleagues [35] proposed a grading system of COCCs based on the morphology of the oocyte cytoplasm, cumulus mass, corona cells, and membrana granulosa cells, for oocytes prior to insemination by conventional IVF. Five grades (*mature group, approximately mature, immature, postmature, and atretic*) were previously described and reported in Table 13.1. The authors reported higher fertilization rates for the oocytes belonging to the mature group compared to those belonging to the other groups. Moreover, the immature group was characterized by a higher incidence of poor morphology day 3 embryos as compared to the mature group.

It has also been suggested that the presence of COCC anomalies such as blood clots or amorphous clumps may be an index of a suboptimal follicular maturation [37, 38] and may impair embryo ability to develop to blastocyst stage. When these oocytes are denuded of their cumulus cells, a significant alteration in cytoplasmic texture has been highlighted [39] that may be related to the reduced fertilization rate obtained when those oocytes are used for insemination [38]. Variation in temperature and pH as well as reactive oxygen species (ROS) induced by the presence of blood clots is pointed to be at the origin of the compromised competence of those oocytes [32].

Although, cumulus–corona mass observation is not sufficient to evaluate oocyte maturity and competence, it is reasonable to hypothesize that ooplasm development is influenced by the action of these cells. In accordance with this hypothesis, it has been suggested that cumulus–corona cells play an important role in the in vitro maturation of oocytes that were immature at the time of retrieval [40, 41]. Therefore, a careful observation of CCOC morphology may be a useful tool for oocyte selection in those circumstances where no direct evaluation of the oocyte is possible. In addition, in our laboratory, where a limited number of oocytes can be inseminated accordingly to the Italian law, we evaluate CCOC prior to denudation for ICSI. In fact, as suggested by Canipari et al. [42], we assume that there is a higher probability to obtain a better quality mature oocyte in a normally expanded cumulus than in a nonexpanded one.

Oocyte Cytoplasmic and Extracytoplasmic Evaluation

It is generally recognized that a "normal" human metaphase II oocyte, at light microscopy level, should have a round, clear zona pellucida; a small perivitelline space containing a single not fragmented polar body; and a pale, moderately granular cytoplasm not containing inclusions [36, 43–48].

However, the majority of the oocytes retrieved after ovarian hyperstimulation exhibit one or more variations of the described "ideal" morphological criteria [36, 44–50]. This is true also for oocytes obtained from proven fertile donors [51]. The actual negative impact of the different oocytes' cytoplasmic and extracytoplasmic "abnormalities" is unclear. Conflicting data have been, in fact, published in the literature concerning oocyte morphology and ICSI outcome [36, 48].

Nuclear Maturity

During oocyte development within the follicle, the nucleus is arrested at the prophase of the first meiotic division. Oocyte nuclear maturation consists in the resumption of the first meiosis, going through the germinal vesicle (GV) breakdown, first meiotic spindle (MS) formation, chromosomal segregation, and IPB extrusion. At this stage, the maturation process is not ended yet; the oocyte has still to enter the second meiotic division where a second arrest occurs at metaphase stage (MII). This stage is characterized by the presence of the MS of the second meiotic division located at the oocyte periphery with one pole attached to the cell cortex. This highly dynamic structure is formed by microtubule, with the chromosomes condensed and aligned at the equatorial region [52–56]. After insemination, this structure plays a crucial role in chromosomal disjunction and segregation and in the correct completion of meiosis and fertilization. MS alteration and dysfunction lead to unbalanced disjunction and/or nondisjunction of chromatids, chromosome scattering, and to the formation of aneuploid embryos [54, 57, 58].

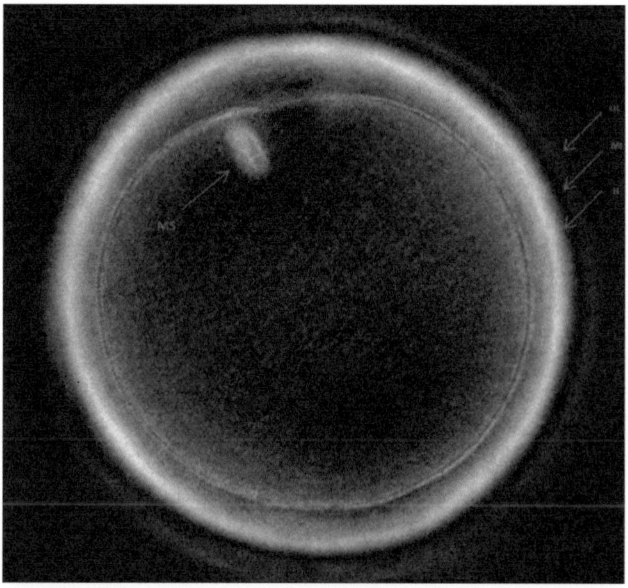

Fig. 13.2 Metaphase II oocyte observed by polarized light microscopy. *MS* meiotic spindle; *IL* zona pellucida inner layer; *ML* zona pellucida middle layer; *OU* zona pellucida outer layer

The presence of the IPB in the perivitelline space is a marker of oocyte meiosis resumption, but not an evidence of MII stage achievement. It is only observing the presence of the MS of the second meiotic division that the oocyte nuclear maturation can be assessed (Fig. 13.2). For this purpose, novel polarized light microscopy systems together with their image processing software (Spindle View Pol-Scope system, CRI, Woburn, MA, USA; OCTAX polarAIDE, MTG, Germany) have been recently introduced in IVF laboratories allowing a noninvasive observation of the MS in living oocytes [59–62]. These systems consist of a microscope equipped with a green filter and a polarizer generating circularly polarized light. Highly ordinate and well-organized structures, such as the parallel-aligned microtubules composing the oocyte MS, are able to shift the vibration plane and retard the polarized light. The induced retardance can be measured (nm), and this parameter is directly related to the microtubules density [60, 63, 64].

The Pol-Scope allows to assess the position and appearance of the spindle and to recognize those oocytes that have not completed the first meiotic division and are still in telophase I [65–67]. At this time of the cell cycle, the oocyte cytoplasm and the cytoplasm of the forming IPB are not yet completely separated by cytokinesis. The MS appears to be interposed between the two separating cells, with its long axis corresponding to the axis connecting the center of the two cells (Fig. 13.3). An oocyte at this stage is usually classified as a "mature MII" when observed with the conventional light microscopy. Although at this stage the presence of the IPB is evident in the perivitelline space, chromosome segregation is not completed. The

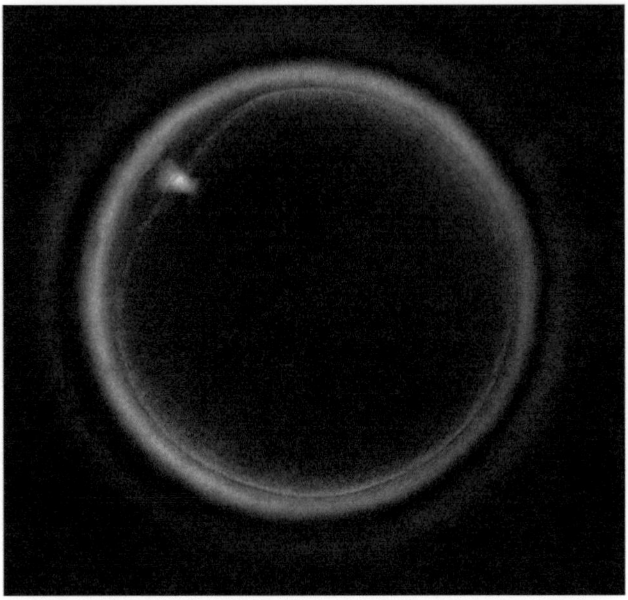

Fig. 13.3 Telophase I oocyte with the meiotic spindle interposed between the polar body and the cytoplasm

use of such immature oocytes for ICSI is unadvisable due to the asynchrony between sperm entry and oocyte nuclear maturity.

The importance of the presence of a detectable MS in the oocyte cytoplasm prior to ICSI has been extensively described in several studies [68–75]. MS visualization has been associated with oocyte fertilization rate, embryo development, and blastocyst progression. However, the percentage of oocytes functionally superior, with a positive MS at visualization, varies substantially between the different studies, between 60 and 90% [69, 70, 72]. These differences have been related to different factors that get involved during laboratory and clinical practices [76].

When studying the MS with the Spindle View systems, these factors must be taken carefully into account in order to keep under control those that may interfere with the visualization of the spindle. First is temperature control during oocytes handling [68, 77]. Secondly, the absence of MS may be due to unfavorable culture conditions and environmental changes [78, 79]. Third factor is the MS orientation during Pol-Scope visualization [70, 72, 73]: oocyte rotation by using a micropipette allows the correct orientation of the MS making it visible at the polarized light, with the long axis oriented perpendicular to the viewer's axis [64, 70, 71].

It has been recently shown, with time-lapse cinematography (Octax EyeWare MX), that at the end of the first meiotic division, the MS takes approximately 40–60 min to reform [67]. Therefore, at least in some cases, the absence of MS signal is due to the oocyte maturation process. Most of the oocytes display the meiotic spindle starting at 38 h after hCG administration, and thereafter [72].

Table 13.2 Parameters that can be considered during MS visualization with polarized light microscopy

Presence/absence of MS, which may be due to		
	Laboratory factors	
		Temperature instability
		Chemical and physical stress during handling and culturing
		Correct oocyte rotation during visualization
	Oocyte maturation, which is related to	
		Time elapsed from hCG administration
		Interval between first and second meiotic divisions
	Maternal factors (i.e., age)	
Position and appearance of MS		
	Allow identification of immature oocytes (late telophase I)	
	Allow assessment of IPB/MS relative position, which affects oocyte fertilization rate and the orientation of the I cleavage plane	
	Allow the correct orientation of MS during ICSI	
Quantitative data		
	MS pole to pole length, which is related to oocyte competence	
	MS mean retardance, which is a measure of MS polimerization	

From Casciani and Rienzi [76], with permission

Polarized light microscopy allows also the evaluation of the appearance (length, shape) and the retardance of the MS in living oocyte. These parameters (Table 13.2) may be considered during oocyte grading and for oocyte selection together with the other morphological parameters that are usually observed with the conventional light microscopy. Although promising, the validity of this approach has not been proven yet, since discrepancies between MS retardance and normal spindle organization and chromosome configuration assessed by confocal microscopy have been reported [80]. This technique is also expensive (due to the cost of the instruments and the time necessary for the additional treatment) and potentially dangerous for the oocytes that may be exposed to injurious environmental conditions during observation. Only specialized laboratories equipped with chamber that allow temperature and atmosphere control on the inverted microscope could, in our opinion, benefit from this technology in the routine work.

Cytoplasmic Aspect

Nuclear maturity is only part of the oocyte maturation process. To acquire full competence for subsequent fertilization and development, the oocyte has to undergo to nuclear and cytoplasmic maturation in a coordinate manner. Disturbances or asynchrony of these two maturation processes are believed to result in a variety of oocyte morphological abnormalities [81–83]. Accordingly, cytoplasmic (vacuoles, refractile bodies, increased cytoplasmic granularity, smooth endoplasmic reticulum clusters) and extracytoplasmic (abnormal zona pellucida, large perivitelline space, abnormal, fragmented, or degenerated IPB) defects potentially reflect oocyte developmental impairments [36, 48, 50, 84–86].

Some authors have suggested that despite normal fertilization and early embryo development that can be achieved in oocytes with "abnormal" cytoplasmic morphology, the resulting embryos have a lower implantation potential [43, 87].

Granular cytoplasm and, in particular, centrally located granular area have been associated with poorer zygote quality and poorer embryo quality [39, 50]. These cytoplasmic alterations may thus be, as suggested, a sign of oocyte immaturity [39]. In agreement with other studies [44, 48, 88], when we investigated the relationship between MII oocyte morphology and ICSI outcome [50], we observed that also oocyte vacuolization has a detrimental effect on fertilization rate. Furthermore, no fertilization has been described when vacuole size above 14 μm was present in the injected oocyte [48, 88]. It is believed that vacuoles arise either spontaneously [89] or by fusion of preexisting vesicles derived from smooth endoplasmic reticulum and/or Golgi apparatus [90]. How vacuolization affects pronuclear formation is still unclear. Probably, the presence of these cytoplasmic inclusions interferes with the cytoskeleton function [48]. A negative effect of these structures on the metaphase II meiotic spindle has also been suggested [89].

Meriano et al. [91] and Otsuki et al. [92] have shown that the presence of smooth endoplasmic reticulum clusters in the oocytes significantly impairs embryo development and implantation. In regard to the presence of SER in the oocyte cytoplasm, we were unable to identify a relationship between the presence of this abnormality and fertilization rate and pronuclear/embryo quality. However, because of the very low number of oocytes treated (only 0.5% of oocytes displaying this feature), no real conclusion can be drawn regarding this particular aspect.

Extracytoplasmic Structure Evaluation

Extracytoplasmic peculiarities are classified as fragmented I polar body, abnormal I polar body (large and/or degenerated), abnormal zona pellucida (with sets and/or thick and/or dark), large perivitelline space, and abnormal oocyte shape (oval).

First polar body morphology has been suggested as a possible indicator of fertilization and embryo quality after ICSI [47, 66, 93–95]. Embryo transfers selected on the basis of I polar body morphology have been associated with increased implantation and pregnancy rates [93]. However, recent studies have failed to demonstrate any relationship between I polar body fragmentation and embryo implantation rate [66, 94]. Moreover, it has been shown that the aneuploidy rate of the metaphase II oocytes is unrelated to the morphology of the first polar body [96].

In our hands, the presence of an abnormal first polar body (degenerated and/or large) in the metaphase II oocytes analyzed was relatively rare (4.4%). However, this feature was associated with a significantly reduced fertilization rate. It has been suggested that degenerated polar body may reflect an asynchrony between nuclear and cytoplasmic maturation [81], which would explain the lower ability of the cell to support pronuclear formation after ICSI. Furthermore, a correspondence between the presence of large polar body and poor embryo development was already

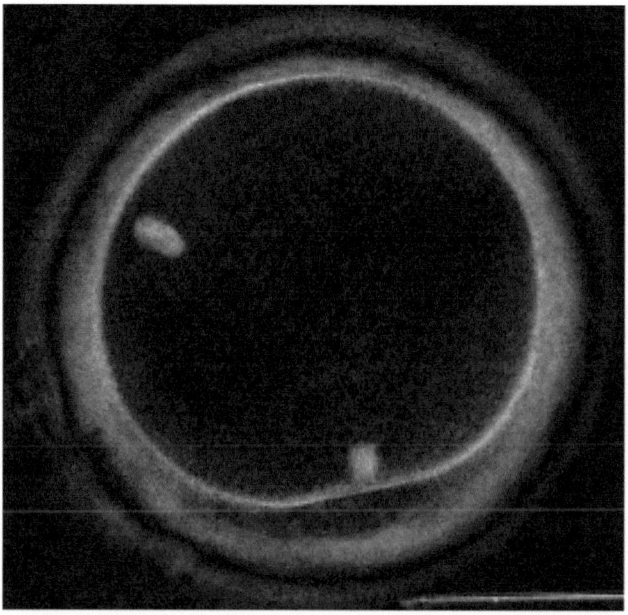

Fig. 13.4 Giant oocyte with two detectable meiotic spindles

described [45, 66, 93]. According to animal experiments [97], it has been postulated that the emission of an abnormally large polar body is due to the inability of the meiotic spindle to migrate correctly at the very periphery of the cell. It is, in fact, the position of the main axis of the meiotic spindle that dictates the orientation of the cleavage furrow. A centrally located meiotic spindle would lead to the formation of enlarged polar body [66]. The polar body morphology, and in particular degenerated and large polar bodies (but not fragmented), may be thus considered a marker of oocyte maturation disturbances [66, 97]. Nevertheless, in our hands, once fertilized, these oocytes did not show an impaired developmental potential in vitro.

A large perivitelline space in the injected oocytes significantly affected fertilization rate and pronuclear morphology [50]. This observation may be ascribed to an overmaturity of these oocytes at the time of ICSI [49].

Special attention should also be focused on giant oocytes. Although the occurrence of these oocytes is relatively rare after ovarian hyperstimulation, the use of these cells for in vitro fertilization is potentially dangerous. These oocytes contain an extra set of chromosomes and therefore two meiotic spindles when observed at the polarized light microscopy (Fig. 13.4). It has been also described that all embryos generated from giant oocytes are chromosomally abnormal, but they may have a normal cleavage and development to blastocyst stage [98]. The transfer of these embryos could thus increase the risk of undesired miscarriages [98].

Possible Damage to the Oocyte

Oocyte Parthenogenetic Activation

In mouse and human oocytes, chemical agents such as ethanol and Ca^{2+} ionophore as well as electrical-field stimulation may initiate a series of events leading to the release of the meiotic arrest at metaphase II and consequent cell divisions of activated oocyte. Although human oocytes seem to be less susceptible to artificial activation in comparison to other mammalian oocytes, several factors related to IVF procedures, such as the high vacuum pressures used for follicles aspiration and the high concentration of hyaluronidase used for cumulus cells stripping as well as oocyte pipetting, may activate mature oocytes and induce parthenogenetic activation [99, 100].

When ICSI has been introduced, a concentration of 760 IU/mL of hyaluronidase was used to denude oocytes, but high parthenogenetic activation rates (17%) were observed [100]. Van Steirteghem et al. [101] were able to reduce the activation rate to 3% by employing lower concentration (78 IU/mL) of enzyme. Moreover, Joris et al. [102] investigated whether a further reduction of hyaluronidase concentration might influence oocyte intactness and its ability to fertilize and support embryo development. Although no significant effect on ICSI outcome was observed, a significant lower degeneration rate was registered when a concentration of 10 IU of enzyme per millilitre was used. This finding would justify the use of lower concentration of enzyme.

Meiotic Spindle

A less perceptible effect but likewise harmful to the oocyte is represented by the potential displacement of the polar body following the denuding procedure. Notwithstanding the intrinsic ability of the polar body to move along the plasma membrane of the oocyte, the mechanical stripping of the cumulus cells may impair the microtubule frame and the actin filament organization, causing the break of the cellular bridges that connect the polar body to the oocyte. This would result in an IPB displacement from its original extrusion site [70].

The use of polarized light microscopy may be helpful in the assessment of the position of the MS in regard to the IPB. It should be underlined that the MS is not only involved in chromosome segregation but it is also a key organelle in the creation of the IPB. MS position at the very periphery of the cell, attached to the oolemma cortex [103], dictates the orientation of the cleavage furrow and thus the site of IPB extrusion. According to different studies, moderate degrees of IPB/MS deviation do not seem to affect ICSI outcome, in terms of fertilization and embryo development rates [69, 70]. However, in our laboratory, we found that a mechanical stress able to induce a dislocation of the IPB $\geq 90°$ with respect of the MS position is related to a lower fertilization rate [70]. MS dislocation has also been reported to affect embryo development since its position determines the correct orientation of the first cleavage plane and therefore of the animal–vegetal pole [71]. It is thus advisable to perform oocyte denudation in gentle manner.

Besides affecting ICSI outcome, a possible drawback of IPB displacement is the potential injury that the MS may undergo during microinsemination. In fact, when performing ICSI, the oocyte is maintained in a fixed position where the IPB is placed at 90° from the injection pipette entry site. Displaced IPB may thus expose the MS to the pipette passageway during sperm injection and hence to mechanical damage. In view of this fact, the Pol-Scope may be a helpful tool during ICSI, allowing the correct orientation of the MS (and not of the IPB) as far as possible from the injection pipette entry spot.

Moreover, it has been widely shown that oocyte exposure to even slight temperature variations dramatically injures the MS structure by inducing microtubules disassembly [68, 104–107]. In fact, MS microtubules are highly sensitive to chemical and physical stress that may occur during oocyte retrieval and handling. Thermal stability is therefore necessary during oocyte denudation, observation, and manipulation.

Mechanical Stress

In order to avoid damage to the oocytes, a meticulous care should be taken during the mechanical removal of cumulus cells. In fact, an excessive or vigorous pipetting of the oocyte may result in zona pellucida fracture and even oocyte degeneration. The stripping of the cumulus cells should be performed gradually by employing decreasing inner diameter denuding pipettes. The use of stripper with a diameter smaller than 140 μm should be avoided since it may induce oocyte deformation and damage the oocyte cytoskeleton impairing its ability to sustain correct pronuclear formation.

Enzyme Type and Concentration

Hyaluronidase or Coronase

Traditionally, the denuding procedure is performed by using a bovine-derived hyaluronidase. Bovine testicular hyaluronidase is an endo-β-*N*-acetyl-D-hexosaminidase that catalyzes the hydrolysis of hexosaminidic linkage contained in hyaluronic acid. Although purified preparations of the enzyme are commercially available, the possibility of animal-derived pathogens or contaminant transmission cannot be excluded [108]. The use of a plant enzyme preparation containing citric acid and papaine as well as NaCl and phosphate (Coronase) has been proposed as an alternative to animal extracted hyaluronidase. Because of the different action mechanism of Coronase that acts by chelating Ca++ ions and inducing a degradation of glycoprotein granules of the hyaluronic matrix, a longer exposure time to the enzyme is required [109]. However, Coronase exhibited similar performance in terms of oocyte integrity and competence preservation when compared to conventional hyaluronidase. Moreover, because of the absence of any human or animal compounds, it may be more suitable for the clinical practice [109].

Enzyme Concentration

In order to minimize any potential toxic effect on oocytes, a reduced enzyme concentration as well as shorter exposure time is advisable. As already mentioned, lower concentrations of the enzyme such as 80 IU/mL, which is generally used in the clinical practice, significantly decrease the rate of parthenogenesis. A concentration as low as 10 IU/mL in combination with a denuding pipette of 1,000 μm diameter has also been shown to be able to denude mature oocytes efficiently [24].

Animal-Derived or Recombinant Human Hyaluronidase

Several concerns arose from the clinical application of the animal origin enzyme that may be affected by a reduced purity and standardization. Human recombinant hyaluronidase (Cumulase) has been proposed to circumvent problems and concerns associated with the animal origin. When De Vos et al. [110] conducted a randomized sibling-oocyte study in order to validate the effectiveness of recombinant human hyaluronidase vs. bovine-derived hyaluronidase, they observed comparable results in terms of oocyte survival and fertilization. Evison [111], who observed a significantly increased rate of normal fertilization coupled to a significantly decreased rate of oocyte damage when the recombinant form of the enzyme was used, confirmed these findings. Following up these observations, the human recombinant form of the enzyme may represent a safer, quality-controlled but likewise effective alternative.

Influence of Microenvironment Condition

A general principle for the physical environment is to keep it free of any insults. The handling of oocytes during the entire IVF procedure should be carried out under conditions of constant pH and stable temperature. In order to prevent the evaporation of the medium and minimize the fluctuations of the pH and the temperature, 4-(2-hydroxyethyl)-1-piperazineethanesulfonic acid (HEPES)-buffered media and temperature-controlled humidified chambers are employed to maintain these parameters in a physiological range.

Temperature

We have already affirmed that temperature fluctuations likely associated with the handling of oocytes may impair the microtubular system. Changes in spindle organization have been observed in human mature oocytes exposed to room temperature even for only few minutes [105]. Notwithstanding the ability of the meiotic spindle to reassemble when the temperature is reestablished, the risk of aneuploidy occurrence is increased after a temperature-induced depolymerization [105].

Because of this extreme meiotic spindle sensitivity to temperature changes, all the equipment in use (Petri dishes and Pasteur pipette) should be prewarmed at 37°C. In order to maintain a constant temperature in the droplets, the working areas (hood and microscope) and the thermo plate must be calibrated regularly. However, it is very difficult to maintain constant temperature without the use of specific chambers.

CO_2 Concentration

Dale et al. demonstrated that the baseline intracellular pH (pHi) of human egg is 7.4 ± 0.1 [112]. Unlike germinal vesicle that is endowed with a robust mechanism of pH regulation, denuded metaphase II oocytes lacking of HCO_3^-/Cl^- and Na^+/H^+ functioning exchangers do not exhibit the ability to control and regulate intracellular pH [113]. It is only 2–3 h after fertilization that the oocyte initiates to recover the exchanger activity and the consequent ability to regulate its pH. To preserve oocyte homeostasis and avoid that pHi fluctuations that may impair developmental competence, HEPES-buffered media are usually employed during the oocytes handling outside the incubator. However, media containing bicarbonate/CO_2 buffers would be preferable, since, although requiring controlled chambers to maintain a 5–7% CO_2 atmosphere, they circumvent the use of HEPES and thus the increased risk of toxicity to the oocyte. In fact, the low percentage of CO_2 entails a low percentage of HCO_3^- in the media that is essential to the functionality of HCO_3^-/Cl^- exchanger and thus the HCO_3^--dependent mechanism that oocytes utilize to defend against acidosis.

O_2 Concentration

Several IVF procedures entail an increase in oxidative stress that may be detrimental to the embryo. Although several physiological events, such as ovulation and fertilization, as well as the implantation process, are modulated by a ROS formation [114–116], a considerable increase in ROS concentration exceeding the oocyte antioxidant defenses may result in cellular structural and functional alterations. It has already been shown that during their journey along female reproductive tract, embryos encountered a decreasing oxygen gradient. Moreover, oxygen levels in oviduct and uterus of several species are considerably lower than in the atmosphere (1.5–6 vs. 21%).

Therefore, it has been suggested that the employment of low oxygen tension (5%) within the incubation atmosphere may improve mammalian embryo development [117–120]. Even if the precise O_2 level is still unknown and may be developmental stage dependent, the low oxygen level should be a principal for all mammalian embryo culture systems including humans.

Incomplete Denudation

In support of a positive effect of cumulus–corona cells on oocyte development, it was proposed that incomplete denudation of oocytes prior to ICSI improves embryo quality and development since it may assist embryonic metabolism, either stimulating gene expression [121] or reducing oxidative stress [122]. A study involving sibling oocytes investigated the actual effect of homologous adhering cumulus cells, resulting in an improvement in terms of preimplantation development when oocytes were cultured with attached cumulus cells [123].

Similar findings were obtained in previous studies, suggesting that the presence of cumulus cells allows better nuclear as well cytoplasmic in vitro maturation, particularly in oocytes that were immature at the time of denudation [124, 125].

Future Direction and Improvement

The involvement of automated systems in IVF procedures is attracting increasing attention. A microfluidic device has been proposed to remove cumulus cells automatically, aiming to minimize physical stresses related to this procedure [126]. The system entails pressure-driven flow to obtain a correct positioning and transit of CCOC into microchannel that allow yielding predictable cumulus removal. Although further studies are required to assess the impact of these procedures on embryo health, several efforts are focusing on the development of a single integrated automated system skilled to perform all the steps from oocyte retrieval to insemination and embryo culture.

References

1. Biggers JD, Whittingham DG, Donahue RP. The pattern of energy metabolism in the mouse oocyte and zygote. Proc Natl Acad Sci USA. 1967;58(2):560–7.
2. Donahue RP, Stern S. Follicular cell support of oocyte maturation: production of pyruvate in vitro. J Reprod Fertil. 1968;17(2):395–8.

3. Brower PT, Schultz RM. Intercellular communication between granulosa cells and mouse oocytes: existence and possible nutritional role during oocyte growth. Dev Biol. 1982;90(1):144–53.
4. Haghighat N, Van Winkle LJ. Developmental change in follicular cell-enhanced amino acid uptake into mouse oocytes that depends on intact gap junctions and transport system Gly. J Exp Zool. 1990;253(1):71–82.
5. Buccione R, Vanderhyden BC, Caron PJ, Eppig JJ. FSH-induced expansion of the mouse cumulus oophorus in vitro is dependent upon a specific factor(s) secreted by the oocyte. Dev Biol. 1990;138:16–25.
6. Salustri A, Ulisse S, Yanagishita M, Hascall VC. Hyaluronic acid synthesis by mural granulosa cells and cumulus cells in vitro is selectively stimulated by a factor produced by oocytes and by transforming growth factor-beta. J Biol Chem. 1990;265(32):19517–23.
7. Canipari R, Epifano O, Siracusa G, Salustri A. Mouse oocytes inhibit plasminogen activator production by ovarian cumulus and granulosa cells. Dev Biol. 1995;167(1):371–8.
8. Eppig JJ, Wigglesworth K, Pendola FL. The mammalian oocyte orchestrates the rate of ovarian follicular development. Proc Natl Acad Sci USA. 2002;99(5):2890–4.
9. Hussein TS, Froiland DA, Amato F, Thompson JG, Gilchrist RB. Oocytes prevent cumulus cell apoptosis by maintaining a morphogenic paracrine gradient of bone morphogenetic proteins. J Cell Sci. 2005;118(Pt 22):5257–68.
10. Dong J, Albertini DF, Nishimori K, et al. Growth differentiation factor-9 is required during early ovarian folliculogenesis. Nature. 1996;383:531–5.
11. Albertini DF, Combelles CM, Benecchi E, Carabatsos MJ. Cellular basis for paracrine regulation of ovarian follicle development. Reproduction. 2001;121:647–53.
12. Testart J, Lassalle B, Frydman R, Belaisch JC. A study of factors affecting the success of human fertilization in vitro. II. Influence of semen quality and oocyte maturity on fertilization and cleavage. Biol Reprod. 1983;28:425–31.
13. Laufer N, Tarlatzis BC, DeCherney AH, et al. Asynchrony between human cumulus–corona cell complex and oocyte maturation after human menopausal gonadotropin treatment for in vitro fertilization. Fertil Steril. 1984;42:366–72.
14. Bar-Ami S, Gitay-Goren H, Brandes JM. Different morphological and steroidogenic patterns in oocyte/cumulus–corona cell complexes aspirated at in vitro fertilization. Biol Reprod. 1989;41:761–70.
15. McKenzie LJ, Pangas SA, Carson SA, et al. Human cumulus granulosa cell gene expression: a predictor of fertilization and embryo selection in women undergoing IVF. Hum Reprod. 2004;19:2869–74.
16. Fatehi AN, Roelen BA, Colenbrander B, et al. Presence of cumulus cells during in vitro fertilization protects the bovine oocyte against oxidative stress and improves first cleavage but does not affect further development. Zygote. 2005;13:177–85.
17. Edwards RG, Steptoe PC, Fowler RE, Baillie J. Observations on preovulatory human ovarian follicles and their aspirates. Br J Obstet Gynaecol. 1980;87(9):69–79.
18. Khamsi F, Roberge S, Lacanna IC, Wong J, Yavas Y. Effects of granulosa cells, cumulus cells, and oocyte density on in vitro fertilization in women. Endocrine. 1999;10:161–6.
19. Rattanachaiyanont M, Leader A, Léveillé MC. Lack of correlation between oocyte-corona-cumulus complex morphology and nuclear maturity of oocytes collected in stimulated cycles for intracytoplasmic sperm injection. Fertil Steril. 1999;71(5):937–40.
20. Khamsi F, Roberge S. Granulosa cells of the cumulus oophorus are different from mural granulosa cells in their response to gonadotropins and IGF-I. J Endocrinol. 2001;170(3):565–73.
21. Palermo G, Joris H, Devroey P, Van Steirteghem AC. Pregnancies after intracytoplasmic injection of single spermatozoon into an oocyte. Lancet. 1992;340(8810):17–8.
22. ESHRE. Intracytoplasmic sperm injection (ICSI) in 2006: evidence and evolution. Hum Reprod Update. 2007;13:515–26.
23. Mahadevan MM, Trounson AO. Removal of the cumulus oophorus from the human oocyte for in vitro fertilization. Fertil Steril. 1985;43(2):263–7.

24. Van de Velde H, Nagy ZP, Joris H, De Vos A, Van Steirteghem AC. Effects of different hyaluronidase concentrations and mechanical procedures for cumulus cell removal on the outcome of intracytoplasmic sperm injection. Hum Reprod. 1997;12(10):2246–50.
25. Trounson AO, Mohr LR, Wood C, Leeton JF. Effect of delayed insemination on in-vitro fertilization, culture and transfer of human embryos. J Reprod Fertil. 1982;64(2):285–9.
26. Van de Velde H, De Vos A, Joris H, Nagy ZP, Van Steirteghem AC. Effect of timing of oocyte denudation and micro-injection on survival, fertilization and embryo quality after intracytoplasmic sperm injection. Hum Reprod. 1998;13(11):3160–4.
27. Rienzi L, Ubaldi F, Anniballo R, Cerulo G, Greco E. Preincubation of human oocytes may improve fertilization and embryo quality after intracytoplasmic sperm injection. Hum Reprod. 1998;13(4):1014–9.
28. Ho JY, Chen MJ, Yi YC, Guu HF, Ho ES. The effect of preincubation period of oocytes on nuclear maturity, fertilization rate, embryo quality, and pregnancy outcome in IVF and ICSI. J Assist Reprod Genet. 2003;20(9):358–64.
29. Yanagida K, Yazawa H, Katayose H, Suzuki K, Hoshi K, Sato A. Influence of oocyte preincubation time on fertilization after intracytoplasmic sperm injection. Hum Reprod. 1998; 13(8):2223–6.
30. Veeck LL. The morphologic estimation of mature oocytes and their preparation for insemination. In: Jones Jr HW, Jones GS, et al., editors. In-vitro fertilization—Norfolk. Baltimore: Williams and Wilkins; 1986. p. 81.
31. Wolf DP. Oocyte quality and fertilization. In: Wolf DP, editor. In-vitro fertilization and embryo transfer. New York: Plenum; 1988. p. 129–38.
32. Daya S, Kohut J, Gunby J, et al. Influence of blood clots in the cumulus complex on oocyte fertilization and cleavage. Hum Reprod. 1990;5:744–6.
33. Veeck LL. The morphological assessment of human oocytes and early conception. In: Keel BA, Webster BW, editors. Handbook of the laboratory diagnosis and treatment of infertility. Boca Raton: CRC Press; 1990. p. 353–69.
34. Ng ST, Chang TH, Wu TC. Prediction of the rates of fertilization, cleavage, and pregnancy success by cumulus-coronal morphology in an in vitro fertilization program. Fertil Steril. 1999;72:412–7.
35. Lin YC, Chang SY, Lan KC, et al. Human oocyte maturity in vivo determines the outcome of blastocyst development in vitro. J Assist Reprod Genet. 2003;20:506–12.
36. Balaban B, Urman B. Effect of oocyte morphology on embryo development and implantation. Reprod Biomed Online. 2006;12:608–15.
37. Motta PM, Nottola SA, Pereda J, et al. Ultrastructure of human cumulus oophorus: a transmission electron microscopic study on oviductal oocytes and fertilized eggs. Hum Reprod. 1995;10:2361–7.
38. Ebner T, Moser M, Shebl O, Sommergruber M, Yaman C, Tews G. Blood clots in the cumulus-oocyte complex predict poor oocyte quality and post-fertilization development. Reprod Biomed Online. 2008;16(6):801–7.
39. Kahraman S, Yakin K, Donmez E, et al. Relationship between granular cytoplasm of oocytes and pregnancy outcome following intracytoplasmic sperm injection. Hum Reprod. 2000; 15:2390–3.
40. Goud PT, Goud AP, Qian C, et al. In-vitro maturation of human germinal vesicle stage oocytes: role of cumulus cells and epidermal growth factor in the culture medium. Hum Reprod. 1998;13:1638–44.
41. Yamazaki Y, Wakayama T, Yanagimachi R. Contribution of cumulus cells and serum to the maturation of oocyte cytoplasm as revealed by intracytoplasmic sperm injection (ICSI). Zygote. 2001;9:277–82.
42. Canipari R, Camaioni A, Scarchilli L, Barberi M, Salustri A. Oocyte maturation and ovulation: mechanism of control. 2PN Attual Scient Biol Reprod. 2004;1:62–8.
43. Alikani M, Palermo G, Adler A, Bertoli M, Blake M, Cohen J. Intracytoplasmic sperm injection in dysmorphic human oocytes. Zygote. 1995;3:283–8.

44. De Sutter P, Dozortsev D, Qian C, Dhont M. Oocyte morphology does not correlate with fertilization rate and embryo quality after intracytoplasmic sperm injection. Hum Reprod. 1996;11:595–7.
45. Xia P. Intracytoplasmic sperm injection: correlation of oocyte grade based on polar body, perivitelline space and cytoplasmic inclusions with fertilization rate and embryo quality. Hum Reprod. 1997;12:1750–5.
46. Balaban B, Urman B, Sertac A, Alatas C, Aksoy S, Mercan R. Oocyte morphology does not affect fertilization rate, embryo quality and implantation rate after intracytoplasmic sperm injection. Hum Reprod. 1998;13(12):3431–3.
47. Ebner T, Yaman C, Moser M, Sommergruber M, Feichtinger O, Tews G. Prognostic value of first polar body morphology on fertilization rate and embryo quality in intracytoplasmic sperm injection. Hum Reprod. 2000;15:427–30.
48. Ebner T, Moser M, Tews G. Is oocyte morphology prognostic of embryo developmental potential after ICSI? Reprod Biomed Online. 2006;12:507–12.
49. Mikkelsen AL, Lindenberg S. Morphology of in-vitro matured oocytes: impact on fertility potential and embryo quality. Hum Reprod. 2001;16:1714–8.
50. Rienzi L, Ubaldi FM, Iacobelli M, Minasi MG, Romano S, Ferrero S, Sapienza F, Baroni E, Litwicka K, Greco E. Significance of metaphase II human oocyte morphology on ICSI outcome. Fertil Steril. 2008;90(5):1692–700.
51. Ten T, Mendiola J, Vioque J, de Juan J, Bernabeu R. Donor oocyte dysmorphism and their influence on fertilization and embryo quality. Reprod Biomed Online. 2006;14:40–8.
52. Longo FJ, Chen DY. Development of cortical polarity in mouse eggs: involvement of the meiotic apparatus. Dev Biol. 1985;107:382–94.
53. Szollosi D, Czolowska R, Soltynska MS, et al. Ultrastructure of cell fusion and premature chromosome condensation (PCC) of thymocyte nuclei in metaphase II mouse oocytes. Biol Cell. 1986;56:239–49.
54. Eichenlaub-Ritter U, Shen Y, Tinneberg HR. Manipulation of the oocyte: possible damage to the spindle apparatus. Reprod Biomed Online. 2002;5:117–24.
55. Ursula E-R, Vogt E, Yin H, Gosden R. Symposium: mitochondria and human conception spindles, mitochondria and redox potential in ageing oocytes. Reprod Biomed Online. 2004;8:45–58.
56. Rienzi L, Ubaldi F, Iacobelli M, Minasi MG, Romano S, Greco E. Meiotic spindle visualization in living human oocytes. Reprod Biomed Online. 2005;10(2):192–8.
57. Battaglia DE, Goodwin P, Klein NA, et al. Influence of maternal age on meiotic spindle assembly in oocytes from naturally cycling women. Hum Reprod. 1996;11:2217–22.
58. Bernard A, Fuller BJ. Cryopreservation of human oocytes: a review of current problems and perspectives. Hum Reprod Update. 1996;2:193–207.
59. Oldenbourg R, Mei G. New polarized light microscope with precision universal compensator. J Microsc. 1995;180:140–7.
60. Oldenbourg R. Polarized light microscopy of spindles. Methods Cell Biol. 1999;61:175–208.
61. Liu L, Trimarchi JR, Oldenbourg R, Keefe DL. Increased birefringence in the meiotic spindle provides a new marker for the onset of activation in living oocytes. Biol Reprod. 2000;63(1): 251–8.
62. Braga D, Madaschi C, Bonetti TC, Iaconelli A, Rodrigues D, Borges E. Meiotic spindle imaging with Octax ICSI guard in in vitro matured human oocytes. Fertil Steril. 2006; 86(3):129.
63. Pelletier C, Keefe DL, Trimarchi JR. Noninvasive polarized light microscopy quantitatively distinguishes the multilaminar structure of the zona pellucida of living human eggs and embryos. Fertil Steril. 2004;81 Suppl 1:850–6.
64. Shen Y, Stalf T, Mehnert C, Eichenlaub-Ritter U, Tinneberg HR. High magnitude of light retardation by the zona pellucida is associated with conception cycles. Hum Reprod. 2005;20(6):1596–606.
65. Rienzi L, Martinez F, Ubaldi F, et al. Polscope analysis of meiotic spindle changes in living metaphase II human oocytes during the freezing and thawing procedures. Hum Reprod. 2004;19:655–9.

66. De Santis L, Cino I, Rabellotti E, et al. Polar body morphology and spindle imaging as predictors of oocyte quality. Reprod Biomed Online. 2005;11(1):36–42.
67. Montag M, Schimming T, van der Ven H. Spindle imaging in human oocytes: the impact of the meiotic cell cycle. Reprod Biomed Online. 2006;12:442–6.
68. Wang WH, Meng L, Hackett RJ, Odenbourg R, Keefe DL. Limited recovery of meiotic spindles in living human oocytes after cooling–rewarming observed using polarized light microscopy. Hum Reprod. 2001;16:2374–8.
69. Moon JH, Hyun CS, Lee SW, et al. Visualization of the metaphase II meiotic spindle in living human oocytes using the Polscope enables the prediction of embryonic developmental competence after ICSI. Hum Reprod. 2003;18:817–20.
70. Rienzi L, Ubaldi F, Martinez F, et al. Relationship between meiotic spindle location with regard to the polar body position and oocyte developmental potential after ICSI. Hum Reprod. 2003;18:1289–93.
71. Cooke S, Tyler JP, Driscoll GL. Meiotic spindle location and identification and its effect on embryonic cleavage plane and early development. Hum Reprod. 2003;18:2397–405.
72. Cohen Y, Malcov M, Schwartz T, et al. Spindle imaging: a new marker for optimal timing of ICSI? Hum Reprod. 2004;19:649–54.
73. Rama Raju GA, Prakash GJ, Krishna KM, Madan K. Meiotic spindle and zona pellucida characteristics as predictors of embryonic development: a preliminary study using PolScope imaging. Reprod Biomed Online. 2007;14:166–74.
74. Zeng HT, Ren Z, Yeung WS, Shu YM, Xu YW, Zhuang GL, Liang XY. Low mitochondrial DNA and ATP contents contribute to the absence of birefringent spindle imaged with PolScope in in vitro matured human oocytes. Hum Reprod. 2007;22(6):1681–6.
75. Petersen CG, Oliveira JB, Mauri AL, Massaro FC, Baruffi RL, Pontes A, Franco Jr JG. Relationship between visualization of meiotic spindle in human oocytes and ICSI outcomes: a meta-analysis. Reprod Biomed Online. 2009;18(2):235–43.
76. Casciani V, Rienzi L. Meiotic spindle visualization prior to ICSI procedure. Alpha Newslett. 2007;37:4–8.
77. Wang WH, Meng L, Hackett RJ, Oldenbourg R, Keefe DL. Rigorous thermal control during intracytoplasmic sperm injection stabilizes the meiotic spindle and improves fertilization and pregnancy rates. Fertil Steril. 2002;77:1274–7.
78. Van Santbrink EJ, Hop WC, Van Dessel TJ, de Jong FH, Fauser BC. Decremental follicle-stimulating hormone and dominant follicle development during the normal menstrual cycle. Fertil Steril. 1995;64:37–43.
79. Wang WH, Meng L, Hackett RJ, Odenbourg R, Keefe DL. The spindle observation and its relationship with fertilization after intracytoplasmic sperm injection in living human oocytes. Fertil Steril. 2001;75:348–53.
80. Coticchio G, Sciajno R, Hutt K, Bromfield J, Borini A, Albertini DF. Comparative analysis of the metaphase II spindle of human oocytes through polarized light and high-performance confocal microscopy. Fertil Steril. 2010;93(6):2056–64.
81. Eichenlaub-Ritter U, Schmiady H, Kentenich H, Soewarto D. Recurrent failure in polar body formation and premature chromosome condensation in oocytes from a human patient: indicators of asynchrony in nuclear and cytoplasmic maturation. Hum Reprod. 1995;10:2343–9.
82. Hassan-Ali H, Hisham-Saleh A, El-Gezeiry D, et al. Perivitelline space granularity: a sign of human menopausal gonadotropin overdose in intracytoplasmic sperm injection. Hum Reprod. 1998;13:3425–30.
83. Loutradis D, Drakakis P, Kallianidis K, et al. Oocyte morphology correlates with embryo quality and pregnancy rate after intracytoplasmic sperm injection. Fertil Steril. 1999;72:240–4.
84. Kahraman S, Yakin K, Donmez E, et al. Relationship between granular cytoplasm of oocytes and pregnancy outcome following intracytoplasmic sperm injection. Hum Reprod. 2000;15:2390–3.
85. Scott LA, Smith S. The successful use of pronuclear embryo transfers the day following oocyte retrieval. Hum Reprod. 1998;13:1003–13.

86. Scott L. Pronuclear scoring as a predictor of embryo development. Reprod Biomed Online. 2003;6:201–14.
87. Serhal PF, Ranieri DM, Kinis A, Marchant S, Davies M, Khadum IM. Oocyte morphology predicts outcome of intracytoplasmic sperm injection. Hum Reprod. 1997;12:1267–70.
88. Ebner T, Moser M, Sommergruber M, Gaiswinkler U, Shebl O, Jesacher K, Tews G. Occurrence and developmental consequences of vacuoles throughout preimplantation development. Fertil Steril. 2005;83(6):1635–40.
89. Van Blerkom J. Occurrence and developmental consequences of aberrant cellular organization in meiotically mature human oocytes after exogenous ovarian hyperstimulation. J Electron Microsc Tech. 1990;16(4):324–46.
90. El Shafie M, Sousa M, Windt ML, Kruger TF. Ultrastructure of human oocytes: a transmission electron microscopy view. In: El Shafie M, Sousa M, Windt ML, Kruger TF, editors. An atlas of the ultrastructure of human oocyte. A guide for assisted reproduction. New York: Parthenon; 2000. p. 151–71.
91. Meriano JS, Alexis J, Visram-Zaver S, Cruz M, Casper RF. Tracking of oocyte dysmorphisms for ICSI patients may prove relevant to the outcome in subsequent patient cycles. Hum Reprod. 2001;16:2118–23.
92. Otsuki J, Okada A, Morimoto K, Nagai Y, Kubo H. The relationship between pregnancy outcome and smooth endoplasmic reticulum clusters in MII human oocytes. Hum Reprod. 2004;19:1591–7.
93. Ebner T, Moser M, Yaman C, Feichtinger O, Hartl J, Tews G. Elective transfer of embryos selected on the basis of first polar body morphology is associated with increased rates of implantation and pregnancy. Fertil Steril. 1999;72:599–603.
94. Ciotti PM, Notarangelo L, Morselli-Labate AM, Felletti V, Porcu E, Venturosi V. First polar body morphology before ICSI is not related to embryo quality or pregnancy rate. Hum Reprod. 2004;19:2334–9.
95. De Santis L, Cino I, Rabellotti E, Calzi F, Persico P, Borini A, et al. Polar body morphology and spindle imaging as predictors of oocyte quality. Reprod Biomed Online. 2005;11: 36–42.
96. Verlinsky Y, Lerner S, Illkevitch N, Kuznetsov V, Kuznetsov I, Cieslak J, et al. Is there any predictive value of first polar body morphology for embryo genotype or developmental potential? Reprod Biomed Online. 2003;7:336–41.
97. Verlhac MH, Lefebvre C, Guillaud P, Rassinier P, Maro B. Asymmetric division in mouse oocytes: with or without MOS. Curr Biol. 2000;10:1303–6.
98. Balakier H, Bouman D, Sojecki A, Librach C, Squire JA. Morphological and cytogenetic analysis of human giant oocytes and giant embryos. Hum Reprod. 2002;17:2394–401.
99. Muechler EK, Graham MC, Huang KE, et al. Parthenogenesis of human oocytes as a function of vacuum pressure. J In Vitro Fert Embryo Transf. 1989;6:335–7.
100. Palermo G, Joris H, Devoroey P, et al. Sperm characteristics and outcome of human assisted fertilization by subzonal insemination and intracytoplasmic sperm injection. Fertil Steril. 1993;59:826–35.
101. Van Steirteghem AC, Nagy ZP, Joris H, et al. High fertilization and implantation rates after intracytoplasmic sperm injection. Hum Reprod. 1993;8:1061–6.
102. Joris H, Nagy Z, Van de Velde H, et al. Intracytoplasmic sperm injection: laboratory set-up and injection procedure. Hum Reprod. 1998;13(Suppl 1):76–86. Review.
103. Maro B, Verlhac MH. Polar body formation: new rules for asymmetric divisions. Nat Cell Biol. 2002;4:E281–3.
104. Sathananthan AH, Trounson A, Freemann L, Brady T. The effects of cooling human oocytes. Hum Reprod. 1988;3:968–77.
105. Pickering SJ, Braude PR, Johnson MH, Cant A, Currie J. Transient cooling to room temperature can cause irreversible disruption of the meiotic spindle in the human oocyte. Fertil Steril. 1990;54:102–8.
106. Almeida PA, Bolton VN. The effect of temperature fluctuations on the cytoskeletal organisation and chromosomal constitution of the human oocyte. Zygote. 1995;3:357–65.

107. Zenzes MT, Bielecki R, Casper RF, Leibo SP. Effects of chilling to 0°C on the morphology of meiotic spindles in human metaphase II oocytes. Fertil Steril. 2001;75:769–77.
108. Truyen U, Parrish CR, Harder TC, Kaaden OR. There is nothing permanent except change. The emergence of new virus diseases. Vet Microbiol. 1995;43:103–22.
109. Parinaud J, Vieitez G, Milhet P, Richoilley G. Use of a plant enzyme preparation (Coronase) instead of hyaluronidase for cumulus cell removal before intracytoplasmic sperm injection. Hum Reprod. 1998;13(7):1933–5.
110. De Vos A, Van Landuyt L, Van Ranst H, Vandermonde A, D'Haese V, Sterckx J, Haentjens P, Devroey P, Van der Elst J. Randomized sibling-oocyte study using recombinant human hyaluronidase versus bovine-derived Sigma hyaluronidase in ICSI patients. Hum Reprod. 2008;23(8):1815–9.
111. Evison M, Pretty C, Taylor E, Franklin C. Human recombinant hyaluronidase (Cumulase) improves intracytoplasmic sperm injection survival and fertilization rates. Reprod Biomed Online. 2009;18(6):811–4.
112. Dale B, Menezo Y, Cohen J, DiMatteo L, Wilding M. Intracellular pH regulation in the human oocyte. Hum Reprod. 1998;13(4):964–70.
113. FitzHarris G, Baltz JM. Regulation of intracellular pH during oocyte growth and maturation in mammals. Reproduction. 2009;138(4):619–27.
114. Heinecke JW, Shapiro BM. The respiratory burst oxidase of fertilization. A physiological target for regulation by protein kinase C. J Biol Chem. 1992;267(12):7959–62.
115. Schomer B, Epel D. Redox changes during fertilization and maturation of marine invertebrate eggs. Dev Biol. 1998;203(1):1–11.
116. Schomer Miller B, Epel D. The roles of changes in NADPH and pH during fertilization and artificial activation of the sea urchin egg. Dev Biol. 1999;216(1):394–405.
117. Dumoulin J, Meijers C, Bras M, Coonen E, Geraedts JP, Evers JL. Effect of oxygen concentration on human in-vitro fertilization and embryo transfer. Hum Reprod. 1999;14:465–9.
118. Kovacic B, Vlaisavljević V. Influence of atmospheric versus reduced oxygen concentration on development of human blastocysts in vitro: a prospective study on sibling oocytes. Reprod Biomed Online. 2008;17(2):229–36.
119. Ciray HN, Aksoy T, Yaramanci K, Karayaka I, Bahceci M. In vitro culture under physiologic oxygen concentration improves blastocyst yield and quality: a prospective randomized survey on sibling oocytes. Fertil Steril. 2009;91(4 Suppl):1459–61.
120. Nanassy L, Peterson CA, Wilcox AL, Peterson CM, Hammoud A, Carrell DT. Comparison of 5% and ambient oxygen during days 3-5 of in vitro culture of human embryos. Fertil Steril. 2010;93(2):579–85.
121. McKenzie LJ, Pangas SA, Carson SA, et al. Human cumulus granulosa cell gene expression: a predictor of fertilization and embryo selection in women undergoing IVF. Hum Reprod. 2004;19:2869–74.
122. Fatehi AN, Roelen BA, Colenbrander B, et al. Presence of cumulus cells during in vitro fertilization protects the bovine oocyte against oxidative stress and improves first cleavage but does not affect further development. Zygote. 2005;13:177–85.
123. Ebner T, Moser M, Sommergruber M, et al. Incomplete denudation of oocytes prior to ICSI enhances embryo quality and blastocyst development. Hum Reprod. 2006;21(11):2972–7.
124. Goud PT, Goud AP, Qian C, Laverge H, Van der Elst J, De Sutter P, Dhont M. In-vitro maturation of human germinal vesicle stage oocytes: role of cumulus cells and epidermal growth factor in the culture medium. Hum Reprod. 1998;13:1638–44.
125. Yamazaki Y, Wakayama T, Yanagimachi R. Contribution of cumulus cells and serum to the maturation of oocyte cytoplasm as revealed by intracytoplasmic sperm injection (ICSI). Zygote. 2001;9:277–82.
126. Zeringue HC, Beebe DJ. Microfluidic removal of cumulus cells from Mammalian zygotes. Methods Mol Biol. 2004;254:365–74.

Chapter 14
Intracytoplasmic Sperm Injection

Gianpiero D. Palermo, Queenie V. Neri, Devin Monahan, Takumi Takeuchi, Peter N. Schlegel, and Zev Rosenwaks

Intracytoplasmic sperm injection (ICSI) involves the insertion of a single spermatozoon into the oocyte, bypassing all the egg coat penetration and gamete fusion steps characteristic of natural fertilization. This was first achieved in the sea urchin [1], in the mouse [2], and later in hamster eggs [3]. This micromanipulation approach was also plagued by oocyte injury and lysis [4], with only about 30% of injected mouse eggs surviving the procedure [5]. Because the sperm-egg fusion step is bypassed in ICSI, male pronucleus development generally required oocyte activation in most species tested. This was achieved by the vigorous suction of ooplasm prior to sperm nucleus insertion [6] or by exposure to A23187 [7, 8].

The first ICSI offspring were obtained in the rabbit following the transfer of sperm-injected eggs into the oviduct of a pseudopregnant female [9], with a bovine live birth reported soon thereafter [10]. Although applied to human gametes some years earlier [11], the first human pregnancies from ICSI was established only in 1992 [12], and since then, hundreds of thousands of ICSI babies have been born [13–15].

ICSI has made conception and parenthood possible for couples with many forms of male factor infertility and at rates similar to those in patients treated by standard in vitro fertilization (IVF) with apparently normal gametes [16, 17].

G.D. Palermo, MD, PhD (✉)
The Ronald O. Perelman and Claudia Cohen Center for Reproductive Medicine, 1305 York Avenue, New York, NY 10021, USA

Weill Cornell Medical College, 1305 York Avenue, 7th Floor, New York, NY 10021, USA
e-mail: gdpalerm@med.cornell.edu

Q.V. Neri, BSc, MSc • D. Monahan, BSc • T. Takeuchi, MD, PhD • Z. Rosenwaks, MD
The Ronald O. Perelman and Claudia Cohen Center for Reproductive Medicine, Weill Cornell Medical College, New York, NY, USA

P.N. Schlegel, MD
Department of Urology, Weill Cornell Medical College, New York Presbyterian/Weill Cornell Hospital, New York, NY, USA

Z.P. Nagy et al. (eds.), *Clinical Embryology: A Practical Guide*,
DOI 10.1007/978-1-4614-8376-2_14,

Indications for Intracytoplasmic Sperm Injection

Despite agreement in some areas, no universal standards for patient selection have been defined. However, there is a general consensus that ICSI be adopted when an extremely poor sperm sample is noted or following fertilization failure using in vitro techniques.

When initial sperm concentration in the ejaculate is $<5 \times 10^6$/mL, the likelihood of fertilization with standard IVF is significantly reduced [18], and therefore, such couples should be considered unsuitable for this procedure, particularly where <1% normal forms are observed. However, fertilization of mature oocytes may still fail to occur in the presence of normal sperm because of a hardening of the zona pellucida [19] or when oocytes reveal ooplasmic inclusions [20, 21]. Abnormalities of the zona pellucida prevent sperm fusion with the oolemma [22], thus justifying sperm injection. In most instances, however, failure of fertilization is due to coexisting sperm abnormalities presenting ICSI as the only treatment option [13].

Early experience showed that isolated nuclei of testicular and epididymal hamster spermatozoa decondensed soon after injection into mature hamster oocytes and formed pronuclei in activated eggs [3]. Although IVF of human oocytes was accomplished in men with epididymal spermatozoa recovered in cases of obstructive azoospermia [23, 24], only with the advent of ICSI was it possible to obtain consistent fertilization with them [16, 25, 26]. Testicular biopsy was employed to obtain sperm cells from men who had a scarred epididymis, and therefore, no chance of retrieval through that route [27–29]. However, the therapeutic possibilities of ICSI go even further since immotile testicular spermatozoa and even spermatids have been successfully used [30].

Some men produce only round-headed spermatozoa which have no acrosome and can neither bind to nor penetrate zona-free hamster oocytes [31, 32]. However, ICSI has enabled even such acrosomeless spermatozoa to establish pregnancies [33–37]. Moreover, ICSI's dependability has broadened its initial use from a technique capable of overriding the dysfunctionality of spermatozoa to one that may partly compensate for problems with the egg. Indeed, ICSI has allowed successful fertilization when only a few and/or abnormal oocytes were available [38]. Stripping cumulus cells from the oocytes allows a direct assessment of maturation, thus offering a woman with a limited number of oocytes a much greater chance of successful fertilization. In fact, the availability of ICSI has been instrumental in some European countries that include Italy and Germany in circumventing restrictive legislation that limits the number of oocytes inseminated or embryos to be replaced [39–41].

ICSI has also made possible a more consistent fertilization of cryopreserved oocytes [42]—overcoming the problem that freezing can lead to a premature exocytosis of cortical granules, resulting in zona hardening and inhibition of natural sperm penetration [43–46]. ICSI is also the preferred conception method during the application of preimplantation genetic diagnosis (PGD). It avoids DNA contamination from additional sperm adhering to the zona, and it enhances the number of fertilizable oocytes and so embryos available for screening [47].

ICSI also has an impact in the arena of HIV infection. Three-quarters of individuals infected by HIV or HCV are in their reproductive years. Male-to-female transmission of HIV is estimated to be only 1/1,000 acts of unprotected intercourse [48] and even fewer in HCV-infected patients [49]. Moreover, because of antiretroviral therapies, the course of HIV-1 infection has shifted from a lethal-acquired immunodeficiency syndrome to a chronic manageable disease. Though many patients infected with HIV-1 show interests in beginning a family, most serodiscordant couples are concerned, nevertheless, with the possibility of both horizontal and vertical transmission of the virus. In such cases, intrauterine insemination (IUI) with spermatozoa processed by double gradient centrifugation followed by swim up has been the preferred method of treating serodiscordant couples with an HIV-1-infected male partner [50]. However, the use of ICSI has been proposed by several groups because of its negligible semen exposure, thereby reducing the risk of viral transmission [51, 52]. Advantages of ICSI over IUI also include the considerably higher success rate [52], requiring fewer attempts to achieve pregnancy while reducing viral exposure [53]. Fortunately, so far, no seroconversions have been reported following ART treatments including IUIs [54].

Finally, because only a single spermatozoon is needed for each egg, ICSI has allowed treatment of men who are virtually azoospermic (also defined as cryptozoospermic) [55]. Such cases of spermatogenic arrest have necessarily involved the injection of immature spermatozoa or even spermatogonia [29, 30, 56, 57]. Nonetheless, where fertilization occurs in such cases, conception is accomplished with embryo implantation following a similar pattern, at least in our experience, to that seen in IVF.

Equipment

- Micromanipulation system (NAI-2P, Narishige International USA, Inc.)
  - Hydrchapteraulic microinjector (IM-6), modified with a metal syringe (SYR-15)
  - Injector (IM-9C), air-filled
  - BDH oil—for loading the injector (BDH Laboratory Supplies, Poole, Dorset, England)
- Inverted microscope with Nikon Polarized Optics CFI S Plan Fluor (20 and ×40 objectives) and CFI Apo (2, 4, and ×10 objectives) (TE2000U, Nikon USA, Melville, NY, USA)
- Vibration-free table (Newport Research Corporation, Irvine, CA, USA)
- Custom-designed horseshoe-shaped heated stage (Easteach Laboratory, Maspeth, NY, USA)
- Microtools (Conception Technologies, San Diego, CA, USA)
  - Injection pipette (IC-SPN-30; 4–6 μL ID)
  - Injection pipette (IC-C1; 5–6 μL ID)
  - Holding pipette (HP-120-30)

- Oocyte transfer and denudation pipettes (hand-pulled, flame-polished Pasteur pipettes)
- ICSI dish (BD Falcon 351006; Becton, Dickinson and Co., Franklin Lakes, NJ, USA)
  - Stereomicroscope (SZX12, Olympus America Inc., Center Valley, PA, USA)
  - Distriman® Repetitive Pipette (F164001, Gilson, Inc., Middleton, WI, USA)—ICSI medium dispenser
  - AutoRep E™ Electronic Repeating Pipette (AR-E1, Rainin Instrument LLC, Oakland, CA, USA)—oil dispenser
  - Pipetman P20 (F123600, Gilson, Inc.)—polyvinylpyrrolidone (PVP) and sperm loading

Reagents

- ICSI Cumulase® (16125000, MediCult, Origio, Mt. Laurel, NJ, USA)
- Embryo culture medium (home-brew, modified Cornell medium based on G1™ and G2™ components [58, 59]).
- ICSI injection medium (G-MOPS™ [10129] supplemented with 6% G-MM™ [10038], Vitrolife, Inc., Englewood, CO, USA).
- Tissue culture oil (ART-4008, SAGE In Vitro Fertilization, Inc. A CooperSurgical Company, Trumbull, CT, USA)
- 7% PVP with HSA (90121, Irvine Scientific, Santa Ana, CA, USA)

Sperm Preparation

Ejaculated Sample

Semen samples are collected by masturbation after at least 3 days of abstinence; they are then allowed to liquefy for about 20 min at 37°C prior to analysis. Other methods of semen collection such as electroejaculation and retrograde ejaculation have been described elsewhere [16].

Semen concentration and motility are assessed in a Makler counting chamber (Sefi Medical Instruments, Haifa, Israel). As might be expected, morphologic quality of the sperm has a significant positive correlation with male infertility. This evaluation is performed using the strict criteria of Kruger et al. [60]. Evaluations are carried out by spreading 10 μL of semen or sperm suspension on prestained slides (Cell-Vu®, Prestained Morphology Slides [DRM-900], Fertility Technology, Marietta, Georgia, USA), which can provide rapid results. At least 200 spermatozoa/slide are categorized microscopically at ×100 under oil immersion. Two counts are performed for both concentration and morphology. Semen quality is considered suboptimal when the sperm concentration is <20 × 10^6/mL, the progressive motility is <40%, or the proportion of spermatozoa with normal morphology is <4% of the spermatozoa.

For selection of spermatozoa, the sample is washed by centrifugation at 600 × *g* for 5 min in HTF medium supplemented with 0.4% HSA. Semen samples with <5 × 10^6/mL spermatozoa or <20% motile spermatozoa are washed in a home-brew medium by a single centrifugation at 600 × *g* for 5 min. The resuspended pellet is layered on a discontinuous density gradient (Isolate®, Irvine Scientific) on two (90 and 50%) or single (90%) layers and then centrifuged at 300 × *g* for 20 min when samples have a sperm density of <5 × 10^6/mL spermatozoa and <20% motile spermatozoa. The sperm-rich fraction is rinsed by adding 4 mL of culture medium and centrifuged at 500–1,800 × *g* for 5 min to remove silica gel particles. For spermatozoa with poor kinetic characteristics, the sperm suspension is exposed to a 3 μM solution of pentoxifylline for 15 min and centrifuged one more time. The concentration of the assessed sperm suspension is adjusted to 1–1.5 × 10^6/mL, when necessary, by the addition of HTF medium and, subsequently, incubated at 37°C in 5% CO_2 in air.

Surgically Retrieved Spermatozoa

Azoospermia can be indicative of epididymal vas obstruction or absence (obstructive azoospermia) or a failure of spermatogenesis (non-obstructive azoospermia). Obstructive azoospermia is characterized by normal sperm production and is often caused by congenital maldevelopment of the vas deferens, often associated with a cystic fibrosis gene mutation(s). The treatment for these men is microsurgical epididymal sperm aspiration (MESA), or when the epididymal access is lacking, direct testicular sampling is undertaken. On the other hand, non-obstructive azoospermia is characterized by a varying degree of spermatogenetic failure and may be associated with certain chromosomal abnormalities [61, 62]. The only method to retrieve spermatozoa from this form of azoospermia is a direct extraction of sperm or germ cells from a testis.

Microsurgical Epididymal Sperm Aspiration

The infertility of men due to irreparable obstructive azoospermia has been treated successfully by MESA [63, 64] or percutaneous testicular retrieval of spermatozoa [65]. In the MESA procedure, 1–5 μL of fluid is aspirated from the lumen of an individual epididymal tubule in the midportion of the obstructed epididymis with a 300–350 μm glass pipette. The epididymal fluid is diluted with 300 μL of culture medium. Additional proximal punctures of the epididymis are performed until enough spermatozoa are obtained. Because sperm concentration in the epididymal fluid often reaches over 1 × 10^6/μL, only microliter quantities generally suffice.

Epididymal fluid is diluted in 500 μL culture medium and processed like ejaculated spermatozoa. After removal of the density gradient medium, a 1 μL aliquot of the final suspension at approximately 1×10^6/mL is placed in the injection dish [16, 66].

Testicular Sperm Extraction

In the case of men with non-obstructive azoospermia, spermatozoa are retrieved directly from the testis in a procedure called testicular sperm extraction (TESE). Typically, multiple biopsies are needed to find the rare spermatogenetic foci that are present within the testes of such men. Biopsies are performed under optical magnification to identify and preserve the subtunical testicular blood supply with biopsy incisions made in avascular regions [63].

Each biopsy specimen is first rinsed in culture medium to remove red blood cells, separated into individual tubules on sterile glass slides, and minced using fine scissors. The resulting suspension of seminiferous tubules is then sequentially passed through a 24-gauge angiocatheter to further disrupt the tubules. Individual testicular samples are distributed in 5.0-mL centrifuge tubes (Falcon, Becton Dickinson and Company, Lincoln Park, NJ, USA) containing an excess of culture medium. To assess for the presence of spermatozoa, a small amount (~5 μL) of suspension medium is carefully studied under a phase contrast microscope at ×200–400. In preparation for ICSI, the shredded testicular tissue is removed and the suspension medium subsequently centrifuged at 500–1,800 × *g* for 5 min, with the pellet being subjected to a single-layer density gradient centrifugation. It has been possible to identify individual and enlarged seminiferous tubules that presumably are supporting spermatogenesis in contrast to the surrounding thin sclerotic tubules. Biopsy samples are placed into 200–300 μL aliquots of culture medium on a glass slide and examined under a phase contrast microscope and repeated until the presence of spermatozoa is documented. The specimen is then placed directly into a 40 μL drop under oil where the tips of two 25-gauge needles on 1-mL syringes are used to shred the testicular tissue. Subsequently, the tissue is removed from the droplet, and 3 μL of the suspension is placed directly onto the injection dish.

Microdissection Testicular Sperm Extraction

In cases of non-obstructive azoospermia, the procedure for direct microscopic identification of functioning seminiferous tubules is referred to as microdissection testicular sperm extraction (micro-TESE) [67]. As with the standard multi-biopsy approach, optical magnification (6–8 power) is used to visualize blood vessels under the surface of the tunica vaginalis, allowing testis biopsy incisions to be made in avascular regions. Instead of planning for multiple incisions in the tunica albuginea, an attempt is made to open it widely by creating the incision on the testis' midportion. This optimizes exposure of the testicular parenchyma without disrupting its blood supply. Direct examination is carried out at ×20–25 under the operating microscope, during which an attempt is made to identify individual seminiferous tubules that were larger than others in the testicular parenchyma. Small (2–10 mg) segments are excised sharply from tubules that are larger and more opaque (whiter). Each excised specimen is further cut into smaller pieces to promote the release of any spermatozoa, with the resulting suspension examined as in standard TESE. Although additional incisions in the same or contralateral testes can be made until spermatozoa are retrieved or when further biopsies would appear to compromise the blood supply of the testes. Once spermatozoa are found, the procedure is terminated and testes sutured.

When no spermatozoa are identified, testicular tissue are placed in 1 mL of prewarmed medium supplemented with 5% HSA, 1.6 mM $CaCl_2$ (Sigma Chemical Co., St Louis, MO), 25 μg/mL DNase (Sigma Chemical Co.), and 1,000 IU/mL collagenase type IV (Sigma Chemical Co.) [68]. DNase is added to the incubation medium to prevent clotting of the resulting cell suspension due to the release of free DNA from apoptotic cells [69, 70]. Testicular tissue is exposed to collagenase and incubated at 37°C for 1 h. The suspension is pipetted every 10–15 min to enhance enzymatic digestion. Large portions of tubular walls are removed with fine tweezers. The digested suspension is then centrifuged twice at 500 × *g* for 5 min. The supernatant is removed and the pellet resuspended in 500 μL of sperm cell medium.

Oocyte Collection

Superovulation is performed by administration of gonadotropins in association with agonist or antagonist protocol [71]. Human chorionic gonadotropin (hCG) is administered when criteria for oocyte maturity are met, and oocyte retrieval by vaginal ultrasound-guided puncture is performed 35 h later. Under the inverted microscope at ×100, the cumulus corona cell complexes are scored as mature, slightly immature, completely immature, or slightly overmature. Thereafter, the oocytes are incubated for more than 4 h. Immediately prior to micromanipulation, the cumulus corona cells are removed by exposure to HTF-HEPES-buffered medium containing 40 IU/mL of ICSI Cumulase®. The removal is necessary for observation of the oocyte and effective use of the holding and/or injecting pipette during micromanipulation. For final removal of the residual corona cells, the oocytes are repeatedly aspirated in and out of a hand-drawn Pasteur pipette with an inner diameter of ~200 μm. Each oocyte is then examined under the microscope to assess the maturation stage and its integrity, metaphase II (MII) being assessed according to the absence of the germinal vesicle and the presence of an extruded polar body. ICSI is performed only in oocytes that have reached this level of maturity.

Intracytoplasmic Sperm Injection Procedure

Loading Tools

The holding and injection pipettes are inserted into the respective micromanipulation tool holders mounted on an inverted microscope. The controllers are pneumatic for the holding pipette and oil-filled for the injection pipette. Using the coarse motorized controllers, the pipettes are positioned in the center of the microscopic field at ×20, then the magnification is gradually increased while maintaining the tools in focus by adjusting the hydraulic controllers. Under the highest magnification (×400), correct pipette positioning is achieved only by the use of the hydraulic joysticks, and both pipettes should be able to course through the entire optical field. With regard to tool-tip angles, the distal bent portions of both microtools should be slightly above parallel to avoid the elbows touching the bottom of the dish and interfering with the control. This also allows prompt immobilization and visual control of the spermatozoon inside the injection pipette. Once properly aligned, the pipettes are raised by means of the coarse motorized controllers to allow placement of the ICSI dish on the microscope stage.

ICSI Dish Preparation

Nine drops containing 8 μL of injection medium are placed in a Petri dish, with one in the center radially surrounded by the other eight (Fig. 14.1). The drops should be as close together as possible to allow full visualization within the 20 mm opening on the heated stage. The drops should then be gently overlaid with culture oil to prevent evaporation. Using a red non-embryo toxic wax pencil, the 12 o'clock

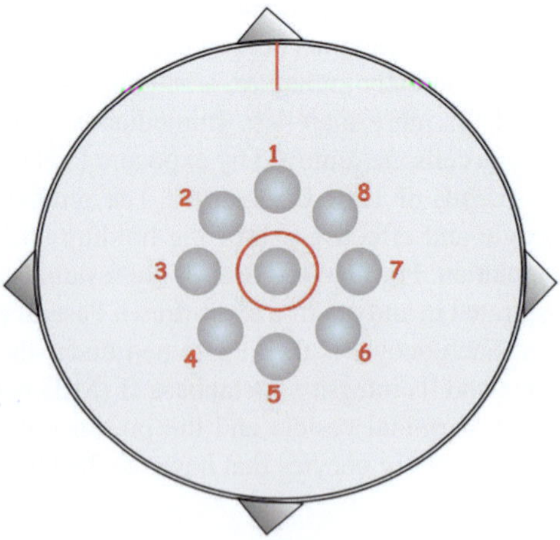

Fig. 14.1 The drawing depicts a Petri dish containing the droplets of medium (8 μL) and sequentially numbered going counter clockwise. The center droplet is removed and replaced with PVP and sperm while in each surrounding droplets, an individual oocyte will be placed

position is marked, a circle drawn around the central drop, and the drops are sequentially numbered starting from the 12 o'clock position, moving counter clockwise. This allows easy navigation between droplets during ICSI. ICSI dishes are stored at 37°C until use.

Loading Gametes into the ICSI Dish

Immediately prior to the injection under a stereomicroscope, the central drop is removed and replaced with 1 μL of sperm suspension diluted in 4 μL of 7% PVP. Using a hand-pulled Pasteur pipette, MII oocytes are aspirated from the culture dish, and a single oocyte is placed in each drop.

Sperm Immobilization

Position the spermatozoon at 90° with respect to the pipettes' tip, gently lower the cylindrical tip to compress the principal piece of the tail, by rolling the posterior flagellum over the bottom of the Petri dish (Fig. 14.2a–c). If initially unsuccessful, the procedure is repeated until the tail is clearly kinked, looped, or convoluted (Fig. 14.2d). It is important to note, however, that a misshapen tail may adhere to the dish or to the inner surface of the pipette. The spermatozoon is aspirated tail first. The injection needle is lifted slightly via the two control knobs of the joystick to avoid damaging the needle spike. The microscope stage is then repositioned until the injection needle enters the oocyte drop. It is important to note that the difference in media consistency (PVP vs. culture medium) may allow the sperm to move distally into the pipette and become loose.

Injection

To find the egg, the magnification is briefly lowered to ×200, and once the egg is centrally in the field, the magnification brought back to ×400. The oocyte is held in place by suction through the holding pipette, and using both tools, the oocyte is rotated slowly to locate the polar body and the area of cortical rarefaction (or polar granularity) (Fig. 14.3a). When the equatorial plane of the oocyte is located, the depth of the holding pipette is adjusted to have its internal opening in the same plane. This allows for greater support of the holding pipette in a position opposite to the injection point. It is ideal to have the inferior pole of the oocyte touching the bottom of the dish, as it affords a better grip of the egg during the injection procedure. The injection pipette is lowered and focused with the outer right border of the oolemma on the equatorial plane at 3 o'clock. Bring the spermatozoon close to the

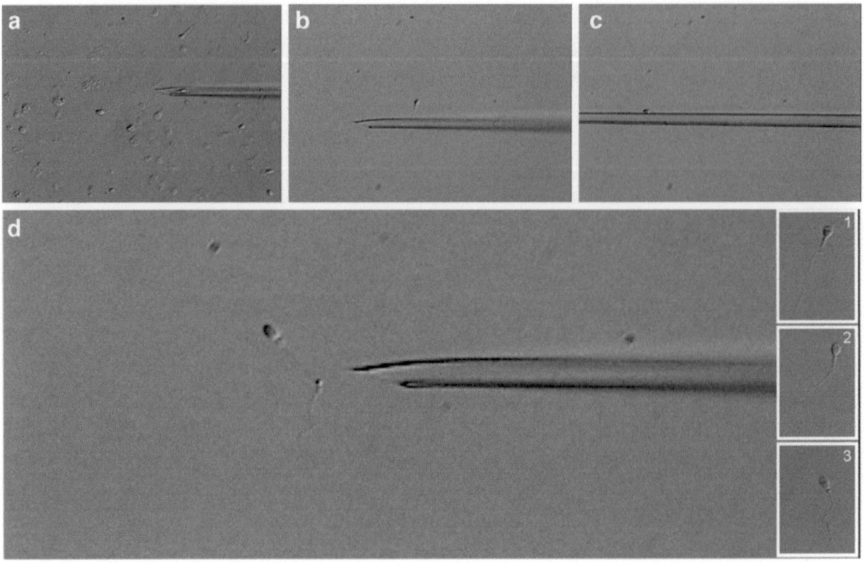

Fig. 14.2 Aggressive immobilization of a testicular spermatozoon prior to intracytoplasmic sperm injection (ICSI). (**a**) A single spermatozoon displaying a satisfactory morphology is aspirated from a sperm droplet. Such droplets are made without PVP in cases where sperm count and motility are poor. (**b**) The chosen spermatozoon is then moved into the PVP droplet, where the injection pipette is gently lowered onto the sperm tail mainpiece, compressing it. Even though the spermatozoon is immotile, immobilization is still carried out to ensure the best chance of fertilization, since a damaged sperm membrane facilitates exposure of the nucleus to the ooplasm. (**c**) While maintaining downward pressure on the flagellum, the injection pipette is moved back and forth, effectively rolling the spermatozoon on the dish bottom. (**d**) Once immobilization is completed, the tail should be permanently distorted—either looped (1), kinked (2), or convoluted (3)

beveled opening of the injection pipette then bring the pipette to the zona, press against it to begin penetration, and thrust forward to the inner surface of the oolemma at 9 o'clock (Fig. 14.3b–d). At this point, a break in the membrane should occur at the approximate center of the egg (Fig. 14.3e). Such a break is indicated by a sudden quivering of the convexities of the oolemma (at the site of invagination) above and below the penetration point (Fig. 14.3f), as well as by the proximal flow of cytoplasmic organelles and the spermatozoon back into the pipette. The spermatozoon is then ejected with the cytoplasmic component (Fig. 14.3g). To optimize its interaction with the cytoplasm, the sperm should be ejected past the tip of the pipette to ensure a close intermingling with the ooplasmic lattices, which help maintain the sperm in place while withdrawing the pipette (Fig. 14.3h). To induce oocyte activation, additional ooplasm is aspirated back and forth with the injection pipette. It is paramount to avoid leaving behind residual medium with the spermatozoon as well as closing the breach of penetration. This is accomplished by generating a mild suction while removing the pipette. To do this, when the pipette is at the approximate center of the egg some surplus medium is reaspirated so that the cytoplasmic structures can envelop the sperm, thereby reducing the size of the breach (Fig. 14.3i).

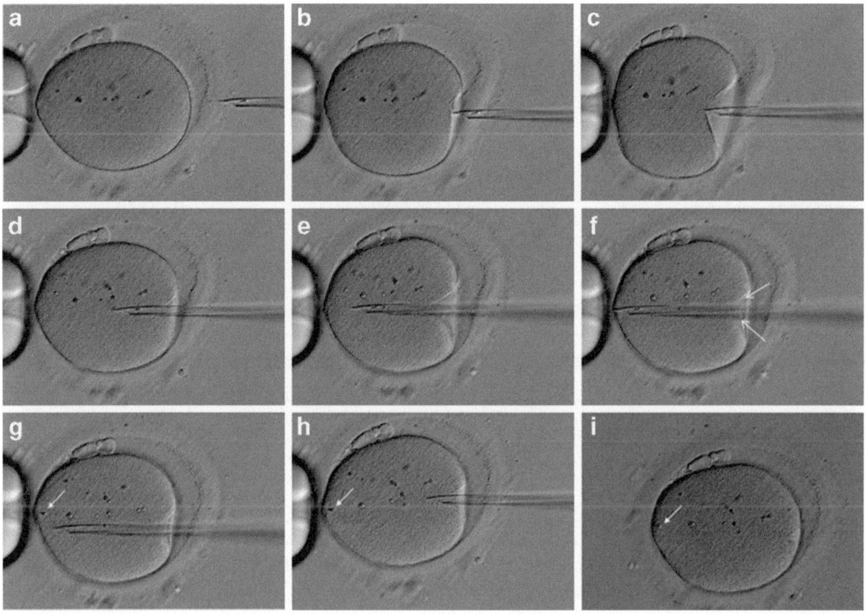

Fig. 14.3 ICSI of a human oocyte. (**a**) The oolemma at the 3 o'clock portion of the oocyte is brought into focus, as are the holding (*left*) and injection pipette (*right*) tips. Suction is applied on the holding pipette to stabilize the oocyte, and the spermatozoon is advanced to the tip of the injection pipette. (**b**) Advancement of the injection pipette through the zona at the oocyte's equatorial plane bypasses the zona and brings the pipette spike into contact with the oocyte membrane. (**c–e**) Its elasticity creates a funnel around the injection pipette as it moves deeper into the oocyte. (**f**) Once the oolemma is penetrated, there is a distinct quivering of the oocyte membrane, which then returns to its original position (*arrows*). (**g**) As the sperm is deposited in the ooplasm (*arrow*), a small amount of cytoplasm is aggressively aspirated and released to facilitate oocyte activation. (**h**) Removal of the injection pipette is accompanied by gentle aspiration from the center of the oocyte outward to facilitate resealing of the membrane by bringing the borders of the injection funnel into closer proximity. (**i**) An injected oocyte with sperm in the cytoplasm (*arrow*) displaying minimal evidence of tool penetration at its 9 o'clock edge

This also expedites the closure of the terminal part of the funnel-shaped opening at 3 o'clock. Once the pipette is extracted, the edges of the entry point should maintain a funnel shape with the tip toward the center of the egg. If the border of the oolemma becomes everted, the cytoplasmic organelles can leak out and the oocyte may lyse. The average time required to accomplish a single oocyte injection is about 30–40 s.

Embryo Development and Clinical Outcome

In the last 16 years at Cornell, we have performed a total of 29,191 ART cycles with an average maternal age for IVF of 37.6 ± 4 years and for ICSI of 35.8 ± 5 years and mean paternal ages of 39.6 ± 6 and 40.8 ± 8 years, respectively. Of those

Table 14.1 ICSI outcome according to semen source

Semen origin	Cycles	Fertilization (%)	Clinical pregnancies (%)
Fresh ejaculate	15,199	92,876/124,774 (74.4)	5,712 (37.6)
Frozen ejaculate	1,531	9,296/12,643 (73.5)	547 (35.7)
Electroejaculate	70	517/681 (75.9)	34 (48.6)
Frozen electroejaculate	9	78/102 (76.5)	3 (33.3)
Retrograde ejaculate	29	231/280 (82.5)	9 (31.0)

Table 14.2 Fertilization and pregnancy rates according to the origin of spermatozoa

	Spermatozoa	
No. of	Ejaculated	Surgically retrieved
Cycles	16,838	1,846
Maternal age (M years ± SD)	37.3 ± 5[a]	34.2 ± 5[a]
Fertilization (%)	102,998/138,480 (74.4)[b]	11,290/17,897 (63.1)[b]
Clinical pregnancies (%)	6,305 (37.5)[c]	849 (46.0)[c]

[a] Student's *t*-test, two independent samples; difference in maternal age, $P < 0.0001$
[b] x^2, 2 × 2, 1 *df*, effect of sperm source on fertilization rate, $P = 0.0001$
[c] x^2, 2 × 2, 1 *df*, effect of sperm source on clinical pregnancy rate, $P = 0.0001$

cycles, 36.0% (10,503) included the standard in vitro insemination of 106,931 oocytes from 5,943 couples with a fertilization rate of 58.9% and a clinical pregnancy rate of 40.4%, the remainder being ICSI cycles. IVF was generally performed in patients with normal semen, while ICSI has been used to treat couples with doubtful spermatozoa, a history of poor fertilization, and/or limited numbers of oocytes. Nonetheless, the two systems consistently generated similar results.

Of 10,922 couples treated by ICSI, the average number of oocytes retrieved was 10.8 per cycle ($n = 201{,}709$), of which 156,377 (77.5%) were at MII and, therefore, subjected to ICSI. Of the oocytes injected, 94.7% (148,089/156,377) survived and 114,288 (73.1%) developed two pronuclei (PN). Of the oocytes that were abnormally fertilized, 4,066 (2.6%) displayed 1PN and 5,004 (3.2%) 3PN.

The types of mature spermatozoa included 15,199 ejaculated samples, 1,531 cryopreserved, 79 obtained by electroejaculation, and 29 by bladder catheterization (Table 14.1). Among the collection/cryopreservation methods, fertilization rates ranged from 73.5 to 82.5%. The clinical pregnancy rate was comparable in all groups.

When more immature forms of spermatozoa were utilized, for example, those surgically retrieved, the fertilization rate of 46.0% was satisfactory but lower than that with ejaculated spermatozoa ($P = 0.0001$) (Table 14.2). While the clinical pregnancy rate was lower in the ejaculated group in comparison to the surgically retrieved spermatozoa, this difference may be attributed to the maternal age. The etiology of the *vas deferens or efferens* obstruction, congenital or acquired, had no effect on fertilization after ICSI giving an overall rate of 70.5% and a clinical pregnancy rate of 53.5%. However, after cryopreservation of epididymal spermatozoa, the clinical pregnancy was dramatically reduced from 62.3 to 48.2% ($P = 0.0001$).

Table 14.3 Pregnancy characteristics of 18,684 ICSI cycles

	No. of (%)	Negative outcomes	
ICSI cycles	18,684		
Embryo replacements	17,337		
Positive ßhCGs	9,435 (50.5)		
		Biochemical pregnancies	1,521
		Blighted ova	681
		Ectopic pregnancies	79
Patients with fetal heartbeats	7,154 (38.3)		
		Miscarriages/therapeutic abortions	708
Deliveries and ongoing pregnancies	6,446		

Table 14.4 The relationship of maternal age to ICSI outcome

	Maternal age		
No. of cycles with (%)	<35	35–39	≥40
Cycles	5,755	6,412	5,533
(a) Embryo replacement	5,318	5,956	5,091
(b) Clinical pregnancy (+FHB) (% on a)	2,823 (53.1)[a]	2,535 (42.6)[a]	1,323 (26.0)[a]
(c) Delivery and ongoing pregnancy (% on a)	2,670 (50.2)[a]	2,297 (38.4)[a]	795,902 (18.8)[a]

[a] x^2, 3 × 2, 2 *df*, effect of maternal age on pregnancy outcome, $P = 0.0001$

In testicular extraction cases, with the compromised spermatogenesis typical of the non-obstructed azoospermic patient, the spermatozoa recovered generated a fertilization rate of 56.9% and a clinical pregnancy rate of 41.2%. When comparing fresh vs. cryopreserved spermatozoa in testicular cycles, the clinical pregnancy rate was comparable between the two groups (42.6 vs. 35.6%).

Of the 18,684 ICSI cycles analyzed, 9,435 resulted in a positive ßhCG (50.5%), and in about 38% of all cycles, the presence of at least one fetal heartbeat was observed (Table 14.3). Among the positive ßhCG, 1,521 (16.1%) were biochemical pregnancies, 681 (7.2%) were anembryonic, and 79 (0.8%) were ectopic. Among the 7,154 cycles with a fetal heart, 708 spontaneously miscarried. This left an ongoing pregnancy rate of 34.5% per retrieval (6,446/18,684) and 37.5% per embryo replacement procedure (6,446/17,337).

When 17,700 ICSI cycles (after exclusion of the donor egg cycles) were plotted as a function of increasing maternal age, there was a progressive decrease in pregnancy ($P = 0.0001$) (Table 14.4) and, consequently, delivery rates ($P = 0.0001$). As predicted, there was a higher incidence of miscarriages, therapeutic abortions, and overall pregnancy losses as a function of the age of the female partner ($P = 0.0001$), pregnancy wastage being 2.4 times greater in women ≥40 years compared to those of <35 years.

A total of 5,922 ICSI patients delivered 8,105 babies comprising 4,051 males and 3,994 females (with 60 unknown genders). A total of 3.3% (268) exhibited congenital abnormalities at birth, of which 130 were major and 138 were minor. IVF children ($n = 4,999$) had a 3.1% overall malformation rate (90 major and 65 minor). Major malformations ranged from cardiac defects to multiorgan diseases including central nervous system anomalies, chromosomal abnormalities (gonosomal trisomies such as 47,XXX; 47,XXY and autosomal trisomies such as chromosomes 7, 18, 21), and urogenital disorders requiring surgery such as severe hypospadias and undescended testes. Examples of minor malformations were café-au-lait spots, urethral defects, and very mild form of clubfoot.

Intracytoplasmic Sperm Injection Failure

ICSI failure can occur on three different levels: a failure to obtain sperm for injection, failure of fertilization after injection, and a failure to establish a pregnancy after embryo transfer.

Failure to Obtain Sperm

In men with non-obstructive azoospermia, rarely, it is impossible to retrieve any spermatozoa from the testes. On the other hand, as might be expected, sperm are recovered in virtually all attempts involving men with obstructive azoospermia.

Failure of Fertilization After ICSI

As noted above, fertilization failure occurs in about 2% of ICSI cycles, whether male infertility is present or not [33, 72]. The reasons for these few failures remain unclear, but probably involve either poor sperm viability or an asynchronous oocyte maturation [47, 73].

Some men carrying acrosomeless (also known as globozoospermic) spermatozoa cannot achieve syngamy even after ICSI [33, 74, 75]. However, successful fertilization, pregnancy, and offspring have resulted after treating the oocytes post-ICSI by either a chemical agent [34, 75–77] or an electrical pulse [76, 78]. Similarly, the chances of fertilization in these problematic cases may sometimes be enhanced by utilizing sperm-derived activating extracts or calcium-releasing compounds [79, 80]. Oocyte activation agents include calcium ionophore [7], electrostimulation [76], and strontium [77]. Such adjunct treatments help to activate the oocyte by increasing the Ca^{2+} permeability of the cell membrane, thereby allowing extracellular Ca^{2+} flow into the oocyte and also inducing Ca^{2+} release from the intracellular calcium stores. In one of the first series of assisted oocyte activations, in patients with previous fertilization failure [34], the authors first injected a spermatozoon together with $CaCl_2$ and, thereafter, a calcium ionophore—this dual exposure resulted in an overall fertilization of >70%. These approaches have been able to trigger oocyte activation, allow concurrent sperm nuclear decondensation, and therefore, zygote development. To further enhance oocyte activation and syngamy, spermatozoa may be exposed to an agent that facilitates sperm membrane permeabilization [81, 82].

The inability to activate an egg has been attributed to the absence of a specific sperm protein that has been investigated in many occasions [79, 83, 84]. More recently, however, one such factor—phospholipase C-ζ1 (PLCζ1)—has been identified in mice. Following its injection into mouse oocytes, PLCζ1 was capable of inducing calcium oscillations that were identical to those observed following fertilization by a sperm [85, 86]. As an interesting correlate, the PLCζ1 isoform was undetectable in sperm of men that experienced fertilization failure with ICSI [87]. Taken together, these findings open a new avenue in the diagnosis and potential treatment of couples whose ICSI cycles terminate abruptly with unexpectedly low or definitive absence of fertilization.

Failure to Conceive After ICSI Fertilization

It must be emphasized finally that the implications of one fertilization failure for subsequent ICSI attempts are not necessarily bleak. When couples with failed ICSI fertilization attempted further ICSI cycles, their success rates were similar to other couples undergoing repeat ICSI cycles [34, 36, 88, 89].

On the other hand, as with IVF, some couples fail to conceive despite repeated ICSI cycles where the causes range from centrosomal dysfunction to DNA abnormalities [79, 90, 91]. Two hundred couples who had 433 cycles of ICSI treatment without success subsequently had 23 (12%) live births with no further treatment within 4 years of the last ICSI cycle [92]. The only predictor of live birth after ICSI failure was a shorter time to pregnancy (the time between seeking infertility treatment and the actual achievement of a pregnancy), suggesting that unknown factors contributing to longer duration of infertility were barriers to success [93].

Safety

Notwithstanding the large number of babies born from the ICSI procedure worldwide, concerns still exist as to whether the use of suboptimal spermatozoa can result in genomic abnormalities in the progeny [94]. These qualms are not only limited to the inheritance of specific traits that bear on fertility, but most importantly, those related to the postnatal well-being of the offspring as reflected in growth [95] or cognitive development [96]. Therefore, follow-up of ART children is highly recommended and is being applied increasingly [97–100]. Parent-administered questionnaire has been proposed as way of doing this, since a routine office assessment is costly and time-consuming [15, 101, 102].

The specific concerns in regard to ICSI, whether real or theoretical [103–106], involve the insemination method, the use of spermatozoa with genetic or structural defects, and the possible introduction of foreign genes. Even if there seems to be no evidence for a higher frequency of congenital abnormalities with ICSI compared to conventional IVF, more subtle effects might become evident in comparison to naturally conceived children. In fact, recent epidemiological studies of ART children report a twofold increase in infant malformations [107], a recurrent reduction in birth weight [108], certain rare syndromes related to imprinting errors [109–114], and even a higher frequency of some cancers [115]. On the other hand, such observations do not prove that there is an increased risk of imprinting disorders and, even less so, childhood cancers in ICSI children [106]. A systematic survey aimed at clarifying imprinting issues suggests that only Beckwith–Wiedemann syndrome (BWS) may have such a link [116].

A shorter gestational age and a lower birth weight have been noted in ART pregnancies irrespective of the conception method [95, 108]. The basis for this could lie in an unclear medical history [117], in the fact that a singleton may result from early in utero loss of a twin [118] or where an ART delivery is performed at the slightest sign of fetal distress [119]. When our Cornell data were stratified according to maternal age, singleton ICSI children had the same mean gestational age and birth weight as those conceived naturally [15]. Similarly, in the study of Lin et al. [120] levels of neonatal distress, NICU admission, and congenital malformations were comparable in both groups. The most unsettling concerns in regard to the health of ART offspring relate to a reported twofold increase in major malformations [107]. However, this study failed to correct for maternal age and for other patient characteristics [121], for the presence of male factor [122], and even in its classification methods [123]. Our follow-up records, beginning in the mid-1990s, have revealed an incidence of malformations within the expected range for the general population of New York State [124]. In another series, ICSI vs. naturally conceived singletons that were matched for maternal age displayed no difference in neonatal outcomes [120], and this was clearly the case when the outcomes of neonates generated by different artificial conception procedure, ICSI vs. IVF, were investigated [125].

In this connection, Bowen et al. [96] evaluated the medical and developmental state of 1-year-old children born after ICSI, IVF, or natural conception. They found that most 1-year-old ICSI children were healthy and developing normally, as measured by the Bayley Scales of Infant Development. However, about 17% displayed learning difficulties compared to those conceived by IVF or naturally. It was a later report that dismissed this concern in 2-year-old ICSI toddlers [126] which inspired our follow-up study in 3-year-olds.

Because of the confounding role of multiple gestations, as part of a multicenter international investigation, we then decided to assess singleton births at 5 years of age. Although this revealed no differences in the full scale IQ between ICSI and NC children, surprisingly, NC parents displayed higher levels of distress and dysfunctional child interactions and had more difficult children compared to the ICSI group ($P < 0.05$) [14]. This study revealed also that ICSI children were indeed characterized by a lower birth weight ($P < 0.05$) and also by a higher proportion of major malformations ($P < 0.05$) than their NC counterparts. The higher proportion of affected children was concentrated in the Belgian center [127]. Another study comprising 1,500 children from five European countries failed to show a higher incidence of major malformation in the ART group compared to NC children despite a clear difference in their parental age [98]. The same Brussels group confirmed a malformation level of 10.0 vs. 3.4% in the same cohort of NC children once they reached 8 years of age [128]. These three additional malformations included of an inguinal hernia and two nevus flammeus that required only minor surgical corrections. Interestingly, when the same ICSI progeny was reassessed for their physical and intellectual performances at 10 years of age, their state matched that of a natural conception group [129]. A prospective match-controlled study was performed to investigate the growth of children in the UK following IVF and ICSI up to 12 years of age. This study showed that height, weight, and head circumference did not differ between IVF and ICSI.

A limited number of studies have addressed the issue of cancer among children conceived by assisted reproduction. A report from the Netherlands identified five cases of retinoblastoma in IVF children—significantly more than expected [115]. A Swedish registry-based study identified five cases of Langerhan's histiocytosis among 16,280 IVF infants in comparison to the 0.9 expected cases in the general population [130]. However, these two reports have not been verified by other investigations, and the overall risk of cancer and the individual incidence of all other recorded cancer were not greater than expected. In fact, since childhood cancers are rare, larger studies are required to reliably observe any increase in risk among ART children.

Questions have been posed also about the effect of the embryo culture medium on the health of ART children in general and whether this can induce imprinting disorders [131]. Imprinting disorders such as Angelman syndrome (AS) [109, 113] and BWS [109, 132, 133] have been described in connection to assisted reproductive technologies. A survey of 1,000 British families raising children afflicted with transient neonatal diabetes mellitus, Prader–Willi syndrome, AS, or BWS revealed that only the latter, where *H19*'s downregulation plays a pivotal role, appeared to maintain an association with the ARTs [116]. Both syndromes have been found to be largely due to epigenetic defects rather than a genetic mutation or uniparental disomy [134], thus suggesting that some aspect of the ARTs may be responsible.

In a recent study in mice, Wilson et al. [135] attempted to assess the role of standard IVF and ICSI on gene expression imbalances, and they compared these two procedures to natural mating. The authors concluded that IVF and ICSI were no different in regard to issues of gene expression but had minor differences observed between the ART procedures and natural conception. Thus, the ART procedure itself does not induce the imprinting imbalances. Another group investigated the basic procedures common to IVF and ICSI such as embryo transfer and in vitro culture [136]. In vitro culture increases the loss of imprinting but even basic techniques, such as embryo transfer, can also lead to misexpression of several imprinted genes during postimplantation development.

In summary, the most important factor that can lead to adverse outcomes in offspring conceived by IVF or ICSI is that of high-order pregnancies. However, the introduction of single embryo transfer has reduced this considerably. Although perinatal outcomes such as prematurity, low birth weight, perinatal mortality, and increased incidence of malformations have been linked to the techniques of IVF and ICSI, the main culprit is related to infertility itself. Overall, no significant long-term neurodevelopmental differences have been found in connection with the ARTs, though the risks associated with childhood cancer and future fertility still require further research.

Acknowledgments We are grateful to the clinicians, scientists, embryologists, and nursing staff of The Ronald O. Perelman and Claudia Cohen Center for Reproductive Medicine. We are most grateful to Professor J Michael Bedford for his critical reading of the manuscript, Jennifer Hu and Qiansheng Alan Zhan for assisting with data entry, and Eugene Ermolovich for his photographic contribution. Queenie Neri was funded by the grant ULI RR024996 of the Clinical and Translational Science Center at Weill Cornell Medical College.

References

1. Hiramoto Y. Microinjection of the live spermatozoa into sea urchin eggs. Exp Cell Res. 1962;27:416–26.
2. Lin TP. Microinjection of mouse eggs. Science. 1966;708:333–7.
3. Uehara T, Yanagimachi R. Microsurgical injection of spermatozoa into hamster eggs with subsequent transformation of sperm nuclei into male pronuclei. Biol Reprod. 1976;4:467–70.
4. Markert CL. Fertilization of mammalian eggs by sperm injection. J Exp Zool. 1983;2:195–201.
5. Thadani VMA. study of hetero-specific sperm-egg interactions in the rat, mouse, and deer mouse using in vitro fertilization and sperm injection. J Exp Zool. 1980;3:435–53.
6. Perreault SD, Zirkin BR. Sperm nuclear decondensation in mammals: role of sperm-associated proteinase in vivo. J Exp Zool. 1982;2:253–7.
7. Hoshi K, Yanagida K, Sato A. Pretreatment of hamster oocytes with Ca^{2+} ionophore to facilitate fertilization by ooplasmic micro-injection. Hum Reprod. 1992;6:871–5.
8. Younis AI, Brackett BG, Fayrer-Hosken RA. Influence of serum and hormones on bovine oocyte maturation and fertilization in vitro. Gamete Res. 1989;2:189–201.
9. Iritani A, Utsumi K, Miyake M, Hosoi Y, Saeki K. In vitro fertilization by a routine method and by micromanipulation. Ann N Y Acad Sci. 1988;541:583–90.
10. Goto K, Kinoshita A, Takuma Y, Ogawa K. Fertilisation of bovine oocytes by the injection of immobilised, killed spermatozoa. Vet Rec. 1990;21:517–20.
11. Lanzendorf S, Maloney M, Ackerman S, Acosta A, Hodgen G. Fertilizing potential of acrosome-defective sperm following microsurgical injection into eggs. Gamete Res. 1988;4:329–37.
12. Palermo G, Joris H, Devroey P, Van Steirteghem AC. Pregnancies after intracytoplasmic injection of single spermatozoon into an oocyte. Lancet. 1992;8810:17–8.
13. Palermo GD, Colombero LT, Schattman GL, Davis OK, Rosenwaks Z. Evolution of pregnancies and initial follow-up of newborns delivered after intracytoplasmic sperm injection. JAMA. 1996;23:1893–7.
14. Ponjaert-Kristoffersen I, Tjus T, Nekkebroeck J, Squires J, Verte D, Heimann M, Bonduelle M, Palermo G, Wennerholm UB. Psychological follow-up study of 5-year-old ICSI children. Hum Reprod. 2004;12:2791–7.

15. Palermo GD, Neri QV, Takeuchi T, Squires J, Moy F, Rosenwaks Z. Genetic and epigenetic characteristics of ICSI children. Reprod Biomed Online. 2008;6:820–33.
16. Palermo GD, Cohen J, Alikani M, Adler A, Rosenwaks Z. Intracytoplasmic sperm injection: a novel treatment for all forms of male factor infertility. Fertil Steril. 1995;6:1231–40.
17. Neri QV, Takeuchi T, Palermo GD. An update of assisted reproductive technologies results in the United States. Ann N Y Acad Sci. 2008;1127:41–8.
18. Yovich JL, Stanger JD. The limitations of in vitro fertilization from males with severe oligospermia and abnormal sperm morphology. J In Vitro Fert Embryo Transf. 1984;3:172–9.
19. De Felici M, Siracusa G. "Spontaneous" hardening of the zona pellucida of mouse oocytes during in vitro culture. Gamete Res. 1982;6:107–13.
20. Bedford JM, Kim HH. Sperm/egg binding patterns and oocyte cytology in retrospective analysis of fertilization failure in vitro. Hum Reprod. 1993;3:453–63.
21. Van Blerkom J, Henry G. Oocyte dysmorphism and aneuploidy in meiotically mature human oocytes after ovarian stimulation. Hum Reprod. 1992;3:379–90.
22. Lalonde L, Langlais J, Antaki P, Chapdelaine A, Roberts KD, Bleau G. Male infertility associated with round-headed acrosomeless spermatozoa. Fertil Steril. 1988;2:316–21.
23. Temple-Smith PD, Southwick GJ, Yates CA, Trounson AO, de Kretser DM. Human pregnancy by in vitro fertilization (IVF) using sperm aspirated from the epididymis. J In Vitro Fert Embryo Transf. 1985;3:119–22.
24. Silber S, Ord T, Borrero C, Balmaceda J, Asch R. New treatment for infertility due to congenital absence of vas deferens. Lancet. 1987;8563:850–1.
25. Silber SJ, Nagy ZP, Liu J, Godoy H, Devroey P, Van Steirteghem AC. Conventional in-vitro fertilization versus intracytoplasmic sperm injection for patients requiring microsurgical sperm aspiration. Hum Reprod. 1994;9:1705–9.
26. Tournaye H, Devroey P, Liu J, Nagy Z, Lissens W, Van Steirteghem A. Microsurgical epididymal sperm aspiration and intracytoplasmic sperm injection: a new effective approach to infertility as a result of congenital bilateral absence of the vas deferens. Fertil Steril. 1994;6:1045–51.
27. Craft I, Bennett V, Nicholson N. Fertilising ability of testicular spermatozoa. Lancet. 1993;8875:864.
28. Schoysman R, Vanderzwalmen P, Nijs M, Segal-Bertin G, van de Casseye M. Successful fertilization by testicular spermatozoa in an in-vitro fertilization programme. Hum Reprod. 1993;8:1339–40.
29. Fishel S, Green S, Bishop M, Thornton S, Hunter A, Fleming S, al-Hassan S. Pregnancy after intracytoplasmic injection of spermatid. Lancet. 1995;8965:1641–2.
30. Tesarik J, Mendoza C, Testart J. Viable embryos from injection of round spermatids into oocytes. N Engl J Med. 1995;8:525.
31. Lanzendorf SE, Maloney MK, Veeck LL, Slusser J, Hodgen GD, Rosenwaks Z. A preclinical evaluation of pronuclear formation by microinjection of human spermatozoa into human oocytes. Fertil Steril. 1988;5:835–42.
32. Lundin K, Sjogren A, Nilsson L, Hamberger L. Fertilization and pregnancy after intracytoplasmic microinjection of acrosomeless spermatozoa. Fertil Steril. 1994;6:1266–7.
33. Liu J, Nagy Z, Joris H, Tournaye H, Devroey P, Van Steirteghem A. Successful fertilization and establishment of pregnancies after intracytoplasmic sperm injection in patients with globozoospermia. Hum Reprod. 1995;3:626–9.
34. Heindryckx B, Van der Elst J, De Sutter P, Dhont M. Treatment option for sperm- or oocyte-related fertilization failure: assisted oocyte activation following diagnostic heterologous ICSI. Hum Reprod. 2005;8:2237–41.
35. Tejera A, Molla M, Muriel L, Remohi J, Pellicer A, De Pablo JL. Successful pregnancy and childbirth after intracytoplasmic sperm injection with calcium ionophore oocyte activation in a globozoospermic patient. Fertil Steril. 2008;4:1202.e1201–5.
36. Egashira A, Murakami M, Haigo K, Horiuchi T, Kuramoto T. A successful pregnancy and live birth after intracytoplasmic sperm injection with globozoospermic sperm and electrical oocyte activation. Fertil Steril. 2037;2009(6):e2035–9.

37. Taylor SL, Yoon SY, Morshedi MS, Lacey DR, Jellerette T, Fissore RA, Oehninger S. Complete globozoospermia associated with PLCzeta deficiency treated with calcium ionophore and ICSI results in pregnancy. Reprod Biomed Online. 2010;4:559–64.
38. Ludwig M, al-Hasani S, Kupker W, Bauer O, Diedrich K. A new indication for an intracytoplasmic sperm injection procedure outside the cases of severe male factor infertility. Eur J Obstet Gynecol Reprod Biol. 1997;2:207–10.
39. Ludwig M, Strik D, Al-Hasani S, Diedrich K. No transfer in a planned ICSI cycle: we cannot overcome some basic rules of human reproduction. Eur J Obstet Gynecol Reprod Biol. 1999;1:3–11.
40. Ludwig M, Schopper B, Al-Hasani S, Diedrich K. Clinical use of a pronuclear stage score following intracytoplasmic sperm injection: impact on pregnancy rates under the conditions of the German embryo protection law. Hum Reprod. 2000;2:325–9.
41. Benagiano G, Gianaroli L. The new Italian IVF legislation. Reprod Biomed Online. 2004;2:117–25.
42. Porcu E, Fabbri R, Seracchioli R, Ciotti PM, Magrini O, Flamigni C. Birth of a healthy female after intracytoplasmic sperm injection of cryopreserved human oocytes. Fertil Steril. 1997;4:724–6.
43. Johnson MH. The effect on fertilization of exposure of mouse oocytes to dimethyl sulfoxide: an optimal protocol. J In Vitro Fert Embryo Transf. 1989;3:168–75.
44. Schalkoff ME, Oskowitz SP, Powers RD. Ultrastructural observations of human and mouse oocytes treated with cryopreservatives. Biol Reprod. 1989;2:379–93.
45. Vincent C, Pickering SJ, Johnson MH. The hardening effect of dimethylsulphoxide on the mouse zona pellucida requires the presence of an oocyte and is associated with a reduction in the number of cortical granules present. J Reprod Fertil. 1990;89(1):253–9.
46. Van Blerkom J, Davis PW, Merriam J. The developmental ability of human oocytes penetrated at the germinal vesicle stage after insemination in vitro. Hum Reprod. 1994;9(4): 697–708.
47. ESHRE. Intracytoplasmic sperm injection (ICSI) in 2006: evidence and evolution. Hum Reprod Update. 2007;6:515–26.
48. de Vincenzi IA. longitudinal study of human immunodeficiency virus transmission by heterosexual partners. European Study Group on Heterosexual Transmission of HIV. N Engl J Med. 1994;6:341–6.
49. Garrido N, Meseguer M, Simon C, Pellicer A, Remohi J. Assisted reproduction in HIV and HCV infected men of serodiscordant couples. Arch Androl. 2004;2:105–11.
50. Bujan L, Daudin M, Pasquier C. Choice of ART programme for serodiscordant couples with an HIV infected male partner. Hum Reprod. 2006;5:1332–3; author reply 1333–4.
51. Sauer MV, Chang PL. Establishing a clinical program for human immunodeficiency virus 1-seropositive men to father seronegative children by means of in vitro fertilization with intracytoplasmic sperm injection. Am J Obstet Gynecol. 2002;4:627–33.
52. Mencaglia L, Falcone P, Lentini GM, Consigli S, Pisoni M, Lofiego V, Guidetti R, Piomboni P, De Leo V. ICSI for treatment of human immunodeficiency virus and hepatitis C virus-serodiscordant couples with infected male partner. Hum Reprod. 2005;8:2242–6.
53. Pena JE, Thornton MH, Sauer MV. Assessing the clinical utility of in vitro fertilization with intracytoplasmic sperm injection in human immunodeficiency virus type 1 serodiscordant couples: report of 113 consecutive cycles. Fertil Steril. 2003;2:356–62.
54. van Leeuwen E, Prins JM, Jurriaans S, Boer K, Reiss P, Repping S, van der Veen F. Reproduction and fertility in human immunodeficiency virus type-1 infection. Hum Reprod Update. 2007;2:197–206.
55. Bendikson KA, Neri QV, Takeuchi T, Toschi M, Schlegel PN, Rosenwaks Z, Palermo GD. The outcome of intracytoplasmic sperm injection using occasional spermatozoa in the ejaculate of men with spermatogenic failure. J Urol. 2008;3:1060–4.
56. Edwards RG, Tarin JJ, Dean N, Hirsch A, Tan SL. Are spermatid injections into human oocytes now mandatory? Hum Reprod. 1994;12:2217–9.

57. Tsai MC, Takeuchi T, Bedford JM, Reis MM, Rosenwaks Z, Palermo GD. Alternative sources of gametes: reality or science fiction? Hum Reprod. 2000;5:988–98.
58. Gardner DK. Mammalian embryo culture in the absence of serum or somatic cell support. Cell Biol Int. 1994;18(12):1163–79.
59. Gardner DK, Lane M. Culture and selection of viable blastocysts: a feasible proposition for human IVF? Hum Reprod Update. 1997;3(4):367–82.
60. Kruger TF, Menkveld R, Stander FS, Lombard CJ, Van der Merwe JP, van Zyl JA, Smith K. Sperm morphologic features as a prognostic factor in in vitro fertilization. Fertil Steril. 1986;6:1118–23.
61. Reijo R, Alagappan RK, Patrizio P, Page DC. Severe oligozoospermia resulting from deletions of azoospermia factor gene on Y chromosome. Lancet. 1996;9011:1290–3.
62. Girardi SK, Mielnik A, Schlegel PN. Submicroscopic deletions in the Y chromosome of infertile men. Hum Reprod. 1997;8:1635–41.
63. Schlegel PN, Berkeley AS, Goldstein M, Cohen J, Alikani M, Adler A, Gilbert BR, Rosenwaks Z. Epididymal micropuncture with in vitro fertilization and oocyte micromanipulation for the treatment of unreconstructable obstructive azoospermia. Fertil Steril. 1994;5:895–901.
64. Schlegel PN, Palermo GD, Alikani M, Adler A, Reing AM, Cohen J, Rosenwaks Z. Micropuncture retrieval of epididymal sperm with in vitro fertilization: importance of in vitro micromanipulation techniques. Urology. 1995;2:238–41.
65. Sheynkin YR, Schlegel PN. Sperm retrieval for assisted reproductive technologies. Contemp Urol. 1997;9:21–36.
66. Palermo G, Joris H, Derde MP, Camus M, Devroey P, Van Steirteghem A. Sperm characteristics and outcome of human assisted fertilization by subzonal insemination and intracytoplasmic sperm injection. Fertil Steril. 1993;4:826–35.
67. Schlegel PN, Li PS. Microdissection TESE: sperm retrieval in non-obstructive azoospermia. Hum Reprod Update. 1998;4:439.
68. Reis MM, Tsai MC, Schlegel PN, Feliciano M, Raffaelli R, Rosenwaks Z, Palermo GD. Xenogeneic transplantation of human spermatogonia. Zygote. 2000;2:97–105.
69. Crabbe E, Verheyen G, Silber S, Tournaye H, Van de Velde H, Goossens A, Van Steirteghem A. Enzymatic digestion of testicular tissue may rescue the intracytoplasmic sperm injection cycle in some patients with non-obstructive azoospermia. Hum Reprod. 1998;1O:2791–6.
70. Crabbe E, Verheyen G, Tournaye H, Van Steirteghem A. The use of enzymatic procedures to recover testicular germ cells. Hum Reprod. 1997;8:1682–7.
71. Dragisic KG, Davis OK, Fasouliotis SJ, Rosenwaks Z. Use of a luteal estradiol patch and a gonadotropin-releasing hormone antagonist suppression protocol before gonadotropin stimulation for in vitro fertilization in poor responders. Fertil Steril. 2005;4:1023–6.
72. Bhattacharya S, Hamilton MP, Shaaban M, Khalaf Y, Seddler M, Ghobara T, Braude P, Kennedy R, Rutherford A, Hartshorne G, Templeton A. Conventional in-vitro fertilisation versus intracytoplasmic sperm injection for the treatment of non-male-factor infertility: a randomised controlled trial. Lancet. 2001;9274:2075–9.
73. Ermolovich E, Monahan D, Neri QV, Rosenwaks Z, Palermo G. Premature removal of cumulus cells results in incomplete maturation of cytoplasmic lattices. Hum Reprod. 2010;1:218.
74. Battaglia DE, Koehler JK, Klein NA, Tucker MJ. Failure of oocyte activation after intracytoplasmic sperm injection using round-headed sperm. Fertil Steril. 1997;1:118–22.
75. Rybouchkin A, Benijts J, De Sutter P, Dhont M. Disintegration of chromosomes in dead sperm cells as revealed by injection into mouse oocytes. Hum Reprod. 1997;8:1693–8.
76. Yanagida K, Katayose H, Yazawa H, Kimura Y, Sato A, Yanagimachi H, Yanagimachi R. Successful fertilization and pregnancy following ICSI and electrical oocyte activation. Hum Reprod. 1999;5:1307–11.
77. Yanagida K, Morozumi K, Katayose H, Hayashi S, Sato A. Successful pregnancy after ICSI with strontium oocyte activation in low rates of fertilization. Reprod Biomed Online. 2006;6:801–6.

78. Mansour R, Fahmy I, Tawab NA, Kamal A, El-Demery Y, Aboulghar M, Serour G. Electrical activation of oocytes after intracytoplasmic sperm injection: a controlled randomized study. Fertil Steril. 2009;1:133–9.
79. Palermo GD, Avrech OM, Colombero LT, Wu H, Wolny YM, Fissore RA, Rosenwaks Z. Human sperm cytosolic factor triggers Ca^{2+} oscillations and overcomes activation failure of mammalian oocytes. Mol Hum Reprod. 1997;4:367–74.
80. Morozumi K, Shikano T, Miyazaki S, Yanagimachi R. Simultaneous removal of sperm plasma membrane and acrosome before intracytoplasmic sperm injection improves oocyte activation/embryonic development. Proc Natl Acad Sci USA. 2006;47:17661–6.
81. Johnson LR, Moss SB, Gerton GL. Maintenance of motility in mouse sperm permeabilized with streptolysin O. Biol Reprod. 1999;3:683–90.
82. Glenn DR, McVicar CM, McClure N, Lewis SE. Sildenafil citrate improves sperm motility but causes a premature acrosome reaction in vitro. Fertil Steril. 2007;5:1064–70.
83. Parrington J, Swann K, Shevchenko VI, Sesay AK, Lai FA. Calcium oscillations in mammalian eggs triggered by a soluble sperm protein. Nature. 1996;6563:364–8.
84. Wolny YM, Fissore RA, Wu H, Reis MM, Colombero LT, Ergun B, Rosenwaks Z, Palermo GD. Human glucosamine-6-phosphate isomerase, a homologue of hamster oscillin, does not appear to be involved in Ca^{2+} release in mammalian oocytes. Mol Reprod Dev. 1999;3:277–87.
85. Saunders CM, Larman MG, Parrington J, Cox LJ, Royse J, Blayney LM, Swann K, Lai FA. PLC zeta: a sperm-specific trigger of Ca(2+) oscillations in eggs and embryo development. Development. 2002;15:3533–44.
86. Swann K, Saunders CM, Rogers NT, Lai FA. PLCzeta(zeta): a sperm protein that triggers Ca^{2+} oscillations and egg activation in mammals. Semin Cell Dev Biol. 2006;2:264–73.
87. Yoon SY, Jellerette T, Salicioni AM, Lee HC, Yoo MS, Coward K, Parrington J, Grow D, Cibelli JB, Visconti PE, Mager J, Fissore RA. Human sperm devoid of PLC, zeta 1 fail to induce Ca(2+) release and are unable to initiate the first step of embryo development. J Clin Invest. 2008;11:3671–81.
88. Moomjy M, Sills ES, Rosenwaks Z, Palermo GD. Implications of complete fertilization failure after intracytoplasmic sperm injection for subsequent fertilization and reproductive outcome. Hum Reprod. 1998;8:2212–6.
89. Heytens E, Parrington J, Coward K, Young C, Lambrecht S, Yoon SY, Fissore RA, Hamer R, Deane CM, Ruas M, Grasa P, Soleimani R, Cuvelier CA, Gerris J, Dhont M, Deforce D, Leybaert L, De Sutter P. Reduced amounts and abnormal forms of phospholipase C zeta (PLCzeta) in spermatozoa from infertile men. Hum Reprod. 2009;10:2417–28.
90. Palermo G, Munne S, Cohen J. The human zygote inherits its mitotic potential from the male gamete. Hum Reprod. 1994;7:1220–5.
91. Evenson D, Wixon R. Meta-analysis of sperm DNA fragmentation using the sperm chromatin structure assay. Reprod Biomed Online. 2006;4:466–72.
92. Osmanagaoglu K, Collins J, Kolibianakis E, Tournaye H, Camus M, Van Steirteghem A, Devroey P. Spontaneous pregnancies in couples who discontinued intracytoplasmic sperm injection treatment: a 5-year follow-up study. Fertil Steril. 2002;3:550–6.
93. Ludwig M. Risk during pregnancy and birth after assisted reproductive technologies: an integral view of the problem. Semin Reprod Med. 2005;4:363–70.
94. Ludwig M, Katalinic A. Malformation rate in fetuses and children conceived after ICSI: results of a prospective cohort study. Reprod Biomed Online. 2002;2:171–8.
95. Schieve LA, Ferre C, Peterson HB, Macaluso M, Reynolds MA, Wright VC. Perinatal outcome among singleton infants conceived through assisted reproductive technology in the United States. Obstet Gynecol. 2004;6:1144–53.
96. Bowen JR, Gibson FL, Leslie GI, Saunders DM. Medical and developmental outcome at 1 year for children conceived by intracytoplasmic sperm injection. Lancet. 1998;9115:1529–34.
97. Papaligoura Z, Panopoulou-Maratou O, Solman M, Arvaniti K, Sarafidou J. Cognitive development of 12 month old Greek infants conceived after ICSI and the effects of the method on their parents. Hum Reprod. 2004;6:1488–93.

98. Bonduelle M, Wennerholm UB, Loft A, Tarlatzis BC, Peters C, Henriet S, Mau C, Victorin-Cederquist A, Van Steirteghem A, Balaska A, Emberson JR, Sutcliffe AG. A multi-centre cohort study of the physical health of 5-year-old children conceived after intracytoplasmic sperm injection, in vitro fertilization and natural conception. Hum Reprod. 2005;2:413–9.
99. Leunens L, Celestin-Westreich S, Bonduelle M, Liebaers I, Ponjaert-Kristoffersen I. Cognitive and motor development of 8-year-old children born after ICSI compared to spontaneously conceived children. Hum Reprod. 2006;11:2922–9.
100. Ombelet W, Peeraer K, De Sutter P, Gerris J, Bosmans E, Martens G, Ruyssinck G, Defoort P, Molenberghs G, Gyselaers W. Perinatal outcome of ICSI pregnancies compared with a matched group of natural conception pregnancies in Flanders (Belgium): a cohort study. Reprod Biomed Online. 2005;2:244–53.
101. Squires J, Carter A, Kaplan P. Developmental monitoring of children conceived by intracytoplasmic sperm injection and in vitro fertilization. Fertil Steril. 2003;2:453–4.
102. Neri QV, Tanaka N, Wang A, Katagiri Y, Takeuchi T, Rosenwaks Z, Palermo GD. Intracytoplasmic sperm injection. Accomplishments and qualms. Minerva Ginecol. 2004;3: 189–96.
103. Cummins JM, Jequier AM. Treating male infertility needs more clinical andrology, not less. Hum Reprod. 1994;7:1214–9.
104. de Kretser DM. The potential of intracytoplasmic sperm injection (ICSI) to transmit genetic defects causing male infertility. Reprod Fertil Dev. 1995;2:137–41; discussion 132–41.
105. De Rycke M, Liebaers I, Van Steirteghem A. Epigenetic risks related to assisted reproductive technologies: risk analysis and epigenetic inheritance. Hum Reprod. 2002;10:2487–94.
106. Edwards RG, Ludwig M. Are major defects in children conceived in vitro due to innate problems in patients or to induced genetic damage? Reprod Biomed Online. 2003;2:131–8.
107. Hansen M, Kurinczuk JJ, Bower C, Webb S. The risk of major birth defects after intracytoplasmic sperm injection and in vitro fertilization. N Engl J Med. 2002;10:725–30.
108. Schieve LA, Meikle SF, Ferre C, Peterson HB, Jeng G, Wilcox LS. Low and very low birth weight in infants conceived with use of assisted reproductive technology. N Engl J Med. 2002;10:731–7.
109. Cox GF, Burger J, Lip V, Mau UA, Sperling K, Wu BL, Horsthemke B. Intracytoplasmic sperm injection may increase the risk of imprinting defects. Am J Hum Genet. 2002; 1:162–4.
110. DeBaun MR, Niemitz EL, Feinberg AP. Association of in vitro fertilization with Beckwith-Wiedemann syndrome and epigenetic alterations of LIT1 and H19. Am J Hum Genet. 2003;1:156–60.
111. Maher ER, Brueton LA, Bowdin SC, Luharia A, Cooper W, Cole TR, Macdonald F, Sampson JR, Barratt CL, Reik W, Hawkins MM. Beckwith-Wiedemann syndrome and assisted reproduction technology (ART). J Med Genet. 2003;1:62–4.
112. Gicquel C, Gaston V, Mandelbaum J, Siffroi JP, Flahault A, Le Bouc Y. In vitro fertilization may increase the risk of Beckwith-Wiedemann syndrome related to the abnormal imprinting of the KCN1OT gene. Am J Hum Genet. 2003;5:1338–41.
113. Orstavik KH, Eiklid K, van der Hagen CB, Spetalen S, Kierulf K, Skjeldal O, Buiting K. Another case of imprinting defect in a girl with Angelman syndrome who was conceived by intracytoplasmic semen injection. Am J Hum Genet. 2003;1:218–9.
114. Halliday J, Oke K, Breheny S, Algar E, David JA. Beckwith-Wiedemann syndrome and IVF: a case-control study. Am J Hum Genet. 2004;3:526–8.
115. Moll AC, Imhof SM, Cruysberg JR, Schouten-van Meeteren AY, Boers M, van Leeuwen FE. Incidence of retinoblastoma in children born after in-vitro fertilisation. Lancet. 2003; 9354:309–10.
116. Sutcliffe AG, Peters CJ, Bowdin S, Temple K, Reardon W, Wilson L, Clayton-Smith J, Brueton LA, Bannister W, Maher ER. Assisted reproductive therapies and imprinting disorders—a preliminary British survey. Hum Reprod. 2006;4:1009–11.
117. Kovalevsky G, Coutifaris C. Low and very low birth weight after use of assisted reproductive technology. N Engl J Med. 2002;18:1451–2; author reply 1451–2.

118. Davies MJ. Low and very low birth weight after use of assisted reproductive technology. N Engl J Med. 2002;18:1451–2; author reply 1451–2.
119. Shwayder JM. Liability in high-risk obstetrics. Obstet Gynecol Clin North Am. 2007;3: 617–25, xiv.
120. Lin K, Kang HJ, Neri QV, Rosenwaks Z, Palermo G. Obstetrical and perinatal outcomes of ICSI versus natural singleton pregnancies. Fertil Steril. 2003;3:109.
121. Steinkampf MP, Grifo J. Major birth defects after assisted reproduction. N Engl J Med. 2002;18:1449–51; author reply 1449–51.
122. Sills ES, Palermo GD. Major birth defects after assisted reproduction. N Engl J Med. 2002;18:1449–51; author reply 1449–51.
123. Sutcliffe AG, Bonduelle M, Taylor BW. Major birth defects after assisted reproduction. N Engl J Med. 2002;18:1449–51; author reply 1449–51.
124. Palermo GD, Cohen J, Rosenwaks Z. Intracytoplasmic sperm injection: a powerful tool to overcome fertilization failure. Fertil Steril. 1996;5:899–908.
125. Neri QV, Takeuchi T, Kang HJ, Lin K, Wang A, Palermo GD. Genetic assessment and development of children that result from assisted reproductive technology. Clin Obstet Gynecol. 2006;1:134–7.
126. Bonduelle M, Wilikens A, Buysse A, Van Assche E, Devroey P, Van Steirteghem AC, Liebaers I. A follow-up study of children born after intracytoplasmic sperm injection (ICSI) with epididymal and testicular spermatozoa and after replacement of cryopreserved embryos obtained after ICSI. Hum Reprod. 1998;13:196–207.
127. Bonduelle M, Bergh C, Niklasson A, Palermo GD, Wennerholm UB. Medical follow-up study of 5-year-old ICSI children. Reprod Biomed Online. 2004;1:91–101.
128. Belva F, Henriet S, Liebaers I, Van Steirteghem A, Celestin-Westreich S, Bonduelle M. Medical outcome of 8-year-old singleton ICSI children (born > or = 32 weeks' gestation) and a spontaneously conceived comparison group. Hum Reprod. 2007;2:506–15.
129. Leunens L, Celestin-Westreich S, Bonduelle M, Liebaers I, Ponjaert-Kristoffersen I. Follow-up of cognitive and motor development of 10-year-old singleton children born after ICSI compared with spontaneously conceived children. Hum Reprod. 2008;1:105–11.
130. Kallen B, Finnstrom O, Nygren KG, Olausson PO. In vitro fertilization in Sweden: child morbidity including cancer risk. Fertil Steril. 2005;3:605–10.
131. Edwards RG. Molecular genetics analyses in basic and clinical embryology. Reprod Biomed Online. 2002;2:220–1.
132. Sutcliffe AG, D'Souza SW, Cadman J, Richards B, McKinlay IA, Lieberman B. Minor congenital anomalies, major congenital malformations and development in children conceived from cryopreserved embryos. Hum Reprod. 1995;12:3332–7.
133. Olivennes F, Mannaerts B, Struijs M, Bonduelle M, Devroey P. Perinatal outcome of pregnancy after GnRH antagonist (ganirelix) treatment during ovarian stimulation for conventional IVF or ICSI: a preliminary report. Hum Reprod. 2001;8:1588–91.
134. Gosden R, Trasler J, Lucifero D, Faddy M. Rare congenital disorders, imprinted genes, and assisted reproductive technology. Lancet. 2003;9373:1975–7.
135. Wilson TJ, Lacham-Kaplan O, Gould J, Holloway A, Bertoncello I, Hertzog PJ, Trounson A. Comparison of mice born after intracytoplasmic sperm injection with in vitro fertilization and natural mating. Mol Reprod Dev. 2007;4:512–9.
136. Rivera RM, Stein P, Weaver JR, Mager J, Schultz RM, Bartolomei MS. Manipulations of mouse embryos prior to implantation result in aberrant expression of imprinted genes on day 9.5 of development. Hum Mol Genet. 2008;1:1–14.

Part IV
Embryo Evaluation and Grading

Chapter 15
Pronuclear Scoring in Human In Vitro Fertilization

Lynette Scott

Historically, the introduction of pronuclear scoring was observational and from two different perspectives, even if the morphological features score resulted in the same outcome and conclusions. Pronuclear scoring involves descriptions of the nucleolar precursor bodies (NPBs) which are clearly visible spherical structures observed in the nuclei of the fertilized oocyte, or for that matter, in the nuclei of any actively dividing cells. The two scoring systems [1, 2] looked at the same parameters of the NPBs, namely, their alignment, number, and relative size in the newly formed male and female nucleus. These parameters were shown to be predictive of continued development and resultant outcome. In the 1999 model from Tesarik et al. [2], the NPBs and their pattern were used as an indicator of sperm decondensation and function during intracytoplasmic sperm injection (ICSI) cases. The model of Scott et al. [1] described patterns of NPBs in the fertilized oocyte and how these changed, how they were related to a halo seen in the oocyte and the dynamic nature of fertilization, and how the patterns correlated with continued embryo viability.

Pronuclear scoring is descriptive and based on NPB and nuclear morphology and accomplished at the time of fertilization check, which should be between 16 and 18 h postinsemination. Although descriptive, the patterns have a biological basis and are predictive of development based on cell cycle and structure and function of the nucleus and nucleolus.

L. Scott, PhD (✉)
Fertility Centers of New England, Reading, MA, USA
e-mail: scottl@fertilitycenter.com

Z.P. Nagy et al. (eds.), *Clinical Embryology: A Practical Guide*,
DOI 10.1007/978-1-4614-8376-2_15, © Springer Science+Business Media New York 2013

Pronuclear/Zygote Scoring

At fertilization, the male and female pronuclei appear on the periphery of the oocyte, early in the process (as early as 6 h after insemination), and rotate into the center by approximately 16–18 h postinsemination, or 56–58 h post-hCG, which is the ideal time for any NPB scoring system [1–6].

In both systems [1, 2], equality of alignment of NPBs in the two nuclei is important, with the numbers of NPBs also being correlated with implantation and development [7]. Where there was equality in both alignment and numbers, there was greater blastocysts development and increased implantation [8–13]. Additionally, the total number of NPBs at the time of scoring is predictive of outcome. There should be between 5 and 7 per nucleus in any mammalian mitotic cell, and for embryos it is also predictive of outcome [7] (Fig. 15.1). From all data, literature, and the consensus meeting [14], an ideal pronuclear score is where there is equality in alignment and numbers between the two nuclei.

The most crucial aspect of pronuclear scoring is the concept of visualizing the oocyte and the nuclei in a three-dimensional state. The oocyte has polarity due to the placement of the spindle, the shape of the spindle, and the attachment of the nuclei to this spindle. This is not in a two-dimensional flat form, but two spheres

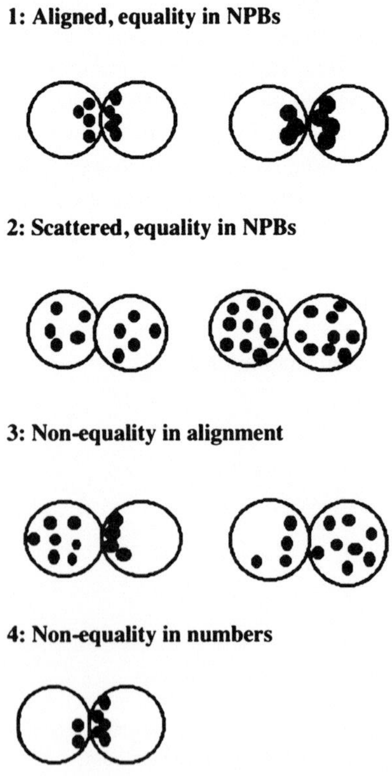

Fig. 15.1 Nucleolar precursor body (NPB) patterns in fertilized oocytes. Patterns 1 and 2 are normal, and 3 and 4 are abnormal

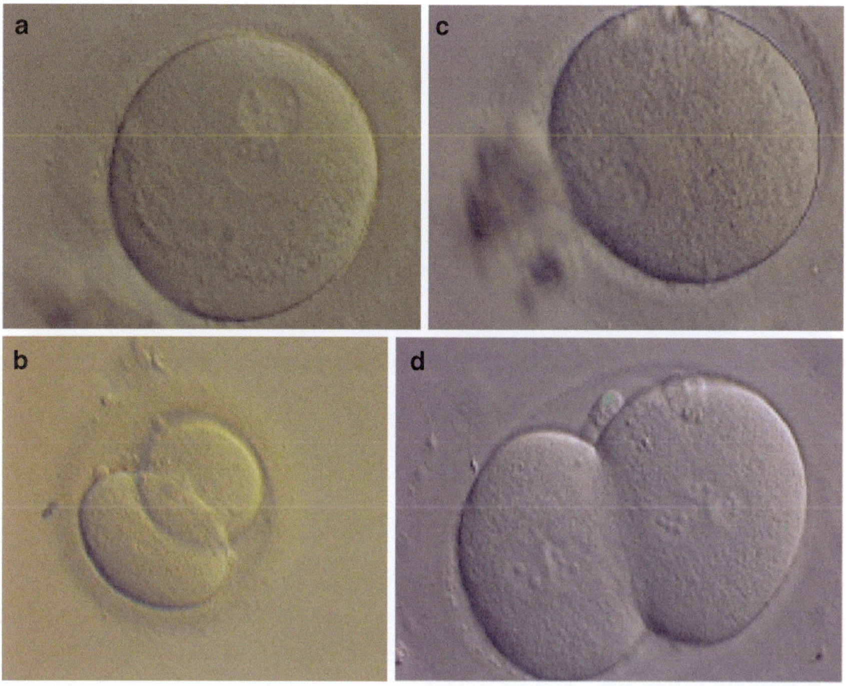

Fig. 15.2 Off-center position of nuclei resulting in abnormal cleavage. (**a**, **b**) Off-center alignment resulting in 2-cell embryo with very unequal cell sizes, which have limited developmental potential. (**c**, **d**) Off-center alignment leading to a 2-cell embryo with severe multinucleation, which results in aneuploidy and abnormal development

aligning on a three-dimensional cone structure (the mitotic spindle) within a sphere. Appreciating that the nuclei and NPBs are juxtaposed onto the spindle and that the spindle may lie in any plane between them, and that the chromatin and then chromosomes need to condense onto the spindle, allows an embryologist to mentally rotate the nuclei in order to look at the NPBs' relative to a slice or 2D plane, between the nuclei. In this way, equality and alignment can be easily assigned.

Pronuclear scoring requires the following observations:

- Appearance of the nuclei in a central position is normal with a peripheral position (or directly under the polar bodies) being abnormal, and the nuclei not being in close contact is highly abnormal, resulting in abnormal first mitotic cleavage (Figs. 15.2 and 15.3).
- Relative size of the two nuclei: they should be approximately the same size with no more than a 30% difference in diameter, which is abnormal (Fig. 15.4).
- Equality in both numbers and distribution of NPBs per nucleus with deviations from this being abnormal (Fig. 15.5).
- Presence or absence of a halo, which is an area of clearing of the cytoplasm in the periphery of the oocyte, which is desirable but not necessary (Fig. 15.6).

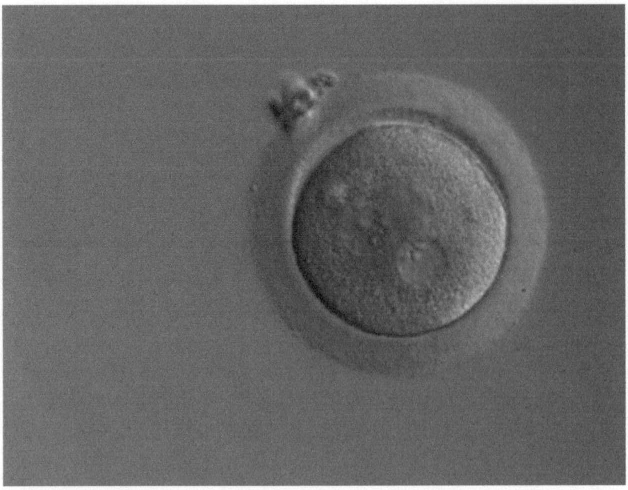

Fig. 15.3 Pronuclear oocyte with nuclei that are not central and juxtaposed

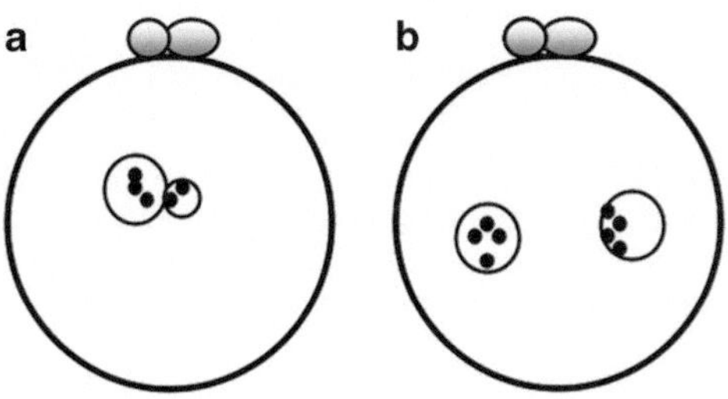

Fig. 15.4 Abnormal alignment or size of nuclei. (**a**) Unequal sizes; (**b**) nuclei not juxtaposed

- Major deviations from these patterns such as ghost pronuclei containing no NPBs or pronuclei with one large central NPB: both conditions are highly abnormal and are associated with imprinting errors, abnormal gene activation, and aneuploidy (Figs. 15.7 and 15.8).

Biology of the Nucleus and Nucleolar Precursor Bodies

The question is why are NPBs and their number and alignment important? What is their function in the early embryo, and what is their contribution to an embryo's ability to form a viable pregnancy? Understanding the biology of the NPBs and the structures they function with makes the concept of PN scoring for use in deselecting certain embryos a viable option in an ART laboratory.

The NPBs are part of the nucleoli, which are present in any actively dividing cells. Nucleoli are the organelles in the cell where all proteins are constructed and

Fig. 15.5 NPB and pronuclear scoring. Representation of scoring

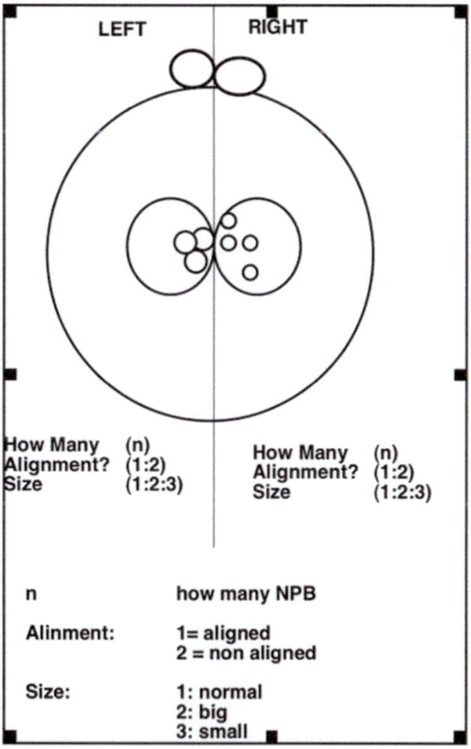

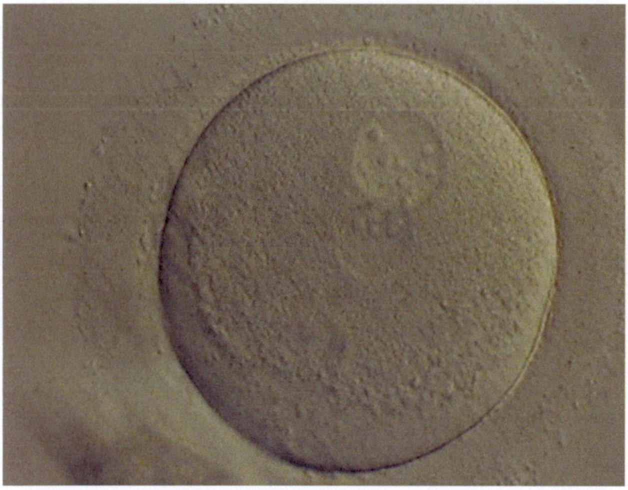

Fig. 15.6 Fertilized oocyte with halo, or clearing of cytoplasm, in the periphery of the cell

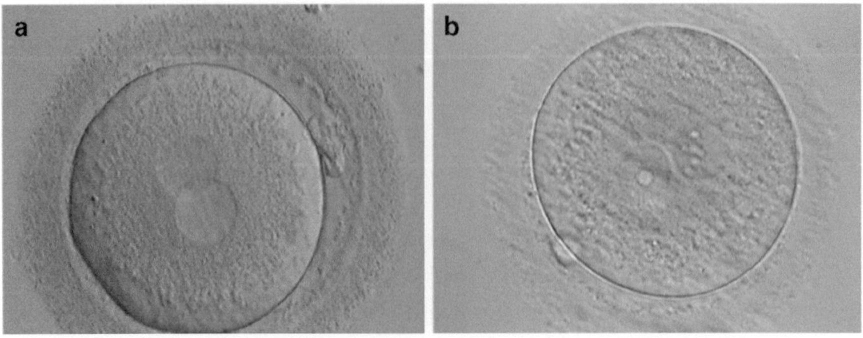

Fig. 15.7 Abnormal fertilized oocytes. (**a**) Ghost nuclei at 16–18 h postinsemination; no NPBs visible, abnormal with risk of imprinting errors. (**b**) Fertilized oocyte presenting with one large central NPB in one nucleus, abnormal sperm nucleus

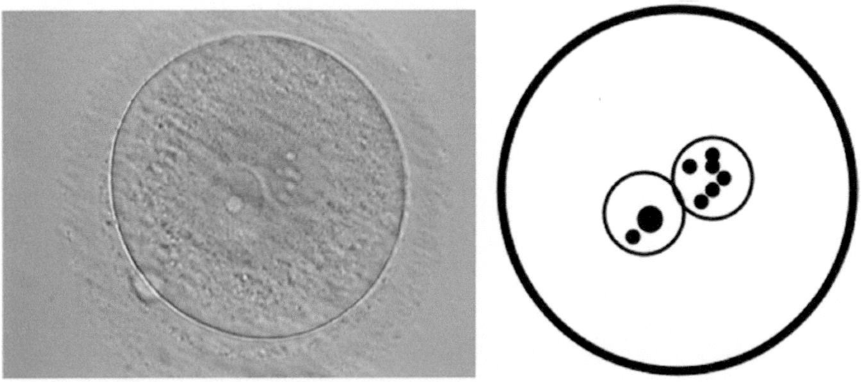

Embryo	XY	13	15	16	17	18	21	22	interpretation
1	0	1	0	0	1	1	2	2	complex
2	X0	1	1	1	1	0	2	1	complex
3	X0	1	2	1	2	1	2	1	complex
4	0	0	2	1	1	1	1	1	complex
5	XXY	2	3	2	1	1	1	1	complex
6	XX	1	1	1	2	2	2	1	complex
7	XY	2	2	2	1	2	1	1	complex

Fig. 15.8 Oocyte with abnormal NPBs in one nucleus, one large central NPB, and the FISH analysis of the resulting 8-cell embryo. The high rates of sex chromosome abnormalities and monosomies result from the abnormal development of the sperm, which fertilized this oocyte

are the site of ribosomal RNA (rRNA) production [15]. The nucleolus has other functions such as nuclear organization, cell growth through protein assembly, and developmental control [16]. Some growth factors and developmental regulatory proteins are also produced within the nucleoli [17].

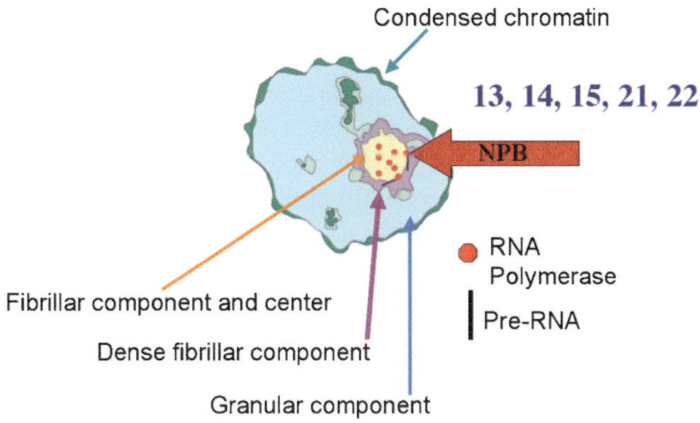

Fig. 15.9 Diagrammatic representation of a nucleolus structure and NPBs and the attachment of chromatin from the five heterochromatic chromosomes onto the spindle

Nucleoli are located on the DNA at sites where the genes for rRNA are located (rDNA) and where ribosomal precursors are constructed. These sites are the nucleolar organizing regions (NORs), and they contain many copies of the genes for the major rRNAs, namely, 18S and 28S—rRNA, in tandem repeats [18, 19]. Small rRNA (5S-rRNA) is synthesized outside the nucleolus, as are other nucleolar proteins, such as the factors and enzymes required for transcription and all the precursor units of the ribosomes [19].

The NORs are clustered on the DNA in areas where there is heterochromatin adjacent to rDNA genes. There are only five NOR-bearing chromosomes: 13, 14, 15, 21, and 22; the heterochromatic chromosomes [20] (Fig. 15.9) are also the chromosomes most likely to be abnormal in any aneuploidy screen [21, 22].

Nucleoli in vertebrates contain three functional components: the dense fibrillar component (DFC) that is required for transcription, the fibrillar center (FC) that is surrounded by the DFC, stores inactive transcription factors, and is the center of the nucleolus, and the granular or cytoplasmic component (GC) [18, 19, 23]. The GC usually lies on the periphery of the nucleolus. rDNA transcription and early ribosome biosynthesis occurs in the DFC, and the subsequent steps of forming the mature rRNA, preribosomes occurs in the GC. When cells are not active, the nucleoli are small, and when active, they are large. During development and at each mitotic event, the nucleoli dissemble into their component parts. When they disassemble, the FC region remains and can be visualized in the mitotic nuclei (or pronuclei) as spheres. It is the FC region (the spheres) that is scored or seen during pronuclear scoring; the NPBs are the FC regions of the nucleoli. Since these only reside on the five heterochromatic chromosomes, what is also being seen, indirectly, is the condensation of chromatin from chromosomes 13, 14, 15, 21, and 22 onto the spindle (Fig. 15.9).

Certain cells have a slightly different arrangement, such as Sertoli cells, in which there is only one nucleolus per cell and only one large FC region. Again, this is important in PN scoring for identifying embryos originating from sperm with defects in their RNA and protein assembly apparatus. Fertilized oocytes which present with nuclei in which there is one large central NPB most likely originated from sperm in which the nucleolar apparatus is abnormal, and during sperm maturation, the number of nucleoli has not increased to the normal 5–7. Embryos with this defect do not develop, are frequently chaotic, and are complex abnormal by FISH screening. Pronuclear scoring can deselect these forms of embryos and also allow a biological diagnosis for the infertility and abnormal sperm maturation (Fig. 15.8).

The development of the oocyte from the primordial to mature MII phase results in a huge growth phase, with the oocyte increasing its size 300 times and requiring vast amounts of new protein. Since new protein production requires nucleoli, nucleoli function is very active in oocyte maturation. As the oocyte reaches the final stages of growth, it goes into a resting phase, waiting for the signal for final maturation through the LH surge. At this stage, the nucleoli dissociate (see above) and only reform when the embryonic genome is in place, and the newly formed embryo is growing and requires the creation of new proteins [3–5].

The nucleoli become active during mitosis. As chromatin begins to condense onto the mitotic spindle (in an oocyte at sperm entry), the NPBs will appear to condense onto the spindle. In PN scoring, the lack of symmetry in this condensation is seen as unequal alignment of NPBs, unequal numbers of NPBs, and different sizes which means delayed or fast condensation in one nucleus. This may indicate abnormal or asynchronous karyo- and cytokinesis, which may result in embryos with little developmental potential, hence the use for PN scoring.

Nucleoli are also associated with the process of aging and begin to fragment, resulting in increased numbers of dense bodies in the cells [23]. Thus, inequality in NPBs between nuclei in oocytes will lead to abnormal development, and increased numbers may indicate fragmentation and aging.

Another aspect of nucleoli formation and delays in this, with implications for embryos, is the evidence from nuclear transfer experiments. In these embryos, there is real evidence of delayed embryonic genome activation. This is due to the late onset of functional nucleoli and NPB formation and activation, indicating that NPBs and nucleoli play an important role in embryonic genome activation and cell cycle [25, 26].

In conclusion, the use of pronuclear scoring is an important part of embryo selection in human IVF since it allows for early elimination of embryos that have fundamental flaws in their nuclei and in aspects of protein production and nuclear remodeling during mitosis and general nuclear function. What is scored in PN scoring is part of the cell that is crucial for normal development. PN scoring, performed at the very early stages of embryo development, reflects the health and normality of the gametes, which is essential as a flawed, biologically abnormal gamete is unlikely to produce a normal embryo with full developmental competence.

References

1. Scott LA, Smith S. The successful use of pronuclear embryo transfers the day following oocyte retrieval. Hum Reprod. 1998;13:1003–13.
2. Tesarik J, Greco E. The probability of abnormal preimplantation development can be predicted by a single static observation on pronuclear stage morphology. Hum Reprod. 1999;14(5): 1318–23.
3. Scott L. Classification of pronuclei and polarity of the zygote: correlations with outcome. In: Patrizio P, Guelman V, Tucker M, editors. A color atlas for human assisted reproduction: laboratory and clinical insights. Philadelphia: Lippincott Williams & Wilkins; 2003.
4. Scott L. Morphological correlates of oocyte and embryo competence-identification. In: Van Blerkom J, editor. Hum Fertil. 2002;5:206–14.
5. Scott L. Pronuclear scoring as a predictor of embryo development. Biomed Online. 2003;6: 57–70.
6. Scott L. The biological basis of non-invasive strategies for selection of human oocytes and embryos. Hum Reprod Update. 2003;9:237–49.
7. Scott L, Finn A, et al. Morphologic parameters of early cleavage-stage embryos that correlate with fetal development and delivery: prospective and applied data for increased pregnancy rates. Hum Reprod. 2007;22:230–40.
8. Ludwig M, Schopper B, et al. Clinical use of a pronuclear stage score following intracytoplasmic sperm injection: impact on pregnancy rates under the conditions of the German embryo protection law. Hum Reprod. 2000;15(2):325–9.
9. Scott L. The origin of monozygotic twinning. Reprod Biomed Online. 2002;5:276–84.
10. Zollner U, Steck T. Pronuclear scoring. Time for international standardization. J Reprod Med. 2003;48:365–9.
11. Borini A, Cattoli M, et al. Predictive factors for embryo implantation potential. Reprod Biomed Online. 2005;10:653–68.
12. Senn A, Urner F, et al. Morphological scoring of human pronuclear zygotes for prediction of pregnancy outcome. Hum Reprod. 2006;21:234–9.
13. Chen C, Kattera S. Comparison of pronuclear zygote morphology and early cleavage status of zygotes as additional criteria in the selection of day 3 embryos: a randomized study. Fertil Steril. 2006;85:347–52.
14. ALPHA Scientists In Reproductive Medicine; ESHRE Special Interest Group Embryology. Istanbul consensus workshop on embryo assessment: proceedings of an expert meeting. Reprod Biomed Online. 2011;22(6):632–46.
15. Leugn A, Lamond A. The dynamics of the nucleolus. Crit Rev Eukaryot Gene Expr. 2003;13: 39–54.
16. Hernandez-Verdun D, Roussel P. Regulators of nucleolar functions. Prog Cell Cycle Res. 2003;5:301–8.
17. Pedersen T. Growth factors in the nucleolus? J Cell Biol. 1998;143:279–81.
18. Goessens G. Nucleolar structure. Int Rev Cytol. 1984;87:107–58.
19. Schwarzacher H, Wachtler F. The nucleolus. Anat Embryol. 1993;188:515–36.
20. Dimitri P, Corradini N, et al. The paradox of functional heterochromatin. Bioessays. 2005;27: 29–41.
21. Gianaroli L, Magli MC, et al. Pronuclear morphology and chromosomal abnormalities as scoring criteria for embryo selection. Fertil Steril. 2003;80(2):341–9.
22. Finn A, Scott L, et al. Sequential embryo scoring as a predictor of aneuploidy in poor-prognosis patients. Reprod Biomed Online. 2010;21:381–90.
23. Schwartz P, Hinney B, et al. Oocyte-sperm interaction in the course of IVF: a scanning electron microscopy analysis. Reprod Biomed Online. 2003;7:192–8.
24. Guarente L. Link between aging and the nucleolus. Genes Dev. 1997;11:2449–55.
25. Laurincik J, Maddox-Hyttel P. Nucleolar remodeling in nuclear transfer embryos. Adv Exp Med Biol. 2007;591:84–92.
26. Svarcova O, Dinnyes A, et al. Nucleolar re-activation is delayed in mouse embryos cloned from two different cell lines. Mol Reprod Dev. 2009;76:132–41.

Chapter 16
Cumulative Morphological Assessment of Embryo Quality

Barry Behr and Aparna Hegde

It is not inconceivable that in the near future legal, financial, and moral obligations arising from concern over the dangers of multiple pregnancy will compel the limitation of the number of embryos transferred in in vitro fertilization (IVF) patients to just one. Some European and Nordic countries have already introduced mandates to limit the number of embryos that can be replaced while others have issued guidelines and recommendations for the number of oocytes to be inseminated or number of embryos cultured and/or the ability to cryopreserve them [1, 2]. Thus, transferring only one embryo represents the ultimate goal of assisted reproductive technologies (ART), and many studies have been dedicated to the choice of the right one [3]. However, an important milestone still to be attained in the practice of ART is the development of a comprehensive, reliable, and definitive selection protocol for the most viable embryo with maximum implantation potential. Since the inception of IVF, the most widely used criteria for selecting the best embryos for transfer have been based on cell number and morphology [4]. Biochemical methods to assess human gamete and embryo quality have been described by analyzing either follicular fluid [5] or metabolic activity of the embryo [6, 7]. These methods, however, are still very complex, time-consuming, and impractical in most busy ART laboratories. Hence, the assessment of morphology has been, and will remain, the first choice for selection as it is quick and, although not foolproof, has consistently been shown to have some predictive value [8].

With all the morphological criteria described, there is still the limit of a maximum implantation rate, leading to the use of multiple embryo transfers. Also, all morphological methods of selection described rely on a single static observation of the embryos, whereas the embryo itself, after fertilization, is on a very strict set of clocks governing division and initiation of key events from gene activation through

B. Behr, PhD, HCLD (✉) • A. Hegde, MD
IVF Laboratory, Department of Obstetrics and Gynecology,
Standord School of Medicine, Stanford, CA 94305-5317, USA
e-mail: Behr1@stanford.edu

Z.P. Nagy et al. (eds.), *Clinical Embryology: A Practical Guide*,
DOI 10.1007/978-1-4614-8376-2_16, © Springer Science+Business Media New York 2013

compaction and blastulation which is a dynamic process [9]. Each stage of the complex developmental process is dependent upon the successful completion of the previous one. This would imply that optimal evaluation of an embryo's potential would necessitate multiple assessments of the embryo at each of the developmental checkpoints as it makes its transition from a single-celled zygote after fertilization of the oocyte to a blastocyst and from maternal to embryonic genome activation, initiation of protein synthesis, and cell differentiation. Thus, conducting noninvasive evaluation of the preimplantation period in a systematic, cumulative fashion should provide for the most predictive information regarding embryo quality. This chapter will outline the various morphological criteria that are currently available for selection within the framework of a continuous model from the oocyte through to the blastocyst. No one selection criteria is better, but if possible a combination of one, two, or even three selection points should lead to more accurate selection [10]. An embryo that does not meet a selection criterion at one point may meet it at another but should be avoided, as it is unlikely that culture can correct an impaired embryo.

Oocyte Quality: Day 0

Mounting evidence that oocyte quality profoundly affects fertilization and subsequent embryo development drives the continued search for reliable predictors of oocyte developmental competence [11]. Five levels of oocyte developmental competence were characterized by Sirard et al. [12], including the ability to resume meiosis, to cleave upon fertilization, to develop into a blastocyst, to induce pregnancy, and to generate a healthy offspring. Cytoplasmic changes accompanying oocyte growth may include messenger RNA (mRNA) transcription, protein translation, and post-translational modification [13, 14]. These activities are necessary for meiotic maturation [15], activation of the zygotic genome [16], and blastocyst formation [17]. Any dysfunction or dislocation of oocyte components, such as meiotic spindle, cortical granules, or mitochondria, can decrease the oocyte viability and has a crucial impact on embryo development and quality [18–20]. Vlaisavljevic et al. have shown that there is potentially a problem with greater than 50% of all oocytes retrieved in human ART cycles [21]. In a study of two groups of patients with unstimulated cycles who underwent day 2 and day 5 transfers, respectively, there was no difference in the fertilization rate in the two groups or the achievement of an embryo on day 2. However, only 55% of embryos placed in extended culture grew to the blastocyst stage. This may indicate an intrinsic problem with a large cohort of retrieved oocytes that is exacerbated by ovarian stimulation, or a deficiency in the culture systems used [22]. Overall the implantation rates per embryo transferred were different between day 2 and day 5 (24 vs. 40%), but per oocyte retrieved, there was no difference (12 vs. 14%). Thus, developmental fate of the embryo is largely dictated by the quality of the oocyte [22].

Although the use of cellular and molecular predictors of oocyte quality may be more precise and objective, and no information can be obtained on the day of

Table 16.1 Morphological parameters to assess quality of oocyte

Criterion	Parameters	References
Cumulus–oocyte complex	Compactness and thickness of the cumulus investment, brightness of the cytoplasm	[25–27]
Cytoplasm	Granularity (large or small granules, homogenous or clustering distribution of granules, in center or in the periphery of oocyte), coloration, regions of organelle clustering (vacuoles, endoplasmic reticulum)	[28–30]
Polar body	Shape (round or ovoid), size (large or small), surface (smooth or rough), cytoplasm (intact or fragmented)	[31, 32]
Zona pellucida	Thickness, structure	[33]
Perivitelline space	Size (normal or increased), the presence or absence of grain	[34, 35]
Meiotic spindle	Location and refraction	[36]

From Lasienë et al. [23]—http://medicina.kmu.lt, with permission

follicle aspiration because cumulus cells impair evaluation in IVF oocytes, morphological parameters may still provide valuable information for the preselection of oocytes with higher developmental competence. Table 16.1 [23–37] describes the morphological parameters of the oocyte that can be assessed.

Historically, the evaluation of oocyte maturity in conventional IVF has been based on the expansion and radiance of the cumulus–corona complex [38]: Expanded cumulus matrix and a "sun-burst" corona radiata denote preovulatory (metaphase II) oocytes, less-expanded complex denotes intermediate maturity, and the absence of an expanded cumulus might indicate oocyte immaturity (prophase I). However, this method is unreliable in case of disparity of maturation process in oocyte and cumulus as can happen when there is a drop in estradiol levels during controlled hyperstimulation [39].

ICSI facilitates morphological assessment of the oocyte due to the inherent requirement for the removal of cumulus and corona cells. Oocytes retrieved from patients following controlled ovarian hyperstimulation show varying stages of meiotic maturity. Only oocytes at metaphase II are suitable for ICSI, whereas oocytes at metaphase I may only be used if only a few MII oocytes are available as their fertilization rate was found to be rather low [40]. Oocytes at prophase I and giant MII oocytes (which mostly result in digynic triploidy) should be discarded [41, 42]. Disturbances or asynchrony in cytoplasmic [30, 35, 43] and nuclear maturation [31, 44] of the oocyte may result in different morphological abnormalities, respectively. Such disturbances may be caused by reduced blood supply of the follicle during controlled hyperstimulation resulting in oxygen deficiency and reduced viability [45] and abnormal oocyte spindle as well as chromosomal defects [46]. In the presence of such an inherent cytoplasmic defect or disorganization, the formation of polar axes which are associated with morphogenesis throughout pre- and postimplantation stages [47] may be impaired. Also, disproportionate segregation of mitochondria and proteins at the first cleavage division can result in cleavage arrest or a limited implantation potential [7].

It has been recognized that MII oocytes of good morphology should have a clear, moderately granulate cytoplasm, a small perivitelline space, an intact first polar body, and a colorless zona pellucida [31, 34, 48]. However, more than half of all oocytes show at least one morphological abnormality [7].

Cytoplasm and Polar Body

According to the morphological criteria described in Table 16.1, human oocytes are classified as (a) normal oocytes; (b) oocytes with extracytoplasmic abnormalities (dark zona pellucida, large perivitelline space with debris, fragmentation of the polar body, and abnormal consistency of the oolemma and the zona pellucida); (c) oocytes with intracytoplasmic abnormalities (dark or granular cytoplasm and cytoplasmic fragments); (d) oocytes with shape abnormalities; and (e) oocytes with multiple abnormalities [29].

Some studies have revealed that the embryos developed from the oocytes of normal cytoplasmic structure undergo the best uterine implantation [29], while three studies [29, 34, 49] were not able to correlate oocyte morphology with fertilization rate or embryo quality. Serhal et al. [28] described a pregnancy rate of 24% in patients with transfers derived solely from normal oocytes compared to 3% in oocytes with cytoplasmic abnormalities. Other studies have reported similar results [43]. Kaharman et al. found ongoing pregnancy rates to be poor (12.8%) in patients with granular cytoplasm [30]. A high frequency of aneuploidy was found in many cells of the developing embryo when the oocyte had cytoplasmic abnormalities [29, 30, 48]. A significant decrease in preclinical pregnancy loss has been found in patients in whom none of the replaced embryos was dysmorphic in origin (20 vs. 58.3% in oocytes with multiple dysmorphism) [50] This may be due to higher rate of aneuploidy found in dysmorphic oocytes [30, 51, 52].

Extrusion of first polar body indicating the end of meiotic maturation can easily be examined [7]. An intact first polar body showing a smooth surface was found to be of positive prognostic value in terms of fertilization and embryo quality, as well as implantation and pregnancy rate [31, 53, 54]. Conversely, oocytes with a fragmented first polar body developed worse (55.1%) after fertilization than those with a normal polar body (60.3%) [48]. Navarro et al. [55] reported that the presence of an enlarged polar body is related to poorer rates of fertilization, cleavage, and top-quality embryos. However, identification of first polar body fragmentation did not seem to interfere with ICSI outcomes [32].

Prognostic relevance of first polar body morphology has also been suggested by data for oocytes matured in vitro [56]. It is thought that aging in vivo in MII before aspiration may lead to degeneration of the first polar body and that the resultant overmaturity of such oocytes may further contribute to a diminished developmental potential [31, 44, 53].

Perivitelline Space and Zona Pellucida

Xia et al. [48] found that oocytes with a large perivitelline space developed worse after intracytoplasmic sperm injection (37.5%) than those with normal perivitelline space (60.3%). Oocytes, which had large grains in the perivitelline space, developed worse (59%) after fertilization than those without grains (71.1%) [35]. The thickness of the zona pellucida varies from 10 to 31 μm [57] and is not related to the cytoplasm diameter. The thickness of the zona pellucida influences sperm penetration. Oocytes are fertilized best in vitro when the thickness of the zona pellucida is less than 18.6 μm [23]. Presence of thick zona pellucida (22 μm and thicker) could be an indication for intracytoplasmic sperm injection for infertile patients [58] as it does not have any influence on embryo development following ICSI.

Meiotic Spindle

Meiotic spindle has a significant influence on the correct alignment of chromosomes in the oocyte and their segregation during meiosis. Parameters of meiotic spindle (location and refraction) may be used to determine the quality of oocytes. Nowadays, meiotic spindle can be examined, and its location can be determined by means of polarizing microscopy, avoiding damage to the oocyte as opposed to confocal microscope, which causes damage [23].

The birefringence of meiotic spindle can be studied with the help of a Polscope microscope. It has been estimated that the oocytes with birefringent spindle have higher developmental potential after fertilization in vitro or intracytoplasmic sperm injection than oocytes without birefringent spindle [24, 36, 59, 60]. Moon et al. [36] estimated by Polscope that the location of meiotic spindle could vary in an oocyte. Therefore, it can be damaged when *blind* intracytoplasmic sperm injection is made into human oocytes. However, no relationship was found between deviation of the meiotic spindle from the polar body within oocytes and oocyte developmental competence [24, 36]. Battaglia et al. [61] reported that the number of oocytes with spindle abnormalities (abnormal placement of tubulin) increased with increasing women's age (40 years and older). This abnormality is associated with displacement of one or more chromosomes from the metaphase plate during second meiotic division and thus can cause aneuploidy [61]. The routine use of a Polscope in the IVF lab is challenging as temperature and orientation of the oocyte during the spindle observation can significantly affect the interpretation of the results.

Rienzi et al. derived an MII (metaphase II) oocyte morphological score (MOMS) by identifying relationships among oocyte appearance, fertilization status, PN score, and day 2 embryo quality [62]. Morphological examination of 1,191 MII oocytes showed that presence of vacuoles, abnormal first polar body, and large perivitelline space were related to a lower fertilization rate. Pronuclear morphology was adversely

Table 16.2 Metaphase II oocyte morphology scoring system (MOMS)

Extracytoplasmic features	Points
Abnormal polar body	2.0
Large perivitelline space	1.4
Cytoplasmic features	
Granular cytoplasm	1.4
Centrally located granular area	2.7
Vacuoles	2.1

From Reinzi et al. [62], with permission

affected by the presence of a large perivitelline space, diffuse cytoplasmic granularity, and/or centrally located granular area. The later characteristic was also found to be negatively related to day 2 embryo quality. According to the odds ratios obtained for each oocyte morphotype, an MII MOMS was calculated (see Table 16.2) [62]. A significant relationship was found between MOMS and female age, female basal FSH, and clinical outcome.

Zygote Quality Day 1: Pronuclear Scoring Systems

There has been a suspicion that major abnormalities of pronuclear development (i.e., pronuclei of unequal sizes, at a distance or not centrally located within the zygote cytoplasm) are incompatible with normally progressive development [63]. Hence, a number of different noninvasive pronuclear scoring systems have been proposed which rely upon one static observation of simple morphological parameters at the pronuclear stage performed at 16–18 h postinsemination with both standard IVF and ICSI. All pronuclear scoring systems [64–67] attempt to classify zygotes based on the following characteristics of the two pronuclei: symmetry (equal vs. unequal), position (in apposition vs. at a distance), and location (central vs. noncentral). The nucleoli are scored based on number (3–7), symmetry (equal vs. unequal sizes), and location (polarized or aligned vs. nonpolarized or nonaligned). Other parameters that may be factored in are polar body morphology and alignment, cytoplasmic morphology (presence or absence of halo), timing of nuclear membrane breakdown, and finally a second embryo evaluation at 25–27 h postinsemination for pronuclear morphology (presence vs. absence of pronuclei) and/or early cell division [63].

The original score of Scott et al. was based on parameters such as pronuclear size and alignment, alignment of nucleoli within the pronuclei, and cytoplasmic morphology such as appearance of cytoplasm, presence of a halo, timing of nuclear membrane breakdown, and early cell division [64]. The total score ranges from 7 to 25 with optimal score equal to or above 15. The revised score included only parameters that could be assessed at the time of fertilization assessment (17–18 h postinsemination), classifying the zygotes into five basic groups denoted as *z* score [66] which were later condensed into four basic categories [67]. They also showed an increase of 1.6-fold in implantation rates when the *z*-scoring system was included in embryo selection [67].

Tesarik and Greco, however, claim that it is possible to predict preimplantation development by focusing exclusively on the number, distribution, and synchrony of development of nucleolar precursor bodies (NPBs) in each pronucleus [65, 68]. These authors considered interpronuclear synchrony, evaluated at 12–20 h after IVF/ICSI, to be more important than the actual NPB polarity at the site of pronuclear apposition as they assumed that polarization of nucleoli was not evident from the beginning of pronuclei formation but appeared progressively with time [68]. The optimal synchronized pattern (pattern 0) yielded 37.3% of good-quality embryos compared with only 27.8% of all other patterns.

Ludwig et al. [69], Zollner et al. [70], Senn et al. [71], Kaharman et al. [72], and Gianaroli et al. [73] developed further systems for scoring pronuclear morphology which are all based on a common theme of the value of symmetry in all of the morphological parameters examined.

Testing of the pronuclear morphology scoring systems by various ART facilities reported inconsistent results in their usefulness in predicting embryonic implantation potential [63]. Various studies have shown strong correlation of pronuclear scoring system with blastocyst development potential [66, 67, 74], implantation rates [64–66, 69, 74–78], pregnancy rate [78], and chromosomal status [72, 73, 79–83].

However, Salumets et al. [84], James et al. [85], Jaroudi et al. [86], and Payne et al. [87] failed to show any correlation between zygote score and pregnancy rate. No agreement also currently exists regarding the utility of using the cytoplasmic halo as a marker of embryo quality [88]. Salumets et al. [84], Scott [22], Ebner et al. [7], and Stalf et al. [89] found a positive association, while Zollner et al. [70] found that a halo of extreme dimensions might have a detrimental effect on blastocyst development.

Undoubtedly, pronuclear scoring is a rapid, simple, early, noninvasive selection technique requiring one static observation of simple morphological parameters at 16–18 h postinsemination. However, no standardized scoring system for zygote grading is currently in use. Hence, comparing success rates between laboratories while controlling for embryo quality is a challenge [63]. Pronuclear morphology is also very fluid, and there is considerable biological variation within normal development with different numbers and dimensions of nucleoli being compatible with development. Given the dynamic nature of PN formation [68], including NPB distribution, migration, coalescence, and dissolution, the timing of evaluation is of critical importance. [Zygotes formed from ICSI reveal their PNs approximately 4 h earlier than those formed by routine examination [88, 90].] The scoring is more time-consuming than the cursory assessment of the zygote that is currently done for determination of fertilization. Accurate assessment of the 3-dimensional disposition and number of NPBs is difficult as it requires the visual memorization of the spatial organization of the structures through multiple focal planes, and this memorization must be done rapidly to avoid prolonged exposure of the zygote to light, to temperature, and to pH shifts [88]. Further refinement of the scoring system is needed, and additional features such as the ratio of the NPBs per nucleus [91]. The orientation of the pronuclei relative to the polar bodies [6, 92] may need to be assessed for possible inclusion of the pronuclear scoring systems due to studies suggesting association with outcomes.

Significance of Timing of First Cleavage

When the final steps of oocyte maturity are triggered by LH surge (hCG injection), a clock is set in the oocyte, which will mark the time since this event all through the development of the preimplantation embryo [9]. Strangely, this time point is seldom used when assessing embryos. Any delay in a developmental event will result in the embryo being out of synchrony with the clock [22]. A 4-cell embryo scored in the morning of day 2 is definitely not the same as one that was scored as 4-cell in the afternoon [6]. Thus, one of the most critical factors in determining selection criteria for embryos is to ascertain strict time points to compare embryos [93]. The first cleavage to the 2-cell stage at 24–27 h after insemination or microinjection has been shown to be one such critical time point for selecting embryos for transfer [94, 95]. Early entry into the first mitotic division accounts for early completion of the final events of fertilization alignment of the pronuclei, alignment of the chromosomes on the metaphase spindle, and finally the first mitotic division. Also, early cleavage is a clearly visible event, whereas pronuclear morphology may vary during the dynamic process of syngamy [68]. Entry into first mitotic division by 22–24 h after insemination has been correlated with increased blastocyst formation [96, 97], increased implantation rates [95, 98–103], increased pregnancy rates [84, 94–96, 102, 103], and presence of a euploid set of chromosomes [100, 104]. Significantly, in the original embryo scoring system described by Scott and Smith [64], embryos that had already cleaved to the 2-cell stage by 25–26 h postinsemination were assigned an additional score of 10. Terriou et al. [105] found that even early first cleavage was strongly associated with good embryo morphology on day one, and multivariate analysis demonstrated that early embryo cleavage and embryo score on day one had strong complementary predictive value for pregnancy.

Interestingly, first cleavage can occur earlier in ICSI zygotes compared to those obtained by IVF [100]. This is because the direct injection of a spermatozoan bypasses most of the fertilization steps and results in a shorter fertilization time [90]. Hence, Lundin et al. [100] suggest that it may be better either to inseminate oocytes earlier or screen IVF zygotes later in order to obtain comparable data. However, until more studies are available on ICSI embryos, checking embryos on day 1 at 22–24 h after insemination can be considered a simple and noninvasive procedure that may help to select embryos in which the time clock is advanced or at least not delayed [22].

Day 2 Scoring: Multinucleation and Blastomere Morphology

During the early years of conventional IVF, oocyte quality could not be estimated, and there were no day 1 scoring systems available [7]. Hence, grading systems for day 2 embryo based on the number (representative of cleavage speed), shape of the blastomeres, and percentage of fragmentation were introduced [7, 38]. The various day 2 scoring systems that have been proposed (see Table 16.3) [3, 4, 38, 88, 106–110]

Table 16.3 Examples of various scoring systems for embryo selection

References	Name	Day of assessment	System type	Scoring range	Best embryo	Cell number	Frag	Symm	Compaction/ expansion	Cytoplasm features	Cleavage rate	Multi nucleation
Cummins et al. [4]	Embryo quality score (EQS)/ embryo development rating (EDR)	2 or 3	Score	1–4	Score 4		+	+		+	+	
Puissant et al. [106]	Embryo scoring	2	Grade	1–4	Grade 4	+	+	+				
Veeck (1991)	Morphological grading	3	Grade	1–4	Grade 1	+	+	+				
Steer et al. [107]	Cumulative embryo score (CES)	3	Grade	1–4	Grade 4	+	+	+				
Giorgetti et al. [108]	4-Point embryo score	2	Point	1–4	4 point	+	+	+				
Ziebe et al. [109]	Embryo quality score	2	Symm or frag score with cell	Symm: 1.0–2.0 Frag: 2.1, 2.2, 3.0, 4.0	≥4 cell +2.1	+	+	+			+	
Van Royen et al. [3]	Top-quality embryo	2 and 3	Score	Frag: A, B, C	Top quality	+	+					+
Desai et al. [110]	Embryo quality store (D3EQ)	3	Score	1–10	Score 10	+	+	+	+/+	Pitting vacuole		

From Ceyhan et al. [88], with permission
+ indicates characteristic included in assessment system; *Frag* fragmentations; *Symm* symmetry

are either exclusive day 2 scores [106, 108, 109] or include grading that can be done on either day 2 or 3 [4] or grading that includes parameters observed on both day 2 and 3 [3]. Van Royen's "top-quality embryo" includes multinucleation on day 2 in addition to day 3 parameters [3]. Though various studies have indicated a positive association of transfer of high-quality embryos as determined by the various scores with improved developmental potential, implantation rate, and pregnancy rate, a major problem with most of these studies was the impossibility of knowing which embryo actually implanted, as the embryo transfers were grouped possibly resulting in contradictory results [7, 111]. However, Guerif et al. [111] cultured more than 4,000 embryos individually in microdrops and sequentially evaluated them from day 1 to day 6, and they found that early cleavage and cell number on day 2 were the most powerful parameters to predict the development of a good morphology blastocyst at day 5. The grading system [111] they used is as follows: Blastomeres were classified into three groups (<4 cells, 4 cells, >4 cells). The degree of fragmentation was expressed as a percentage of the total oocyte volume occupied by anucleate cytoplasmic fragments. The rate of fragmentation was scored (<20% of the volume of embryo, between 20 and 50% of the volume of the embryo, >50% of the volume of the embryo). Embryos with one or more multinucleated blastomeres were excluded from extended embryo culture. Embryos with pattern 0, early cleavage, four regular blastomeres, <20% of fragmentation, and no multinucleated blastomeres were classified as *top quality* [111]. Scott et al. [91] also found that in addition to pronucleate morphology, day 2 morphology of cleaving embryos is stronger positive predictors of implantation than day 3 morphology or the ability to achieve the blastocyst stage of development. Parameters that were most consistently correlated with no delivery were lack of pronuclear symmetry and abnormal day 2 morphology parameters, multinucleation, and uneven cell size (defined as >20% difference in size/volume of the cells [91]).

Multinucleation

Day 2 state of nucleation has proven to be highly significant in terms of fetal development and delivery [91]. Multinucleation is a common phenomenon with the presence of multinucleation reported in 79.4% of all cycles by Van Royen et al. [112] and 74% by Jackson et al. [113]. Significantly, the observed multinucleation is an underestimation of the actual rate as the percentages reported in literature only reflect multinucleation at the interphase stage when the nucleus is visible [112].

Day 2 after insemination/injection seems to be the most rewarding and practical for nuclear observations. Multinucleation was discovered in 27.4% of the embryos on day 2 vs. only 15.1% on day 3 in a study by Van Royen et al. [112]. This may be partly due to the larger dimensions of day 2 cells and also their better optical accessibility (less overlap) due to the smaller number of cells [112]. Also, Staessen and Van Steireghem [114] reported that 30% of embryos with multinucleation in the 2-cell stage did not show multinucleation in the 3 to 8-cell stage.

Multinucleation indicates a breakdown of one or more cellular events. Multinucleation occurring during the first mitotic event is most likely due to chromosome segregation error and/or mitotic error in the first cleavage [22]. Supporting this contention is the study by Kligman et al. [115] in which more than 70% of embryos displaying multinucleation had aneuploidy when analyzed by FISH. Many studies have correlated the occurrence of multinucleation with an increased rate of aneuploidy and chromosomal abnormalities [115–118]. Multinucleation occurring in embryos while proceeding through the second and third mitotic event may be due to presence of karyokinesis without cytokinesis, accounting for about 30% of multinucleated blastomeres or due to errors in chromosome segregation or other mitotic errors [117].

Various studies have documented the occurrence of reduced in vitro development [104, 119, 120] and lower implantation rate [104, 120–123] when multinucleation is present on day 2. Coupled with day-3 morphology, multinucleation screening on day 2 has enabled the use of single-embryo transfers without any decrease in pregnancy rates compared to the use of more than one embryo and a single selection criterion [121, 123]. Van Royen et al. [112] found that the incidence of multinucleation was positively correlated with factors such as shorter than average stimulations, higher than average number of oocytes retrieved, and higher than average FSH dose for stimulation, and hence, they hypothesized that multinucleation is due to the developmental failure of the oocyte. Also, they found that there is a significant relationship between multinucleation and other negative morphological characteristics of early-cleaving embryos like fragmentation and cleavage rate, and the lowest incidence of multinucleation coincides with minimal fragmentation and optimal cleavage rate [112].

Blastomere Morphology

In human embryos, it has been proposed that the blastomeres in the 4-cell stage differ from each other: The second polar body which remains attached to the embryo until the blastocyst stage is adherent to only one cell, the progeny of which ends up on the outside of the blastocyst at the junction between the inner cell mass (ICM) and the trophectoderm and determines the embryonic axis [22]. Only one cell is capable of forming hCG at the blastocyst stage. Thus, both the tetrahedron shape of the 4-cell embryo and the need for all the cells to be intact are necessary aspects of normal embryonic development [22]. Screening for abnormal day-2 embryos, i.e., 4-cell embryos without the correct orientation, size of blastomeres, or number, is potentially simple and may eliminate embryos that have no potential for later development.

Cell Number

More than 25 years ago, Edwards et al. [124] performed intermittent evaluations of the growing human embryos to determine if they progress through preimplantation development along a predictable timeline, with 95% of them estimated to reach the 2-cell stage by 33.2 h, the 4-cell stage by 49.0 h, the 8-cell stage by 64.8 h, and the 16-cell stage 80.7 h after insemination. Data from single [108] and homogeneous double and triple embryo transfers [109] have confirmed that on day 2, 4-cell embryos, even when showing minor fragmentation, should be preferred for transfer to good-quality 2-cell embryos. Many studies have reported the existence of optimal cleavage rates, with those embryos cleaving either too quickly or too slowly being associated with compromised development [108, 109, 119]. Scott et al. [91] retrospectively considered the impact of day 2 morphometrics on developmental potential and found that when the cell number is considered at 42–44 h post-hCG, even (two and four cells) rather than uneven (three, five, and greater) cell numbers were significantly associated with positive outcome. The 2-cell embryo proceeds through an intermediate 3-cell stage before rapidly cleaving again to form a 4-cell tetrahedron embryo [125–127]. An embryo, which is an even-sized 3-cell, or a 3-cell that is not progressing fast to a 4-cell, is most likely abnormal or has cytokinetic delays [91]. In the study by Scott et al. [91], no embryo scored as 3-cell on day 2 resulted in a successful delivery. Guerif et al. [111] also found that the blastocyst formation rate was higher for 4-cell embryos on day 2 compared to faster cleaving (5–8 cells) or slower cleaving (2–3 cells) embryos. Other studies have also seconded the contention that the presence of greater than 4 cells on day 2 has a negative impact on blastocyst formation [128–130]. Two hypotheses have been suggested to explain this finding [111]: (i) Some blastomeres in these embryos might be rather large anucleate fragments [109], thus explaining the overestimation of their numbers, and (ii) accelerated division might be an indicator of developmental instabilities that would affect the embryo's ability to develop to a blastocyst. Fast developing embryos have been reported to exhibit higher levels of aneuploidy compared to synchronous embryos [131].

Cell Size and Symmetry

Blastomere size and symmetry are relevant parameters that are often underestimated. In embryos with an even number of blastomeres (i.e., 4, 6, or 8 cells) that are, however, asymmetric, the asymmetry likely arises from an uneven distribution of proteins, mRNA, and various organelles, including mitochondria, between the two sister cells. In embryos having an uneven number of blastomeres (i.e., 5 or 7 cells), the asymmetry is more likely to reflect an asynchrony of cell division than an uneven distribution of cytoplasm [88]. It must be remembered though that in normal human development, there is a degree of cleavage asynchrony [22], resulting in 3-, 5-, and 7-cell embryos. This is a normal phenomenon and allows the correct spatial arrangement of the cells in the embryo as it divides [125]. Thus, at any one point, not all cells would be of the same size. However, in an embryo, there can be only three sizes from the 3 to 8-cell stage, and any deviation from this rule will mean that the embryo is fragmented or that one blastomere has arrested [22].

Though there is a need for more studies on the impact of cell asymmetry on embryo development, a few have shown that asymmetry is associated with poor development potential of embryos [104, 123, 132], a markedly reduced implantation rate [104, 108], and a higher incidence of aneuploidy [108]. In the study by Scott et al. [91], no deliveries were recorded when transferred embryos presented with unequal cell size on day 2, regardless of day 1, 3, or 5 morphology. In another group of patients in the same study, only 12 of 132 clinical pregnancies (9%) were from the transfer of at least one embryo with uneven cell size on day 2. Hence, Scott et al. [91] have stated that cell symmetry is a highly significant scoring parameter that has biological significance and should be incorporated into any gated/sequential embryo selection system.

Blastomere cell size has been linked to fragmentation [132] where the degree of fragmentation was correlated with the extent of unevenness of blastomeres. However, the study by Scott et al. [91] did not second this finding, and uneven cell size on day 2 in their study appeared to be more inherent to the embryo and related to cleavage rather than to fragmentation.

It remains to be definitively determined whether spatial arrangement of the blastomeres bears any relationship to developmental competency of the embryos though one study failed to show any significance [133].

Fragmentation

Fragmentation in the embryo refers to the presence of extracellular cytoplasmic fragments not associated with the blastomeres per se [88]. These fragments need to be differentiated from normal *blebs* that occur transiently during cell division [92]. The etiology of fragmentation appears to be linked to abnormalities in the link between nuclear and cytoplasmic cell division [88] that may be associated with apoptosis [134, 135] or anomalies in chromosomal segregation [88]. Antczak and Van Blerkom [92] have questioned the contention that a direct association between fragmentation and apoptosis exists but speculated that fragments per se may provide a trigger for apoptosis if a certain level of developmentally important proteins is eliminated from their polarized domains. The distorted link between nuclear and cytoplasmic cell division may arise from intrinsic problems within the embryo, and/or from developmental abnormalities caused by poor culture conditions [88].

Scoring Systems for Fragmentation

Fragmentation has many phenotypes described which differ in the sizes of the fragments described, the percentage of the volume of the embryo occupied by fragments, and the distribution of this anomaly among the blastomeres [136].

Table 16.4 Classification of fragmentation

Pattern	Description	Degree	% Of fragmentation
Type 1	Minimal in volume, and fragments are associated with one blastomere	W1	0–5
Type 2	Localized fragments predominantly occupying the perivitelline space	W2	6–15
Type 3	Small, scattered fragments may be in the cleavage cavity or peripherally positioned	W3	16–25
Type 4	Large fragments distributed throughout the embryonic mass and are associated with asymmetric cells	W4	26–35
Type 5	Fragments appear neurotic, with characteristic granularity and cytoplasmic contraction within the intact blastomeres	W5	>35

From Ceyhan et al. [88], with permission

The simple scoring system for fragmentation is based on the volume of the embryo occupied by fragments (1, score 0 = 0%, score 1 = <10%, score 2 = 10–25%, score 3 = >25%) [137]. Alikani et al. [136] proposed a more detailed classification system that took into account the size and location of the fragments relative to the size and position of the nucleated cell (see Table 16.4) [88, 136].

Fragmentation in the embryo is significant as it has been observed that the rate of blastocyst formation decreases significantly with fragmentation on day 2 [111, 119, 138].

Several hypotheses have been suggested to explain the detrimental effects of fragments on embryo development [111]. Van Blerkom et al. [139] suggested that fragments might physically impede cell–cell interactions, interfering with compaction, cavitation, and blastocyst formation. In addition, ultrastructural observations of degeneration in blastomeres adjacent to fragments [140] suggest that fragments might release toxic substances and therefore damage nearby cells [136]. Alternatively, fragments might also reduce the volume of cytoplasm and deplete the embryos of essential organelles or polarized domains [92]. Heavily fragmented embryos are known to present a higher rate of chromosome abnormalities, in particular mosaicism [116, 141, 142]. In the case of moderate fragmentation, it has been suggested that more than the occurrence of fragments per se, the different temporal or spatial patterns of fragmentation have a more profound effect on embryo development [50, 92, 139]. On the other hand, certain phenotypes of minor fragmentation may disappear during in vitro culture, either by lysis or by resorption [104, 139], thereby providing for a high-quality, stage-appropriate embryo on the day of transfer. Interestingly, Alikani et al. [136] showed that microsurgical removal of small fragments can improve implantation potential of embryos by restoring spatial relationship of cells within the embryo and prevention of secondary degeneration, thus mimicking normal embryonic development in the presence of minor fragmentation. This approach to morphology improvement is controversial.

Day 3 Scoring

There have been many different day 3 scoring systems for selecting cleavage stage embryos, all of which have shown a correlation with implantation [107, 110, 143, 144]. As on day 2, cell number (representing cleavage rate), blastomere morphology and fragmentation on day 3 have been correlated with embryo developmental potential. Various studies have shown a positive correlation of the number of cells in day 3 embryos (up to 8) with implantation rates following day 3 transfer [106, 107], rate of blastocyst formation [145], and pregnancy rates [145, 146] when compared to embryos with less than eight cells. Alikani et al. [119] too found that embryos with 7–9 cells on day 3 converted to blastocysts at a significantly higher rate than day 3 embryos with <7 cells or >9 cells. Racowsky et al. [137] demonstrated that those embryos with exactly eight cells on day 3 had the highest implantation rates. They also found that embryos with more than eight cells had a significantly lower implantation rate than those with eight cells (18.1 vs. 24.9%), which may be related to an increased incidence of aneuploidy [147]. The extent of fragmentation on day 3 has been found to be closely related to both implantation following day 3 transfer [137] and also the likelihood of progressing to blastocyst formation and subsequent implantation [88]. Perinatal outcome of such pregnancies with greater than 50% fragmentation has been found to be poor [148].

Van Royen et al. [3, 123] defined a "top-quality embryo" for transfer on day 3 using the following strict criteria: combining day 2 and 3 morphology, four or five blastomeres on day 2 and at least seven blastomeres on day 3 after fertilization, absence of multinucleated blastomeres, and <20% of fragments on day 2 and day 3 after fertilization. In a prospective randomized trial using these criteria, it was found that implantation rate of 42.3% and an ongoing pregnancy rate of 38.5% were obtained for single top-quality embryo transfers as compared to 48.1 and 74%, respectively, for double top-quality embryo transfers [121]. However, the patients in the study were heavily selected: Less than 25% of patients during the time of the study had embryos of sufficient quality to have a single-embryo transfer [6]. The same group [10] conducted a retrospective analysis of single-embryo transfers using the strict top-quality criteria, and they found that the average number of embryos transferred decreased from 2.265 (in 1998) to 1.79 (in 2001), and the multiple pregnancy and twinning rates dropped from 33.6 and 29.5% (in 1998) to 18.6 and 16.3% (in 2001), respectively, while still maintaining the average ongoing pregnancy rate (33.5% per transfer).

Day 4 Scoring

Compaction and morula formation, phenomena which are best seen on day 4 of embryonic development, have been found to be useful indicators of developmental competence [149, 150]. Though compaction begins as early as the 8–16-cell stage on day 3, it is typically observed as a prelude to morula formation on day 4 [88].

The degree of compaction on day 4 has been found to be associated with implantation potential [149], and hence, it is plausible that early compaction on day 3 may also be an important positive predictor of embryonic development [88]. The day 3 score created by Desai et al. [110] included compaction as one of the parameters. Though the association of compaction with pregnancy rate was not found to be significant in the study by Desai et al. [110], Skiadas et al. [150] found that early compaction was significantly associated with implantation depending upon the degree of fragmentation: In optimal embryos on day 3 (≥8 cells and displaying <10% fragmentation), early compaction was associated with a significantly higher implantation rate as compared to embryos with ≥ fragmentation [150].

There are only two studies that have studied the impact of embryo morphology parameters on day 4 such as compaction, degree of fragmentation, and cytoplasmic vacuolization on further embryonic development [150], and both suggest that these parameters could be useful markers. A potentially informative scoring system for day 4 of embryonic development is the one suggested by Feil et al. [151]: grade 1, early blastocyst, with cavitation or compacted embryo; grade 2, grade 1 compacted morula with one or more morphological anomaly; grade 3, partially compacted embryo with vacuoles or excessive fragmentation present or embryo with eight cells or more and without any signs of compaction; and grade 4, embryos with eight cells or more, with no signs of compaction and having vacuoles or excess fragments, or embryos with less than eight cells and with no sign of compaction. In their study [151], day 4 and 5 single-embryo transfers resulted in similar ongoing pregnancy rates of 38.7 and 32.1%, respectively. More studies are needed before this day 4 grading system can be accepted as a viable option to the accepted day 5/6 scoring system of Gardner et al. [152]. Also, though D4 evaluation may be potentially valuable, generally leaving embryos undisturbed in culture on day 4 is a more standard approach, relying primarily on earlier parameters or blastocyst development.

Day 5 or 6 Scoring of the Blastocyst

The assessment of the embryo at either the pronucleate or cleavage stage can be at best considered an assessment of the oocyte, and thus, it provides limited information regarding true embryonic developmental potential. There is a strong paternal effect on development that is mainly evident after the 8-cell stage [153, 154]. Seli et al. [155] have established that a significant negative correlation exists between DNA damage in ejaculated spermatozoa and subsequent blastocyst development.

There is evidence that embryo selection on day 2 or 3 based on morphological criteria may be imprecise, resulting in transfer of embryos that are abnormal or arrest at later developmental stages [156–158]. Consequently, extended culture till blastocyst stage and day 5 or 6 scoring of the blastocyst for the selection of the best embryo may be beneficial.

The blastocyst is very dynamic and since it grows rapidly, ideally, it should be assessed and scored sequentially. At approximately 154 h after hCG or 112–114 h after insemination, the blastocyst should have a defined blastocoel, a distinct ICM protruding into the blastocoel cavity, and a ring of evenly spaced and sized trophectoderm cells [22]. Any discrepancy in this sequence of events could lead to developmental problems.

If compaction, which normally begins at the 8–16-cell stage, starts too early, it can lead to the formation of a trophoblastic vesicle, where all the cells are allocated on the outside, leaving none for the ICM [159]. As compaction progresses, refractile bodies in the cells begin to fuse in defined areas to form the blastocoel. If these vesicles form too early, there is the appearance of a paving-stone formation which has a negative impact on blastocyst formation and implantation [22]. If the blastocysts are very expanded by this stage, they may have lowered viability [160]. Also, blastocysts that have finger-like projections across the blastocoel which do not break down with time should be avoided [22].

ICM dimensions have also been found to be highly indicative of blastocyst implantation potential [161]. Richter et al. [161] found that day 5 expanded blastocysts with ICMs of >4,500 μm^2 implanted at a higher rate than those with smaller ICMs (55 vs. 31%). Day 5 expanded blastocysts with slightly oval ICMs implanted at a higher rate (58%) compared with those with either rounder ICMs (7%) or more elongated ICMs (33%). Implantation rates were highest (71%) for embryos with both optimal ICM size and shape [161].

A number of scoring systems for blastocysts have been proposed that take into account some of the above concerns and show correlations with implantation [128, 152, 162]. However, the score devised by Gardner et al. [152] is most commonly used and will be described here. It was determined in the mouse model that total cell number, ICM cell number, and glycolysis had the strongest correlation with embryo viability [6]. Blastocyst formation and hatching, however, were poorly correlated with pregnancy outcome [6]. An alphanumeric scoring system was therefore developed that takes into account three aspects of blastocyst morphology: degree of expansion, ICM development, and trophectoderm development (Fig. 16.1) [163]. In a retrospective analysis of the blastocyst score and subsequent implantation rates, it was determined that when a patient received two top-scoring blastocysts, i.e., 3AA or higher, an implantation rate of 70% was attained [152]. Conversely, when a patient received slow or low-scoring blastocysts, i.e., <3AA, the implantation rate fell to 28% [152].

Interestingly, Richter et al. [161] found that blastocyst diameter and trophectoderm cell numbers were unrelated to implantation rates. In their study, pregnancy rates were higher for day 5 transfers of optimally shaped ICMs compared with day 5 transfers of optimally sized ICMs. They have suggested that this lack of association between trophectoderm cell numbers and implantation rates casts doubts on the appropriateness of inclusion of the trophectoderm grade in the scoring system defined by Gardner et al. [152]. However, this lack of association is surprising, given that it is the trophectoderm that forms the initial connection to the uterine wall and develops into the placenta and associated tissues supporting embryonic development [161]. It may be that the sample sizes used in the study were insufficient to detect existing relationships. It is also possible that some as yet undetermined characteristic of the trophectoderm layer could be indicative of blastocyst viability and implantation potential [161].

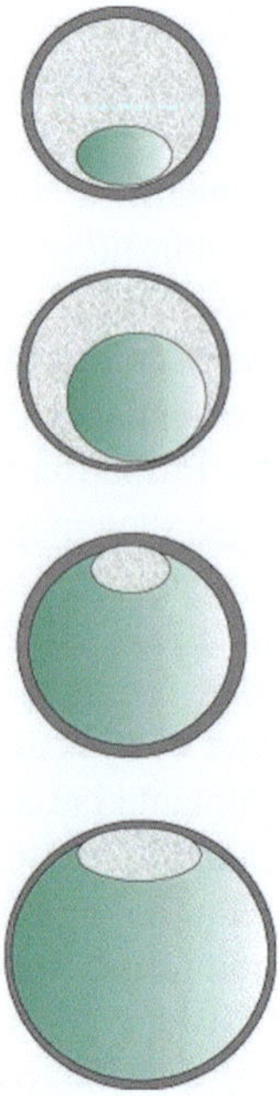

Fig. 16.1 Blastocyst scoring system used to select embryos for transfer. Initially, blastocysts are given a numerical score from 1 to 6 based upon their degree of expansion and hatching status: (1) early blastocyst, the blastocoels being less than half the volume of the embryo; (2) blastocyst, the blastocoels being greater than or equal to half of the volume of the embryo; (3) full blastocyst, the blastocoel completely fills the embryo; (4) expanded blastocyst, the blastocoel volume is now larger than that of the early embryo and the zona is thinning; (5) hatching blastocyst, the trophectoderm has started to herniated though the zona; and (6) hatched blastocyst, the blastocyst has completely escaped from the zona. The initial phase of the assessment can be performed on a stereo microscope. The second step in scoring the blastocysts should be performed on an inverted microscope. For blastocysts graded as 3–6 (i.e., full blastocysts onwards), the development of the inner cell mass (ICM) and trophectoderm can then be assessed; ICM grading: (A) tightly packed, many cells; (B) loosely grouped, several cells; (C) very few cells. Trophectoderm grading: (A) many cells forming a tightly knit epithelium, (B) few cells, and (C) very few cells forming a loose epithelium (from Gardner and Schoolcraft [163], with permission)

Sequential Multiday Scoring Systems

A concept that includes many of the above morphological factors is one that attempts to have a continuous scoring system whereby multiple multiday parameters are used to select the best embryo as opposed to a single evaluation performed shortly before transfer. The possibility of combining or integrating findings from observations at different periods of time to improve the assessment of embryo viability has been explored in many studies [111], and several numerical scoring systems have been proposed. Racowsky et al. [164] have classified these systems as follows: morphological observations and the allotment of scores [3, 108, 110, 165, 166], the

Table 16.5 Graduated embryo score of cleavage stage embryos

Evaluation	Hours after insemination	Developmental milestone	Score
1	16–18	Nucleoli aligned along pronuclear axis	20
2	25–27	Cleavage regular and symmetrical	30
		Fragmentation[a]	30
		Absent	25
		<20%	0
		>20%	
3	64–67	Cell number and grade[b] 7CI, 8CI, 8CII, 9CI	20
Total score			100

From Neuber et al. [177], with permission

[a] If the embryo was not cleaved at 25–27 h, grading of fragmentation should occur at the 64- to 67-h evaluation if the embryo reached the 7-cell stage and had <20% fragmentation

[b] Grade I = symmetrical blastomeres and absent fragmentation, grade II = slightly uneven blastomeres and <20% fragmentation, grade III = uneven blastomeres and >20% fragmentation. Grade A embryos are seven or more cells with <20% fragmentation

application of logistic regression analysis [105, 111, 167–169], class probability tree analysis [170], a case-based reasoning system [171], decision tree data mining [172], and automated pattern analysis [173].

Fisch et al. [174] proposed the graduated embryo score (GES) to evaluate parameters from the first 3 days of development (pronuclear morphology, early cleavage, and day 3 morphology) following a study using 1,245 embryos (see Table 16.5) [165, 174]. Using the GES score, they found that embryos scoring 90–100 had 64% blastocyst formation compared with 31% scoring 70–85 and with 11% scoring 30–65 [174]. In patients with at least one transferred embryo scoring ≥70, the pregnancy rate was 59% compared with 34% if all embryos scored <70. Among embryos scoring 70–100, an implantation rate of 39% was seen, compared with 24% among embryos scoring 0–65. In later studies, they further validated their score and found prospectively that transfer of one or more embryos with GES ≥ 70 predicts pregnancy and implantation rates better than a single morphological evaluation on day 3 [165]. Also, they found that day 3 transfers using GES and sHLA-G improve predictive accuracy of ART outcome, allowing single-embryo transfers, with age ≤37 years being an important qualifier [175].

Neuber et al. [176] examined morphological parameters of 1,550 individually cultured embryos, on all 5 days of development, and proposed a multistep sequential embryo assessment scoring system. Figure 16.2 shows a number of scenarios for sequential assessment predicting blastocyst development [176]. They found a significant positive relationship between early-cleaving 2-cell embryos and subsequent good-quality ≥4-cell, ≥7-cell, and blastocyst development. Combining all parameters, they found that a developing embryo showing PN symmetry with early cleavage, and subsequent good ≥4-cell and ≥7-cell cleavage, has a one in two chance of developing into a good-quality blastocyst [176]. Neuber et al. [177] later developed a computer algorithm based on the sequential assessment tool which took into account quantifiable visual characteristics of multiple stages of development,

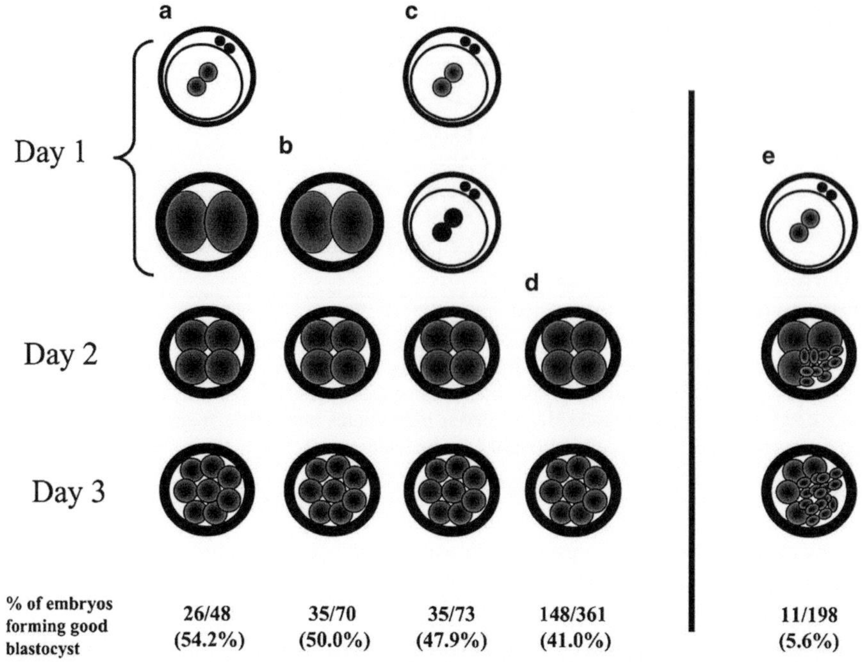

Fig. 16.2 Sequential assessment of individual embryos and their ability to reach the blastocyst stage on day 5. Percentage development to the blastocyst stage is calculated from the number of blastocysts divided by the number of embryos showing the sequential cleavage characteristics. (**a**) All embryos showing PN alignment, early cleavage, and good-quality >4- and >7-cell development. (**b**) All embryos showing early cleavage and good-quality >4- and >7-cell development. (**c**) All embryos showing PN alignment, PN breakdown, and good-quality >4- and >7-cell development. (**d**) All embryos showing good-quality >4- and >7-cell development only. (**e**) All embryos showing intact PN and poor quality >4- and >7-cell development (from Neuber et al. [177], with permission)

beginning with pronuclear alignment, the length of the first cell cycle, and cleavage stages (cell number and morphological appearance) up to day 3 of insemination.

Rienzi et al. [178] used a combined pronuclear, cleavage-stage, and day 3 scoring system to state that in a selected population of good prognosis patients, implantation potential of day 3 and day 5 embryos is equal. Using a multiple-step scoring system, Rienzi [179] later reported 77% blastocyst formation on day 5 for embryos with normal pronuclear stage and early cleavage on day 1; 4–5 cells with equal blastomere size, <10% fragmentation and no multinucleation on day 2; and >6 cells with equal blastomere size, <10% fragmentation, and no multinucleation on day 3. However, the proposed values that defined these scores were attributed quite arbitrarily since they were only based on observed frequencies [111].

Gardner and Sakkas [6] too have proposed a multiday scoring system combining morphological parameters evaluated 18–19 h (pronuclear, cytoplasm, NPB, and polar body morphology), 25–26 h (early cleavage and nuclear membrane breakdown), 42–44 h (multinucleation, cell number, and fragmentation), 66–68 h (multinucleation, cell number, and fragmentation), 94–96 h (compaction, signs of blastocoels formation), and 106–108 h (trophectoderm, ICM, and blastocoel cavity) postinsemination/ICSI. The maximum score for a perfect embryo over 5 days would be 180. This score needs to be prospectively studied for its efficacy.

Key Issues Regarding Sequential Morphological Assessment

Though the idea of sequentially assessing embryos seems promising, conflicting results exist overall, and there is currently no consensus on (1) the optimum day(s) for evaluation, (2) the optimum set of variables that should be used in a predictive model, (3) the statistical methods used for data analyses and interpretation, (4) the scoring system to be used for embryo selection, and (5) the model performance benchmarks for future comparison. Answers to these questions are necessary so that quantitative comparisons can be made about the relative efficacies of the different evaluation protocols [88, 164].

There are several concerns regarding the various morphological grading systems:

1. Most studies evaluating embryo viability using pronuclear stage [65, 66], early-cleaving 2-cell embryos [95, 99, 102], and culture until the blastocyst stage [152] have involved grouped embryos. Since the developmental fate of each embryo was not traceable to a viable implantation and there is no proof that the predicted top-quality embryo was the one that implanted out of all the embryos transferred, the conclusions made must be interpreted with caution [88].
2. Results of the various studies may be contradictory due to the multifactorial situations in which nearly all of these studies were performed, namely, the use of different culture media, stimulation protocols, and differences in timing of fertilization assessments, for example, the inclusion of early cleavage in the scoring system used [64].
3. Early development especially the pronuclear stage is very dynamic, and evaluation of early-stage embryo requires testing to be accomplished within strict time windows. In a busy laboratory, adherence to such strict timelines is difficult. Moreover, evaluations are usually accomplished during regular work hours that may not coincide with the optimal or most predictive times to evaluate an embryo.
4. A *numerical scoring system* for selection is frequently based on assignment of seemingly arbitrarily weighted values [88] without multivariate analyses or Spearman's correlation being performed [133, 178]. And hence, it is plausible that the obtained score does not precisely predict the implantation potential. Also, categorical grouping of continuous variables (e.g., fragmentation) may lead to contradictory results.
5. Most of the studies on which the scoring systems are based are retrospective with very few reporting prospective assessment with demonstrated improvement in

selection [102, 165]. Rigorous prospective testing of any specific algorithm is necessary to prove that its application does improve embryo selection [88].

6. Many studies have involved datasets involving both day 3 and day 5 transfers [91, 165], an approach likely to reduce utility of the analyses due to various confounders relating to patient selection bias, culture influences (e.g., probable improved overall quality of embryos cultured to day 5, possible loss of developmentally competent day 3 embryos not supported by extended culture conditions), and variances in uterine receptivity [88].
7. Studies based on multiple embryo transfers may introduce further confounding factors due to the possible interembryo cooperation/interaction whereby a poorer-quality embryo may either increase or decrease the likelihood of a better quality embryo implanting or, conversely, a better quality embryo may enhance the independent implantation potential of one considered of poorer quality [88, 180].
8. Precision and consistency of scoring systems among embryologists (particularly for embryos of marginal quality) within and across laboratories must be taken into consideration [88, 133] as it may reduce the accuracy of the system.
9. The potential benefits of the multiday scoring systems must be weighed against the possible detrimental effects of environmental perturbations (light exposure, temperature, pH shifts, etc.) caused due to increased time taken for conducting the strict evaluations.

Racowsky et al. [164] have called into question the need for a sequential system of assessment. They assert that logically, an embryo that shows normal development on day 3 is likely to have exhibited normal development earlier in culture [88]. They have claimed that unpublished preliminary data from their group, utilizing multivariate analysis of a dataset of single-embryo transfers of embryos cultured individually, suggest that no additional benefit is accrued from early cleavage and day 2 assessments over that obtained exclusively from evaluation on day 3. They found that there is considerable overlap in the morphological appearance of those embryos that successfully implant vs. those that fail. Guerif et al. [111] have also advocated the need to search for additional criteria, including the ability of the blastocyst to develop. They prospectively and sequentially evaluated (pronuclear morphology on day 1; early cleavage, cell number, and fragmentation rate on day 2) in 4,042 individually grown embryos and found that the combination of all four parameters allowed the prediction of blastocyst development with an area under the receiver operating characteristics curve of 0.688, which represents a fairly low prediction of embryo viability.

However, it is plausible that early developmental insults resulting in morphological defects that can be seen on day 0 or 1 may not be visually apparent when the embryo is examined on day 3 or 5 but may manifest later in the form of lowered implantation potential and reduced pregnancy rate. More stringent studies comparing sequential assessment with single assessment are required before any definitive conclusions can be made.

Summary

Selecting embryos for transfer is a large part of the *art* in assisted reproductive technology. [165]. A future in which single-embryo transfers are the norm due to legal or ethical issues is well within sight. Hence, development of a universally accepted accurate, noninvasive, easy, simple, and quick grading system to select the best possible embryo with maximum implantation potential is one of the greatest challenges in in vitro fertilization today. A significant number of human preimplantation embryos undergo deviant development in vitro, failing to follow the expected normal developmental timeline. Hence, it would appear prudent to incorporate as much information gathered at the pronuclear and cleavage stages into the final assessment as possible. This realization has prompted the hypothesis that multiple evaluations through early preimplantation development may improve selection compared with a single evaluation performed shortly before transfer. Such an evaluation would logically take into account every developmental hurdle in the preimplantation development period of the embryo, thus improving predictive accuracy. Various scoring systems, that include various different combinations of multiday evaluations, have been proposed. Most have been found to be associated with improved developmental competency of the embryo. However, consensus on most aspects of sequential analysis remains elusive, including the parameters used in the different scoring systems, optimal day(s) or time for evaluation, predictive accuracy of the various scores and intergrader consistency of evaluation, and lastly appropriate study design and statistical analysis. There are also issues regarding the reliability of the results due to inability to determine the exact developmental fate of the selected *best embryo* due to grouping of the embryos in most studies. Various metabolic methods of embryo evaluation are now proving to offer precise, objective information about the embryo. However, in the absence of alternatives, the development of a universally accepted sequential scoring system that does a multifactorial analysis of various morphological parameters at each defined hurdle of embryonic development is still an enticing proposition.

References

1. Ludwig M, Schopper B, Katalinic A, Sturm R, Al-Hasani S, Diedrich K. Experience with the elective transfer of two embryos under the conditions of the German embryo protection law: results of a retrospective data analysis of 2573 transfer cycles. Hum Reprod. 2000;15:319–24.
2. Montag M, Van der Ven H. Evaluation of pronuclear morphology as the only selection criterion for further embryo culture and transfer: results of a prospective multicentre study. Hum Reprod. 2001;16:2384–9.
3. Van Royen E, Mangelschots K, De Neubourg D, Valkenburg M, Meerssche M, Ryckaer G, Masterminds W, Gerris J. Characterization of a top quality embryo, a step towards single-embryo transfer. Hum Reprod. 1999;14:2345–9.
4. Cummins J, Breen T, Harrison K, Shwan J, Wilson L, Hennessey J. A formula for scoring human embryo growth rates in vitro fertilization: its value in predicting pregnancy and in

comparison with visual estimates of embryo quality. J In Vitro Fert Embryo Transf. 1986; 3(5):284–95.
5. Mendoza C, Ruiz-Requena E, Ortega E, Cremades N, Martinez F, Bernabeu R, Greco E, Tesarik J. Follicular fluid markers of oocyte developmental potential. Hum Reprod. 2002;17:1017–22.
6. Gardner D, Sakkas D. Assessment of embryo viability: the ability to select a single embryo for transfer—a Review. Placenta. 2003;24:S5–12.
7. Ebner T, Moser M, Sommergruber M, Tews G. Selection based on morphological assessment of oocytes and embryos at different stages of preimplantation development: a review. Hum Reprod. 2003;9:251–62.
8. Sakkas D, Gardener D. Noninvasive methods to assess embryo quality. Curr Opin Obstet Gynecol. 2005;17:283–8.
9. Johnson M, Day M. Egg timers: how is developmental time measured in the early vertebrate embryo? Bioessays. 2000;22:57–63.
10. Gerris J, De Neubourg D, Mangelschots K, Van R, Vercruyssen M, Barudy-Vasquez J, Valkenburg M, Ryckaert G. Elective single day 3 embryo transfer halves the twinning rate without decrease in the ongoing pregnancy rate of an IVF/ICSI programme. Hum Reprod. 2002;17:2626–31.
11. Wang Q, Sun Q. Evaluation of oocyte quality: morphological, cellular and molecular predictors. Reprod Fertil Dev. 2007;2007(19):1–12.
12. Sirard M, Richard F, Blondin P, Robert C. Contribution of the oocyte to embryo quality. Theriogenology. 2006;65:126–36.
13. Sirard M, Florman H, Leibfried-Rutledge M, Barnes F, Sims M, First N. Timing of nuclear progression and protein synthesis necessary for meiotic maturation of bovine oocytes. Biol Reprod. 1989;40:1257–63.
14. Kastrop P, Bevers M, Destree O, Kruip T. Protein synthesis and phosphorylation patterns of bovine oocytes maturing in vivo. Mol Reprod Dev. 1991;29:271–5.
15. Hunter A, Moor R. Stage-dependent effects of inhibiting ribonucleic acids and protein synthesis on meiotic maturation of bovine oocytes in vitro. J Dairy Sci. 1987;70:1646–51.
16. Barnes F, First N. Embryonic transcription in in vitro cultured bovine embryos. Mol Reprod Dev. 1991;29:117–23.
17. De Souza P, Caveney A, Westhusin M, Watson A. Temporal patterns of embryonic gene expression and their dependence on oogenetic factors. Theriogenology. 1998;49:115–28.
18. Sun Q, Wu G, Lai L, Park K, Cabot R, Cheong H, et al. Translocation of active mitochondria during pig oocyte maturation, fertilization and early embryo development in vitro. Reproduction. 2001;122:155–63.
19. Coticchio G, Sereni E, Serrao L, Mazzone S, Iadarola I, Borini A. What criteria for the definition of oocyte quality? Ann N Y Acad Sci. 2004;1034:132–44.
20. Combelles C, Racowsky C. Assessment and optimization of oocyte quality during assisted reproductive technology treatment. Semin Reprod Med. 2005;23:277–84.
21. Vlaisavljevic V, Kovacic B, Reljic M, Garvric L, Cizek S. Is there any benefit from the culture of a single oocyte to a blastocyst-stage embryo in unstimulated cycles. Hum Reprod. 2001;16:2279–383.
22. Scott L. The biological basis of non-invasive strategies for selection of human oocytes and embryos. Hum Reprod. 2003;9(3):237–49.
23. Lasiene K, Vitkus A, Valanciute A, Lasysy V. Morphological criteria of assessment of oocyte quality. Medicina (Kaunas). 2009;45(7):505–15.
24. Wang W, Meng L, Hackett R, Keefe D. Developmental ability of human oocytes with or without birefringent spindles imaged by Polscope before insemination. Hum Reprod. 2001;16:1464–8.
25. Blondin P, Sirard MA. Oocyte and follicular morphology as determining characteristics for developmental competence in bovine oocytes. Mol Reprod Dev. 1995;41(1):54–62.
26. Warriach HM, Chohan KR. Thickness of cumulus cell layer is a significant factor in meiotic competence of buffalo oocytes. J Vet Sci. 2004;5(3):247–51.

27. Nagano M, Katagiri S, Takahashi Y. Relationship between bovine oocyte morphology and in vitro developmental potential. Zygote. 2006;14(1):53–61.
28. Serhal P, Ranieri D, Kinis A, Marchant S, Davies M, Khadum I. Oocyte morphology predicts outcome of intracytoplasmic sperm injection. Hum Reprod. 1997;12:1267–70.
29. Balaban B, Urman B, Sertac A, Alatas C, Aksoy S, Mercan R. Oocyte morphology does not affect fertilization rate, embryo quality and implantation rate after intracytoplasmic sperm injection. Hum Reprod. 1998;13(12):3431–3.
30. Kahraman S, Yakin K, DoÈnmez E, Samli H, Bahce M, Cengiz C, Sertyel S, Samli M, Imirzalioglu N. Relationship between granular cytoplasm of oocytes and pregnancy outcome following intracytoplasmic sperm injection. Hum Reprod. 2000;15:2390–3.
31. Ebner T, Yaman C, Moser M, Sommergruber M, Feichtinger O, Tews G. Prognostic value of first polar body morphology on fertilization rate and embryo quality in intracytoplasmic sperm injection. Hum Reprod. 2000;15:427–30.
32. Ciotti P, Notarangelo L, Morselli-Labate A, Felletti V, Porcu E, Venturoli S. First polar body morphology before ICSI is not related to embryo quality or pregnancy rate. Hum Reprod. 2004;19(10):2334–9.
33. Gabrielsen A, Lindenberg S, Petersen K. The impact of the zona pellucida thickness variation of human embryos on pregnancy outcome in relation to suboptimal embryo development. A prospective randomized controlled study. Hum Reprod. 2001;16(10):2166–70.
34. De Sutter P, Dozortsev D, Qian C, Dhont M. Oocyte morphology does not correlate with fertilization rate and embryo quality after intracytoplasmic sperm injection. Hum Reprod. 1996;11:595–7.
35. Hassan-Ali H, Hisham-Saleh A, El-Gezeiry D, Baghdady I, Ismaeil I, Mandelbaum J. Perivitelline space granularity: a sign of human menopausal gonadotrophin overdose in intracytoplasmic sperm injection. Hum Reprod. 1998;13:3425–30.
36. Moon J, Hyun C, Lee S, Son W, Yoon S, Lim J. Visualization of the metaphase II meiotic spindle in living human oocytes using the Polscope enables the prediction of embryonic developmental competence after ICSI. Hum Reprod. 2003;18:817–20.
37. Rienzi L, Ubaldi F, Martinez F, Iacobelli M, Minasi MG, Ferrero S, Tesarik J, Greco E. Relationship between meiotic spindle location with regard to the polar body position and oocyte developmental potential after ICSI. Hum Reprod. 2003;18(6):1289–93.
38. Veeck L. The morphological assessment of human oocytes and early conception. In: Keel BA, Webster BW, editors. Handbook of the laboratory diagnosis and treatment of infertility. Boca Raton: CRC Press; 1990. p. 353–69.
39. Laufer N, Tarlatzis B, DeCherney A, Masters J, Haseltine F, MacLusky N, Naftoline F. Asynchrony between human cumulus-corona cell complex and oocyte maturation after human menopausal gonadotropin treatment for in vitro fertilization. Fertil Steril. 1984;42:366–72.
40. De Vos A, Van de Velde H, Joris H, Van Steirteghem A. In vitro matured metaphase-I oocytes have a lower fertilization rate but similar embryo quality as mature metaphase-II oocytes after intracytoplasmic sperm injection. Hum Reprod. 1999;14:1859–63.
41. Balakier H, Bouman D, Sojecki A, Librach C, Squire J. Morphological and cytogenetic analysis of human giant oocytes and giant embryos. Hum Reprod. 2002;17:2394–401.
42. Rosenbusch B, Schneider M, GlaÈser B, Brucker C. Cytogenetic analysis of giant oocytes and zygotes to assess their relevance for the development of digynic triploidy. Hum Reprod. 2002;17:2388–93.
43. Loutradis D, Drakakis P, Kallianidis K, Milingos S, Dendrinos S, Michalas S. Oocyte morphology correlates with embryo quality and pregnancy rate after intracytoplasmic sperm injection. Fertil Steril. 1999;72:240–4.
44. Eichenlaub-Ritter U, Schmiady H, Kentenich H, Soewarto D. Recurrent failure in polar body formation and premature chromosome condensation in oocytes from a human patient: indicators of asynchrony in nuclear and cytoplasmic maturation. Hum Reprod. 1995;9:2343–9.
45. Chui D, Pugh N, Walker S, Gregory L, Shaw R. Follicular vascularity—the predictive value of transvaginal power Doppler ultrasonography in an in-vitro fertilization programme: a preliminary study. Hum Reprod. 1997;12:191–6.

46. Van Blerkom J, Antczak M, Schrader R. The developmental potential of the human oocyte is related to the dissolved oxygen content of follicular fluid: association with vascular endothelial growth factor levels and perifollicular blood flow characteristics. Hum Reprod. 1997;12:1047–55.
47. Edwards R. The role of embryonic polarities in preimplantation growth and implantation of mammalian embryos. Hum Reprod. 2000;15 Suppl 6:1–8.
48. Xia P. Intracytoplasmic sperm injection: correlation of oocyte grade based on polar body, perivitelline space and cytoplasmic inclusions with fertilization rate and embryo quality. Hum Reprod. 1997;12:1750–5.
49. Hammah S. Oocyte and embryo quality: is their morphology a good criterion? J Gynecol Obstet Biol Reprod. 2005;34(7):5S38–41.
50. Alikani M, Palermo G, Adler A, Bertoli M, Blake M, Cohen J. Intracytoplasmic sperm injection in dysmorphic human oocytes. Zygote. 1995;3:283–8.
51. Plachot M, De Grouchy J, Junca A, Mandelbaum J, Cohen J, Salat-Baroux J. Chromosome analysis of ovocytes and human embryos collected after fertilization in vitro. A model of natural selection against aneuploidy. Rev Fr Gynecol Obstet. 1988;83(10):613–7.
52. Van Blerkom J, Henry G. Oocyte dysmorphism and aneuploidy in meiotically—mature human oocytes after ovarian stimulation. Hum Reprod. 1992;7:379–90.
53. Ebner T, Moser M, Yaman C, Feichtinger O, Hartl J, Tews G. Elective embryo transfer selected on the basis of first polar body morphology is associated with increased rates of implantation and pregnancy. Fertil Steril. 1999;72:599–603.
54. Ebner T, Moser M, Sommergruber M, Yaman C, Peger U, Tews G. First polar body morphology and blastocyst formation rate in ICSI patients. Hum Reprod. 2002;17:2415–8.
55. Navarro P, Araujo M, de Araújo C, Rocha M. Relationship between first polar body morphology before intracytoplasmic sperm injection and fertilization rate, cleavage rate, and embryo quality. Int J Gynaecol Obstet. 2009;104(3):226–9.
56. Mikkelsen A, Lindenberg S. Morphology of in-vitro matured oocytes: impact on fertility potential and embryo quality. Hum Reprod. 2001;16:1714–8.
57. Wang Q, Sun Q. Evaluation of oocyte quality: morphological, cellular and molecular predictors. Reprod Fertil Dev. 2007;2007(19):1–12.
58. Bertrand E, Van den Bergh M, Englert Y. Does zona pellucida thickness influence the fertilization rate? Hum Reprod. 1995;10(5):1189–93.
59. Shen Y, Stalf T, Mehnert C, De Santis L, Cino I, Tinneberg H, et al. Light retardance by human oocyte spindle is positively related to pronuclear score after ICSI. Reprod Biomed Online. 2006;12(6):737–51.
60. Fang C, Tang M, Li T, Peng W, Zhou C, Zhuang G, et al. Visualization of meiotic spindle and subsequent embryonic development in in vitro and in vivo matured human oocytes. J Assist Reprod Genet. 2007;24(11):495–9.
61. Battaglia D, Goodwin P, Klein N, Soules M. Influence of maternal age on meiotic spindle in oocytes from naturally cycling women. Hum Reprod. 1996;11:2217–22.
62. Rienzi L, Ubaldi F, Iacobelli M, Minasi M, Romano S, Ferrero S, Sapienza F, Baroni E, Litwicka K, Greco E. significance of metaphase II human oocyte morphology on ICSI outcome. Fertil Steril. 2008;90(5):1692–700.
63. James A. Human pronuclei as a mode of predicting viability. In: Elder K, Cohen J, editors. Human preimplantation embryo selection. London: Informa UK Ltd; 2007. p. 31–40.
64. Scott L, Smith S. The successful use of pronuclear embryo transfers the day following oocyte retrieval. Hum Reprod. 1998;13:1003–13.
65. Tesarik J, Greco E. The probability of abnormal preimplantation development can be predicted by a single static observation on pronuclear stage morphology. Hum Reprod. 1999; 14:1318–23.
66. Scott L, Alvero R, Leondires M, Miller B. The morphology of human pronuclear embryos is positively related to blastocyst development and implantation. Hum Reprod. 2000; 15:2394–403.
67. Scott L. Pronuclear scoring as a predictor of embryo development. Reprod Biomed Online. 2003;6:57–60.

68. Tesarik J, Kopecny V. Development of human male pronucleus: ultrastructure and timing. Gamete Res. 1989;24:135–49.
69. Ludwig M, Schopper B, Al-Hasani S, Diedrich K. Clinical use of a pronuclear stage score following intracytoplasmic sperm injection: impact on pregnancy rates under the conditions of the German embryo protection law. Hum Reprod. 2000;15:325–9.
70. Zollner U, Zollner KP, Hartl G, Dietl J, Steck T. The use of a detailed zygote score after IVF/ICSI to obtain good quality blastocysts: the German experience. Hum Reprod. 2002; 17:1327–33.
71. Senn A, Urmer F, Chanson A, et al. Morphological scoring of human pronuclear zygotes for prediction of pregnancy outcome. Hum Reprod. 2006;21:234–9.
72. Kahraman S, Kumtepe Y, Sertyel S, Donmez E, Benkhalifa M, Findikli N, Vanderzwalmen P. Pronuclear morphology scoring and chromosomal status of embryos in severe male infertility. Hum Reprod. 2002;17:3193–200.
73. Gianaroli L, Magli M, Ferraretti A, et al. Pronuclear morphology scoring and chromosomal status of embryos in severe male infertility. Fertil Steril. 2003;80:341–9.
74. Balaban B, Urman B, Isklar A, Alatas C, Aksoy S, Mercan R, Mumcu A, Nunhglu A. The effects of pronuclear morphology on embryo quality parameters and blastocyst transfer outcome. Hum Reprod. 2001;16:2357–61.
75. Tesarik J, Junca A, Hazout A, Aubriot F, Nathan C, Cohen-Bacrie P, Dumont-Hassan M. Embryos with high implantation potential after intracytoplasmic sperm injection can be recognized by a simple, non-invasive examination of pronuclear morphology. Hum Reprod. 2000;15:1396–9.
76. Tesarik J, Mendoza C, Greco E. Paternal effects acting during the first cell cycle of human preimplantation development after ICSI. Hum Reprod. 2002;17:184–7.
77. Wittemer C, Bettahar-Lebugle K, Ohl J, Rongieres C, Nisand I, Gerlinger P. Zygote evaluation: an efficient tool for embryo selection. Hum Reprod. 2000;15:2591–7.
78. Scott L. Embryologic strategies for overcoming recurrent ART treatment failure. Hum Fertil. 2002;5:206–14.
79. Sadowy S, Tomkin G, MunneÂ S, Ferrara-Congedo T, Cohen J. Impaired development of zygotes with uneven pronuclear size. Zygote. 1998;63:137–41.
80. Balaban B, Yakin K, Urman B, Isiklar A, Tesarik J. Pronuclear morphology predicts embryo development and chromosome constitution. Reprod Biomed Online. 2004;8(6):695–700.
81. Gamiz P, Rubio C, de los Santos M, et al. The effect of pronuclear morphology on early development and chromosomal abnormalities in cleavage-stage embryos. Hum Reprod. 2003;18:2413–9.
82. Chen C, Shen G, Horng S, Wang C, Huang H, Wang H, Soong Y. The relationship of pronuclear state morphology and chromosome status at cleavage stage. J Assist Reprod Genet. 2003;20(10):413–20.
83. Edirisinghe W, Jemmott R, Smith C, Allan J. Association of pronuclear Z score with rates of aneuploidy in in vitro-fertilised embryos. Reprod Fertil Dev. 2005;17(5):529–34.
84. Salumets A, HydeÂn-Granskog C, Suikkari A, Tiitinen A, Tuuri T. The predictive value of pronuclear morphology of zygotes in the assessment of human embryo quality. Hum Reprod. 2001;16:2177–81.
85. James A, Hennessy S, Reggio B, Wiemer K, Larsen F, Cohen J. The limited importance of pronuclear scoring of human zygotes. Hum Reprod. 2006;21(6):1599–604.
86. Jaroudi K, Al-Hassan S, Sieck U, et al. Zygote transfer on day 1 versus cleavage stage embryo transfer on day 3: a prospective randomized trial. Hum Reprod. 2004;2004(19):645–8.
87. Payne J, Raburn D, Couchman G, Price T, Jamiso M, Walmer D. Relationship between pre- embryo pronuclear morphology (zygote score) and standard day 2 or 3 embryo morphology with regard to assisted reproductive technique outcomes. Fertil Steril. 2005;84(4) :900–9.
88. Ceyhan S, Jackson K, Racowsky C. Section III: Assisted reproduction techniques. Selecting the most competent embryo (Chap. 10); Elective single-embryo transfer (Chap.11). In: Carrell D, Racowsky C, Schlegel P, Van Voorhis B, editors. Biennial review of infertility, Vol. 1. New York: Humana; 2009. p. 143–84.

89. Stalf T, Herrero J, Mehnert C, Manolopoulos K, Lenhard A, Gips H. Influence of polarization effects in ooplasma and pronuclei on embryo quality and implantation in an IVF program. J Assist Reprod Genet. 2002;19(8):355–62.
90. Nagy Z, Janssenswillen C, Janssens R, De Vos A, Staessen R, Van de Velde H, Van Steirteghem A. Timing of oocyte activation, pronucleus formation, and cleavage in humans after intracytoplasmic sperm injection (ICSI) with testicular spermatozoa and after ICSI or in vitro fertilization on sibling oocytes with ejaculated spermatozoa. Hum Reprod. 1998; 13:1606–12.
91. Scott L, Finn A, O'Leary T, McLellan S, Hill J. Morphological parameters of early cleavage—stage embryos that correlate with fetal development and delivery: prospective and applied data for increased pregnancy rates. Hum Reprod. 2007;22(1):230–40.
92. Antczak M, Van Blerkom J. Temporal and spatial aspects of fragmentation in early human embryos: possible effects on developmental competence and association with the differential elimination of regulatory proteins from polarized domains. Hum Reprod. 1999;14:429–47.
93. Bavister B. Culture of preimplantation embryos: facts and artifacts. Hum Reprod Update. 1995;1:91.
94. Sakkas D, Shoukir Y, Chardonnens D, Bianchi P, Campana A. Early cleavage of human embryos to the two-cell stage after intracytoplasmic sperm injection as an indicator of embryo viability. Hum Reprod. 1998;13:182–7.
95. Shoukir Y, Campana A, Farley T, Sakkas D. Early cleavage of in-vitro fertilized human embryos to the 2-cell stage: a novel indicator of embryo quality and viability. Hum Reprod. 1997;12:153–6.
96. Van Montfoort A, Dumoulin J, Kester A, Evers J. Early cleavage is a valuable addition to existing embryo selection parameters: a study using single embryo transfers. Hum Reprod. 2004;19:2103–8.
97. Fenwick J, Platteau P, Murdoch A, Herbert M. Time from insemination to first cleavage predicts developmental competence of human preimplantation embryos in vitro. Hum Reprod. 2002;17:407–12.
98. Edwards R, Steptoe PC, Purdy J. Establishing full term human pregnancies using cleaving embryos grown in vitro. Br J Obstet Gynecol. 1980;87:737–57.
99. Bos-Mikich A, Mattos A, Ferrari A. Early cleavage of human embryos: an effective method for predicting successful IVF/ICSI outcome. Hum Reprod. 2001;16:2658–61.
100. Lundin K, Bergh C, Hardarson T. Early embryo cleavage is a strong indicator of embryo quality in human IVF. Hum Reprod. 2001;16:2652–7.
101. Petersen C, Mauri A, Ferreira R, Baruffi R, Franco Junior J. Embryo selection by the first cleavage parameter between 25 and 27 h after ICSI. J Assist Reprod Genet. 2001;18:209–12.
102. Sakkas D, Percival G, D'Arcy Y, Sharif K, Afnan M. Assessment of early cleaving in vitro fertilized human embryos at the 2- cell stage before transfer improves embryo selection. Fertil Steril. 2001;76:1150–6.
103. Giorgetti C, Hans E, Terriou P, Salzmann J, Barry B, Chabert-Orsini V, Chinchole J, et al. Early cleavage: an additional predictor of high implantation rate following elective single embryo transfer. Reprod Biomed Online. 2007;14(1):85–91.
104. Hardarson T, Hanson C, Sjogren A, Lundin K. Human embryos with unevenly sized blastomeres have lower pregnancy and implantation rates: indications for aneuploidy and multinucleation. Hum Reprod. 2001;16:313–8.
105. Terriou P, Giorgetti C, Hans E, Salzmann J, Charles O, Cignetti L, Avon C, Roulier R. Relationship between even early cleavage and day 2 embryo score and assessment of their predictive value for pregnancy. Reprod Biomed Online. 2007;14(3):294–9.
106. Puissant F, Van Rysselberge M, Barlow P, et al. Embryo scoring as a prognostic tool in IVF treatment. Hum Reprod. 1987;2:705–8.
107. Steer C, Mills C, Tan S, Campbell S, Edwards R. The cumulative embryo score: a predictive embryo scoring technique to select the optimal number of embryos to transfer in an in-vitro fertilization and embryo transfer programme. Hum Reprod. 1992;7:117–9.

108. Giorgetti C, Terriou P, Auquier P, Hans E, Spach J, Salzmann J, Roulier R. Embryo score to predict implantation after in vitro fertilization: based on 957 single embryo transfers. Hum Reprod. 1995;10(9):2427–31.
109. Ziebe S, Petersen K, Lindenberg S, Andersen A, Gabrielsen A, Andersen A. Embryo morphology or cleavage stage: how to select the best embryos for transfer after in-vitro fertilization. Hum Reprod. 1997;10(9):2427–31.
110. Desai N, Goldstein J, Rowland D, Goldfarb J. Morphological evaluation of human embryos and derivation of an embryo quality scoring system specific for day 3 embryos: a preliminary study. Hum Reprod. 2000;15(10):2190–6.
111. Guerif F, Le Gouge A, Giraudeau B, Poindron J, Bidault R, Gasnier O, Royere D. Limited value of morphological assessment at days 1 and 2 to predict blastocyst developmental potential: a prospective study based on 4042 embryos. Hum Reprod. 2007;22:1973–81.
112. Van Royen E, Mangelschots K, Vercruyssen M, De Neubourg D, Valkenburg M, Ryckaert G, Gerris J. Multinucleation in cleavage stage embryos. Hum Reprod. 2003;18(5):1062–9.
113. Jackson K, Ginsburg E, Hornstein M, Rein M, Clarke R. Multinucleation in normally fertilized embryos is associated with an accelerated ovulation induction response and lower implantation and pregnancy rates in in vitro fertilization—embryo transfer cycles. Fertil Steril. 1998;70:60–6.
114. Staessen C, Van Steirtegham A. Genetic constitution of multinuclear blastomeres and their derivative daughter blastomeres. Hum Reprod. 1998;13:1625–31.
115. Kligman I, Benadiva C, Alikani M, Munne S. The presence of multinucleated blastomeres in human embryos is correlated with chromosomal abnormalities. Hum Reprod. 1996;11:1492–8.
116. Munne A, Cohen J. Chromosome abnormalities in human embryos. Hum Reprod Update. 1998;4:842–55.
117. Pickering S, Taylor A, Johnson M, Braude P. An analysis of multinucleated blastomere formation in human embryos. Hum Reprod. 1995;10:1912–22.
118. Laverge H, De Sutter P, Verschraegen-Spae M, De Paepe A, Dhont M. Triple colour fluorescent in-situ- hybridization for chromosomes X, Y and 1 on spare human embryos. Hum Reprod. 1997;12:1492–8.
119. Alikani M, Calderon G, Tomkin G, Garrisi G, Kokot M, Cohen J. Cleavage anomalies in early human embryos and survival after prolonged culture in-vitro. Hum Reprod. 2000;15: 2634–43.
120. Levy R, Benchaib M, Cordonier H, Souchier C, Guerin J. Laser scanning confocal imaging of abnormal arrested human preimplantation embryos. J Assist Reprod Genet. 1998;15: 485–95.
121. Gerris J, De Neubourg D, Mangelschots K, Van Royen E, Van de Meerssche M, Valkenburg M. Prevention of twin pregnancy after in-vitro fertilization or intracytoplasmic sperm injection based on strict embryo criteria: a prospective randomized clinical trial. Hum Reprod. 1999;14:2581–7.
122. Pelinck M, De Vos M, Dekens M, Van der Elst J, De Sutter P, Dhont M. Embryos cultured in vitro with multinucleated blastomeres have poor implantation potential in-vitro fertilization and intracytoplasmic sperm injection. Hum Reprod. 1998;13:960–3.
123. Van Royen E, Mangelschots K, De Neubourg D, Laureys I, Ryckaert G, Gerris J. Calculating the implantation potential of day 3 embryos in women younger than 38 years of age: a new model. Hum Reprod. 2001;16(2):326–32.
124. Edwards R, Purdy J, Steptoe P, Walters D. The growth of human preimplantation embryos in vitro. Am J Obstet Gynecol. 1981;141(4):408–16.
125. Roux C, Joanne C, Agnani G, Fromm M, Clavequin M, Bresson J. Morphometric parameters of living human in-vitro fertilized embryos: importance of the asynchronous division process. Hum Reprod. 1995;10:1201–7.
126. Hiragi T, Solter D. Mechanisms of first cleavage specification in the mouse egg: is our body plan set at day 0? Cell Cycle. 2005;4:661–4.
127. Gardner R, Davies T. An investigation of the origin and significance of bilateral symmetry of the pronuclear zygote in the mouse. Hum Reprod. 2006;21:492–502.

128. Dokras A, Sargent I, Barlow D. Human blastocyst grading: an indicator of developmental potential. Hum Reprod. 1993;8:2119–27.
129. Shapiro B, Harris D, Richter K. Predictive value of 72-hr blastomere cell number on blastocyst development and success of subsequent transfer based on the degree of blastocyst development. Fertil Steril. 2000;73:582–6.
130. Langley M, Marek D, Gardner D, Doody K, Doody K. Extended embryo culture in human assisted reproduction treatments. Hum Reprod. 2001;16(5):902–8.
131. Magli M, Gianaroli L, Munne S, Ferraretti A. Incidence of chromosomal abnormalities from a morphologically normal cohort of embryos in poor-prognosis patients. J Assist Reprod Genet. 1998;15(5):297–301.
132. Hnida C, Engenheiro E, Ziebe S. Computer-controlled, multilevel, morphometric analysis of blastomere size as biomarker of fragmentation and multinuclearity in human embryos. Hum Reprod. 2004;19:288–93.
133. Carrell D, Peterson C, Jones K, Hatasaka H, Udoff L, Cornwell C, et al. A simplified coculture system using homologous attached cumulus tissue results in improved human embryo morphology and pregnancy rates during in vitro fertilization. J Assist Reprod Genet. 1999;16(7):344–9.
134. Jurisicova A, Varmuza S, Casper R. Programmed cell death and human embryo fragmentation. Mol Hum Reprod. 1996;2(2):93–8.
135. Perez G, Tao X, Tilly J. Fragmentation and death (a.k.a. apoptosis) of ovulated oocytes. Mol Hum Reprod. 1999;5(5):414–20.
136. Alikani M, Cohen J, Tomkin G, Garrisi G, Mack C, Scott R. Human embryo fragmentation in vitro and its implications for pregnancy and implantation. Fertil Steril. 1999;71:836–42.
137. Racowsky C, Combelles C, Nureddin A, et al. Day 3 and day 5 morphological predictors of embryo viability. Reprod Biomed Online. 2003;6:323–31.
138. Hardy K, Stark J, Winston R. Maintenance of the inner cell mass in human blastocysts from fragmented embryos. Biol Reprod. 2003;68(40):1165–9.
139. Van Blerkom J, Davis P, Alexander S. A microscopic and biochemical study of fragmentation phenotypes in stage-appropriate human embryos. Hum Reprod. 2001;16:719–29.
140. Sathanathan H, Trounson A, Freeman L, Brady T. The effects of cooling human oocytes. Hum Reprod. 1988;3:968–77.
141. Plachot M, De Grouchy J, Junca A, et al. Chromosome analysis of ovocytes and human embryos collected after fertilization in vitro. A model of natural selection against aneuploidy. Rev Fr Gynecol Obstet. 1987;83(910):613–7.
142. Pellester F, Girardet A, Andreo B, Arnal F, Hueau C. Relationship between morphology and chromosomal constitution in human preimplantation embryo. Mol Reprod Dev. 1994;39(2):141–6.
143. Tan S, Royston P, Cambell S. Cumulative conception and live birth rates after in-vitro fertilization. Lancet. 1992;339:1390–4.
144. Dawson K, Conaghan J, Ostera G, Winston R, Hardy K. Delaying transfer to the third day post-insemination, to select nonarrested embryos, increases development to the fetal heart stage. Hum Reprod. 1995;10:177–82.
145. Jones GM, Trounson AO, Lolatgis N, Wood C. Factors affecting the success of human blastocyst development and pregnancy following in vitro fertilization and embryo transfer. Fertil Steril. 1998;70(6):1022–9.
146. Carillo A, Lane B, Pridham D, et al. Improved clinical outcomes for in vitro fertilization with delay of embryo transfer from 48 to 72 hours after oocyte retrieval: use of glucose and phosphate free media. Fertil Steril. 1998;69:329–34.
147. Munne A, Cohen J. Unsuitability of multinucleated human blastomeres for preimplantation genetic diagnosis. Hum Reprod. 1993;8:1120–5.
148. Ebner T, Yaman C, Moser M, Sommergruber M, PoÈ lz, W W, Tews G. Embryo fragmentation in vitro and its impact on treatment and pregnancy outcome. Fertil Steril. 2001;76:281–5.
149. Della Ragione T, Verheyen G, Papanikolaou E, Van Landuyt L, Devroey P, Van Steirteghem A. Developmental stage on day-5 and fragmentation rate on day-3 can influence the implantation

potential of top-quality blastocysts in IVF cycles with single embryo transfer. Reprod Biol Endocrinol. 2007;5:2.
150. Skiadas C, Jackson K, Racowsky C. Early compaction on day 3 may be associated with increased implantation potential. Fertil Steril. 2006;86(5):1386–91.
151. Feil D, Henshaw R, Lane M. Day 4 embryo selection is equal to Day 5 using a new embryo scoring system validated in single embryo transfers. Hum Reprod. 2008;23(7): 1505–10.
152. Gardner R. Flow of cells from polar to mural trophectoderm is polarized in the mouse blastocyst. Hum Reprod. 2000;15:694–701.
153. Janny L, Menezo Y. Evidence for a strong paternal effect on human preimplantation embryo development and blastocyst formation. Mol Reprod Dev. 1994;38:36–42.
154. Miller J, Smith T. The effect of intracytoplasmic sperm injection and semen parameters on blastocyst development in vitro. Hum Reprod. 2001;16:918–24.
155. Seli E, Gardner D, Schoolcraft W, Moffatt O, Sakkas D. The extent of nuclear DNA damage in ejaculated spermatozoa impacts on blastocyst development after IVF. Fertil Steril. 2002;78 Suppl 1:S61.
156. Rijnders P, Jansen C. The predictive value of day 3 embryo morphology regarding blastocyst formation, pregnancy and implantation rate after day 5 transfer following in-vitro fertilization or intracytoplasmic sperm injection. Hum Reprod. 1998;13:2869–73.
157. Graham J, Han T, Porter R, Levy M, Stillman R, Tucker J. Day 3 morphology is a poor predictor of blastocyst quality in extended culture. Fertil Steril. 2000;74:495–7.
158. Milki A, Hinckley MD, Gebhardt J, Dasig D, Westphal L, Behr B. Accuracy of day 3 criteria for selecting the best embryo. Fertil Steril. 2002;77:1191–5.
159. Johnson M, Ziomek C. The foundation of two distinct cell lineages within mouse morula. Cell. 1981;24:71–80.
160. Racowsky C, Jackson K, Cekleniak N, Fox J, Hornstein M, Ginsburg E. The number of eight-cell embryos is a key determinant for selecting day 3 or day 5 transfer. Fertil Steril. 2000;73:558–64.
161. Richter K, Harris D, Daneshmand S, Shapiro B. Quantitative grading of a human blastocyst: optimal inner cell mass size and shape. Fertil Steril. 2001;76(6):1157–67.
162. Balaban B, Urman B, Sertac A, Alatas C, Aksoy S, Mercan R. Blastocyst quality affects the success of blastocyst-stage embryo transfer. Fertil Steril. 2000;74:282–7.
163. Gardner D, Schoolcraft W. In-vitro culture of human blastocysts. In: Jansen R, Mortimer D, editors. Towards reproductive certainty: fertility and genetics beyond 1999. Carnforth: Parthenon Press; 1999. p. 378–88.
164. Racowsky C, Ohno-Machado L, Kim J, Biggers J. Is there an advantage in scoring early embryos on more than one day? Hum Reprod. 2009;24(9):2104–13.
165. Fisch J, Sher G, Adamowicz M, Keskintepe L. The graduated embryo score predicts the outcome of assisted reproductive technologies better then a single day 3 evaluation and achieves results associated with blastocyst transfer from day 3 embryo transfer. Fertil Steril. 2003;80(6):1352–8.
166. Sjoblom P, Menezes J, Cummins L, Mathiyalagan B, Costello M. Prediction of embryo developmental potential and pregnancy based on early stage morphological characteristics. Fertil Steril. 2006;86:848–61.
167. Terriou P, Sapin C, Gioretti C, Hans E, Spach J, Roulier R. Embryo score is a better predictor of pregnancy than the number of transferred embryos or female age. Fertil Steril. 2001;75:525–31.
168. Holte J, Berglund I, Milton K, Garello C, Gennarelli G, Revelli A, Bergh T. Construction of an evidence-based integrated morphology cleavage embryo score for implantation potential of embryos scored and transferred on day 2 after oocyte retrieval. Hum Reprod. 2007;22:548–57.
169. Vergouw C, Botros L, Roos P, Lens J, Schats R, Hompes P, Burns D, Lambalk C. Metabolomic profiling by near-infrared spectroscopy as a tool to assess embryo viability: a novel, non-invasive method for embryo selection. Hum Reprod. 2008;23:1499–504.

170. Saith R, Srinivasan A, Michie D, Sargent I. Relationships between the developmental potential of human in-vitro fertilization embryos and features describing the embryo, oocyte and follicle. Hum Reprod. 1998;4:121–34.
171. Jurisica I, Mylopoulos J, Glasgow J, Shapiro H, Casper R. Case-based reasoning in IVF: prediction and knowledge mining. Artif Intell Med. 1998;12:1–24.
172. Trimarchi J, Goodside J, Passmore L, Silberstein T, Hamel L, Gonzalez L. Comparing data mining and logistic regression for predicting IVF outcome. Fertil Steril. 2003;80:S100.
173. Patrizi G, Manna C, Moscatelli C, Nieddu L. Pattern recognition methods in human-assisted reproduction. Int Trans Oper Res. 2004;11:365–79.
174. Fisch J, Rodriguez H, Ross R, Overby G, Sher G. The Graduated Embryo Score (GES) predicts blastocyst formation and pregnancy rate from cleavage-stage embryos. Hum Reprod. 2001;16(9):1970–5.
175. Fisch J, Keskintepe L, Ginsburg M, Adamowicz M, Sher G. Graduated Embryo score and soluble human leukocyte antigen-expression improve assisted reproductive technology outcomes and suggest a basis for elective single-embryo transfer. Fertil Steril. 2006;87(4):757–63.
176. Neuber E, Rinaudo P, Trimarchi J, Sakkas D. Sequential assessment of individually cultured human embryos as an indicator of subsequent good quality blastocyst development. Hum Reprod. 2003;18:1307–12.
177. Neuber E, Mahutte N, Arici A, Sakkas D. Sequential embryo assessment investigator—driven morphological assessment at selecting a good quality blastocyst. Fertil Steril. 2006; 85(3):794–6.
178. Rienzi L, Ubaldi F, Iacobelli M, Ferrero S, Minasi M, Martinez F, Tesarik J, Greco E. Day 3 embryo transfer with combined evaluation at the pronuclear and embryo stages compares favourably with day 5 blastocyst transfer. Hum Reprod. 2002;17:1852–5.
179. Rienzi L. Significance of morphological attributes of the early embryo. Reprod Biomed Online. 2005;10:669–81.
180. Hunault C, Eijkemans M, Pieters M, te Velde E, Habbema J, Fauser B, Macklon N. A prediction model for selecting patients undergoing in vitro fertilization for selecting patients undergoing in vitro fertilization for elective single embryo transfer. Fertil Steril. 2002;77(40):725–32.

Chapter 17
Metabolomics: The *ViaMetrics-E* ™ Procedure for Assessing Embryo Viability

D. Sakkas, L. Botros, M. Henson, K. Judge, and P. Roos

Assisted Reproduction Technology

Success of ART

The treatment of infertility has been a technological challenge as far back as the fourteenth century when there are accounts of Arab peoples using artificial insemination on horses. Even in the third century AD, records show that Jewish thinkers were discussing the possibility of accidental or unintentional human insemination by artificial means. In 1978, the culmination of knowledge in the technologies associated with IVF led to the first IVF birth in the world [1]. Further improvements in the early 1980s by groups in Australia led to births after drug-induced superovulation in the mother, the world's first frozen embryo baby [2], and the first donor egg baby [3].

Utilization of assisted reproductive technologies (ART) continues to increase annually, with over 140,000 treatment cycles being initiated in the United States alone in 2008. This trend is driven by the steady improvement in ART delivery rates, the improved access to care in many areas, and the relative ineffectiveness of other treatment options. At the current time, more than 1% of all children born in the United States and Europe are from ART-related conceptions, and in Denmark, for example, the proportion of ART births out of all births is at 3.9%.

D. Sakkas, PhD (✉)
Department of Obstetrics, Gynecology and Reproductive Sciences, Yale University School of Medicine, New Haven, CT, USA
e-mail: denny.sakkas@yale.edu

L. Botros, MSc • M. Henson, PhD • K. Judge, PhD • P. Roos, PhD
Molecular Biometrics, Inc., Norwood, MA, USA

Z.P. Nagy et al. (eds.), *Clinical Embryology: A Practical Guide*,
DOI 10.1007/978-1-4614-8376-2_17,

Risks of ART Related to Multiple Embryo Transfers

The ability to induce superovulation in the mother has led to the availability of numerous embryos per treatment cycle. As a consequence, however, the success rates established through IVF are attained, in many cases, only through the simultaneous transfer of multiple embryos. For the <35 age group in 2008 in the United States, an average of 2.2 embryos per patient were transferred leading to a 41.3% delivery rate per initiated IVF cycle and an overall multiple birth rate of 35.2%. The live birth results for older age groups decrease dramatically even though more embryos are transferred. The relative risk for multiple births in the 35–40 age group, however, remains above 25% [data from www.sart.org].

The risks related to multiple gestations are well known and include preterm delivery, low birth weight, and dramatic increase in the relative risk for cerebral palsy [reviewed by [4]]. These complications lead to a higher incidence of medical, perinatal, and neonatal complications and a tenfold increase in healthcare costs compared to a singleton delivery [5]. Decreasing the prevalence of multiple gestations while maintaining or improving overall pregnancy rates remains the most significant contemporary goal of infertility research.

Toward Single Embryo Transfer

In a number of countries, including Norway, Sweden, Denmark, Belgium, and England, the dangers associated with multiple pregnancies have been allayed by legal restrictions on the number of embryos that can be transferred in a single IVF cycle. For example, in most Scandinavian countries and Belgium, the government has set a legal limit of single embryo transfer (SET) (i.e., only one embryo to be transferred per cycle) for specific patient groups, while many other European countries have restricted the number of transferred embryos to a maximum of two. In other parts of the world, where no legal restrictions exist, the onus is on the individual clinic (as well as the patient) to decrease the number of embryos transferred so that an acceptable balance can be achieved between the risks associated with multiple gestations and "acceptable" pregnancy rates. This approach has worked well in countries such as Finland and Australia which enjoy remarkably high rates of SET. Current indications are that in the future clinics in the United States and other countries, currently lacking legislation, will be compelled via legal, financial, and/or moral obligation to restrict the number of embryos transferred in order to minimize the risk of multiple gestations.

Implementing SET in the Laboratory

A major issue in limiting the number of embryos transferred is the apparent inability to accurately estimate the reproductive potential of individual embryos within a cohort of embryos. Great progress has been made using the existing selection techniques, which largely encompasses morphological evaluation, but many limitations exist. Morphological assessment has been a stalwart in the armory of the embryologist for selecting which embryo(s) to replace. Since the early years of IVF, it was noted that embryos cleaving faster and those of better morphological appearance were more likely to lead to a pregnancy [6, 7]. Morphological assessment systems have evolved over the past decade and in addition to the classical parameters of cell number and fragmentation, numerous other characteristics have been examined including pronuclear morphology, early cleavage to the 2-cell stage, top quality embryos on successive days, and various forms of sequential assessment of embryos [see reviews by [8–10]]. In addition, the ability to culture and assess blastocyst-stage embryos has also significantly improved the ability to select embryos on the basis of morphology [11].

Faced with the scenario that the worldwide IVF community, will, in the future, have to select only one or two embryos for transfer, we will be forced to make certain changes. The first may be to rely on less aggressive stimulation protocols, hence generating a lower number of eggs at collection [12, 13]. The second is to improve the selection process for defining the quality of individual embryos so that the ones we choose for transfer are more likely to implant.

Assessing the Embryo for Transfer

Noninvasive Assessment of Embryo Culture Media

Historically, it is accepted that there is a relationship between metabolic parameters and embryo viability. In 1980, Renard et al. [14] observed that day-10 cattle blastocysts which had an elevated glucose uptake developed better, both in culture and in vivo after transfer than those blastocysts with a lower glucose uptake. Subsequently, in 1987, using noninvasive microfluorescence, Gardner and Leese [15] measured glucose uptake by individual day-4 mouse blastocysts prior to transfer to recipient females. Those embryos that went to term had a significantly higher glucose uptake in culture than those embryos that failed to develop after transfer. Further animal studies by Lane and Gardner [16] showed that glycolytic rate of mouse blastocysts could be used to select embryos for transfer prospectively. Morphologically identical mouse blastocysts with equivalent diameters were identified using metabolic criteria, as "viable" prior to transfer and had a fetal development of 80%. In contrast, those embryos that exhibited an abnormal metabolic profile (compared to in vivo developed controls) developed at a rate of only 6%. Clearly, such data provide dramatic evidence that metabolic function is linked to embryo viability.

Human Embryo Studies Assessing Metabolism

A limited number of studies have been performed on nutrient uptake and the subsequent viability of the human embryo. In a retrospective analysis, Conaghan et al. [17]

observed an inverse relationship between pyruvate uptake by 2- to 8-cell embryos and subsequent pregnancy. In a study on human morulae and blastocysts of different degrees of expansion, no conclusive date was generated on the ability of nutrient consumption of utilization to predict pregnancy outcome [18]. Unfortunately, in both the above studies, the medium used to assess embryo metabolism was a simple one and was not reflective of current commercial media which are more complex in nature. In contrast, Van den Bergh et al. [19] showed that in patients who conceived following blastocyst transfer, embryos had an elevated glucose uptake and a higher oxidative rate compared to those blastocysts which failed to establish a pregnancy. Significantly, in the work of Van den Bergh et al. [19], a complete medium was used for the metabolic assessment, thereby alleviating the culture-induced metabolic stress.

Furthermore, two studies have determined the relationship between embryo nutrition and subsequent development in vitro [20, 21]. Gardner et al. [20] determined that glucose consumption on day 4 by human embryos was twice as high in those embryos that went on to form blastocysts. They also found that blastocyst quality affected glucose uptake. Poor quality blastocysts consumed significantly less glucose than top-scoring embryos. In studies on amino acid turnover by human embryos, Houghton et al. [21] determined that alanine release into the surrounding medium on day 2 and day 3 was highest in those embryos that did not form blastocysts. Brison et al. [22] have reported that changes in concentration of amino acids in the spent medium of human zygotes cultured for 24 h in an embryo culture medium containing a mixture of amino acids using high-performance liquid chromotography. They found that aspargine, glycine, and leucine were all significantly associated with clinical pregnancy and live birth.

Other Noninvasive Assessment Techniques

Other techniques have also been reported to measure metabolic parameters in culture media; however, they have yet to be tested in a clinical IVF setting. These include the self-referencing electrophysiological technique, which is a noninvasive measurement of the physiology of individual cells and monitors the movement of ions and molecules between the cell and the surrounding media [23, 24]. An alternative approach measures oxygen consumption of developing embryos using a microsensor system. Interestingly, although this technology has been shown to correlate with bovine blastocyst development, it was less successful in predicting mouse embryo development [25, 26]. The technology has yet to be assessed in a clinical IVF setting however. Recently, more emphasis has been placed on the relationship between reactive oxygen species (ROS) levels in culture media to the outcome of in vitro fertilization cycles. This idea was first introduced by Nasr-Esfahani and Johnson in 1990 as an explanation of abnormal development of mouse embryos in vitro. In the human, a recent study by Bedaiwy et al. [27] has shown that increasing levels of ROS generation in day-3 in vitro embryo culture media may have a detrimental effect on in vitro embryo growth parameters, as well as clinical pregnancy rates in IVF and ICSI cycles.

Criteria for Adopting Noninvasive Embryo Assessment in the Laboratory

The inherent ease for the laboratory to assess various morphological markers makes it the preferred assessment technique to transfer embryos. Even with the adoption of more complex forms of assessment, it will still remain as one of the main tools we have in our armory for assessment. For a new technique to be acceptable in a laboratory setting, it must satisfy a number of criteria. It should be able to:

1. Measure a difference in predicting embryo viability without damaging the embryo
2. Measure the change quickly
3. Measure the change consistently and accurately

Metabolomics

The chemical reactions of metabolism are organized into metabolic pathways, in which one chemical is transformed through a series of steps into another chemical, by a sequence of enzymes. A new and emerging technology which allows us to measure factors in embryo culture media is metabolomics. The complete array of small-molecule metabolites that are found within a biological system constitutes the metabolome and reflects its functional phenotype [28]. Metabolomics is the systematic study of this dynamic inventory of metabolites, as small molecular biomarkers representing the functional phenotype in a biological system. Using various forms of spectral and analytical approaches, metabolomics attempts to determine metabolites associated with physiologic and pathologic states [29]. Metabolic studies of embryos indicate that embryos that result in pregnancy are different in their metabolomic profile compared to embryos that do not lead to pregnancies [30].

Investigation of the metabolome of embryos, as detected in the culture media they grow in using targeted spectroscopic analysis and bioinformatics, may therefore divulge these differences. In a recent study, Seli et al. [30] established that these differences are detectable in the culture media using both Raman and near-infrared (NIR) spectroscopy. In this study, a total of 69 day-3-spent embryo culture media samples from 30 patients with known outcome (0 or 100% sustained implantation rates) were evaluated using Raman and/or NIR spectroscopy. A regression formula was developed to calculate a relative "embryo viability score"—relating to embryo reproductive potential—which correlated implantation outcome to both Raman and NIR spectral metabolomic profiles. Both Raman and NIR spectroscopic analysis of the spent culture media of embryos with proven reproductive potential demonstrated significantly higher viability scores than those that failed to implant. Interestingly, when human embryos of similar morphology are examined using the same NIR spectral profile, their viability scores vary remarkably in relation to morphology, indicating that the metabolome of embryos that look similar differ significantly. This observation is in agreement with the study of Katz-Jaffe et al. [31, 32], who revealed that the proteome of individual human blastocysts of the same grade differed between embryos, again indicating that embryo morphology is not completely linked to its physiology.

The algorithm established was subsequently used to predict the likelihood of pregnancy from blinded embryo culture media samples. When the algorithm developed was used to blindly test a subgroup of 16 day-3 embryo samples collected at a different centers and cultured using a different type of commercial media, viability scores of embryos with proven reproductive potential were significantly higher compared to embryos that failed to implant [33]. A larger analysis of SET cycles has also been undertaken whereby NIR spectral analysis of frozen day-2 and day-3 embryo culture media samples was performed blinded to outcome. Individual metabolic profiles were established from 7 μL of the samples with each measurement taking less than 1 min. Statistical analysis performed on the metabolic profiles established a viability score (as generated above) that was significantly different ($P < 0.001$) between the pregnant and nonpregnant patients. A cutoff value for predicting pregnancy was taken at >0.3. When this cutoff was used to examine embryos of excellent and good morphology that underwent SET, a significant difference was found in the establishment of pregnancy [34].

More recent data have used a semiquantitative approach to apply this technology. A series of studies have been undertaken whereby algorithms for predicting outcomes of days 2, 3, and 5 SETs have been developed and tested blindly against samples unrelated to those used to develop the algorithms. The data confirmed that as the Viability Scores™ generated by the algorithms increase the tendency for the assessed embryo to implant and display fetal cardiac activity (FCA) also increases (Fig. 17.1). Subsequent data have also shown that this pattern is independent of morphology as the ability of the Viability Score™ to relate to FCA is maintained within groups of embryos with the same morphology.

The ViaMetrics-E ™ *Procedure*

ViaMetrics-E™ is a rapid, noninvasive procedure which, when used as an adjunct to morphology, provides an objective measure of embryo viability, thereby helping clinicians and embryologists identify embryos of the highest reproductive potential. Through the use of a highly sensitive method of metabolomic analysis by NIR spectroscopy, the *ViaMetrics-E*™ procedure can be performed on-site in just minutes, requiring only a small amount of spent embryo culture media (i.e., embryo-conditioned media normally discarded after an embryo's culture period).

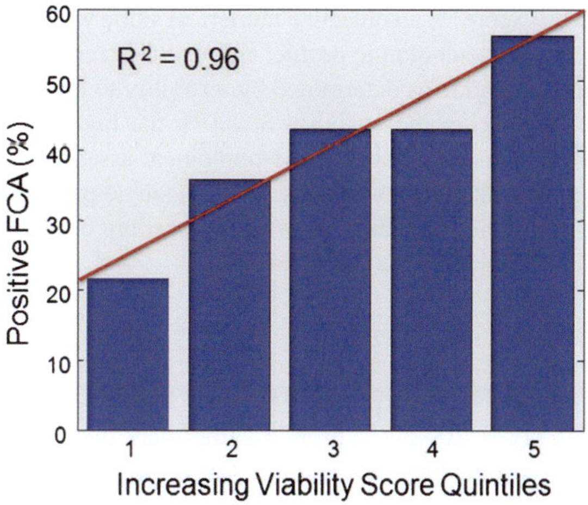

Viability Score Quintile	FCA Positive Rate (%)
1	21.4
2	35.7
3	42.9
4	42.9
5	56.3

Fig. 17.1 Prediction of positive fetal cardiac activity (FCA) in relation to increasing Viability Scores™ when blindly assessing day-5 SET media samples using a preestablished day-5 algorithm. The data analysis includes 72 SET samples from four different clinics using four different embryo culture media. Columns 1–5 contain 14, 14, 14, 15, and 15 SETs, respectively, in each column and represent the SETs with the lowest viability scores in column 1 and increasing Viability Scores™ in columns 2 through to 5, which contains the 15 highest Viability Scores™ (Molecular Biometrics Inc., unpublished data)

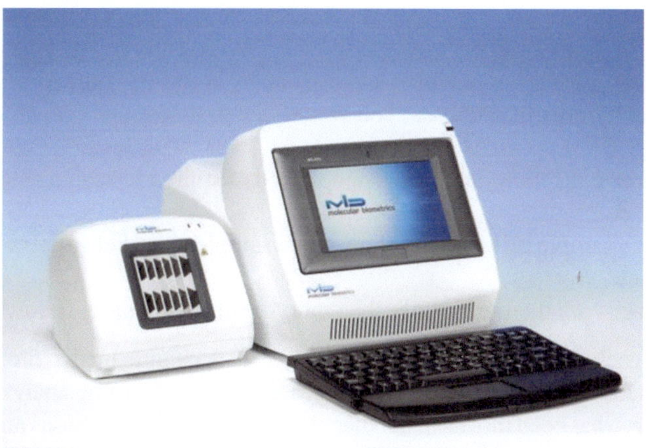

Fig. 17.2 The ViaMetrics™ instrumentation. The temperature stabilizer is on the *left*, and instrument is on the *right* (courtesy of Molecular Biometrics, ©2010 Molecular Biometrics, Inc.)

After an embryo has been removed from a culture media droplet but prior to transfer, a small volume of the spent culture media is sampled and injected into a single-use sample cell. The sample cell is then placed into the *ViaMetrics*™ instrument (Fig. 17.2), which analyzes the sample using NIR biospectroscopy-based metabolomics and proprietary bioinformatics.

The procedure reports a Viability Score™, an objective numerical value which is a quantification of the culture media's metabolomic profile, and which is representative of an embryo's reproductive potential, as determined by its ability to implant and display FCA at 12 weeks. The higher the Viability Score™, the higher the reproductive potential of the embryo. As an adjunct to morphological assessment, the Viability Score™ can be used to rank embryo viability within a single patient's cohort of embryos with similar morphology grades. The entire procedure outlined below will take approximately 15–20 min to scan five embryos.

Embryo Culture

1. Embryos are cultured individually in 20–25 μL droplets. Important note: Any commercially available embryo culture media can be used for the technique.
2. In parallel to the preparation of embryo culture droplets, prepare up to 100 μL of the same media in a separate petri dish or a test tube and place in an incubator for the same period of time as the embryo.
3. The *ViaMetrics-E*™ procedure is able to determine viability when performing days 2, 3, or 5 transfers.

To Prepare Samples for the *ViaMetrics-E* ™ Procedure

1. Perform a routine morphological assessment of the embryos on your chosen day of transfer and determine which and how many embryos you will assess.
2. Select the number of embryos, you would like to assess and prepare the sample cells (Fig. 17.3).
3. First, retrieve the total number of sample cells required to scan a single patient's cohort of embryos.
4. Label each sample cell with the appropriate sample identifier (patient ID, embryo number, etc.).
5. Sample cells are then filled with the embryo culture media as follows:
   (a) For each individually cultured embryo in a culture media droplet, collect between 10 and 14 μL of the embryo culture media to be analyzed after the embryo has been moved to another media droplet. All collections are performed with a gel-loading pipette.
   (b) Perform the media collection under a stereomicroscope. Verify that media are collected and that collection of any of the oil overlay is avoided.
   (c) Once the sample has been collected, wipe the pipette tip with an unused Kimwipe® to remove any oil residue from the outside of the pipette tip and verify that there are no bubbles in the sample.
6. Insert the gel-loading tip fully into either of the 2-cell injection ports on the side of the sample cell and slowly deposit the embryo culture media sample into the cell channel.

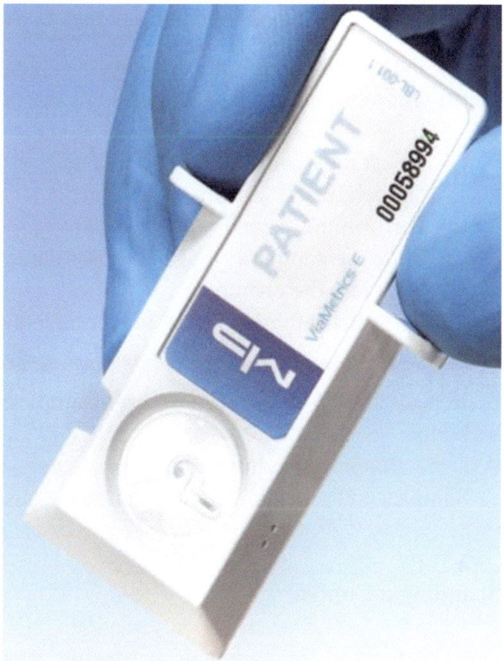

Fig. 17.3 A sample cell that is used to scan the embryo culture media and control media. There are two small injection ports on the side

7. Insert the loaded sample cell into the temperature stabilizer (Fig. 17.2) for 4 min before initiating the *ViaMetrics-E*™ procedure.
8. Repeat the above sample cell-loading procedure for each embryo within the patient's cohort.

Scanning a Sample

1. A quality control is performed daily prior to scanning samples by completing three separate scans: a dark cell scan (that blocks the light path), an empty chamber scan, and a reference standard scan.
2. Select the *ViaMetrics-E*™ button on the graphical user interface to initiate the embryo viability assessment procedure (Fig. 17.2).
3. The patient ID and the day of transfer must be entered [culture media type and droplet volume are optional data fields].
4. Retrieve a filled sample cell from the temperature stabilizer. Insert the sample cell into the cell chamber of the instrument (Fig. 17.2) and slide the door shut.
5. Select the Scan button.
6. The sample is first stabilized for 30 s to equilibrate sample temperature before scanning.

7. The sample is then scanned three times to generate three replicate spectra:
   (a) Perform the first replicate scan.
   (b) Slide the sample cell to the top of the cell chamber and then lower it again fully into the chamber.
   (c) Select the Scan Again button. (The scan will be initiated immediately as the temperature is already equilibrated.)
   (d) Perform the second replicate scan.
   (e) Slide the sample cell to the top of the cell chamber and then lower it again fully into the chamber.
   (f) Perform the third replicate, thus completing the embryo culture media scanning process.
8. Repeat steps 5–8 for each embryo sample by pressing the Scan Next Sample button.
9. Once all embryo culture media sample cells have been scanned, select No More Samples and proceed with the Control Scans.

Scanning a Control

1. The Control Scans enable a baseline to be established for each individual embryo's metabolism as the control media never contained an embryo.
2. All embryo culture media samples are now removed from each sample cell by aspiration.
3. Insert a gel-loading tip fully into the sample cell injection port and initiate the aspiration. Alternate from one injection port to the other until the sample cell is empty and dry.
4. Sample cells are then filled with the control culture media as follows:
   (a) For each individual sample cell, collect between 10 and 14 μL of the control culture media.
   (b) Insert the gel-loading tip fully into either of the 2-cell injection ports on the side of the sample cell and slowly deposit the control culture media sample into the cell channel.
   (c) Insert the loaded sample cell into the temperature stabilizer for 4 min before finalizing the *ViaMetrics-E*™ procedure.
5. Repeat the above control procedure for each sample cell within the patient's cohort.
6. Retrieve a filled control sample cell from the temperature stabilizer. Insert the sample cell into the cell chamber and slide the door shut.
7. The instrument will recognize which embryo scan to pair with the control sample cell scan as each individual sample cell is tracked with an electronic tag or radio frequency identification (RFID) tag.
8. Select the Scan button.
9. The control sample is first stabilized for 30 s to equilibrate sample temperature before scanning.

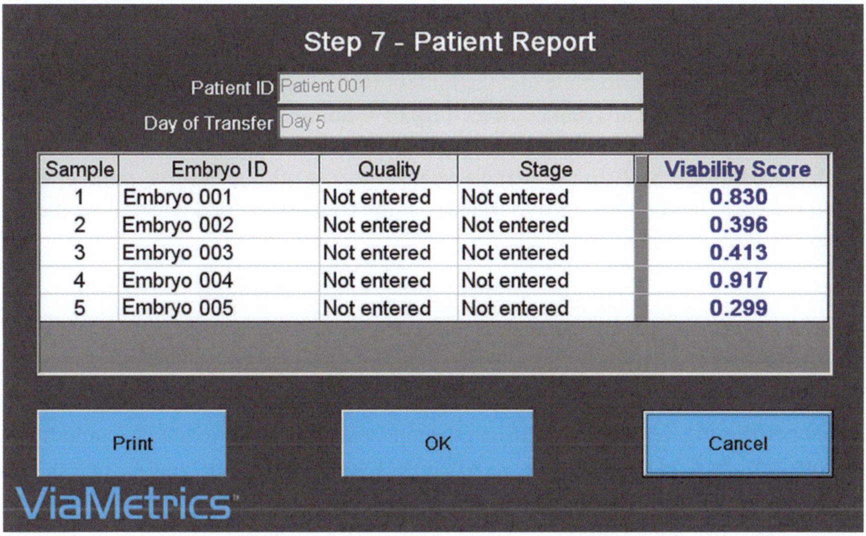

Fig. 17.4 A patient report featuring the patient ID, day of transfer, and the Viability Score™ generated for each individual embryo (Embryo ID) (courtesy of Molecular Biometrics, ©2010 Molecular Biometrics, Inc.)

10. The control sample is then scanned three times to generate three replicate spectra:
    (a) Perform the first replicate scan.
    (b) Slide the sample cell to the top of the cell chamber and then lower it again fully into the chamber.
    (c) Select the Scan Again button. (The scan will be initiated immediately as the temperature is already equilibrated.)
    (d) Perform the second replicate scan.
    (e) Slide the sample cell to the top of the cell chamber and then lower it again fully into the chamber.
    (f) Perform the third replicate scan, thus completing the control culture media scanning process.
11. After each control scan is completed, the Viability Score™ will be displayed for each embryo.
12. Repeat steps 7–12 for each control sample cell until the patient's cohort of embryos is complete.
13. Once all control scans are complete, a patient report screen (Fig. 17.4) will appear that provides information about all completed scans. The instrument provides five columns of data:
    (i) Sample number
    (ii) Embryo ID
    (iii) Embryo quality (optional data entered by user)
    (iv) Embryo stage (optional data entered by user)
    (v) *ViaMetrics-E* ™ Viability Score™

Choosing the Embryo for Transfer

1. Once all scans are complete and the Patient Report screen has been provided, the cohort of embryos are ranked according to Viability Score™. The embryo with good morphology and the highest Viability Score™ can be selected for transfer in the case of a SET. In the scenario below, this would be embryo number 004. In the case of a double embryo transfer, embryo numbers 004 and 001 would be selected for transfer.

Conclusion

When performing an embryo assessment using these new technologies, two important factors must be kept in mind. Firstly, whatever the embryo assessment technique the inherent quality of the embryo is responsible for the score or assessment characteristics. Hence, a poor embryo is not improved by these technologies; it is only assessed as having lower reproductive potential. Secondly, the values obtained by a diagnostic platform are only important for an individual patient. Therefore, it is important to be able to pick the best embryo from an individual patient's cohort; it is this assessment which can potentially improve a couple's chance of achieving a pregnancy per cycle. If the scores are overlaid onto the quintile graph of Fig. 17.1, the following scenario could be envisaged for an individual couple (Fig. 17.5).

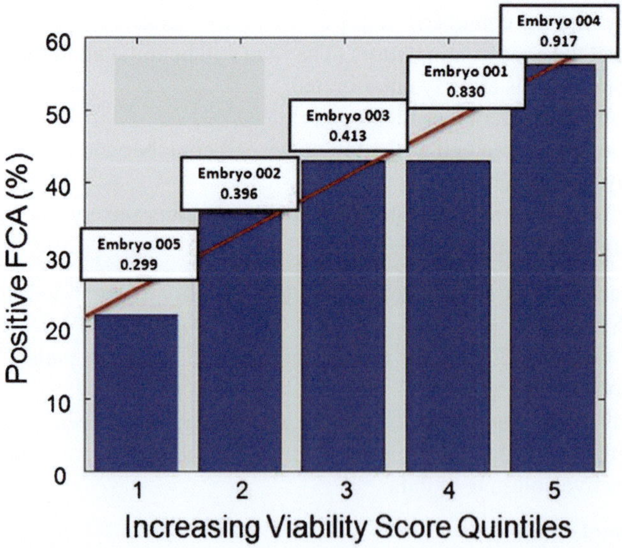

Fig. 17.5 A ranking of the cohort of five embryos displayed in the patient report above in relation to their chance of achieving a positive FCA. Embryo 004 which ranks in the highest quintile of Viability Scores™ has more than double the chance of establishing a positive FCA outcome compared to Embryo 005 which ranks in the lowest quintile

For example in the above scenario where five embryos were assessed from a cohort of equivalent morphological embryos, transferring the highest scoring embryo vs. the lowest scoring embryo could potentially improve the couples chance of achieving pregnancy by more than 20%. Therefore, if an assessment technique could help to choose embryos number 001 or 004 instead of number 005, the benefits for a couple's cycle would be significant.

In the near future, the ability to perform a metabolomic assessment, in addition to other forms of assessment, may provide both a benefit in selecting the best single embryo for transfer and also a diagnostic assessment when there are only poor embryos within a cohort.

Addendum Following a limited clinical release their was a voluntary market withdrawal of ViaMetrics-E due to an inability of the instruments to perform measurements consistently and accurately. This parameter is crucial for adopting this type of assessment in the clinical laboratory. It is hoped that an upgraded version of this technology will be released in the future.

References

1. Steptoe PC, Edwards RG. Birth after the reimplantation of a human embryo [Letter]. Lancet. 1978;2(8085):366.
2. Trounson A, Mohr L. Human pregnancy following cryopreservation, thawing and transfer of an eight-cell embryo. Nature. 1983;305:707–9.
3. Lutjen P, Trounson A, Leeton J, Findlay J, Wood C, Renou P. The establishment and maintenance of pregnancy using in vitro fertilization and embryo donation in a patient with primary ovarian failure. Nature. 1984;307:174–5.
4. Adashi EY, Barri PN, Berkowitz R, Braude P, Bryan E, Carr J, Cohen J, Collins J, Devroey P, Frydman R, Gardner D, Germond M, Gerris J, Gianaroli L, Hamberger L, Howles C, Jones Jr H, Lunenfeld B, Pope A, Reynolds M, Rosenwaks Z, Shieve LA, Serour GI, Shenfield F, Templeton A, Van Steirteghem A, Veeck L, Wennerholm UB. Infertility therapy-associated multiple pregnancies (births): an ongoing epidemic. Reprod Biomed Online. 2003;7:515–42.
5. Ledger WL, Anumba D, Marlow N, Thomas CM, Wilson EC. The costs to the NHS of multiple births after IVF treatment in the UK. BJOG. 2006;113:21–5.
6. Cummins J, Breen T, Harrison K, Shaw J, Wilson L, Hennessey J. A formula for scoring human embryo growth rates in in vitro fertilization: its value in predicting pregnancy and in comparison with visual estimates of embryo quality. J In Vitro Fert Embryo Transf. 1986;3:284–95.
7. Edwards R, Fishel S, Cohen J. Factors influencing the success of in vitro fertilization for alleviating human infertility. J In Vitro Fert Embryo Transf. 1984;1:3–23.
8. De Neubourg D, Gerris J. Single embryo transfer—state of the art. Reprod Biomed Online. 2003;7:615–22.
9. Sakkas D. Evaluation of embryo quality. London: Martin Dunitz Press; 2001.
10. Sakkas D, Gardner DK. Noninvasive methods to assess embryo quality. Curr Opin Obstet Gynecol. 2005;17:283–8.
11. Gardner DK, Surrey E, Minjarez D, Leitz A, Stevens J, Schoolcraft WB. Single blastocyst transfer: a prospective randomized trial. Fertil Steril. 2004;81:551–5.
12. Inge GB, Brinsden PR, Elder KT. Oocyte number per live birth in IVF: were Steptoe and Edwards less wasteful? Hum Reprod. 2005;20:588–92.
13. Patrizio P, Sakkas D. From oocyte to baby: a clinical evaluation of the biological efficiency of in vitro fertilization. Fertil Steril. 2009;91(4):1061–6.

14. Renard JP, Philippon A, Menezo Y. In-vitro uptake of glucose by bovine blastocysts. J Reprod Fertil. 1980;58:161–4.
15. Gardner DK, Leese HJ. Assessment of embryo viability prior to transfer by the noninvasive measurement of glucose uptake. J Exp Zool. 1987;242:103–5.
16. Lane M, Gardner DK. Selection of viable mouse blastocysts prior to transfer using a metabolic criterion. Hum Reprod. 1996;11:1975–8.
17. Conaghan J, Hardy K, Handyside AH, Winston RM, Leese HJ. Selection criteria for human embryo transfer: a comparison of pyruvate uptake and morphology. J Assist Reprod Genet. 1993;10:21–30.
18. Jones GM, Trounson A, Vella PJ, Thouas GA, Lolatgis N, Wood C. Glucose metabolism of human morula and blastocyst-stage embryos and its relationship to viability after transfer. Reprod Biomed Online. 2001;3:124–32.
19. Van den Bergh M, Devreker F, Emiliani S, Englert Y. Glycolytic activity: a possible tool for human blastocyst selection. Reprod Biomed Online. 2001;3 Suppl 1:8.
20. Gardner DK, Lane M, Stevens J, Schoolcraft WB. Noninvasive assessment of human embryo nutrient consumption as a measure of developmental potential. Fertil Steril. 2001;76: 1175–80.
21. Houghton FD, Hawkhead JA, Humpherson PG, Hogg JE, Balen AH, Rutherford AJ, Leese HJ. Non-invasive amino acid turnover predicts human embryo developmental capacity. Hum Reprod. 2002;17:999–1005.
22. Brison DR, Houghton FD, Falconer D, Roberts SA, Hawkhead J, Humpherson PG, Lieberman BA, Leese HJ. Identification of viable embryos in IVF By non-invasive measurement of amino acid turnover. Hum Reprod. 2004;19:2319–24.
23. Trimarchi JR, Liu L, Porterfield DM, Smith PJ, Keefe DL. A non-invasive method for measuring preimplantation embryo physiology. Zygote. 2000;8:15–24.
24. Trimarchi JR, Liu L, Smith PJ, Keefe DL. Noninvasive measurement of potassium efflux as an early indicator of cell death in mouse embryos. Biol Reprod. 2000;63:851–7.
25. Lopes AS, Larsen LH, Ramsing N, Lovendahl P, Raty M, Peippo J, Greve T, Callesen H. Respiration rates of individual bovine in vitro-produced embryos measured with a novel, non-invasive and highly sensitive microsensor system. Reproduction. 2005;130:669–79.
26. Ottosen LD, Hindkjaer J, Lindenberg S, Ingerslev HJ. Murine pre-embryo oxygen consumption and developmental competence. J Assist Reprod Genet. 2007;24:359–65.
27. Bedaiwy MA, Mahfouz RZ, Goldberg JM, Sharma R, Falcone T, Abdel Hafez MF, Agarwal A. Relationship of reactive oxygen species levels in day 3 culture media to the outcome of in vitro fertilization/intracytoplasmic sperm injection cycles. Fertil Steril. 2010;94(6):2037–42.
28. Oliver SG, Winson MK, Kell DB, Baganz F. Systematic functional analysis of the yeast genome. Trends Biotechnol. 1998;16:373–8.
29. Ellis DI, Goodacre R. Metabolic fingerprinting in disease diagnosis: biomedical applications of infrared and Raman spectroscopy. Analyst. 2006;131:875–85.
30. Seli E, Sakkas D, Scott R, Kwok SH, Rosendahl S, Burns DH. Non-invasive metabolomic profiling of embryo culture media using Raman and near infrared spectroscopy correlates with reproductive potential of embryos in women undergoing in vitro fertilization. Fertil Steril. 2007;88(5):1350–7.
31. Katz-Jaffe MG, Gardner DK, Schoolcraft WB. Proteomic analysis of individual human embryos to identify novel biomarkers of development and viability. Fertil Steril. 2006;85:101–7.
32. Katz-Jaffe MG, Schoolcraft WB, Gardner DK. Analysis of protein expression (secretome) by human and mouse preimplantation embryos. Fertil Steril. 2006;86:678–85.
33. Scott R, Seli E, Miller K, Sakkas D, Scott K, Burns DH. Non-Invasive metabolomic profiling of human embryo culture media using Raman spectroscopy predicts embryonic reproductive potential: a prospective blinded pilot study. Fertil Steril. 2008;90(1):77–83.
34. Seli E, Vergouw CG, Morita H, Botros L, Roos P, Lambalk CB, Yamashita N, Kato O, Sakkas D. Noninvasive metabolomic profiling as an adjunct to morphology for noninvasive embryo assessment in women undergoing single embryo transfer. Fertil Steril. 2010;94(2):535–42.

Chapter 18
Oxygen Consumption as an Indicator of Oocyte and Embryo Viability

Ana S. Lopes

Oxygen consumption has been regarded as the best indicator of overall metabolic activity [1] and as a valuable parameter for evaluating oocyte and embryo quality [2–6]. Oxygen is essential for the generation of cellular energy (ATP) in the mitochondria, via oxidative phosphorylation. In the oocyte, ATP production depends mostly on the number and activity of mitochondria present in the ooplasm, which increase exponentially with oocyte maturation during follicular growth [7, 8]. Mitochondrial number and function seem to be strongly related to developmental competence, with lower mitochondrial activity and number associated with premature arrest of the oocyte, fertilization failure and reduced embryo development [9–13]. Mitochondrial respiratory activity accounts for 30% of all the oxygen consumed by the embryo at early cleavage stages, a figure that increases to 60–70% at the blastocyst stage [14]. Thus, changes in mitochondrial activity should be directly reflected on the oxygen consumption by the developing embryo. Furthermore, oxygen is a key element of the oviductal and uterine environment, having important roles in regulating embryonic development [15–17]. Therefore, the measurement of oxygen consumption is a promising alternative or complementary approach to the assessment of oocyte and embryo viability.

Measurements of Oxygen Consumption

History

Several approaches have been used for the measurement of oxygen consumption in oocytes and preimplantation embryos. The first studies used a Cartesian diver technique to measure the oxygen consumption of rabbit ova and mouse embryos [18, 19].

A.S. Lopes, DVM, PhD (✉)
Reproductive Medicine Unit - Heilig Hart Hospital, Leuven Institute for Fertility and Embryology (LIFE), Naamsestraat 105, Leuven 3000, Belgium
e-mail: ana.lopes@lifeleuven.be

Z.P. Nagy et al. (eds.), *Clinical Embryology: A Practical Guide*,
DOI 10.1007/978-1-4614-8376-2_18, © Springer Science+Business Media New York 2013

Subsequent studies on human and mice embryos [20, 21] employed spectrophotometric methods to indirectly measure oxygen consumption, and Overström et al. [2, 22] employed a multichannel apparatus with oxygen electrodes to assess the oxygen consumption of single mouse and cattle embryos. More recently, the oxygen consumption of mouse and cattle embryos has been measured by ultramicrofluorescence [4, 23], by an automatic scanning electrode [14, 24] and by a scanning electrochemical microscopic technique [25]. However, most of the described techniques are invasive, technically challenging and time consuming or require the use of ultraviolet (UV) illumination, radioactive probes or fluorescent dyes. All of these may have toxic side effects and thus are not suitable for the assessment of embryo viability prior to transfer [26, 27]. The ideal method for measuring oxygen consumption of single embryos should be non-invasive, rapid, simple, accurate, reproducible, and capable of the measurement of oocytes and embryos at different developmental stages, all without interfering with their subsequent viability.

The Use of Oxygen Microsensors

The Nanorespirometer: Single Measurements

The Nanorespirometer (Unisense Fertilitech A/S, Aarhus, Denmark) was developed for measuring the oxygen consumption of individual oocytes/embryos at a specific time or stage of development.

Measurement principle and equipment. The production of linear steady-state oxygen gradients was considered the most fundamental requirement for calculating the oxygen-consumption rates of individual oocytes and embryos [28]. The required equipment has been previously described [27]. The measuring unit is composed of seven fused glass capillaries with a closed glass bottom attached to a Udel® polysulfone disc. It is mounted in a holder and submerged in a beaker containing culture medium, which is maintained in a semi-closed system at 38.5°C (or 37°C, depending on the species)and under a constant flow of humidified air (5% CO_2 in 20% O_2). The beaker containing the culture medium is placed in a large glass incubation chamber filled with distilled water at the right temperature to maintain stable temperature conditions during measurements.

Oxygen measurements. An individual oocyte or embryo is placed into the bottom of each glass capillary while two glass capillaries in the rosette are left empty to serve as reference measurement without respiratory activity (=control). The system is left undisturbed for 1 h until a steady-state linear oxygen gradient is established inside the glass capillaries of the measuring unit. The oxygen concentration gradient generated by the respiration of the embryo (Fig. 18.1) is subsequently determined by measuring the oxygen concentration at consecutive equidistant measurement points in the capillary with an oxygen microsensor (Clark-type oxygen microelectrode). The recordings are made by moving the tip of the microsensor down through

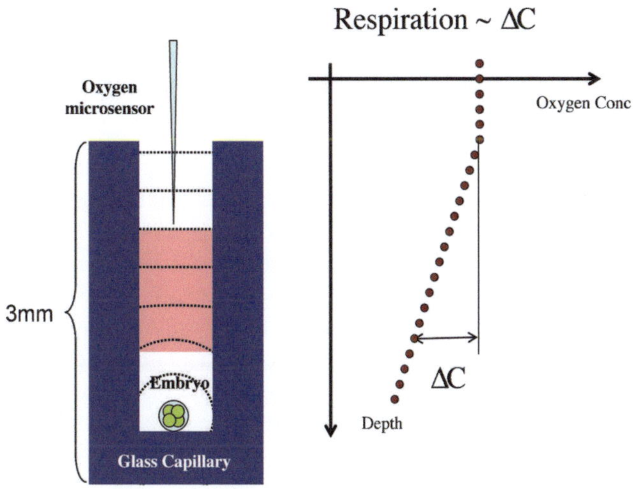

Fig. 18.1 The oxygen-consumption measuring principle. On the *left*, the schematic representation of a glass capillary of the measuring unit (inner diameter 0.68 mm, length 3 mm) with an embryo. On the *right*, an oxygen concentration gradient generated by the oxygen consumption of the embryo and determined by the oxygen microsensor, at consecutive points in the glass capillary. From the slope of the gradient, individual oxygen-consumption rates can be calculated (from Lopes et al. [60], with permission)

the media-filled glass capillary, and the oxygen-consumption rates are calculated from the slope of the linear steady-state oxygen concentration gradients measured for each oocyte or embryo (Fig. 18.1) [27].

Evaluation of the nanorespirometer. The Nanorespirometer directly measures the oxygen consumption of an individual intact oocyte or embryo, which distinguishes this approach from those described earlier [4, 24]. Additionally, the Nanorespirometer measures the overall oxygen-consumption rate of an individual embryo lying freely at the bottom of a glass capillary, overcoming the problem of heterogeneity of the blastocyst surface, encountered by Shiku et al. [25] when using the scanning electrochemical microscopy technique. The oxygen gradients resulting from the consumption of oxygen by individual embryos show nearly complete linearity, and first and second oxygen-consumption measurements of the same embryos are highly correlated, demonstrating the consistency of the results. Evaluation of pregnancy rates following transfer of measured embryos [5] was used to assess the effect of employing the Nanorespirometer on subsequent embryo viability. The results showed that pregnancy rates are similar for measured and non-measured embryos.

The EmbryoScope, Version C : Repeated Measurements

The EmbryoScope, Version C (Unisense Fertilitech) allows for repeated and automated measurements of oxygen consumption with simultaneous acquisition of digital images from individual oocytes or embryos during culture for as long as 7 days. The EmbryoScope, Version C is continuously being developed and consists of a modified version of the Nanorespirometer technology combined with time-lapse videomicrography.

Measurement principle and equipment. The measuring principle used in the EmbryoScope, Version C is similar to that described above for the Nanorespirometer. The equipment has been previously described [5, 6, 29–32]. The EmbryoScope, Version C is built inside a standard in vitro fertilization (IVF) CO_2 incubator (5% CO_2, 19% O_2) and combines a high-resolution microscope system (Leica ×20 LMPLFL objective) with an oxygen microsensor (with a laser positioning system). The microsensor is guided by computer-controlled microcontrollers that guide the alignment of the tip of the microsensor with the wells of the culture dish. The culture dish is an embryo-tested polymer slide with 12 gas-impermeable wells (depth 0.3 mm, diameter 0.7 mm), which is filled with culture medium, overlaid with mineral oil and equilibrated at the right temperature with 5% CO_2 in humidified air for 18 h.

Oxygen-consumption measurements and acquisition of digital images. Oocytes or embryos are loaded into the bottom of each well of the equilibrated culture dish, and the oxygen supply is maintained through molecular diffusion from the overlaying culture medium down through the well. As for the Nanorespirometer, two or three wells of the culture dish should contain only culture medium, in order to serve as reference measurement without respiratory activity (blank). The culture dish is inserted in the incubator 1 h before the start of the measurements so that the oxygen concentration gradient can be established. Calibration of the microsensors is always performed before the measurements as earlier described [29]. Linear oxygen concentration gradients over the oocytes or embryos are repeatedly measured by the oxygen microsensor in all wells of the slide, and calculation of individual oxygen consumption is based on the measured oxygen gradients. The final oxygen-consumption rates of individual oocytes or embryos can be obtained by subtracting the mean value of the blanks in each measurement session from the calculated oxygen-consumption rates.

During embryo development in the EmbryoScope, Version C digital images can be acquired between oxygen-consumption measurements at intervals of 20–120 min. Subsequent analysis of the images allows monitoring the individual embryo development and identifying the time of cell division on embryos that developed beyond the one-cell stage. From the analysis of the time-lapse images, an activity pattern is generated for each individual embryo.

Evaluation of the Embryoscope, Version C. The EmbryoScope™ has been validated using cattle, mouse and human embryos [6,32–34]. For all three species, the embryos reached the blastocyst stage at rates similar to those normally observed using standard in vitro culture systems. Parallel to the measurements with the EmbryoScope, Version C mouse embryos were measured by *closed respirometry*, and similar mean oxygen-consumption rates were obtained using this approach, which indicates that measurements performed with the EmbryoScope, Version C are accurate and consistent with other systems.

Oxygen Consumption of Oocytes and Embryos

Oxygen Consumption, Morphological Quality and Developmental Stage

The oxygen consumption of human oocytes appears to differ between oocytes and between patients [6, 32, 35]. Oxygen consumption of healthy-looking metaphase II (MII) oocytes on the day of retrieval (day 0) ranges from 0.4 to 0.6 nL/h [6, 20, 32, 35, 36], with fragmented and morphologically abnormal oocytes having lower and higher oxygen consumption, respectively. Correlations between oxygen consumption of human MII oocytes and subsequent fertilization and development in vitro show that higher oxygen consumption is associated with higher rates of correct fertilization (2PN formation), higher implantation rates and a slightly but not statistically significant better embryo quality at 48 and 72 h after fertilization [6, 36]. Nevertheless, the correlation between oxygen consumption, fertilization and development might not be linear, as previously suggested by Leese et al. [37], and this needs to be further investigated. The best developmental potential seems to be associated with MII oocytes with an oxygen consumption of approximately 0.5 nL/h on day of retrieval [36].

During embryo development in vitro, a similar pattern of oxygen consumption has been observed for all species studied (human, cattle and mouse embryos): at the early cleavage stages, oxygen consumption is low and constant, rising gradually at the morula stage and then increasing significantly at the expanded blastocyst stage. A two- to threefold increase between early cleavage stages and expanding blastocyst stage has been reported in the literature [4, 6, 14, 19, 23, 27, 29, 33, 34, 38] (Fig. 18.2). This increase is associated with a higher ATP demand at the time of compaction and blastulation [14, 23, 39, 40], in order to accommodate increased protein synthesis and activity of the plasma membrane Na^+/K^+-dependent ATPase [16, 23], as well as changes in mitochondria morphology and number. Thus, an increase in oxidative phosphorylation at the blastocyst stage is reflected by the oxygen consumed by the developing embryo.

In a study involving cattle embryos, correlations among morphological quality, stage of development and oxygen consumption during the 5 days of culture have revealed four distinct respiratory profiles: (a) an abrupt or gradual drop in oxygen consumption for embryos that did not develop beyond the one-cell or early cleavage stages; (b) stable oxygen consumption (range 0.3–0.4 nL/h), for embryos that do not develop beyond the one-cell or early cleavage stages; (c) a small increase in oxygen consumption for a heterogeneous group of embryos (one-cell embryos, embryos at the early cleavage and poor quality blastocysts) and (d) marked increase in oxygen consumption for high-quality expanding blastocysts, with stable rates at the early cleavage stages (approximately 0.4 nL/h) and a significant increase at the expanding blastocyst (approximately 1.2 nL/h). Two pilot studies with human embryos have revealed similar patterns, with embryos that develop to blastocysts showing oxygen-consumption rates ranging between 1.0 and 1.3 nL/h [32] (Ziebe and Lemmen, unpublished data).

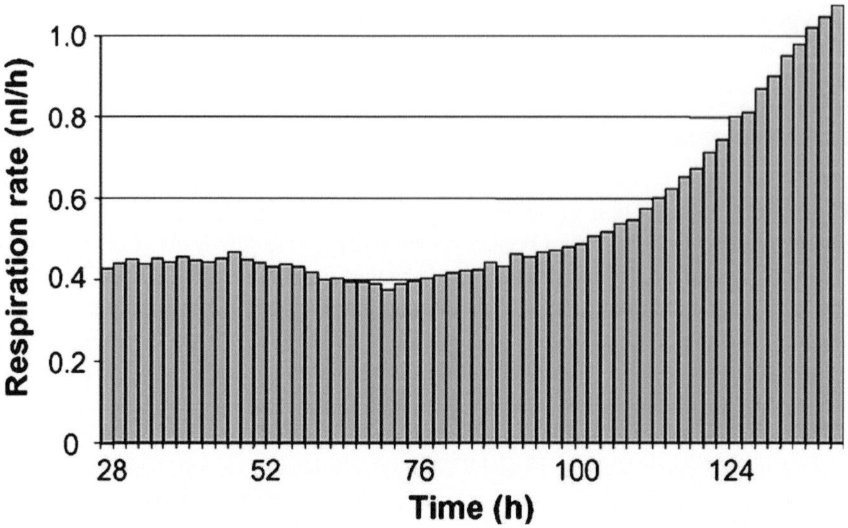

Fig. 18.2 Oxygen-consumption profile of one cattle embryo, measured repeatedly at 2-h intervals from the zygote to the expanding blastocyst stage (from Lopes et al. [60], with permission)

In mouse embryos, higher oxygen-consumption rates at each day or stage were seen in embryos that continued development to the immediately subsequent period [6, 29]. On the contrary, in human embryos a significant decrease in oxygen consumption has been observed from the time of ICSI until transfer on day 3 [29, 32, 41].

An earlier study that assessed the oxygen-consumption rates of individual cattle embryos at short intervals between fertilization and the first division provided evidence of the existence of a major peak of oxygen consumption at the time of fertilization, between 7 and 11 h after sperm penetration. Furthermore, a small respiratory peak was consistently present immediately before or at the exact time of cleavage for every presumptive zygote (Fig. 18.3) [31, 38].

The relationship between oxygen consumption and embryo morphological quality has not been consistent among studies. Some studies suggest that oxygen consumption is higher for embryos judged to be of superior quality, based on morphology [20, 25, 27, 41, 42]. Others showed no correlation between oxygen consumption and morphological evaluation [22, 32], or that blastocysts with a high oxygen consumption have reduced developmental potential [37, 43, 44]. It might be reasonable to assume that the morphologic appearance of an embryo would be linked to its metabolic activity, mainly after major activation of the embryonic genome. This assumption is supported by the fact that oxygen consumption has been correlated with cell number and function [45, 46] and the number of mitochondria [14], which have been shown to be associated with embryo quality. However, the greatest oxygen consumption might not necessarily reflect the most viable embryo. According to Leese et al. [44], less oxygen and nutrients are consumed by a viable embryo, as opposed to a

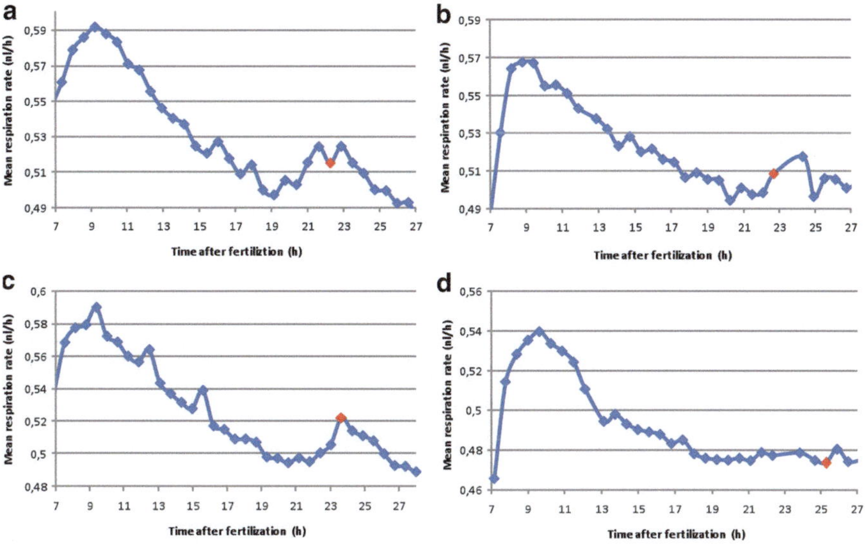

Fig. 18.3 Mean oxygen-consumption rates of cattle embryos that first cleaved at (**a**) 22, (**b**) 23, (**c**) 24 and (**d**) 25 h after IVF. Time-lapse images were acquired during the measurements with the Embryoscope, Version C at intervals of approximately 36 min and used for evaluation of developmental progress. The time of the first cleavage is indicated in each graphic by the *red symbol* (from Lopes et al. [31], with permission)

less viable embryo, that needs higher oxygen consumption to repair molecular/cellular damage in developing embryos. Very high oxygen uptake by an embryo can also result directly from damage to the mitochondria, as leakage of the inner membrane results in increased oxygen consumption, but decreased ATP production. Thus, embryos with mitochondria damage have reduced developmental potential regardless of the high oxygen consumption. Considerable variation in oxygen-consumption rates within each morphological category have also been reported [22, 25, 27], further supporting the hypothesis that measurements of the metabolism of individual oocytes or embryos provide additional and valuable information about their subsequent viability and allow for a more accurate evaluation.

Oxygen Consumption, Culture Conditions and Cryopreservation

Oxygen consumption is significantly affected by culture conditions, namely, by glucose [46], serum [47], amino acids and protein content in the culture media [43, 48] and by the oxygen concentration [49]. For instance, the presence of glucose in the culture media has been shown to significantly reduce the oxygen consumption of the embryo [46]. The oxygen consumption of cattle embryos in serum-free media is higher than that in serum-supplemented media, apparently due to a larger proportion of immature mitochondria in embryos cultured under the latter conditions [47]. Alterations in oxygen-consumption rates associated with the addition of exogenous protein to the medium are another example of how culture conditions can interfere with embryonic oxidative metabolism [48].

In vivo- and in vitro-produced embryos develop in distinctly different conditions, and thus, differences at the metabolic level would be expected. For in vivo-produced cattle embryos, oxygen consumption ranged from 0.7 to 0.9 nL/h at the blastocyst stage [5, 23]. At first sight, these rates would seem significantly lower than those observed for in vitro-produced embryos. However, when these two embryo types were measured with the Nanorespirometer, significant differences could not be detected. The discrepancy was attributed to differences in the proportion of embryos within each morphological quality and stage of development. (Day 7 in vivo-produced cattle embryos have fewer cells and are at less advanced stages of development than day 7 in vitro-produced embryos).

As far as cryopreservation is concerned, results are contradictory. Preliminary results suggest that the oxygen consumption of frozen/thawed embryos is comparable to, and follows a pattern that is similar to, that seen during in vitro development of fresh human embryos [32]. Sakagami et al. [50] observed that oxygen consumption was similar before and after vitrification, as long as the vitrification protocol would ensure a high percentage of cell survival. In contrast to these results, Yamanaka et al. [51] showed that the oxygen consumption rate of vitrified blastocysts just after warming was significantly lower than that of non-vitrified blastocysts (blastocysts derived from culture of embryos vitrified at the pronuclear stage).

Oxygen Consumption, Diameter and Sex of the Embryos

The diameter of in vitro-produced blastocysts appears to be related to oxygen consumption, with significantly larger embryos having higher oxygen-consumption rates [2, 25, 27]. Oxygen consumption does not appear to be dependent on the sex of the embryo [27, 30, 42]. Thus, it seems that sexual dimorphism does not occur at the level of oxidative phosphorylation, and oxygen consumption is mostly associated with quality rather than with the sex of the embryos.

Oxygen Consumption and Chromosomal and Genetic Background

The characterization of the expression of key genes involved in embryo metabolism can provide insight on how genetic patterns affect metabolism and thereby embryo viability. In embryos, ATP is produced by glycolysis and by oxidative phosphorylation, processes which require oxygen and glucose uptake, together with the expression and translation of *Glut1* and *G6PD*. One study showed that the expression of *Glut1* and *G6PD* was directly correlated with oxygen consumption [30], which implies that more metabolically active embryos have increased both oxygen and glucose uptake, indicating that oxidative phosphorylation and glycolysis are jointly involved in the maximization of ATP production.

The analyses of aneuploid morulae and blastocysts indicated that alterations in chromosome number were not related to oxygen-consumption rates [32].

Oxygen Consumption and Reactive Oxygen Species Production

Oxidative phosphorylation, essential for ATP production, was an evolutionary breakthrough but came at a cost with the production of reactive oxygen species (ROS). ROS can induce oxidative modifications of the cell components but, when present under physiological concentrations, they participate in normal cell processes as major factors of growth and developmental regulation [52]. Oxygen consumption and ROS were found to be increased at the time of fertilization of cattle embryos, leading to the suggestion that mitochondrial activity is stimulated by Ca^{2+} waves around the time of sperm penetration. A small peak of oxygen uptake was seen to coincide with the first cell cleavage and with increased ROS production [31]. This increase in oxygen consumption is likely associated with a higher energy requirement for the initiation of cell division and a consequence of increased mitochondrial activity. Thus, there are some specific events during embryo development that appear to be associated with a change in oxygen consumption and REDOX state, indicating that both have a role in sperm-mediated oocyte activation and cell cleavage in cattle embryos.

Oxygen Consumption, Age of the Patients and Hormonal Levels

High doses of gonadotrophins, premature LH surges and advanced age of the female patient negatively affect oocyte quality [53–57], which may consequently affect the metabolism of the matured oocyte. This has been confirmed by the lower oxygen consumption measured in human oocytes of patients with high concentrations of baseline FSH [6]. Furthermore, significantly higher oxygen consumption was measured in oocytes of younger patients, which may be related to the higher number and activity of mitochondria in these oocytes. Finally, oxygen consumption of MII oocytes seems to vary according to the type of gonadotrophin used in the stimulation protocol, (high oxygen consumption was observed in oocytes of donors stimulated with FSH, when compared to oocytes of donors stimulated with FSH + hMG or hMG alone) [36], the length of the stimulation protocol (longer stimulations combined with a lower dose of gonadotrophins are associated with higher oxygen consumption by the oocyte) [36] and serum estradiol on the day of hCG administration (higher serum estradiol was associated with less oxygen consumption) [58].

Table 18.1 Pregnancy status according to category of oxygen consumption (high vs. medium vs. low) of bovine in vivo-produced cattle embryos

Oxygen consumption	Pregnant	Non-pregnant
High (>1.10 nL/h)	25% (n = 1)	75% (n = 3)
Medium (0.78–1.10 nL/h)	100% (n = 13)	0% (n = 0)
Low (<0.78 nL/h)	48% (n = 11)	52% (n = 12)

From Lopes et al. [5], with permission

Oxygen Consumption and Viability Following Embryo Transfer

The oxygen consumption of single oocytes or embryos will only become an important evaluation parameter if a direct correlation with subsequent viability can be demonstrated. The correlation between oxygen-consumption rates and subsequent embryo viability, assessed by the pregnancy status of recipients following transfer of pre-measured embryos, has previously been investigated [5, 22, 36, 41, 59]. Overström et al. [22, 59] proposed that embryonic oxygen-consumption rates are positively related to survival rates, but blastocysts were pooled before transfer. Lopes et al. [5] detected a correlation between individual oxygen consumption and pregnancy status of the recipients following single transfer of the pre-measured embryos. Nevertheless, the mean oxygen consumption for embryos producing a pregnancy was only slightly (but not significantly) higher than that observed for embryos which did not produce a pregnancy. Instead, the authors have proposed that an optimal range of oxygen-consumption rates would be associated with a good pregnancy prognosis. It was suggested that three biologically meaningful categories may exist, with a range of oxygen-consumption rates associated with normal development and too low or too high rates related with developmental problems and reduced developmental potential (Table 18.1). Further investigations are currently being carried out using human oocytes and embryos. Preliminary data shows that higher implantation rates are observed with embryos deriving from oocytes with higher, but not greatest, oxygen-consumption rates [36]. Similarly human embryos that subsequently implanted seem to have a significantly higher oxygen consumption from the time of ICSI until transfer, when compared to embryos that did not implant [41].

Conclusions, Practical Applications and Future Perspectives

Mammalian oocytes and embryos exhibit a high degree of heterogeneity of metabolic activity and developmental capacity. The evaluation of oocyte and embryo quality is controversial, but the measurement of oxygen consumption seems to provide a feasible approach to the assessment of their developmental potential. The EmbryoScope, Version C is a high-resolution device, which provides a non-invasive, fast, accurate and consistent measurement of the oxygen consumption of individual oocytes and embryos throughout their development in culture, without affecting their subsequent viability. These characteristics make the EmbryoScope, Version C a promising tool for assessing oocyte and embryo quality. The combination of oxygen measurements and digital images acquired during embryo development have revealed the general pattern of oxygen consumption from the one-cell stage until the expanded blastocyst stage and have shown common oxygen patterns for embryos arresting during development. Furthermore, the possibility of detection of a respiratory peak at fertilization (signaling sperm-mediated oocyte activation) and at the time of the first cleavage may provide another useful approach to non-invasive evaluation of embryo quality.

The use of oxygen consumption as a diagnostic tool for selection of the most viable embryos has not yet been completely demonstrated. It is still crucial to define and confirm the association between oxygen consumption of individual oocytes and embryos and subsequent fetal development in order to be able to define the optimal oxygen-consumption range.

The oxygen consumption of oocytes and embryos seems to be only partly associated with morphology, suggesting that the embryonic oxygen consumption is a quality indicator on its own. Thus, combining oxygen consumption with morphological evaluation can provide new information on the subsequent viability of oocytes and embryos. The use of oxygen as a parameter of viability may lead to a substantial improvement in the selection of superior oocytes and embryos with higher developmental potential before transfer, which is increasingly required as elective single embryo transfer being progressively implemented worldwide.

Acknowledgment I thank Dr. Don Rieger for his critical review of the manuscript.

References

1. Leese H. What does an embryo need? Hum Fertil. 2003;6:180–5.
2. Overström EW. In vitro assessment of blastocyst differentiation. In: Bavister BD, editor. The mammalian preimplantation embryo. 1st ed. New York: Plenum Press; 1987. p. 95–116.
3. Barnett DK, Bavister BD. What is the relationship between the metabolism of preimplantation embryos and their developmental competence? Mol Reprod Dev. 1996;43:105–33.
4. Houghton FD, Thompson JG, Kennedy CJ, Leese HJ. Oxygen consumption and energy metabolism of the early mouse embryo. Mol Reprod Dev. 1996;44:476–85.
5. Lopes AS, Madsen SE, Ramsing N, Løvendahl P, Greve T, Callesen H. Respiration of individual bovine in vivo and in vitro-produced embryos: correlation with viability following transfer. Hum Reprod. 2007;22:558–66.
6. Scott L, Berntsen J, Davies D, Gundersen J, Hill J, Ramsing N. Symposium: innovative techniques in human embryo viability assessment. Human oocyte respiration-rate measurement—potential to improve oocyte and embryo selection? Reprod Biomed Online. 2008;17: 461–9.
7. Jansen RP, de Boer K. The bottleneck: mitochondrial imperatives in oogenesis and ovarian follicular fate. Mol Cell Endocrinol. 1998;145:81–8.
8. Motta PM, Nottola SA, Makabe S, Heyn R. Mitochondrial morphology in human fetal and adult female germ cells. Hum Reprod. 2000;15:129–47.
9. Dumollard R, Ward Z, Carroll J, Duchen MR. Regulation of redox metabolism in the mouse oocyte and embryo. Development. 2007;134:455–65.

10. May-Panloup P, Chretien MF, Malthiery Y, Reynier P. Mitochondrial DNA in the oocyte and the developing embryo. Curr Top Dev Biol. 2007;77:51–83.
11. Shoubridge EA, Wai T. Mitochondrial DNA and the mammalian oocyte. Curr Top Dev Biol. 2007;77:87–111.
12. Van Blerkom J. Mitochondria in human oogenesis and preimplantation embryogenesis: engines of metabolism, ionic regulation and developmental competence. Reproduction. 2004; 128:269–80.
13. Van Blerkom J. Mitochondria as regulatory forces in oocytes, preimplantation embryos and stem cells. Reprod Biomed Online. 2008;16:553–69.
14. Trimarchi JR, Liu L, Porterfield DM, Smith PJ, Keefe DL. Oxidative phosphorylation-dependent and -independent oxygen consumption by individual preimplantation mouse embryos. Biol Reprod. 2000;62:1866–74.
15. Fischer B, Bavister BD. Oxygen tension in the oviduct and uterus of rhesus monkeys, hamsters and rabbits. J Reprod Fertil. 1993; 99:673–9.
16. Leese HJ. Metabolic control during preimplantation mammalian development. Hum Reprod Update. 1995;1:63–72.
17. Harvey A. Expression of hypoxia-inducible factors during bovine preimplantation embryo development. Ph.D. Thesis, Faculty of Heath Sciences, University of Adelaide. Adelaide, Australia: The University of Adelaide Press; 2003.
18. Fridhandler I, Hafez ESE, Pincus G. Developmental changes in the respiratory activity of rabbit ova. Exp Cell Res. 1957; 13:132–9.
19. Mills RM, Brinster RL. Oxygen consumption of preimplantation mouse embryos. Exp Cell Res. 1967;47:337–44.
20. Magnusson C, Hillensjo T, Hamberger L, Nilsson L. Oxygen consumption by human oocytes and blastocysts grown in vitro. Hum Reprod. 1986;1:183–4.
21. Nilsson BO, Magnusson C, Widehn S, Hillensjo T. Correlation between blastocyst oxygen consumption and trophoblast cytochrome oxidase reaction at initiation of implantation of delayed mouse blastocysts. J Embryol Exp Morphol. 1982;71:75–82.
22. Overström EW, Duby RT, Dobrinsky J, Roche JF. Viability and oxidative metabolism of the bovine blastocyst. Theriogenology. 1992;37:269 (abstract).
23. Thompson JG, Partridge RJ, Houghton FD, Cox CI, Leese HJ. Oxygen uptake and carbohydrate metabolism by in vitro derived bovine embryos. J Reprod Fertil. 1996;106:299–306.
24. Trimarchi JR, Liu L, Porterfield DM, Smith PJ, Keefe DL. A non-invasive method for measuring preimplantation embryo physiology. Zygote. 2000;8:15–24.
25. Shiku H, Shiraishi T, Ohya H, Matsue T, Abe H, Hoshi H, Kobayashi M. Oxygen consumption of single bovine embryos probed by scanning electrochemical microscopy. Anal Chem. 2001;73:3751–8.
26. Donnay I. Metabolic markers of embryo viability. In: Van Soom A, Boerjan M, editors. Assessment of mammalian embryo quality: invasive and non-invasive techniques. 1st ed. Dordrecht, The Netherlands: Kluwer Academic Publishers; 2002. p. 57–94.
27. Lopes AS, Larsen LH, Ramsing N, Løvendahl P, Räty M, Peippo J, Greve T, Callesen H. Respiration rates of individual bovine in vitro produced embryos measured with a novel, non-invasive and rapid microsensor system. Reproduction. 2005;130:669–79.
28. Ottosen LDM. Oxygen and embryo transfer techniques. Aahrus, Denmark: Unisense; 2002.
29. Ottosen LD, Hindkjaer J, Lindenberg S, Ingerslev HJ. Murine pre-embryo oxygen consumption and developmental competence. J Assist Reprod Genet. 2007;24:359–65.
30. Lopes AS, Wrenzychi C, Ramsing N, Herrmann D, Niemann H, Løvendahl P, Greve T, Callesen H. Respiration rates correlate with mRNA expression of G6PD and GLUT1 genes in individual bovine in vitro-produced blastocysts. Theriogenology. 2007;68:223–36.
31. Lopes AS, Lane M, Thompson JG. Oxygen consumption and ROS production are increased at the time of fertilization and cell cleavage in bovine zygotes. Hum Reprod. 2010;25(11): 2762–73.
32. Scott L, Hill J, Ramsing N, Gundersen J. Respiration measurements of human oocytes and embryos: Potential for selection? In: New approaches for non-invasive embryo quality

assessment—proceedings of the ESHRE campus 2008. Tours, France: European Society of Human Reproduction and Embryology; 2008. p. 93–105.
33. Gundersen JK, Ramsing NB, Callesen H. Embryo quality assessment by respiration rate measurements and image analysis of time-lapse images during embryo development. Acta Obstet Gynecol Scand. 2006;86:119 (abstract).
34. Ramsing NB, Callesen H. Embryo quality assessment by respiration rate measurements and image analysis of time-lapse images during embryo development. J Reproduktionsmed Endokrinol. 2006;3:267 (abstract).
35. Tejera A, Herreros J, Romero P, De los Santos MJ, Remohí J, Meseguer M. Análisis de la calidad ovocitaria mediante el consumo de oxígeno; relación con fecundación, desarrollo y calidad embrionaria. Asebir. 2009;14:90 (abstract).
36. Tejera A, Herrero J, De los Santos MJ, Garrido N, Ramsing N, Meseguer M. Oxygen consumption is a quality marker for human oocyte competence conditioned by ovation stimulation regimens.Fertil Steril. 2011;96:618–23.
37. Leese HJ, Sturmey RG, Baumann CG, McEvoy TG. Embryo viability and metabolism: obeying the quiet rules. Hum Reprod. 2007;22:3047–50.
38. Callesen H, Larsen LH, Damgaard L, Gundersen JK, Lopes AS, Greve T, et al. Improved embryo selection using respirometry. Hum Reprod. 2005;20:75 (abstract).
39. Harvey AJ, Kind KL, Thompson JG. REDOX regulation of early embryo development. Reproduction. 2002;123:479–86.
40. Harvey AJ, Kind KL, Pantaleon M, Armstrong DT, Thompson JG. Oxygen-regulated gene expression in bovine blastocysts. Biol Reprod. 2004;71:1108–19.
41. Tejera A, Herrero J, Ramsing N, Garrido N, Grau N, Meseguer M. Time-dependent embryo respiration patterns from 47741 measurements in 575 human embryos showed increasing differences between implanting and non-implanting embryos. Hum Reprod. 2011;26(Suppl 1):61 (abstract).
42. Agung B, Otoi T, Abe H, Hoshi H, Murakami M, Karja NW, Murakami MK, Wongsrikeao P, Watari H, Suzuki T. Relation between oxygen consumption and sex of bovine in vitro fertilized embryos. Reprod Domest Anim. 2005;40:51–6.
43. Manser RC, Leese HJ, Houghton FD. Effect of inhibiting nitric oxide production on mouse preimplantation embryo development and metabolism. Biol Reprod. 2004;71:528–33.
44. Leese HJ, Baumann CG, Brison DR, McEvoy TG, Sturmey RG. Metabolism of the viable mammalian embryo: quietness revisited. Mol Hum Reprod. 2008;14:667–72.
45. Kaidi S, Bernard S, Lambert P, Massip A, Dessy F, Donnay I. Effect of conventional controlled-rate freezing and vitrification on morphology and metabolism of bovine blastocysts produced in vitro. Biol Reprod. 2001;65:1127–34.
46. Donnay I, Feugang JM, Bernard S, Marchandise J, Pampfer S, Moens A, Dessy F. Impact of adding 5.5 mM glucose to SOF medium on the development, metabolism and quality of in vitro produced bovine embryos from the morula to the blastocyst stage. Zygote. 2002;10:189–99.
47. Abe H, Shiku H, Aoyagi S, Matsue T, Hoshi H. Respiration activity of bovine embryos cultured in serum-free and serum-containing media. Reprod Fertil Dev. 2005;17:215 (abstract).
48. Eckert J, Pugh PA, Thompson JG, Niemann H, Tervit HR. Exogenous protein affects development competence and metabolic activity of bovine pre-implantation embryos in vitro. Reprod Fertil Dev. 1998;10:327–32.
49. Hooper K, Lane M, Gardner DK. Reduced oxygen concentration increases mouse embryo development and oxidative metabolism. Theriogenology. 2001;55:334 (abstract).
50. Sakagami N, Yamamoto T, Akiyama K, Nakazawa Y, Kojima N, Nishida K, et al. Viability of porcine embryos after vitrification using water-soluble pullulan films. J Reprod Dev. 2010;56(2):279–84.
51. Yamanaka M, Hashimoto S, Amo A, Ito-Sasaki T, Abe H, Morimoto Y. Developmental assessement of human vitrifed-warmed blastocysts based on oxygen consumption. Hum Reprod. 2011;26: 3366–71.
52. Hancock JT, Desikan R, Neill SJ. Role of reactive oxygen species in cell signalling pathways. Biochem Soc Trans. 2001; 29:345–50.

53. Navot D, Bergh PA, Williams MA, Garrisi GJ, Guzman I, Sandler B, Grunfeld L. Poor oocyte quality rather than implantation failure as a cause of age-related decline in female fertility. Lancet. 1991;337:1375–7.
54. Gordon K. Gonadotrophin-releasing hormone antagonists implications for oocyte quality and uterine receptivity. Ann N Y Acad Sci. 2001;943:49–54.
55. Baart EB, Martini E, Eijkemans MJ, Van Opstal D, Beckers NG, Verhoeff A, Macklon NS, Fauser BC. Milder ovarian stimulation for in-vitro fertilization reduces aneuploidy in the human preimplantation embryo: a randomized controlled trial. Hum Reprod. 2007;22:980–8.
56. Hazout A. Oocyte quality and ovarian reserve. J Gynecol Obstet Biol Reprod (Paris). 2006;35:2S35–6.
57. Alviggi C, Humaidan P, Howles CM, Tredway D, Hillier SG. Biological versus chronological ovarian age: implications for assisted reproductive technology. Reprod Biol Endocrinol. 2009; 7:101.
58. Tejera A, Herrero J, Ramsing N, Pellicer A, Garrido N, Garu N, De los Santos MJ, Meseguer M. Quantification of oocyte quality through respiration patterns correlates oxygen consumption with fertilization and subsequent implantation Hum Reprod. 2010; 25(Suppl 1):13–14 (abstract).
59. Overström EW, Burke PA, Hagopian SS, Selgraph JP. Blastocyst oxidative metabolism and embryo viability. J Cell Biol. 1989;107:607 (abstract).
60. Lopes AS, Greve T, Callesen H. Quantification of embryo quality by respirometry. Theriogenology. 2007;67:21–31.

Chapter 19
Gene Expression Changes During Human Early Embryo Development: New Applications for Embryo Selection

Samir Hamamah, Said Assou, Imène Boumela, and Hervé Dechaud

Early embryo development is a complex process that includes a series of important developmental events: final maturation of the oocyte, fertilization, and early preimplantation embryo development. Morphological changes during preimplantation development can be categorized into three main stages: cleavage (increase in cell number), compaction (polarization and cellular flattening), and blastulation (formation of blastocoels). After fertilization, a zygote is formed—the ultimate totipotent cell that can be seen as the most undifferentiated cell type as it gives rise to all cell types and live offspring. Totipotency persists for the very first cell doublings, from the single cell zygote to at least the 4-cell preembryo. The maternal to zygotic transition serves two important purposes: degradation of maternal RNA and protein and activation of the embryonic genome (Fig. 19.1). At morula stage, the preembryo undergoes compaction, with the loss of the cellular distinction between the blastomeres. This is followed by differentiation of the morula into a blastocyst (approximately 64 cells), composed of inner cell mass (ICM) that will give rise to

S. Hamamah, MBD, PhD (✉)
INSERM U 1040, University Hospital of Montpellier,
Arnaud de Villeneuve Hospital, 34295 Montpellier, Cedex, France

Medical School of Montpellier, University Hospital of Montpellier,
Montpellier, Cedex, France

ART/PGD Department, University Hospital of Montpellier, Montpellier, Cedex, France

Sperm Bank (CECOS), University Hospital of Montpellier, Montpellier, Cedex, France
e-mail: s-hamamah@chu-montpellier.fr

S. Assou, PhD • I. Boumela
CHU Montpellier, Institute for Research in Biotherapy, Hôpital Saint-Eloi,
80, av. Augustin Fliche, 34000 Montpellier, Cedex, France
e-mail: said.assou@inserm.fr

H. Dechaud, MD
Department of Gynecology and Obstetrics and Reproductive Medicine,
CHU Montpellier, Montpellier, Cedex, France

Z.P. Nagy et al. (eds.), *Clinical Embryology: A Practical Guide*,
DOI 10.1007/978-1-4614-8376-2_19,

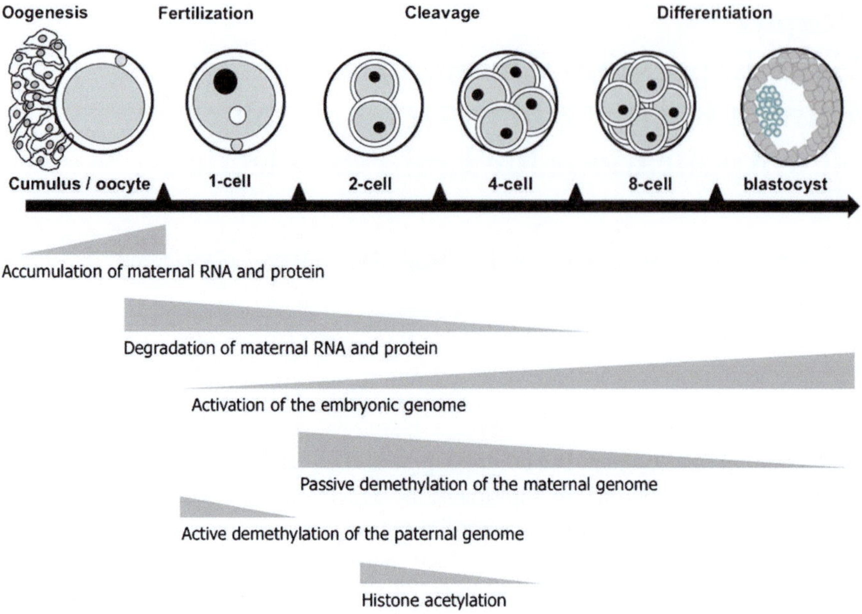

Fig. 19.1 Summary of events in human preimplantation development. Major trends of gene expression changes during early embryonic development. Morphologic transition of preimplantation human embryo and changes in the DNA modification, transcription of maternal and embryonic RNA has been shown at different stages after fertilization

an embryo proper and differentiated cell of the trophectoderm (TE) that will give rise to extra embryonic tissues. ICM contains the cells retaining pluripotency by which they are able to generate three germinal layers: ectoderm, mesoderm, and endoderm. Pluripotent cells can be isolated, adapted, and propagated indefinitely in vitro in an undifferentiated state as human embryonic stem cells (hESCs) [1, 2]. hESCs must retain pluripotency while rapidly proliferating in culture. A group of transcriptional regulatory genes are known to be critical for pluripotency such as *POU5F1/OCT4*, *NANOG*, and *SOX2* [3, 4]. hESCs are remarkable in their ability to generate virtually any cell type, hence carrying many hopes for cell therapy. These cells as well as human mature MII oocytes are both able to achieve the feat of cell reprogramming toward pluripotency, either by somatic cell nuclear transfer or by cell fusion, respectively [5–8]. Comprehending their molecular mechanisms is therefore crucial for better understanding of human development and refinement of assisted reproductive technology (ART) and for regenerative medicine. Significant efforts were made in order to understand the genes expression during the first stages of development until the blastocyst formation. The recent progress in RNA amplification methods and microarray platforms allows us to apply global gene expression profiling to the studies of the oocytes and preimplantation embryos. DNA microarray technology is a major technical breakthrough that can monitor the expression of whole genome within a single experience. This technology provides a unique tool for the determination of gene expression at the level of messenger RNA (mRNA) at a genomic scale. Microarrays have been successfully applied to the high performance expression of many thousands of genes in a single assay. Monitoring changes in gene transcription on a genome-wide basis allows identification of groups or clusters of genes that are functionally related to a cell or tissue phenotype. This technological capacity has opened new paths for biological investigation and generated a large number of applications [9], including the analysis of early embryo development transcriptomic profile.

Recently, there was an important number of reported papers relate to the use of microarrays in ART program [10–13]. The application of this technology to the analysis of early embryonic development poses specific challenges associated with the picogram levels of mRNA in a single oocyte and embryo, the plasticity of the embryonic transcriptome, the scarcity of the material, and ethical considerations. Microarrays on early embryonic development have allowed us to (1) advance our knowledge of the basic biology of oogenesis, fertilization, and preimplantation embryo development; (2) characterize the gene expression profiles of oocyte; and (3) assess the effect of various ART on global patterns of gene expression in the resulting embryos [14]. This technology also has the potential to identify key molecular biomarkers to assess the quality of oocyte and preimplantation embryo. Finally, early embryonic development offers a relatively homogeneous biological system that is well adapted to expression profiling studies. This chapter highlights the recent advances in elucidating the molecular mechanism complexity in early embryonic development. The knowledge of the global pattern of gene expression is important for understanding critical regulatory pathways that are necessary for early embryonic development. Certain gene expression profiles help to unravel the mystery of these developmental stages. Further understanding of the biological role of these genes may expand our knowledge of the oocyte maturation, fertilization, chromatin remodeling, totipotency, pluripotency, and cell reprogramming. The practical implications of compiling gene expression information on human oocytes and embryos would be enormous since it would enhance the already existing efforts to solve problems related to infertility.

Gene Expression Changes During Oocyte Maturation

Embryo development in mammalian is largely dependent on maternal stored mRNAs and proteins produced during oocyte growth phase [15]. During follicle growth, the nuclear maturation of oocytes is arrested at meiotic prophase-I. Transcriptional activity decreases as the oocyte reaches its maximal size [16]. However, the cytoplasm progresses through a series of maturational stages, accumulating mRNAs and proteins that will enable the oocyte to be fertilized and progress through the first cleavage divisions until embryonic genes begin to be expressed. For improving oocyte maturation, microarray technology permits to assess global gene expression changes of mouse and human oocytes. Therefore, differences in the global mRNA transcript profile have been reported in both mouse and human (1) between mature and immature oocytes [10, 17–20], (2) between younger and older oocytes [21–23], (3) between oocytes developed in vitro or in vivo conditions [24–26], and (4) in oocytes from polycystic ovary syndrome (PCOS) patients [27]. A global transcriptome comparison of germinal vesicle (GV)-stage and mature (MII)-stage mouse oocytes revealed that 2,000 genes were upregulated in MII-stage [17]. The authors reported a higher representation of genes associated with protein metabolism, the mitotic cell cycle, electron transport, fertilization, DNA replication, microtubule/cytoskeletal protein family, G-protein-coupled receptors, and expression signaling in mature oocytes (MII). Similarly, the genome-wide gene expression of human immature (GV and metaphase I [MI]) and mature oocytes (MII) reported minor modification of transcript profiles between GV and MI oocytes, while MII oocytes showed overexpression of more than 400 genes and a striking underexpression of more than 800 genes in comparison with the less matures oocytes [10]. Thus, major modifications of the transcript profile appear to occur during the final stage of the oocyte maturation. Components of the M-phase promoting factor, the anaphase-promoting complex, and a number of oocyte specific genes were overexpressed in MII oocytes [10]. A recent study has indicated that old age alters the expression of mouse oocyte genes involved in oxidative stress, chromatin structure, mitochondrial function, DNA methylation, and genome stability [21]. In addition, the expression profiling of young and old oocytes revealed changes in the expression of several kinetochore components of the spindle assembly checkpoint (SAC), including Cdc20: a critical activator of the anaphase-promoting complex and protein kinases (e.g., Bub1, Aurora kinase) [22]. In human, the expression of genes implicated in stress responses, cell cycle regulation, cytoskeletal structure, energy pathways, and transcription control is affected with age [23]. Recently, a substantial difference between younger and older oocyte at the transcriptional level of genes involved in establishment and organization of the meiotic spindle checkpoint, DNA repair, regulation of meiotic cycle, and cell cycle has been reported by a microarray analysis performed on individual oocytes of advanced age women [28]. Microarray technologies were applied to identify the differences between developments in vitro vs. in vivo. The differences in gene expression detected may assist in the design of optimized protocols for ovarian stimulation and in further refining media formulations for in vitro maturations (IVM). In human, Jones et al. [24] compared the transcriptome of oocytes matured in vivo (with relatively high developmental competence) with the transcriptome of oocytes under in vitro IVM conditions (with low developmental competence) and identified an overabundance of a large number of genes in oocytes matured in vitro compared with in vivo. This study suggested that the increase in gene expression detected in vitro could be due to either a deregulation in gene transcription or the posttranscriptional modification of genes, causing an inadequate temporal utilization of transcripts which could be translated as a developmental incompetence of any embryos resulting from these oocytes. Wells and Patrizio [26] elegantly differentiated the mRNA expression in human oocytes at different maturational stages under IVM. They observed that high levels of mRNAs, proteins, substrates, and nutrients are accumulated in the oocyte during maturation and are associated with oocyte developmental competence. In addition, IVM seems to alter the abundance of certain MII oocyte mRNAs compared with in vivo MII oocytes [29, 30]. Studies comparing gene expression arrays in tissues from patients with PCOS compared with normal responders have reported similar pathways for differentially expressed genes in whole ovaries [31, 32] and oocytes [27]. Wood's group identified 374 genes with different mRNA transcripts when analyzing morphologically indistinguishable oocytes from ovulatory normal women and from patients with PCOS [27]. Sixty-eight of the differentially expressed genes involved chromosome alignment and segregation; other genes contained putative androgen receptors. These differences could provide a partial explanation for the reduced fecundity observed in PCOS.

Gene Expression Changes During Embryo Development

The early stages of the embryo manifest an autonomous form of developmental resources by different products, which are provided by the oocyte and subsequent from the activation of embryo genome. Despite this autonomy, they are highly sensitive to the environment under in vitro culture condition. The culture condition can influence the gene expression pattern [33]. Comprehensive analysis of gene expression using microarray approach has recently been achieved for minute samples, such as single embryos. The insight gained from such investigations promises to revolutionize the understanding of embryo biology and to identify new molecular biomarkers of embryo quality and abnormal gene expression in embryo with reduced competence. Most studies have examined global gene expression changes in mice [18, 34–36] as well as in human embryos [14, 37–40]. Gene expression profiling of early mouse embryos showed characteristic patterns of maternal RNA depletion and revealed embryonic genome activation (EGA) [41]. Using a cDNA microarray comprised of 6,144 genes, Chen et al. [42] observed global gene expression changes during the hatching of mouse blastocysts, an essential process for implantation [42]. This study determined that 85 genes were upregulated as blastocysts at the hatching stage. These genes included cell adhesion molecules, epigenetic regulators, stress response regulators, and immunoresponse regulators. Dobson et al. [40] studied the global patterns of gene expression in eight human embryos on days 2 and 3 by using DNA microarray analysis. This study revealed that the first few days of embryo development and oocyte maturation were characterized by a significant decrease in transcript levels, suggesting that decay of RNAs associated with gamete identity is integral to embryo development [40]. In addition, this study revealed that developmental arrest and activation of the embryonic genome are unrelated events. Wells et al. [38] used reverse transcription and real-time fluorescent PCR to quantify the expression patterns of nine known genes (*BRCA1*, *BRCA2*, *BUB1*, *RB1*, *ATM*, *APC*, *TP53*, *MAD2*, and *beta-Actin*) at the early stage of human embryos. Their data has suggested the characterization of gene expression profiles for the different stages of early embryo development [38]. Li et al. [39] used a cDNA microarray containing

9,600 transcripts to investigate 631 differential gene expressions in oocytes, as well as the 4-cell and 8-cell human embryo stages. The expression of 184, 29, and 65 genes was found to have a value higher than two times the median value of all genes expressed in oocytes, 4-cell, and 8-cell embryos, respectively, indicating the expression of some zygotic genes had already occurred at the 4-cell embryo stage [39]. Furthermore, Adjaye and Lehrach, by using a cDNA microarray where 15,529 cDNA were spotted, identified biomarker transcripts specific to ICM when comparing gene expression profiles of ICM and trophectoderm cells (TE) from human blastocysts [43]. This data has shown that 1,324 genes were overexpressed at the blastocyst stage, including a proteasome (*PSMA1*, *PSMB3*), cellular trafficking (*SLC2A14*, *SLC1A3*), protein modifications, and turnover (*TNK1*, *UBE3A*). On the other hand, damage to DNA can have severe cellular consequences. These consequences are even worse when the damage occurs in the cells which are the origin of all cells of the future human being. Hence, DNA repair systems play a crucial role in the early embryo development [44]. The importance of DNA repair gene products during development is highlighted by the phenotypes observed for human genetic disorders associated with DNA damage response defects (reviewed in ref. [45]). Recently, DNA repair gene expression was investigated [46] in human oocytes and blastocysts to identify the pathways involved at these stages and detect potential differences in repair mechanisms pre- and postembryonic genome activation. Large numbers of repair genes were detected indicating that all DNA repair pathways are potentially functional in human oocytes and blastocysts [46]. Finally, transcriptome analysis within the context of embryos can be used to understand a physiological process, mainly done in a research environment with human samples, or it can be used for diagnostic purposes where the goal is to select the best embryo [12, 14, 47].

Comparative Molecular Signature of Metaphase II Oocyte and Inner Cell Mass

Early human embryo development results in the reprogramming of highly specialized germinal cells into pluripotent. The somatic cell can be reprogrammed to a pluripotent state by factors in the oocyte and embryonic stem cells (ESCs) cytoplasm [5, 48]. In this context, the cytoplasmic environments of oocytes and ESC share the capacity to reprogram a somatic nucleus. It is important to determine what events lead to the reprogramming a somatic nuclei after fusion with an oocyte or ESC from the ICM. This issue has been the subject of intense investigation, and studies have focused predominantly on gene expression. The comparison of the gene expression program of these two cell types (oocyte/ESC) could contribute to the understanding of these cell reprogramming properties. To identify these genes, gene expression profiling data of human oocytes and human ES cells were explored [49, 50]. Kocabas et al. [49] compared the transcriptome of human metaphase II oocytes and hESC with reference samples, 1,626 transcripts are significantly upregulated in hESC, and 5,331 transcripts are upregulated in oocytes. The comparison of these transcripts shows that 388 common genes are believed to play an important role in oocyte reprogramming and early events associated with human embryo development. This list of genes includes *POU5F1/OCT4*, *DAZL*, and *DNMT3b* [49]. Assou et al. compared the gene expression profile of mature MII oocytes and hESC and both to somatic tissues [50]. This analysis revealed 652 transcripts conserved in both, oocytes and hESCs, with 1,970 transcripts (2009) detected specifically in the oocyte, in contrast to 1,140 transcripts in the hESCs. These included a significant number of novel genes. The *oocytes signature* comprised *DAZL*, *SOX30*, *ZP2*, *GDF9*, and *AURKC*, which have previously been identified as overexpressed by oocytes [10]. Similarly, the *hESC signature* displayed numerous genes known to be specifically overexpressed in hESC such as *POU5F1/OCT4*, *NANOG*, and *DPPA4*. Genes associated with pluripotency such as *LIN28* and *TDGF1* and a large chromatin remodeling network (*DNMT3B*, *TOP2A*, *JARID2*, *SMARCA5*, *CBX1*, *CBX5*) were found in both oocyte and hESCs. Interestingly, a large set of genes were also found to code for proteins involved in the ubiquitination and proteasome pathway were overexpressed in MII oocytes and hESC. The proteasome is known to interact with chromatin and function at multiple steps in transcription, both through proteolytic and nonproteolytic activities [51]. These results shed light on the molecular mechanisms of early human development and suggest that the proteasome pathway may play a role in initiating and maintaining pluripotency and be used as criteria for oocyte competence. Finally, the comparison of human mature oocytes and hESC helps to understand the early embryo development and pluripotency and is therefore relevant for therapeutics, including improvement of the pregnancy success rate in IVF and regenerative medicine applications such as those involving cell reprogramming.

Apoptotic Events During Embryo Development

The preimplantation period is a critical time for embryo development. More than 50% of the human embryos cultured in vitro fail to reach the blastocyst stage [52]. They exhibit fragmentation and/or arrest their development. Classical apoptotic features have been observed in human and animal preimplantation embryos produced both in vivo and in vitro [52–56]. Apoptosis is a normal mechanism involved in fundamental processes of life, like embryonic development and tissue homeostasis. Detection of apoptosis processes has a big importance for understanding many biological events. It has been proposed that apoptosis may play an important role in eliminating zygotes or embryonic cells carrying chromosomal anomalies or presenting nuclear and/or cytoplasmic defects [57]. However, the degree of apoptosis cannot exceed a certain threshold without leading to the disruption of embryonic homeostasis and developmental arrest. Thus, the balance between pro- and anti-apoptotic factors is crucial in determining the fate of the embryo. Bcl-2 family proteins are key regulators of apoptosis; they can be subdivided into two groups: anti- (such as Bcl-2, Bcl-xl, Mcl-1, and Bcl2l10) and proapoptotic (such as Bax, Bak, Bik, and Hrk) members. They act at the mitochondrial level by controlling the release of apoptogenic factors such as cytochrome C, allowing the activation of the downstream executional phase, including the activation of caspases. Transcriptomic

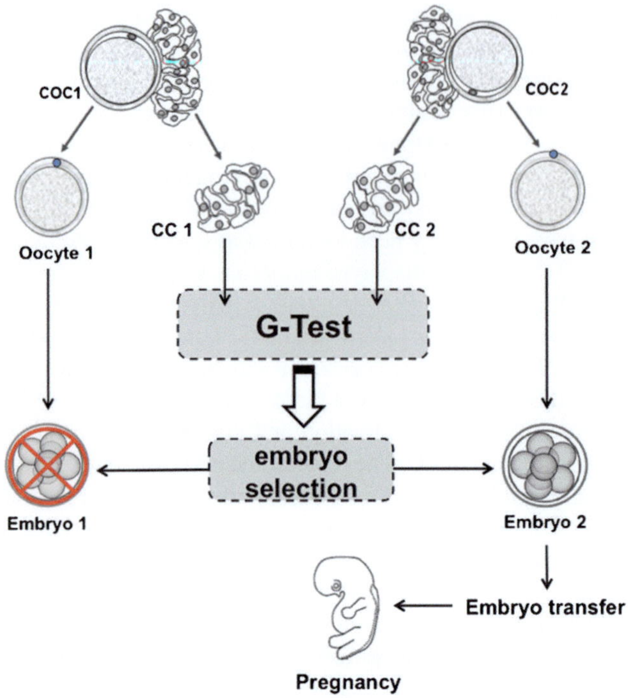

Fig. 19.2 Assessment of embryo quality and pregnancy outcome by *G-test*-based transcriptomic analysis of cumulus cells. *COC* cumulus-oocyte complex; *CC* cumulus cells

analysis revealed a dynamic expression profile of various Bcl-2 family members during early embryonic development (Fig. 19.2) (such as Mcl-1, Bcl2l10, and Bax) [54, 58, 59]. However, the precise role of these proteins in embryo survival needs to be clarified. Caspase 2 and 3 transcripts are expressed at all preimplantation developmental stages [54, 60], and increased caspase 3 activity has been reported in fragmented 4-cell embryos [54]. Finally, survivin plays a key role in embryonic development. It inhibits apoptosis by binding activated caspases (especially caspases 3, 7, and 9). Transgenic embryos, lacking survivin expression, die in utero between the morula and blastocyst stage due to massive apoptosis [61]. Apoptosis of hESCs is considered to be a dynamic process influenced by the culture conditions. Molecular mechanisms controlling the apoptosis of stem cells are still poorly understood and are only hypothetical.

Epigenetic Event During Early Embryonic Development

DNA methylation is an important epigenetic event, regulating gene expression in any developmental processes including gene imprinting and embryogenesis [62]. The paternal genome is actively demethylated in the few hours after fertilization in human zygote. The mechanism responsible for active demethylation in mammals is currently unknown; however, various DNA repair enzymes have been proposed to accomplish this function [63], while the maternal genome is passively demethylated after the 2-cell embryo stage. To maintain methylated DNA, DNA methyltransferases (DNMTs) are necessary. Recently, our team indicated that *DNMT1* transcript was upregulated in human mature oocytes and decreased progressively in embryos day 3, and in hESC [14], *DNMT3A* was enriched in undifferentiated hESC [4], and *DNMT3B* mRNA was detected in both mature oocyte and hESC [50]. Thus, providing a mechanism for the maintenance of DNA methylation and indicating that the *DNMT3* family methyltransferases are candidate epigenetic regulator during early embryonic development. Imprinted genes are genes whose expression is determined by the parent that contributed them. The majority of imprinted genes have been found to have roles in the control of embryonic development [64]. Studies made have established that genetic imprinting is highly conserved among mammals. As imprinting is related to early embryonic development, our team analyzed the expression of 40 imprinted genes and revealed that distinct sets of imprinting genes appear to be involved in human early embryonic development [14]. The imprinted genes can offer new insights into the mechanisms of gene regulation. Gene imprinting provides a form of control of a gene expression. The study of the epigenome is important because minor defects can lead to serious human diseases. Indeed, several syndromes are associated with imprinting defects during early embryonic development [65]. In addition, not only are genes encoding proteins involved in the control and regulation of early embryonic development but also small noncoding RNAs such as microRNAs (miRNAs) that function to regulate gene expression [66]. MiRNAs are approximately 22 nucleotides in length. These are thought to function as repressors of gene expression by blocking mRNA translation [67]. Their normal activities help to coordinate multicellular life, and their dysregulation can contribute to a variety of diseases. The importance of miRNAs regulatory roles is underscored by literature evidence that miRNA function is involved in almost all biological processes, including stem cell regulation [68], cancers [69], and others. The expression patterns of miRNA have been exploited as a new class of biomarkers for disease phenotypes and tissue classifications [67]. To date, the global effect of miRNA during early embryonic development is still undiscovered.

Clinical Applications for Human Embryo Selection

Our understanding of molecular determinants of embryo viability is limited; consequently, current embryo assessment strategies in clinical settings largely rely on embryo morphology. However, most studies suggest that embryos with proper morphological appearance alone are not sufficient to predict a successful implantation. Considering the limitation of morphologic evaluation, there is now a movement toward more sophisticated technologies, such as microarray. This method, involve the analysis of whole embryos, represents a valuable approach to biomarker development, rendering them useless for purposes of clinical testing. Both technical and statistical advances are currently facilitating the application of this approach in ART program. Microarray technology has been used experimentally in humans from trophoblastic biopsies performed on blastocysts. This makes it possible to identify candidate genes involved in adherence or cellular communication with a level expression related to implantation [47]. An indirect and attractive approach for predicting embryo quality and pregnancy outcome has been recently reported by using transcriptomic data of cumulus cells (CCs) [11, 12]. This approach is noninvasive based on the major role of the dialogue between oocyte and surrounding CCs during oocyte maturation. Oocytes and CCs communicate in the follicles through locally secreted factors and neuroendocrine signals. Many studies provide evidence [11, 70] that CCs (1) coordinate follicle development with oocyte maturation, (2) provide energy substrate for oocyte meiotic resumption, (3) regulate oocyte transcription, (4) promote nuclear and oocyte molecular maturation, (5) stimulate amino acid transport and sterol biosynthesis, (6) promote glycolysis [71], and (7) protect the oocyte from the harsh environment. The CCs metabolize alternative substrates, such as amino acids, cholesterol, and glucose, which are essential for the development and function of oocyte [72–74]. CCs share the same follicular environment as the oocyte and both control early as well as delay follicular development. In addition, oocyte quality is a major determinant of the embryo's developmental capacity. Thus, analysis of gene expression in CCs may provide an undirected indication of the microenvironment in which the oocyte matured and will help biologists to achieve a better capability of selecting embryos competent for transfer. Since CCs can be obtained easily during intracytoplasmic sperm injection (ICSI) procedure, and regarding the physiological relevance of the oocyte-CC dialogue during the oocyte maturation process, several groups used microarrays technologies, RT-PCR and quantitative RT-PCR analyses to associate CCs gene expression profile with oocyte competence [75, 76], embryo quality [75–77], and pregnancy outcome [11, 12, 78]. By comparing gene expression profiles of CCs according to embryonic quality and pregnancy outcome, our group reported for the first time a specific transcriptomic signature including 630 genes associated with pregnancy outcome. The majority of the genes differentially expressed were upregulated, suggesting that transcriptional activation in CCs is essential to acquire embryonic competence. Interestingly, genes in CCs resulting in a successful pregnancy were predominantly upregulated, including *BCL2L11* and *PCK1*, respectively involved in apoptosis and gluconeogenesis. Some genes were nevertheless found down regulated in CCs associated with a good pregnancy outcome, such as the transcription factor *NFIB* [12]. In addition, we developed a new potential method "genomic test (G-test)" for competent embryo selection, comprising a step of measuring the expression level of potential biomarkers in CCs (Fig. 19.3). Recently, we conducted a prospective study including 45 biomarkers in CCs associated with embryo and pregnancy outcomes and young (<36 years) normal responder patients referred to our center for cIVF or for ICSI. The embryo selection occurred either according to biomarker profile in CCs (group 1) or to morphological aspects (group 2 used as control). In each group, two embryos were replaced. Our preliminary data of embryo outcome shows the absence of relationship between morphological aspects of embryo and gene expression

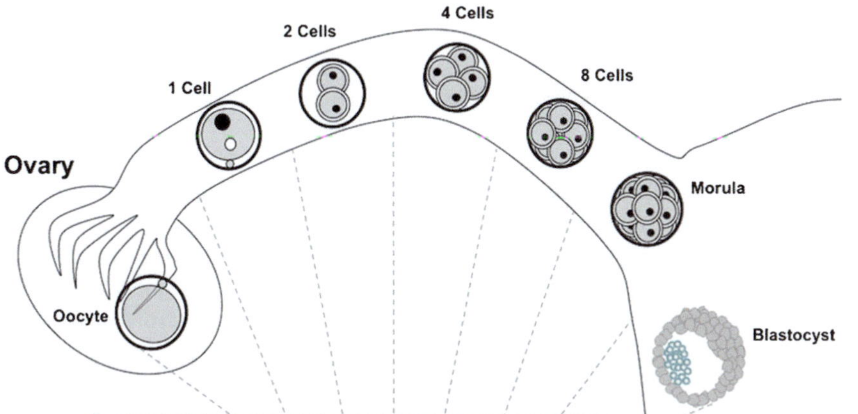

Pro-apoptotic	Bcl2l11	+	nd	nd	nd	+++	nd	-
	Bik	-	-	-	-	+++	nd	-
	Bcl2l13	+++	nd	nd	nd	+++	nd	++
	Bcl2l14	+	nd	nd	nd	+	nd	+
	Bax	+++	+++	+++	+++	+++	+++	+++
Anti-apoptotic	Bcl2l10	+++	-	nd	nd	+++	-	-
	Mcl-1	+++	+++	+++	+++	+++	+++	+++
	Bcl-x	+	+	+	+	+	+	+
	Bfl-1	+	+	+	+	+	+	+

Fig. 19.3 Expression of Bcl-2 family members during early embryonic development. Early embryogenesis stages are presented schematically. The expression levels of the different members are relative, derived from our data and the synthesis of several studies. Very high (+++), high (++), medium (+), low (−), not detected (nd)

profiles in CCs [11]. It is time to reconsider the notion that embryos presenting a low grade according to morphological aspects are able to achieve pregnancy. To date, several of our biomarkers are actually validated in larger clinical trials to assess their predictive value. We have established a mathematical model to identify embryo with high implantation potential. Additionally, measurement of nutrients and metabolites extracted into media surrounding the embryo provides information concerning viability. A multitude of studies proposed that the change in the levels of their metabolites would reflect embryo viability and assessed these metabolites as potential biomarkers [79, 80]. Other studies showed that metabolomic profiling of embryo culture media was independent of morphology, providing an independent parameter in embryo viability assessment [81,82]. Finally, transcriptomics on CCs and metabolomics on culture media techniques are noninvasive, and once adopted, they will allow us to maximize the success of IVF treatment options and should improve in the near future the embryo selection for fresh replacement that is based in part on morphological criteria. Each technique is powerful in itself, but the combination of these techniques will probably revolutionize the success of IVF.

Conclusions

Knowledge of the global pattern of gene expression is important for understanding critical regulatory pathways and key biological process governing human reproduction such as oocyte maturation, embryo development, and ESCs biology. Many studies provided evidence that genes involved with intracellular signaling, cell survival/death, pluripotency, transcription and translation, methylation/demethylation, and nuclear reprogramming are the main cellular processes that control the early embryonic development [14]. In this chapter, we did try to relate for readers the recent advances about the dynamic genes changes of human early embryo development and the application of DNA microarray as a new emergent technology for embryo selection. The use of gene expression of CCs as biomarkers can predict indirectly embryo quality and pregnancy outcome. Investigations on biomarkers offer new and exciting opportunities for embryologists with bioengineering expertise. Techniques of this type may ultimately lead to noninvasive tests for oocyte or embryo quality, revealing previously hidden information concerning both oocyte and embryonic developmental competence. This chapter will be great to those interested on early embryo development; these findings are relevant for therapeutics, including improving the regenerative medicine applications involving pluripotent cells (hESC). Most importantly, our increased knowledge of genes and related transcriptional networks operative during early embryonic development should lead to advances in ART and preimplantation genetic diagnosis.

Acknowledgment This work was partially supported by Ferring pharmaceutical company.

References

1. Reubinoff BE, Pera MF, Fong CY, Trounson A, Bongso A. Embryonic stem cell lines from human blastocysts: somatic differentiation in vitro. Nat Biotechnol. 2000;18:399–404.
2. Thomson JA, Itskovitz-Eldor J, Shapiro SS, Waknitz MA, Swiergiel JJ, Marshall VS, Jones JM. Embryonic stem cell lines derived from human blastocysts. Science. 1998;282:1145–7.
3. Boyer LA, Lee TI, Cole MF, Johnstone SE, Levine SS, Zucker JP, Guenther MG, Kumar RM, Murray HL, Jenner RG, et al. Core transcriptional regulatory circuitry in human embryonic stem cells. Cell. 2005;122:947–56.
4. Assou S, Le Carrour T, Tondeur S, Strom S, Gabelle A, Marty S, Nadal L, Pantesco V, Reme T, Hugnot JP, et al. A meta-analysis of human embryonic stem cells transcriptome integrated into a web-based expression atlas. Stem Cells. 2007;25:961–73.
5. Cowan CA, Atienza J, Melton DA, Eggan K. Nuclear reprogramming of somatic cells after fusion with human embryonic stem cells. Science. 2005;309:1369–73.
6. Hochedlinger K, Blelloch R, Brennan C, Yamada Y, Kim M, Chin L, Jaenisch R. Reprogramming of a melanoma genome by nuclear transplantation. Genes Dev. 2004;18:1875–85.
7. Saito S, Sawai K, Murayama Y, Fukuda K, Yokoyama K. Nuclear transfer to study the nuclear reprogramming of human stem cells. Methods Mol Biol. 2008;438:151–69.
8. Sung LY, Gao S, Shen H, Yu H, Song Y, Smith SL, Chang CC, Inoue K, Kuo L, Lian J, et al. Differentiated cells are more efficient than adult stem cells for cloning by somatic cell nuclear transfer. Nat Genet. 2006;38:1323–8.

9. Stoughton RB. Applications of DNA microarrays in biology. Annu Rev Biochem. 2005; 74:53–82.
10. Assou S, Anahory T, Pantesco V, Le Carrour T, Pellestor F, Klein B, Reyftmann L, Dechaud H, De Vos J, Hamamah S. The human cumulus—oocyte complex gene-expression profile. Hum Reprod. 2006;21:1705–19.
11. Assou S, Haouzi D, De Vos J, Hamamah S. Human cumulus cells as biomarkers for embryo and pregnancy outcomes. Mol Hum Reprod. 2010;16:531–8.
12. Assou S, Haouzi D, Mahmoud K, Aouacheria A, Guillemin Y, Pantesco V, Reme T, Dechaud H, De Vos J, Hamamah S. A non-invasive test for assessing embryo potential by gene expression profiles of human cumulus cells: a proof of concept study. Mol Hum Reprod. 2008;14:711–9.
13. Gasca S, Pellestor F, Assou S, Loup V, Anahory T, Dechaud H, De Vos J, Hamamah S. Identifying new human oocyte marker genes: a microarray approach. Reprod Biomed Online. 2007;14:175–83.
14. Assou S, Boumela I, Haouzi D, Anahory T, Dechaud H, De Vos J, Hamamah S. Dynamic changes in gene expression during human early embryo development: from fundamental aspects to clinical applications. Hum Reprod Update. 2011;17(2):272–90.
15. Moor RM, Dai Y, Lee C, Fulka Jr J. Oocyte maturation and embryonic failure. Hum Reprod Update. 1998;4:223–36.
16. Fair T, Hyttel P, Greve T. Bovine oocyte diameter in relation to maturational competence and transcriptional activity. Mol Reprod Dev. 1995;42:437–42.
17. Cui XS, Li XY, Yin XJ, Kong IK, Kang JJ, Kim NH. Maternal gene transcription in mouse oocytes: genes implicated in oocyte maturation and fertilization. J Reprod Dev. 2007;53: 405–18.
18. Wang QT, Piotrowska K, Ciemerych MA, Milenkovic L, Scott MP, Davis RW, Zernicka-Goetz M. A genome-wide study of gene activity reveals developmental signaling pathways in the preimplantation mouse embryo. Dev Cell. 2004;6:133–44.
19. Yoon SJ, Kim KH, Chung HM, Choi DH, Lee WS, Cha KY, Lee KA. Gene expression profiling of early follicular development in primordial, primary, and secondary follicles. Fertil Steril. 2006;85:193–203.
20. Zhang P, Kerkela E, Skottman H, Levkov L, Kivinen K, Lahesmaa R, Hovatta O, Kere J. Distinct sets of developmentally regulated genes that are expressed by human oocytes and human embryonic stem cells. Fertil Steril. 2007;87:677–90.
21. Hamatani T, Falco G, Carter MG, Akutsu H, Stagg CA, Sharov AA, Dudekula DB, VanBuren V, Ko MS. Age-associated alteration of gene expression patterns in mouse oocytes. Hum Mol Genet. 2004;13:2263–78.
22. Pan H, Ma P, Zhu W, Schultz RM. Age-associated increase in aneuploidy and changes in gene expression in mouse eggs. Dev Biol. 2008;316:397–407.
23. Steuerwald NM, Bermudez MG, Wells D, Munne S, Cohen J. Maternal age-related differential global expression profiles observed in human oocytes. Reprod Biomed Online. 2007;14:700–8.
24. Jones GM, Cram DS, Song B, Magli MC, Gianaroli L, Lacham-Kaplan O, Findlay JK, Jenkin G, Trounson AO. Gene expression profiling of human oocytes following in vivo or in vitro maturation. Hum Reprod. 2008;23:1138–44.
25. Pan H, O'Brien MJ, Wigglesworth K, Eppig JJ, Schultz RM. Transcript profiling during mouse oocyte development and the effect of gonadotropin priming and development in vitro. Dev Biol. 2005;286:493–506.
26. Wells D, Patrizio P. Gene expression profiling of human oocytes at different maturational stages and after in vitro maturation. Am J Obstet Gynecol. 2008;198:455e1–9; discussion 55e9–11.
27. Wood JR, Dumesic DA, Abbott DH, Strauss III JF. Molecular abnormalities in oocytes from women with polycystic ovary syndrome revealed by microarray analysis. J Clin Endocrinol Metab. 2007;92:705–13.
28. Grondahl ML, Yding Andersen C, Bogstad J, Nielsen FC, Meinertz H, Borup R. Gene expression profiles of single human mature oocytes in relation to age. Hum Reprod. 2010;25: 957–68.

29. Lee YS, Latham KE, Vandevoort CA. Effects of in vitro maturation on gene expression in rhesus monkey oocytes. Physiol Genomics. 2008;35:145–58.
30. Zheng P, Patel B, McMenamin M, Moran E, Paprocki AM, Kihara M, Schramm RD, Latham KE. Effects of follicle size and oocyte maturation conditions on maternal messenger RNA regulation and gene expression in rhesus monkey oocytes and embryos. Biol Reprod. 2005;72:890–7.
31. Jansen E, Laven JS, Dommerholt HB, Polman J, van Rijt C, van den Hurk C, Westland J, Mosselman S, Fauser BC. Abnormal gene expression profiles in human ovaries from polycystic ovary syndrome patients. Mol Endocrinol. 2004;18:3050–63.
32. Oksjoki S, Soderstrom M, Inki P, Vuorio E, Anttila L. Molecular profiling of polycystic ovaries for markers of cell invasion and matrix turnover. Fertil Steril. 2005;83:937–44.
33. Lonergan P, Fair T, Corcoran D, Evans AC. Effect of culture environment on gene expression and developmental characteristics in IVF-derived embryos. Theriogenology. 2006;65:137–52.
34. Hamatani T, Carter MG, Sharov AA, Ko MS. Dynamics of global gene expression changes during mouse preimplantation development. Dev Cell. 2004;6:117–31.
35. Rinaudo P, Schultz RM. Effects of embryo culture on global pattern of gene expression in preimplantation mouse embryos. Reproduction. 2004;128:301–11.
36. Zeng F, Baldwin DA, Schultz RM. Transcript profiling during preimplantation mouse development. Dev Biol. 2004;272:483–96.
37. Zhang P, Zucchelli M, Bruce S, Hambiliki F, Stavreus-Evers A, Levkov L, Skottman H, Kerkela E, Kere J, Hovatta O. Transcriptome profiling of human pre-implantation development. PLoS One. 2009;4:e7844.
38. Wells D, Bermudez MG, Steuerwald N, Thornhill AR, Walker DL, Malter H, Delhanty JD, Cohen J. Expression of genes regulating chromosome segregation, the cell cycle and apoptosis during human preimplantation development. Hum Reprod. 2005;20:1339–48.
39. Li SS, Liu YH, Tseng CN, Singh S. Analysis of gene expression in single human oocytes and preimplantation embryos. Biochem Biophys Res Commun. 2006;340:48–53.
40. Dobson AT, Raja R, Abeyta MJ, Taylor T, Shen S, Haqq C, Pera RA. The unique transcriptome through day 3 of human preimplantation development. Hum Mol Genet. 2004;13:1461–70.
41. Hamatani T, Ko M, Yamada M, Kuji N, Mizusawa Y, Shoji M, Hada T, Asada H, Maruyama T, Yoshimura Y. Global gene expression profiling of preimplantation embryos. Hum Cell. 2006;19:98–117.
42. Chen HW, Chen JJ, Yu SL, Li HN, Yang PC, Su CM, Au HK, Chang CW, Chien LW, Chen CS, et al. Transcriptome analysis in blastocyst hatching by cDNA microarray. Hum Reprod. 2005;20:2492–501.
43. Adjaye J, Huntriss J, Herwig R, et al. Primary differentiation in the human blastocyst: comparative molecular portraits of inner cell mass and trophectoderm cells. Stem Cells. 2005;23(10):1514–25.
44. Jaroudi S, SenGupta S. DNA repair in mammalian embryos. Mutat Res. 2007;635:53–77.
45. Hales BF. DNA repair disorders causing malformations. Curr Opin Genet Dev. 2005;15:234–40.
46. Jaroudi S, Kakourou G, Cawood S, Doshi A, Ranieri DM, Serhal P, Harper JC, SenGupta SB. Expression profiling of DNA repair genes in human oocytes and blastocysts using microarrays. Hum Reprod. 2009;24:2649–55.
47. Jones GM, Cram DS, Song B, Kokkali G, Pantos K, Trounson AO. Novel strategy with potential to identify developmentally competent IVF blastocysts. Hum Reprod. 2008;23:1748–59.
48. Rideout III WM, Eggan K, Jaenisch R. Nuclear cloning and epigenetic reprogramming of the genome. Science. 2001;293:1093–8.
49. Kocabas AM, Crosby J, Ross PJ, Otu HH, Beyhan Z, Can H, Tam WL, Rosa GJ, Halgren RG, Lim B, et al. The transcriptome of human oocytes. Proc Natl Acad Sci USA. 2006;103:14027–32.
50. Assou S, Cerecedo D, Tondeur S, Pantesco V, Hovatta O, Klein B, Hamamah S, De Vos J. A gene expression signature shared by human mature oocytes and embryonic stem cells. BMC Genomics. 2009;10:10.

51. Collins GA, Tansey WP. The proteasome: a utility tool for transcription? Curr Opin Genet Dev. 2006;16:197–202.
52. Hardy K, Spanos S, Becker D, Iannelli P, Winston RM, Stark J. From cell death to embryo arrest: mathematical models of human preimplantation embryo development. Proc Natl Acad Sci U S A. 2002;98:1655–60.
53. Jurisicova A, Varmuza S, Casper RF. Programmed cell death and human embryo fragmentation. Mol Hum Reprod. 1996;2:93–8.
54. Jurisicova A, Antenos M, Varmuza S, Tilly JL, Casper RF. Expression of apoptosis-related genes during human preimplantation embryo development: potential roles for the Harakiri gene product and Caspase-3 in blastomere fragmentation. Mol Hum Reprod. 2003;9:133–41.
55. Levy R, Benchaib M, Cordonier H, Souchier C, Guerin JF. Annexin V labelling and terminal transferase-mediated DNA end labelling (TUNEL) assay in human arrested embryos. Mol Hum Reprod. 1998;4:775–83.
56. Yang HW, Hwang KJ, Kwon HC, Kim HS, Choi KW, Oh KS. Detection of reactive oxygen species (ROS) and apoptosis in human fragmented embryos. Hum Reprod. 1998;13:998–1002.
57. Jurisicova A, Acton BM. Deadly decisions: the role of genes regulating programmed cell death in human preimplantation embryo development. Reproduction. 2004;128:281–91.
58. Metcalfe AD, Hunter HR, Bloor DJ, Lieberman BA, Picton HM, Leese HJ, Kimber SJ, Brison DR. Expression of 11 members of the BCL-2 family of apoptosis regulatory molecules during human preimplantation embryo development and fragmentation. Mol Reprod Dev. 2004;68:35–50.
59. Guillemin Y, Lalle P, Gillet G, Guerin JF, Hamamah S, Aouacheria A. Oocytes and early embryos selectively express the survival factor BCL2L10. J Mol Med. 2009;87:923–40.
60. Spanos S, Rice S, Karagiannis P, Taylor D, Becker DL, Winston RM, Hardy K. Caspase activity and expression of cell death genes during development of human preimplantation embryos. Reproduction. 2002;124:353–63.
61. Uren AG, Wong L, Pakusch M, Fowler KJ, Burrows FJ, Vaux DL, Choo KHA. Survivin and the inner centromere protein INCENP show similar cell-cycle localization and gene knockout phenotype. Curr Biol. 2000;10:1319–28.
62. Kafri T, Ariel M, Brandeis M, Shemer R, Urven L, McCarrey J, Cedar H, Razin A. Developmental pattern of gene-specific DNA methylation in the mouse embryo and germ line. Genes Dev. 1992;6:705–14.
63. Gehring M, Reik W, Henikoff S. DNA demethylation by DNA repair. Trends Genet. 2009;25:82–90.
64. Isles AR, Holland AJ. Imprinted genes and mother-offspring interactions. Early Hum Dev. 2005;81:73–7.
65. Yamazawa K, Kagami M, Fukami M, Matsubara K, Ogata T. Monozygotic female twins discordant for Silver-Russell syndrome and hypomethylation of the H19-DMR. J Hum Genet. 2008;53: 950–5.
66. Edson MA, Nagaraja AK, Matzuk MM. The mammalian ovary from genesis to revelation. Endocr Rev. 2009;30:624–712.
67. Bartel DP, Chen CZ. Micromanagers of gene expression: the potentially widespread influence of metazoan microRNAs. Nat Rev Genet. 2004;5:396–400.
68. Gangaraju VK, Lin H. MicroRNAs: key regulators of stem cells. Nat Rev Mol Cell Biol. 2009;10:116–25.
69. Visone R, Croce CM. MiRNAs and cancer. Am J Pathol. 2009;174:1131–8.
70. Sugiura K, Pendola FL, Eppig JJ. Oocyte control of metabolic cooperativity between oocytes and companion granulosa cells: energy metabolism. Dev Biol. 2005;279:20–30.
71. Sugiura K, Su YQ, Diaz FJ, Pangas SA, Sharma S, Wigglesworth K, O'Brien MJ, Matzuk MM, Shimasaki S, Eppig JJ. Oocyte-derived BMP15 and FGFs cooperate to promote glycolysis in cumulus cells. Development. 2007;134:2593–603.
72. Sutton-McDowall ML, Gilchrist RB, Thompson JG. Cumulus expansion and glucose utilisation by bovine cumulus–oocyte complexes during in vitro maturation: the influence of glucosamine and follicle-stimulating hormone. Reproduction. 2004;128:313–9.

73. Preis KA, Seidel Jr G, Gardner DK. Metabolic markers of developmental competence for in vitro matured mouse oocytes. Reproduction. 2005;130:475–83.
74. Eppig J. Mouse oocytes control metabolic cooperativity between oocytes and cumulus cells. Reprod Fertil Dev. 2005;17:1–2.
75. McKenzie LJ, Pangas SA, Carson SA, Kovanci E, Cisneros P, Buster JE, Amato P, Matzuk MM. Human cumulus granulosa cell gene expression: a predictor of fertilization and embryo selection in women undergoing IVF. Hum Reprod. 2004;19:2869–74.
76. Van Montfoort AP, Geraedts JP, Dumoulin JC, Stassen AP, Evers JL, Ayoubi TA. Differential gene expression in cumulus cells as a prognostic indicator of embryo viability: a microarray analysis. Mol Hum Reprod. 2008;14:157–68.
77. Zhang X, Jafari N, Barnes RB, Confino E, Milad M, Kazer RR. Studies of gene expression in human cumulus cells indicate pentraxin 3 as a possible marker for oocyte quality. Fertil Steril. 2005;83 Suppl 1:1169–79.
78. Hamel M, Dufort I, Robert C, Gravel C, Leveille MC, Leader A, Sirard MA. Identification of differentially expressed markers in human follicular cells associated with competent oocytes. Hum Reprod. 2008;23:1118–27.
79. Brison DR, Houghton FD, Falconer D, Roberts SA, Hawkhead J, Humpherson PG, Lieberman BA, Leese HJ. Identification of viable embryos in IVF by non-invasive measurement of amino acid turnover. Hum Reprod. 2004;19:2319–24.
80. Botros L, Sakkas D, Seli E. Metabolomics and its application for non-invasive embryo assessment in IVF. Mol Hum Reprod. 2008;14:679–90.
81. Seli E, Vergouw CG, Morita H, Botros L, Roos P, Lambalk CB, Yamashita N, Kato O, Sakkas D. Noninvasive metabolomic profiling as an adjunct to morphology for noninvasive embryo assessment in women undergoing single embryo transfer. Fertil Steril. 2010;94(2):535–42.
82. Vergouw CG, Botros LL, Roos P, Lens JW, Schats R, Hompes PG, Burns DH, Lambalk CB. Metabolomic profiling by near-infrared spectroscopy as a tool to assess embryo viability: a novel, non-invasive method for embryo selection. Hum Reprod. 2008;23: 1499–504.

Suggested Reading

Haouzi D, Hamamah S. Pertinence of apoptosis markers for the improvement of in vitro fertilization (IVF). Curr Med Chem. 2009;16:1905–16.
Seli E, Botros L, Sakkas D, Burns DH. Noninvasive metabolomic profiling of embryo culture media using proton nuclear magnetic resonance correlates with reproductive potential of embryos in women undergoing in vitro fertilization. Fertil Steril. 2008;90:2183–9.

Chapter 20
Amino Acid Turnover as a Biomarker of Embryo Viability

Christine Leary, Danielle G. Smith, Henry J. Leese, and Roger G. Sturmey

Most of the rise in multiple births observed since the 1980s has been attributed to the increased use of IVF and the practice of replacing more than one embryo into the uterus in order to improve the chances of success. In response to the unacceptably high risks associated with multiple births, several countries have introduced single embryo transfer policies. However, to maintain acceptable pregnancy rates, the pressure to identify the most viable embryo for transfer has intensified.

The most widely used method of embryo selection has been to assign scores on day 2 or day 3 postinsemination on the basis of the embryos cleavage rate and morphological appearance. Studies have shown that correlations exist between these observational cues of embryo quality and their capacity for continued development and subsequent implantation. However, appropriate temporal developmental patterns are critical to predicting embryo viability. For example, Cummins et al. [1] assigned scores based on the ratio between the time at which an embryo was observed at a given stage of development and the expected time taken to reach that particular stage and showed that pregnancy rates were lower for those with above or below average scores. In a powerful study based on observations from single embryo transfer, Giorgetti et al. [2] demonstrated the additional benefit of including a

C. Leary, BSc
Hull IVF Unit, East Riding Fertility Services, The Women and Children's Hospital, Hull Royal Infirmary, Hull, UK

D.G. Smith, BMedChem, PhD
Leeds Institute of Molecular Medicine, University of Leeds, St James's University Hospital, Leeds, UK

H.J. Leese, BSc, PhD
Hull York Medical School, University of Hull, Hertford Building, Hull, UK

R.G. Sturmey, BSc, PhD (✉)
Centre for Cardiovascular and Metabolic Research, Hull York Medical School, University of Hull, Hertford Building, Cottingham Road, Hull, HU6 7RX, UK
e-mail: Roger.sturmey@hyms.ac.uk

Z.P. Nagy et al. (eds.), *Clinical Embryology: A Practical Guide*,

DOI 10.1007/978-1-4614-8376-2_20,

morphology score. Morphological markers linked with implantation include blastomere size, regularity [3] and the presence of fragmentation [2], multinucleation [4], granulation, and zona thickness. Fragmentation is the most commonly reported observation, and >20% fragmentation is regarded by many as biologically deleterious. The caveat is that morphological assessment is highly subjective, and there is evidence that the pattern of fragmentation may be more important than fragmentation per se [5].

Blastocyst formation occurs between day 5 and day 7 and is a critical developmental milestone. Approximately 50% of human zygotes have the potential to reach this stage [6]. Aneuploidy is commonly associated with developmental arrest; hence the proportion of embryos with chromosomal abnormalities is lower in blastocysts compared to cleavage-stage embryos. The method of grading blastocysts is similar to that of grading cleavage-stage embryos; blastocysts are scored on how similar they are to the *morphological ideal*. This involves grading according to presence of a cavity, a visible inner cell mass (ICM), regular trophoblast (TE) cells, degree of expansion, and zona thinning. The ICM and TE are graded according to how tightly cells are packed and the number of cells, particularly in the ICM.

Selection of the most viable embryo to transfer and at which stage of development remains one of the most challenging aspects of in vitro practices. There is little consensus regarding the observations to make and how frequently to record them. Many schemes use a combination of criteria, including the addition of pronuclear morphological scores, early cleavage, and more controversially aneuploidy screening, as adjuncts to those used routinely as described in this section.

Attempts to draw conclusions on the effectiveness of current observational embryo grading and selection tools have been hampered by a lack of generic terminology and methodology. There is a clear need for a standard embryo scoring/selection system, and attempts to introduce external quality assessment schemes are currently being piloted in the UK. It is hoped that with the introduction of consistent terminology and reduced operator scoring variability, this will permit large-center studies and allow more definitive correlations to be drawn leading us closer to defining what indicates a viable embryo.

Why the Need for Objective Markers of Viability?

Embryo selection is currently based on operator observations of embryo developmental and morphology score on the assumption that these two features are affected by intrinsic factors and as such are a reflection of genetic viability of an embryo. They may also be influenced by extrinsic factors such as the culture environment. For example, Lane et al. [7] showed that media composition can affect cleavage rates, and improvements to embryo culture systems have supported the increased development rate of embryos to the blastocyst stage such that extended culture and blastocyst formation is now frequently used to select competent embryos for transfer.

Blastocyst transfer is not a suitable strategy for all patients as it may result in fewer embryos being available for freezing and an increased risk of canceled cycles. Furthermore, embryos are able to adapt to their environment, and if the in vitro environment is suboptimal, prolonged culture may reduce embryo viability or have other more subtle effects such as an undesired modification of epigenetic changes or metabolic dysregulation, although further rigorous evaluation is required. In other words, there is a need to find the safest most effective method to help patients achieve a single healthy pregnancy. An accurate system for assessment of embryo viability will enable practitioners to counsel patients on their chances of conception and reduce the numbers of embryos transferred.

Amino Acid Profiling

The search for biomarkers of embryo viability in spent embryo culture medium has a long history. Potential markers have included the consumption of glucose, lactate, pyruvate, oxygen, and glutamine and the appearance of proteins such as sHLAG and PIF. However, there is increasing evidence to support the proposition that *amino acid profiling* reflects the developmental capacity of early embryos. By measuring a group of 18 compounds, amino acid profiling provides a snapshot of embryo phenotype by virtue of the many roles played by amino acids during embryo development, some of which are considered below. Thus, amino acid profiling differs from conventional metabolic assays, where typically, only one or two metabolites are measured.

Since the first application of amino acid profiling of mouse embryos was published in 1994 by Lamb et al. [8], the technique has been applied to bovine [9–12], porcine [13], and critically, human embryos [14–16]. Without exception, in those studies in which it was addressed, the research has demonstrated that the amino acid composition of spent culture medium i.e., amino acid profile (AAP) of *viable* embryos differs from that given by subviable embryos. These studies have used different indicators of embryo quality, from blastocyst formation [14], through molecular scale observations of DNA damage [15], to correlation with clinical pregnancy [16]. Crucially, the link between AAP and viability is independent of embryo morphological grade and is apparent from day 1–2 or day 2–3 postinsemination.

The Biology of Amino Acids

It is well recognized that amino acids have a variety of roles in the cell in addition to their traditional function as constituents of proteins. Some such roles are listed below with a brief consideration of their contribution in the early embryo.

Protein Synthesis

Protein synthesis is relatively low during the cleavage stages of preimplantation development but increases sharply with blastocyst formation [17, 18]. This is consistent with the observation that the protein content of preimplantation embryos is relatively stable during cleavage before increasing in the blastocyst, with the onset of true growth [19]. This is reflected in the uptake of certain amino acids from within a mixture when provided in culture, as seen in bovine [9], porcine [20], and human [14] embryos.

Energy Sources

Approximately 14% of human energy needs are provided by the oxidation of protein, ultimately provided by the diet, and it is likely that early embryos cultured with a physiological mixture of amino acids will exhibit a similar figure. When cells are provided with an excess of protein or amino acids, then once the requirement for the synthesis of protein and other amino acid-derived products has been met, they will first tend to be oxidized, in preference to carbohydrate and fat, since mammalian cells have no capacity to store amino acids or protein. In most mammalian cells, protein synthesis is one of two major consumers of energy, the other being the Na+, K+, ATPase; their contributions to the energy budget being ~25% each, though with considerable variation depending on the cell type and physiological state. [21–23].

This issue was addressed for mouse blastocysts by Leese et al. [24] who reported considerable variation in the energy cost of protein synthesis depending on methodology and assumptions. Despite these caveats, it is most likely that the protein synthesis will be a major component of energy homeostasis and, in the context of the present discussion, provide a good marker of the overall nutritional requirements of the early embryo.

Nucleotide Synthesis

Glutamine, aspartic acid, and glycine provide carbon and nitrogen atoms for purine and pyrimidine de novo synthesis—metabolic pathways which are essential to mouse preimplantation development [25]. A key amino acid is thought to be glutamine, which is readily consumed by rapidly dividing cells, and in early embryos [19] where in addition to providing purine and pyrimidine nucleotide precursors it acts as an energy source.

Osmolytes

Notable among amino acids which act as osmolytes during mouse preimplantation development are glycine, betaine, glutamine, and proline [26].

Provision of 1-Carbon Units

Methylation reactions, which are integral to appropriate gene silencing by methylation pathways, require functioning methyl group cycling, in which the amino acid methionine is a key component together with derivatives of the vitamin folic acid.

Signaling Molecule Precursors

In the context of the early embryo, perhaps, the best-characterized example of the function of amino acids as precursors of signal transducers is the formation of nitric oxide from arginine. The role of NO has been the subject of a number of studies in the early embryo. For example, Manser et al. [27] reported data consistent with NO having an obligatory role in mouse preimplantation development, in terms of Ca^{2+} signaling in mitochondria [28], and Lipari et al. [29] reported an association between human embryo-mediated NO production and subsequent blastocyst formation.

Thus, the biological rationale for the ability of amino acids to act as biomarkers of early embryo viability is compelling. The practicalities of assaying amino acid metabolism by early embryos are now considered.

How to Measure Amino Acids

Principle of Chromatography/High-Performance Liquid Chromatography

High-performance liquid chromatography (HPLC) is a form of column chromatography, in which compounds of interest are separated according to their chemical and physical properties. A sample containing a mixture of compounds of interest, in the present context, amino acids, is diluted into a liquid carrier, the *mobile phase*, and pumped under high pressure onto a *solid-phase* column. The column impedes the passage of the amino acids as they interact with the packing substrate within the column. By modifying the conditions of the mobile phase, the amino acids are washed off, or *eluted*, from the column and detected by an appropriate system.

Each amino acid differs in terms of structure and chemistry and on this basis interacts with the column in a different way such that it is *retained* on the column for a different length of time. Using this concept of *retention time*, each amino acid may be identified as it is eluted sequentially from the column. Each amino acid generates a quantifiable signal, which is directly proportional to the signal given by a standard mixture of amino acids at known concentration. Using this simple approach, it has been possible to measure changes in the amino acid content of spent embryo culture droplets to a very high degree of sensitivity.

Chemical Properties of Amino Acids

When most of us think of amino acids, we are generally referring to a subset known as the protein amino acids, of which there are 20 naturally occurring L-isomers and are the constituents of proteins. This section will refer to only these naturally occurring amino acids as these are the only relevant subset in the current context. All amino acids share a common structural scaffold, consisting of an amino group, a carboxyl group, and a distinctive side chain denoted as R with each side chain unique to each amino acid. An exception to this general scaffold rule however is proline where the side chain forms a five-membered ring with backbone. Amino acids can be categorized into four main subgroups based on their general chemical nature: weakly acidic, weakly basic, hydrophobic, and polar hydrophilic. These chemical features can be exploited to isolate individual amino acids.

The pI value of most amino acids is approximately six meaning that at neutral pH, amino acids ionize and are typically zwitterionic. That is, they exhibit both a positive charge on the amine and a negative charge on the carboxylate; however, the pI of the side chains of the amino acids varies which affects the overall charge of the particle. It is the chemical and structural properties of the side chain that dictate which subgroup an amino acid falls into, affecting charge, reactivity, and hydrogen-bonding capacity of the amino acid. Therefore, changing the pH and ionic strength of the mobile phase can be used to separate amino acids during chromatography allowing individual amino acids to be isolated. To give one example, under chromatographic conditions of pH 5.9, the solvent, or mobile phase, is positively charged; thus, the first amino acids to elute are *acidic* amino acids: aspartate and glutamate (conjugate bases for aspartic acid and glutamic acid). At this pH, the acidic side chains are deprotonated meaning they are carrying a negative charge and therefore interact with the positively charged mobile phase rather than the uncharged column substrate and so elute very rapidly. Aspartate has a shorter retention time than glutamate because it has shorter hydrocarbon chain therefore slightly less hydrophobicity and thus can pass through the column substrate more rapidly than glutamate.

This one example illustrates how on the basis of their chemical and physical properties amino acids may be separated from the mixture present in embryo culture media. It is also important to emphasize that this is an example of r*everse phase*

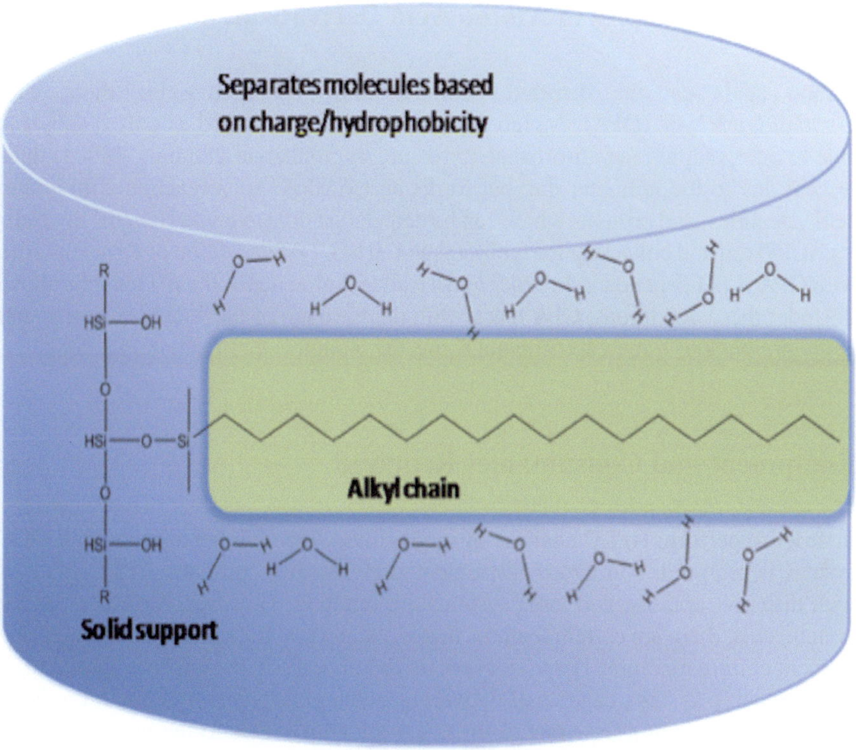

Fig. 20.1 Reverse phase column. The solid support of the column is usually made of chemically inert material of a large pH range, for example, silica. Attached to the inert core are hydrophobic fingers (*green*) made of up alkyl chains. Hydrophillic pockets are formed between the alkyl chains as the column is hydrated with aqueous phase (H_2O) (*blue*). The degree of hydrophilicity of the mobile phase dictates the size of the hydrophilic pockets which in turn affects the ability of the molecules passing through the column to interact with the alkyl chains. These hydrophilic pockets allow charged particles to be retained in the column and separated by manipulating the amount of hydrophilic component in the mobile phase

HPLC, distinguished from conventional HPLC because the mobile rather than solid phase in the column is charged (Fig. 20.1). This small distinction is vital as RP-HPLC offers an extra dimension of flexibility with regard to separation parameters since combinations of mobile phases can be run, according to *gradient* method chromatography. Thus, aspartate and glutamate mentioned above can be eluted in a positively charged mobile phase. Conversely, hydrophobic amino acids such as leucine will not elute from a column when the mobile phase is predominantly aqueous and must therefore be eluted in a nonaqueous mobile phase, for example, consisting predominantly of methanol. Gradient HPLC allows the composition of the mobile phase to be changed gradually from a positively charged aqueous buffer, allowing the rapid elution of small acidic amino acids, to a nonaqueous mobile phase which will enable the elution of the hydrophobic amino acids, such at leucine.

Chemical Principles of Amino Acid Derivatization

Amino acids can be detected fluorometrically by derivatizing them with *o-phthaldialdehyde* (OPA). Amino acids need to be derivatized as only a subset is able to detect ultraviolet absorbance (tyrosine, tryptophan at 280 nm). OPA is fluorescent due to the aromatic ring but forms an isoindole upon reaction with amino acids, peptides, and proteins which can be detected at different wavelengths by exciting at 350 nm and collecting the emission at 430 nm. Derivatization of these moieties with OPA is pH dependant. In order to derivatize amino acids, the pH must be above 9. Under these conditions, OPA reacts with the nitrogen of the backbone amine and in the presence of b-mercaptoethanol forms the isoindole as shown in Fig. 20.2.

Equipment and Consumables Required

In order to perform HPLC analysis of spent culture medium, an appropriate HPLC system is required. Numerous instrumentation suppliers produce HPLC systems with different options, and most systems are modular. However, regardless of the system used, there are certain features that are important for analysis of amino acids in spent culture medium. The system employed to perform the analysis should have a binary pump system, capable of delivering a changing gradient of elution buffers, and able to pump at a flow rate of up to 2.5 mL min^{-1}. Due to the vast number of samples and controls analyzed, an autosampler, with the capacity to carry out automatic derivatization, is also essential. The autosampler also needs to be temperature controlled and able to maintain the samples at 4°C to minimize sample degradation during analysis. A column oven is required to ensure that the chemistry on the column is performed at a standard temperature, usually 25°C. The final component required is the detection system. Since derivatization with OPA yields a fluorescently labeled amino acid, a fluorescent detector is capable of exciting the eluted samples at around 300 nm and detecting emission at approximately 450 nm.

In addition to the system, selecting an appropriate column is fundamental to efficient separation of amino acids with a mixture. Columns commonly used for this type of separation are silica-based; that is, they are packed with inert silica beads.

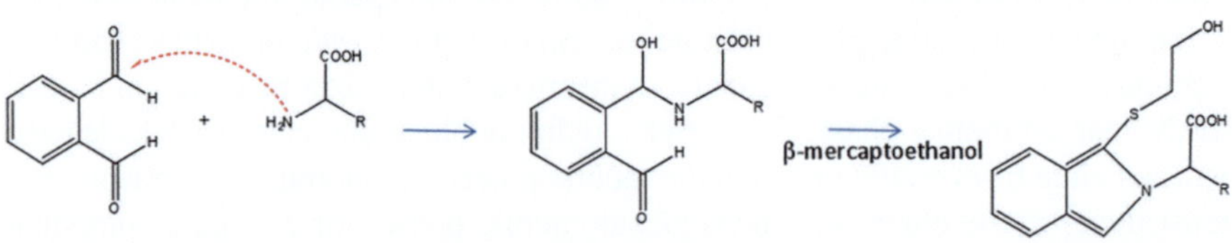

Fig. 20.2 Amino acid derivatization with OPA. The carbonyl of the OPA undergoes nucleophilic attack by the nitrogen of the amine of an amino acid generating intermediate B. In the presence of mercaptoethanol, intermediate B will rapidly convert to the fluorescently detectable isoindole product C

The mean diameter of the particles used to pack the column is given in the column information. Particle size is important since it affects column separation efficiency; a smaller particle size gives superior separation and smaller interparticle space; that is, the column is *more tightly packed*. However, this will lead to a corresponding increase in the pressure applied to the column, termed the *back pressure*. Prolonged exposure to elevated back pressure (in excess of 250 bar) will significantly impact on column lifetime; thus, it is necessary to maintain back pressure below 250 bar, preferably below 200 bar. In other words, the choice of particle size is a compromise between separation efficiency and acceptable back pressure. In addition to particle size, the size and volume of the pores on the packing particles must be considered. Pore size is relevant with respect to the size of analytes; separation of small analytes is optimum with smaller pore sizes; a small analyte in a large pore will have more space to fill as it traverses the column; thus, retention times will increase. The pore volume gives an indication of the surface area of the particle; the smaller the pore size and the higher the volume of pores, the higher the overall surface area of the column packing material, which has the effect of increasing column volume and compound retention times.

Next, one needs to consider the physical dimensions of the column; the internal diameter and the length which combined can be used to calculate the overall column volume, known as the bed volume. As a general rule, a smaller column diameter will lead to improved sensitivity and will enable chromatography to be performed at a lower mobile phase flow rate without any effect on linear flow rate of mobile phase through the column. However, this will lead to a reduction in analyte loading capacity. Similarly, a longer column will improve peak resolution, but at the cost of increased analysis time.

The final key consideration when choosing the column is the carbon load. Typically for amino acid analysis of spent culture medium, octadecyl silane or *ODS* columns are most commonly used, which are chemically bonded to the silica particles within the column, producing $C_{18}H_{37}$ chains. The length of the carbon chain is an important consideration; as a general rule, the longer the carbon chains, the higher the retention of the analytes. C18 is commonly used in RP-HPLC and is suitable for the separation and detection of amino acids in spent culture medium. This is above the *critical chain length* of ten C molecules [28] and is preferable over an alternative C8 column available from many column manufacturers. The carbon chain length, along with the particle size, number of particles, and pore size (i.e., surface area), influences the efficiency of the column.

It is wise to include a precolumn filter. This is a device through which the samples are passed prior to being loaded onto the column and which retains large contaminants. Precolumn filters are an inexpensive option ensuring column protection from blockages and improving column life-span. Normally, these consist of the same material used in the separating column with a lower packing density.

For the separation of amino acids from spent embryo culture medium, there are a number of key considerations; peak resolution must be maintained, as must repeatability and confidence in repeated assays. A series of five identical standards should be run prior to the loading of any samples to account for interrun variability. The variation between areas given on each of these runs should be less than 5%. However, analysis time needs to be kept to a minimum to ensure sufficient sample throughput. It is therefore necessary to make a suitable compromise, based on the factors described above, to ensure that column properties are suitable for a given application.

It is also necessary to consider the components of the mobile phase. Solvents, such as methanol and tetrahydrofuran (THF), should be *HPLC grade*. These are confirmed as high-purity solvents that have been tested to ensure adherence to strict specifications relating to spectral properties and ionic interactions. Solvents must be stored appropriately but not for prolonged periods as the quality can diminish as the solvents react with the containers in which they are stored. It is therefore preferable to store mobile phases in glass bottles rather than those made of plastic. HPLC-grade water is commercially available; however, it is sufficient to use ultrapure water collected from a suitable water purification system that is capable of producing water with a resistance of 18 Ω. This is preferential to using HPLC water stored for prolonged periods as the impurities arising from the storage container are minimized.

The mobile phase of the HPLC system will contain dissolved gases, and it is important to degas the solvents. This is commonly achieved by the inclusion of an in-line degasser in the HPLC system. The removal of dissolved gases is important to ensure consistent chromatographic performance.

How to Prepare Samples and *Do* the High-Performance Liquid Chromatography

Embryos should be placed into small droplets of culture medium containing amino acids; typically, these droplets are 4 μL in volume, placed under oil to minimize evaporation. This is an optimum volume, since it contains amino acids at a concentration low enough to enable detection of small changes, but is sufficiently high to ensure that no single nutrient becomes limiting. At the end of the incubation, typically 24 h, the embryo is removed from the droplet, and the droplet is diluted, at a ratio of 1:12.5 in HPLC-appropriate water. In practice, 2 μL of sample is added to 23 μL of water in an HPLC vial. This gives a convenient 25 μL sample volume that is loaded onto the autosampler. At this stage, the samples are derivatized with OPA (see above), using the autosampler device to inject 25 μL of OPA in solution from a reservoir into the sample. After a suitable reaction time, typically 2 min, the sample is injected onto the column commencing separation of the analytes. The eluted peaks are then quantified.

Data Interpretation

The method of amino acid profiling offers significant promise in predicting embryo viability. At present, with conventional scoring methods, even when strict criteria are applied, approximately 25% of embryos graded as top quality will be aneuploid [8], and there is a clear need for improvement. The assignment of embryo *viability scores* based on their amino acid metabolism may provide a superior, more objective, quantitative selection method. Patients may have a cohort of embryos of differing morphology grades and cleavage rates, as well as embryos that exhibit different amino acid profiles indicative of differing embryo viability. The challenge is to discover the biological basis of these differences.

Statistics and Power

The amino acid profile data generated from animal and human models has been related retrospectively to various outcome measures, including blastocyst development and clinical pregnancy. Data from the analysis of 18 amino acids must be interpreted with care. The utilization of individual amino acids is unlikely to be independent of one another; each must be considered as a latent variable where each amino acid will have a unique contribution to the outcome. One must therefore consider how the specific contribution of any given amino acid differs from the remaining amino acids. For this purpose, the technique of principal components analysis is often used to combine the data into a single index that can serve as a measure of embryo viability [16].

Within any dataset, there will be sample variability and measuring errors. The question that needs to be addressed is whether ordinary sampling variance can account for the differences in viability indices between the pregnant and nonpregnant groups. If the possibility of measuring errors is reduced, only then will we be able to ascertain how much of the variability in outcome can be apportioned to variance in the amino acid data. For instance, if leucine utilization is compared in a pregnant and nonpregnant group, and the variability between the two groups is higher than the within group variance, we can then say with some confidence that any differences are due to more than sampling variability, and the null hypothesis can be rejected. However, a strength of the system used to quantify amino acid metabolism is the inclusion of an internal reference standard, for example, D-A-AMINO-butyric acid (DABA), a nontoxic, chemically inert compound incapable of being metabolized by mammalian cell enabling sampling variance to be corrected.

In significance testing, there are two opposite risks; a type I error is the acceptance of a difference as significant when it is not, i.e., rejecting the null hypothesis when it is true. The converse is a type II error, i.e., accepting the null hypothesis when it is false. The emphasis is generally placed on avoiding type I errors—i.e., false claims. In order to reduce the likelihood of this occurring, emphasis is often placed on significance at the 1% level. However, a balance needs to be struck between statistical significance and clinical relevance, and clinically relevant end points need to be defined. The test may aid embryo selection but may not translate to an immediate difference in clinical pregnancy rates. It could, however, improve cumulative pregnancy rates by enhanced selection criteria for cryopreservation. Rigorous follow-up is therefore required to test the merits of amino acid testing.

Relating to Outcome

The question of *cause or effect* poses a challenge, and confounding variables may bias the results. Statistical modeling has been applied to investigate the relationship with known predictors of pregnancy, such as female age and embryo quality, and in the human, amino acid turnover is a powerful, independent predictor of outcome [16]. However, in order to draw further conclusions from these types of approaches, full randomized prospective clinical trials are now required.

References

1. Cummins JM, Breen TM, Harison KL, et al. A formula for scoring human embryo growth rates in in vitro fertilization: its value in predicting pregnancy and in comparison with visual estimates of embryo quality. J In Vitro Fert Embryo Transf. 1986;3:284–95.
2. Giorgetti C, Terriou P, Auquier P, et al. Embryo score to predict implantation after in-vitro fertilization: based on 957 single embryo transfers. Hum Reprod. 1995;10:2427–31.
3. Hardarson T, Hanson C, Sjogren A, Lundin K. Human embryos with uneven sized blastomeres have lower pregnancy and implantation rates: indications for aneuploidy and multinucleation. Hum Reprod. 2001;16:313–8.
4. Munne S, Cohen J. Unsuitability of multinucleated human blastomeres for preimplantation genetic diagnosis. Hum Reprod. 1998;8:1120–5.
5. Alikani M, Cohen J, Tomkin G, et al. Human embryo fragmentation in vitro and its implications for pregnancy and implantation. Fertil Steril. 1999;71:836–42.
6. Magli M, Jones G, Gras L, et al. Chromosome mosaicism in day 3 aneuploid embryos that develop to morphologically normal blastocysts in vitro. Hum Reprod. 2000;15(8):1781–6.
7. Lane M, Gardner D. Selection of viable mouse blastocysts prior to transfer using metabolic criterion. Hum Reprod. 1996;11:1975–8.
8. Lamb V, Leary C, Herbert M, Murdoch A. Embryo selection in assisted conception. Curr Obstet Gynaecol. 2004;14:291–3.
9. Partridge RJ, Leese HJ. Consumption of amino acids by bovine preimplantation embryos. J Reprod Fertil. 1996;102(2):299–306.
10. Orsi NM, Leese HJ. Amino acid metabolism of preimplantation bovine embryos cultured with bovine serum albumin or polyvinyl alcohol. Theriogenology. 2004;61:561–72.
11. Gopichandran N, Leese HJ. Metabolic characterization of the bovine blastocyst, inner cell mass, trophectoderm and blastocoel fluid. Reproduction. 2003;126:299–308.
12. Sturmey RG, Bermejo-Alvarez P, Gutierrez-Adan A, Rizos D, Leese HJ, Lonergan P. Amino acid metabolism of bovine blastocysts: a biomarker of sex and viability. Mol Reprod Dev. 2010;77:285–96.
13. Humpherson PG, Leese HJ, Sturmey RG. Amino acid metabolism of the porcine blastocyst. Theriogenology. 2005;64:1852–66.
14. Houghton FD, Hawkhead JA, Humpherson PG, Hogg JE, Balen AH, Rutherford AJ, Leese HJ. Non-invasive amino acid turnover predicts human embryo developmental capacity. Hum Reprod. 2002;17:999–1005 [Erratum in: Hum Reprod. 2003;18: 1756–7].
15. Sturmey RG, Hawkhead JA, Barker EA, Leese HJ. DNA damage and metabolic activity in the preimplantation embryo. Hum Reprod. 2009;24:81–91.
16. Brison DR, Houghton FD, Falconer D, Roberts SA, Hawkhead JA, Humpherson PG, Lieberman BA, Leese HJ. Identification of viable embryos in IVF by non-invasive measurement of amino acid turnover. Hum Reprod. 2004;19:2319–24.

17. Epstein CJ, Smith SA. Amino acid uptake and protein synthesis in preimplantation mouse embryos. Dev Biol. 1973;33:171–84.
18. Leese, H.J. (1991). Metabolism of the preimplantation mammalian embryo. In SR Milligan ed. Oxford reviews of reproductive biology, Vol. 13, pp 35-72 Oxford University Press.
19. Leese HJ. Energy metabolism in preimplantation development. In: Bavister BD, editor. Preimplantation embryo development. New York: Springer; 1993. p. 73–82.
20. Booth PJ, Humpherson PG, Watson TJ, Leese HJ. Amino acid depletion and appearance during porcine preimplantation embryo development in vitro. Reproduction. 2005;130:655–68.
21. Buttgereit F, Brand MD. A hierarchy of ATP-consuming processes in mammalian cells. Biochem J. 1995;312:163–7.
22. Rolfe DF, Brown GC. Cellular energy utilization and molecular origin of standard metabolic rate in mammals. Physiol Rev. 1997;77:731–58.
23. Wieser W, Krumschnabel G. Hierarchies of ATP-consuming processes: direct compared with indirect measurements and comparative aspects. Biochem J. 2001;355:389–95.
24. Leese HJ, Donnay I, Macmillan D, Houghton F. Metabolism of the early embryo: energy production and utilisation. In: Gardner DK, Lane M, editors. ART and the human blastocyst. New York: Springer; 2001. p. 61–6.
25. Alexiou M, Leese HJ. Purine utilization, de novo synthesis and degradation in mouse preimplantation embryos. Development. 1992;114:183–92.
26. Anas MK, Hammer MA, Lever M, Stanton JA, Baltz JM. The organic osmolytes betaine and proline are transported by a shared system in early preimplantation mouse embryos. J Cell Physiol. 2007;210:266.
27. Manser RC, Leese HJ, Houghton FD. Effect of inhibiting nitric oxide production on mouse preimplantation embryo development and metabolism. Biol Reprod. 2004;71:528–33.
28. Manser RC, Houghton FD. Ca^{2+}-linked upregulation and mitochondrial production of nitric oxide in the mouse preimplantation embryo. J Cell Sci. 2006;119:2048–55.
29. Lipari CW, Garcia JE, Zhao Y, Thrift K, Vaidya D, Rodriguez A. Nitric oxide metabolite production in the human preimplantation embryo and successful blastocyst formation. Fertil Steril. 2009;91:1316–8.

Further Reading

Fallon A, Booth RF, Bell LD. Applications of HPLC in biochemistry. In: Burdon RH, van Knippenberg PH, editors. Laboratory techniques in biochemistry and molecular biology. Amsterdam: Elsevier Science; 1987. p. 89.

Blake D, Farquhar C, Johnson N, Proctor M. Cleavage stage versus blastocyst stage embryo transfer in assisted conception. Cochrane Database Syst Rev. 2007;(4):CD002118.

Bolton V, Hawes S, Taylor C, et al. Development of spare human preimplantation embryos in vitro: an analysis of the correlations among gross morphology, cleavage rates and development to the blastocyst. J In Vitro Fert Embryo Transfer. 1989;6:30–5.

Khalaf Y, El-Toukhy T, Coomarasamy A, et al. Selective single blastocyst transfer reduces the multiple pregnancy rate and increases pregnancy rates: a pre and post intervention study. BJOG. 2008;115:385–90.

Papanikoloau E, D'haeseleer E, Verheyen G, et al. Live birth rate is significantly higher after blastocyst transfer than after cleavage stage embryo transfer when at least 4 embryos are available on day 3 of embryo culture. A randomized prospective study. Hum Reprod. 2005;20:3198–203.

Chapter 21
Real-Time Embryo Monitoring Device for Embryo Selection

Gábor Vajta and Thorir Hardarson

Noninvasive methods for evaluation of the quality and prediction of developmental competence of in vitro-produced preimplantation-stage embryos are of crucial importance in human-assisted reproduction. Currently, one of the most demanding tasks in this field is to find the optimal solution between two partially contradicting requirements: to achieve the highest pregnancy (and live birth) rates and to keep the proportion of multiple pregnancies at a minimum level. The most feasible approach to meet these requirements is the extended culture and decreased number of transferred embryos; the former may result in the survival of the best embryos, while the latter decreases the chance of multiple implantation [1]. The ultimate realization of this strategy is the single blastocyst transfer [2–4]. Former concerns related to the compromised cryosurvival of blastocysts and decreased chances of a subsequent cryocycle have been mostly eliminated with the introduction of highly efficient vitrification techniques [5–7].

This strategy, however, is not always applicable to all patients. Although conditions of embryo culture have improved considerably, they are still regarded as handicapped compared to the in vivo situation. Accordingly, the best place for preimplantation development is the maternal oviduct and uterus, and extended culture may endanger the success of the assisted reproductive cycle, especially when the number of available oocytes is limited and/or the development at the early cleavage stages is compromised. The growing application of minimal stimulation may result in developmentally more competent oocytes and more appropriate in vivo environment for implantation, but decreases the number of obtainable oocytes. Accordingly, the decision regarding the most optimal timing of embryo transfer may become even more complicated.

G. Vajta, MD, PhD, DSc (✉)
Vajta Embryology Consulting, Rakosi and Vajta Trust, Brinsmead, QLD, Australia
e-mail: gabor.vajta@hotmail.com

T. Hardarson, PhD
Fertility Center Scandinavia, Gothenburg, Sweden

Z.P. Nagy et al. (eds.), *Clinical Embryology: A Practical Guide*,
DOI 10.1007/978-1-4614-8376-2_21,

At present, the only routine method for this prediction and selection is the bi-daily light microscopic evaluation of the morphology. The limits of this approach are widely acknowledged and are related to the snapshot type analysis of dynamic processes [8, 9]. Accordingly, there is an increasing need for alternative methods. Possibilities include specific investigation of certain structures or combined evaluation of morphological features, and sophisticated indirect analysis of intracellular processes by measuring changes in certain parameters in surrounding media [10–16]. A third approach is the real-time light microscopic monitoring of embryo development by using time-lapse photography.

Development of Methods for Time-Lapse Investigations

The idea to apply time-lapse techniques in mammalian embryology is almost as old as the successful embryo culture itself. The first time-lapse investigations on preimplantation embryos were performed in rabbits as early as in 1929 by Lewis and Gregory, followed by investigations in mice [17–19] and in cattle [20, 21], with the purpose to observe some changes in structure elements or to analyze mechanism of dynamic processes including expansion and hatching. These studies were extended later to measurements of cell cycle length, investigation of compaction, blastocoel formation, and compare the effects of various culture conditions [22, 23]. As a more complex task, time-lapse observations were also used to predict developmental competence and sex in golden hamster and mouse embryos [24, 25]. In humans, oocyte activation, pronuclear formation, and cleavage after intracytoplasmic sperm injection were studied with this technology [16]. Time-lapse investigation has helped to understand the mechanism of polar body extrusion and pronuclear formation [26] and provided a direct evidence about the reversible nature of fragmentations [7, 27]. Early disappearance of pronuclei and onset of the first cleavage were found to be correlated with a higher number of blastomeres on Day 2 after oocyte retrieval, proving the predictive potential of time-lapse investigations regarding early-stage development of human embryos [28].

In spite of the demonstrated value of this technique, so far investigations were restricted to the experimental level, and application in an unselected cohort of patients in a routine infertility program was not reported due to the high costs, complicated structure, and the limited capacity of available equipments. Almost all previous studies have used individually designed or specially modified systems; commercial production of various time-lapse equipment has started only recently. However, the principle was the same at all: either to build up an incubator over the stage of a commercially available inverted microscope or to put a modified microscope into a commercially available incubator.

Requirements for a Time-Lapse System for Routine Application in a Standard Human Infertility Program

According to our present knowledge, a real-time light microscopic system to monitor preimplantation-stage human embryo development should meet the following criteria:

1. Provide an optically satisfactory picture suitable for safe diagnosis of key milestones and important features of preimplantation development including the size and shape of the embryo; the intactness, density, and approximate thickness of the zona pellucida; the size of the perivitelline space; intactness of the oolemma; cytoplasmic abnormalities (color, vacuoles, inclusions, granulations), formation, and number of pronuclei; cleavages; number and size of blastomeres; compaction; blastulation; size and shape of the inner cell mass; morphology of the trophectodermal layer; expansion; and hatching.
2. Enable individual identification of embryos, while monitoring in parallel at least 12–16 embryos (in most cycles, this is enough to control the development of all intact zygotes from one patient).
3. Make pictures with a reasonable frequency (the usually applied and acknowledged parameter is 4–6 pictures per hour) during the whole preimplantation period (0–6 days).
4. Due to the commonly used culture systems, enable medium changes and safe repositioning without mixing up embryos. The removal and replacement of dishes as well as the medium change itself should not be more demanding than the present routine in ART laboratories.
5. At any time point, provide pictures about the actual state of all embryos and all previous events without disturbing the safe incubation and the monitoring process. Optimally, this information should be accessible remotely by the internet for selected staff.
6. Assemble pictures into time-lapse videos, enable morphometric analysis of individual pictures, and archive files with the documentations of patients.
7. Eventually, software may also be added for automatic analysis of measurable parameters, to create quality scores of individual features or the whole embryo.
8. The real-time monitoring system should be free of any measurable or potential harm that may implement more dangers to the embryos than the routine acknowledged embryo culture procedure of the accredited ART unit.

The latter primum nil nocere (first, do not harm—Latin) principle is the basis of all medical interventions and is a key condition when new methods are introduced, even if it is an in vitro procedure and is related to preimplantation-stage embryos. Unfortunately, as also applicable to most diagnostic and therapeutic procedures, it is very difficult to meet strictly this requirement in the ART laboratory. However, efforts should be made to find the optimal solution to keep the unavoidable risks at the minimum level, and the potential benefits should highly outbalance the accidental negative effects that may occur. As real-time monitoring is not indispensable for a successful routine ART program, and its potential benefits are not supported with convincing evidences, any risks related to its application should be seriously considered and eliminated or radically minimized.

Potential sources of damage may include the following:

Frequent exposition to visible light: For most embryologist, this is the primary concern, although this factor may be controlled relatively easily. The sensitivity of mammalian embryos to light is a widely acknowledged fact, although the consensus regarding the quantitative characteristics of the harmful dose including intensity, length, and wavelength is still missing [29, 30]. Some exposition to visible light is part of the routine handling of oocytes and embryos in ART procedures both under the microscopes and in the laboratory room. A safe limit for real-time monitoring may be a maximum 10% increase in the cumulative dose, and the potential damage should also be reduced by using longer, supposedly less harmful wavelengths. These goals are relatively easy to achieve with low-intensity light, appropriate filters, and limiting illumination strictly to the period of exposition.

Physical, chemical, and biological damages related to the applied instruments: Theoretically, a stationary microscope equipped with a camera should not mean a major risk to embryo development. However, this arrangement is insufficient for a routine human infertility program where parallel investigation of different dishes, each one containing the embryos of a single patient is required. The most demanding task was to make the real-time monitoring instruments capable for parallel investigation of multiple embryos, or groups of embryos with a safe individual identification possibility for comparative evaluation.

Sophisticated automatic forwarding and focusing systems were installed both for the "incubator on the microscope" or the "microscope in the incubator" design. Unfortunately, even with the latest technical solutions, systems require complicated mechanical arrangements and advanced electronic regulations. Loading of dishes may be more demanding than placing them on the shelves of the incubator. Accordingly, this may increase the inconsistence of temperature and gas atmosphere of all investigated dishes. Additional heat from motors, electrosmog, volatile compounds of lubricants, seals, and other applied material may also cause detectable or hidden but existing damage on embryos. Sterilization and especially maintenance of sterility of these instruments is difficult or impossible; accordingly, the risk of infection is increased and, once occurs, it may hamper further investigations for long. Moreover, the required constant movement of dishes, and the consequent shear stress may compromise the development [31].

Potential risk of malfunction or breakdown: Optimally, routine application of real-time monitoring systems for human embryos would need the unachievable 100% stability or warranty that an accident occurring in the mechanical or electronic part does not make any harm in the development of observed embryos. This requirement is very difficult to fulfill. Even in commercially available carbon dioxide incubators hidden cable contact problems and related minuscule fumes may result in compromised development without detectable malfunction for months (Vajta, unpublished). The probability of such accidents increases in parallel with the complexity of instruments, number of cable contacts, motors, and moving parts.

Potential Benefits of Real-Time Video Monitoring of Embryos

As none of the available technical solutions can entirely fulfill all technical requirements including elimination of potential dangers, the benefits of application of real-time monitoring in routine human infertility programs should exceed the curiosity of professionals and patients and commercial interests by advertising services with live images from the very first moments of life of the future child. As mentioned earlier, determination of the optimal time point of transfer and selection of the developmentally most competent embryo may justify the application. However, no prospective randomized trial has been performed to investigate if using the time-lapse technique may be an independent predictor of birth. Until such trials are published, the use of the time-lapse technique remains only promising.

Time-lapse investigation may provide more precise data about the morphology and developmental kinetics than the routine bi-daily microscopic control that was reported insufficient for accurate evaluation [8, 9, 25, 28]. Some previous studies have demonstrated strong correlation between short initial cleavage cycles and the subsequent development potential of individual embryos. [31–42], although other studies alerted that extremely rapidly cleaving embryos in humans may be potentially compromised because of inappropriate imprinting and chromosomal abnormalities [43–46]. These data indicate that the more accurate the determination of the time points of cleavages, the better prediction of embryo development is possible. According to a recent investigation in mice, the most important are the first and second cleavage (to the two- and three-cell stage), respectively, while the time point of the third cleavage (to the four-cell stage) is indifferent [47].

Another crucial feature is fragmentation that may dramatically reduce pregnancy rates [48, 49], and transfer of fragmented human embryos was reported to increase rates of malformations [50]. However, in contrast to the common opinion, fragmentation is a reversible process and a fragment may disappear by resorption as rapidly as within 10 min [7], although the reabsorption does not modify the compromised developmental competence of these embryos. The chance for a fragmented mouse embryo to reach the blastocyst stage might be reduced by up to 60%, compared to non-fragmented embryos, but the average duration for fragmentation and reabsorption was only 9.1 h; accordingly, 36 or 73% of these fragmentations would not had been noticed in daily or bi-daily monitoring [47].

Real-time investigations may also be used as overall quality control measures for the actual level of embryo production of the IVF unit and may also provide early alarm of any extraordinary events that happen inside the incubators or culture dishes including infection, toxic damage of embryos, or other harmful events that are not detected by sensors or routine quality control investigations.

Finally, real-time investigations accompanied with the use of single media without medium change may eliminate the need of routine bi-daily removing of dishes from the incubator. Although most producers still suggest medium change on Day 3, routinely used highly efficient culture systems in large domestic species [51] indicate that the medium change may not be indispensable, and its disadvantages may outnumber the benefits. Slowly increasing number of human data also proves the feasibility of this approach [47]. With the application of routine time-lapse video monitoring, embryos may remain for 4 or 5 days undisturbed in the strictly regulated environments of the incubators that—according to our present knowledge—provides them optimal conditions for preimplantation development in vitro.

Latest Technical Solutions for Real-Time Monitoring

Recent devices produced individually or industrially are mostly based on the earlier principles and consist of either an incubator build above a microscope, or a microscope placed into an incubator. Variations of the former solutions included a small flat gassed and heated incubator chamber, a large box surrounding most part of the microscope, or the combined application of the two to provide even higher stability ([7, 27, 51–54]; Stage-top Incubator, Tokai-hit, Japan; references have been selected only for illustration and without any commercial or other suggestions or preference). To avoid extensive light exposition from the laboratory environment, some of these boxes have been made from nontransparent material.

No problems with the ambient light occurs when the microscope/camera is placed inside the incubator, but commercially available microscopes are not designed for this purpose and require modifications and additional equipment for applicability [25] (InCu-Cell Live, Sanyo, Japan; Bio-Station, Nikon, Japan). Some of the latest solutions combine the two approaches: a purpose-built incubator accompanied by a purpose-built microscope (Embryoscope, Unisense FertiliTech A/S, Denmark). Typically, these devices are equipped with turntables or other mechanical devices powered by electric motors to enable investigation of multiple embryos, and require also individual focusing before each photograph. Consequently, there is a possibility to expose embryos to shear stress, heat, lubricant fumes, and electromagnetic fields, and the complicated structure may also mean an increased risk of infection.

Another approach for the "microscope into the incubator" principle is a simplified compact digital inverted microscope designed to observe all embryos of a patient in one view field, by using the Well-of-the-Well culture system to locate safely the embryos (Primo-Vision, Cryo-Innovation Ltd, Hungary). The small, sealed digital microscopes are placed inside the regular incubators. The transfer of the images and the control of the microscope units are managed by a PC software through an electric controlling unit that is located outside the incubator and connected to the microscope with a shielded firewire cable through the factory-made side port of the incubator. All electricity is switched off completely in between the image acquisitions, so no potentially harmful continuous electromagnetic effects are present.

With the simplified construction and lack of movement of dishes during observation, the dangers mentioned above are eliminated, and an accidental breakdown would not influence at all the normal culture environment. The system has proved its value for prediction of in vitro developmental competence of mouse embryos [52], and the first human pregnancy after continuous monitoring to the blastocyst stage has also been achieved [55].

Future applications of time-lapse equipment may include observation of embryo development in new culture systems including microfluidic-microchannel devices that will allow for media change/gradient coupled with the possibility of analyzing the spent culture media using advanced diagnostic techniques.

Another potential advancement may include automatic analysis of several patters including cleavages, size of blastomeres, fragmentation, or other features with potential predictive value. Some time-lapse devices are already equipped with programs that are capable for limited automatic evaluations. Further development of these softwares and their widespread application may considerably increase the predictive value regarding implantation potential and full-term development.

Acknowledgment The authors wish to say thanks to Csaba Pribenszky for his extensive support in creation and correction of this manuscript.

References

1. Quea G, Romero K, Garcia-Velasco JA. Extended embryo culture to increase implantation rate. Reprod Biomed Online. 2007;14:375–83.
2. Gardner DK, Lane M. Towards a single embryo transfer. Reprod Biomed Online. 2003;6: 470–81.
3. Bhattacharya S, Templeton A. What is the most relevant standard of success in assisted reproduction?: Redefining success in the context of elective single embryo transfer: evidence, intuition and financial reality. Hum Reprod. 2004;19:1939–42.
4. Pandian Z, Templeton A, Serour G, et al. Number of embryos for transfer after IVF and ICSI: a Cochrane review. Hum Reprod. 2005;20:2681–7.
5. Loutradi KE, Kolibianakis EM, Venetis CA, et al. Cryopreservation of human embryos by vitrification or slow freezing: a systematic review and meta-analysis. Fertil Steril. 2008;90:186–93.
6. Youssry M, Ozmen B, Zohni K, et al. Current aspects of blastocyst cryopreservation. Reprod Biomed Online. 2008;16:311–20.
7. Hardarson T, Löfman C, Coull G, et al. Internalization of cellular fragments in a human embryo: time-lapse recordings. Reprod Biomed Online. 2002;5:36–8.
8. Cummins JM, Breen TM, Harrison KL, et al. A formula for scoring human embryo growth rates in *in-vitro* fertilization: its value in predicting pregnancy and in comparison with visual estimates of embryo quality. J In Vitro Fert Embryo Transf. 1986;3:284–95.
9. Emiliani S, Fasano G, Vandamme B, et al. Impact of the assessment of early cleavage in a single embryo transfer policy. Reprod Biomed Online. 2006;13:255–60.
10. Booth PJ, Watson TJ, Leese HJ. Prediction of porcine blastocyst formation using morphological, kinetic, and amino acid depletion and appearance criteria determined during the early cleavage of *in vitro*-produced embryos. Biol Reprod. 2007;77:765–79.
11. Singh R, Sinclair KD. Metabolomics: approaches to assessing oocyte and embryo quality. Theriogenology. 2007;68S:S56–62.

12. Montag M, van der Ven H. Symposium: innovative techniques in human embryo viability assessment. Oocyte assessment and embryo viability prediction: birefringence imaging. Reprod Biomed Online. 2008;17:454–60.
13. Scott L, Berntsen J, Davies D, et al. Symposium: innovative techniques in human embryo viability assessment. Human oocyte respiration-rate measurement—potential to improve oocyte and embryo selection? Reprod Biomed Online. 2008;17:461–9.
14. Sturmey RG, Brison DR, Leese HJ. Symposium: innovative techniques in human embryo viability assessment. Assessing embryo viability by measurement of amino acid turnover. Reprod Biomed Online. 2008;17:486–96.
15. Katz-Jaffe MG, McReynolds S, Gardner DK, et al. The role of proteomics in defining the human embryonic secretome. Mol Hum Reprod. 2009;15(5):271–7.
16. Nagy ZP, Jones-Colon S, Roos P, et al. Metabolomic assessment of oocyte viability. Reprod Biomed Online. 2009;18:219–25.
17. Lewis WH, Gregory PW. Cinematographs of living developing rabbit eggs. Science. 1929;69: 226–9.
18. Cole RJ. Cinemicrographic observations on the trophoblast and zona pellucida of the mouse blastocyst. J Embryol Exp Morphol. 1967;17:481–90.
19. Mulnard JG. Analyse microcinématographique du développement de l'oeuf de souris du stade II au blastocyte. Archs Biol. 1967;78:107–38.
20. Wright RW, Anderson GB, Cupps PT, Drost M. Blastocyst expansion and hatching of bovine ova cultured *in vitro*. J Anim Sci. 1976;43:170–4.
21. Massip A, Mulnard J. Time-lapse cinematographic analysis of hatching of normal and frozen—thawed cow blastocysts. J Reprod Fertil. 1980;58:475–8.
22. Morgan K, Wiemer K, Steuerwald N, Hoffman D, Maxson W, Godke IL. Use of videocinematugraphy to assess morphological qualities of conventionally cultured and cocultured embryos. Hum Reprod. 1995;10:2371–6.
23. Van Langendonckt A, Auquier P, Dormay I, Massip A, Dessy F. Acceleration of in vitro bovine embryo development in the presence of calf serum. Theriogenology. 1996;45:194.
24. Gonzales DS, Pinherio JC, Bavister BD. Prediction of the developmental potential of hamster embryos in vitro by precise timing of the third cell cycle. J Reprod Fertil. 1995;105:1–8.
25. Arav A, Aroyo A, Yavin S, et al. Prediction of embryonic developmental competence by time-lapse observation and 'shortest half' analysis. Reprod Biomed Online. 2008;17:669–75.
26. Payne D, Flaherty SP, Barry MF, et al. Preliminary observations on polar body extrusion and pronuclear formation in human oocytes using time-lapse video cinematography. Hum Reprod. 1997;12:531–41.
27. Van Blerkom J, Davis P, Alexander S. A microscopic and biochemical study of fragmentation phenotypes in stage-appropriate human embryos. Hum Reprod. 2001;16:719–29.
28. Lemmen JG, Agerholm I, Ziebe S. Kinetic markers of human embryo quality using time-lapse recordings of IVF/ICSI-fertilized oocytes. Reprod Biomed Online. 2008;17:385–91.
29. Takenaka M, Horiuchi T, Yanagimachi R. Effects of light on development of mammalian zygotes. Proc Natl Acad Sci USA. 2007;104:14289–93.
30. Oh SJ, Gong SP, Lee ST, Lee EJ, Lim JM. Light intensity and wavelength during embryo manipulation are important factors for maintaining viability of preimplantation embryos in vitro. Fertil Steril. 2007;88:1150–7.
31. Xie Y, Wang F, Zhong W, et al. Shear stress induces preimplantation embryo death that is delayed by the zona pellucida and associated with stress-activated protein kinase-mediated apoptosis. Biol Reprod. 2006;75:45–55.
32. Edwards R, Fishel S, Cohen J. Factors influencing the success of *in vitro* fertilization for alleviating human infertility. J In Vitro Fert Embryo Transf. 1984;1:3–23.
33. Fenwick J, Platteau P, Mucdoch AP, et al. Time from insemination to first cleavage predicts developmental competence of human preimplantation embryos *in vitro*. Hum Reprod. 2002;17:407–12.
34. Bos-Mikich A, Mattos ALG, Ferrari AN. Early cleavage of human embryos: an effective method for predicting successful IVF/ICSI outcome. Hum Reprod. 2001;16:2658–61.

35. Giorgettic C, Hans E, Terriou P, et al. Early cleavage: an additional predictor of high implantation rate following elective single embryo transfer. Reprod Biomed Online. 2007;14:85–91.
36. Lundin K, Bergh C, Hardarson T. Early embryo cleavage is a strong indicator of embryo quality. In: Third Biennial Alpha Conference, New York, NY, USA; 2001, Vol 3, Suppl 1, p. 52 [abstract].
37. Rienzi L, Ubaldi F, Iacobelli M, et al. Significance of morphological attributes of the early embryo. Reprod Biomed Online. 2005;10:669–81.
38. Hesters L, Prisant N, Fanchin R, et al. Impact of early cleaved zygote morphology on embryo development and *in vitro* fertilization-embryo transfer outcome: a prospective study. Fertil Steril. 2008;89:1677–84.
39. Luna M, Copperman AB, Duke M, et al. Human blastocyst morphological quality is significantly improved in embryos classified as fast on day 3 (>or = 10 cells), bringing into question current embryological dogma. Fertil Steril. 2008;89:358–63.
40. Montfoort A, Dumoulin J, et al. Early cleavage is a valuable addition to existing embryo selection parameters: a study using single embryo transfers. Hum Reprod. 2004;19:2103–8.
41. Petersen CG, Mauri AL, Ferreira R, et al. Embryo selection by the first cleavage parameter between 25 and 27 hours after ICSl. J Assist Reprod Genet. 2001;18:209–12.
42. Windt M-L, Krueger TF, Coetzee K, et al. Comparative analysis of pregnancy rates after the transfer of early dividing embryos versus slower dividing embryos. Hum Reprod. 2004; 19:1155–62.
43. Harper J, Robinson F, Duffy S. Detection of fertilization in embryos with accelerated cleavage by fluorescence *in situ* hybridization. Hum Reprod. 1994;9:1733–7.
44. Ziebe S, Peterson K, Lindenberg S, et al. Embryo morphology or cleavage stage: how to select the best embryos for transfer after *in vitro* fertilization. Hum Reprod. 1997;12:1545–9.
45. Magli M, Gianaroli L, Munne S, et al. Incidence of chromosomal abnormalities from a morphological normal cohort of embryos in poor prognosis patients. J Assist Reprod Genet. 1998;15:297–301.
46. Alikani M, Calderon G, Tomkin G, et al. Cleavage anomalies in early human embryos and survival after prolonged culture *in vitro*. Hum Reprod. 2000;15:2634–43.
47. Pribenszky C, Losonczi E, Molnár M, Lang Z. Prediction of in-vitro developmental competence of early cleavage-stage mouse embryos with compact time-lapse equipment. Reprod Biomed Online. 2010;20(3):371–9.
48. Elder K, Cohen J. Human preimplantation embryo selection. Boca Raton: CRC; 2007.
49. Ragione T, Verheyen G, Papanikolaou EG, et al. Developmental stage on day-5 and fragmentation rate on day-3 can influence the implantation potential of top-quality blastocysts in IVF cycles with single embryo transfer. Reprod Biol Endocrinol. 2007;5:2.
50. Ebner T, Yaman C, Moser M, et al. Embryo fragmentation *in vitro* and its impact on treatment and pregnancy outcome. Fertil Steril. 2001;76:281–5.
51. Holm P, Booth PJ, Callesen H. Kinetics of early *in vitro* development of bovine *in vivo*- and *in vitro*-derived zygotes produced and/or cultured in chemically defined or serum-containing media. Reproduction. 2002;123:553–65.
52. Bavister BD. A mini-chamber device for maintaining a constant carbon dioxidein air atmosphere during prolonged culture of cells on the stage of an inverted microscope. In Vitro Cell Dev Biol. 1988;24:759–63.
53. Holm P, Shukri NN, Vajta G, Booth P, Bendixen C, Callesen H. Developmental kinetics of the first cell cycles of bovine in vitro produced embryos in relation to their in vitro viability and sex. Theriogenology. 1998;50:1285–99.
54. Mio Y, Maeda K. Time-lapse cinematography of dynamic changes occurring during in vitro development of human embryos. Am J Obstet Gynecol. 2008;199:660.e1–5.
55. Pribenszky C, Kovács P, Mátyás S, Molnár M, Rajczy K, Molnár K, Nagy P, Losonczi E, Zádori J, Sprőber P, Kaáli SG, Vajta G. Pregnancy achieved by transfer of a single blastocyst selected by timelapse monitoring. Reprod Biomed Online. 2010;21(4):533–6.

Chapter 22
Predicting Embryo Developmental Potential and Viability Using Automated Time-Lapse Analysis (Eeva Test)

Alice A. Chen and Shehua Shen

Introduction

In in vitro fertilization (IVF) practice, technologies or tests that can help assess the viability and developmental competence of embryos may not only improve IVF success rates; they may also enable broader adoption of single embryo transfer, which would in turn reduce multiple gestation pregnancies and lower associated maternal/fetal risks [1]. Currently, standard embryo assessment methods depend on morphological evaluation by microscope at a few static points in time (e.g., Day 1, Day 2, Day 3, and Day 5 post-insemination) [2, 3]. Morphological evaluation and selection, however, has lacked underlying biological understanding and sufficient predictability for implantation due to the inherent subjectivity of morphological grading [4–6] and the weak correlation between morphology and embryonic health [7–9]. Without predictive and objective tools that can supplement morphology, clinical embryologists are routinely forced to make their best guess of which embryo(s) to transfer among morphologically similar embryos.

New research in embryo assessment promises to provide additional information to help discriminate among morphologically similar embryos and improve the likelihood of selecting the single embryo that will successfully develop, implant, and result in a live birth. However, before new tools and technologies can be introduced into the IVF laboratory, several validation steps should be taken to ensure their safety, accuracy, and efficacy. These steps, which follow the initial discovery and development phases, may include biological validation, clinical validation, performance characterization, and comparison to standard of care [10]. Increasingly, clinical

Note: The *Eeva™* Test is CE Mark approved in Europe and limited to investigational use only in the USA as of the date of publication.

A.A. Chen, Ph.D. (✉) • S. Shen, M.D.
Auxogyn, Inc., 1490 O'Brien Drive, Suite A, Menlo Park, CA 94025, USA
e-mail: achen@auxogyn.com

Z.P. Nagy et al. (eds.), *Clinical Embryology: A Practical Guide*,
DOI 10.1007/978-1-4614-8376-2_22,

practitioners and patients also expect successful validation to result in approval from a regulatory body [11]. In this case, the regulatory body would require the intended use of the new tool or technology to be clearly stated and validated.

The objective of this chapter is to describe the development, validation, and practical application of the first noninvasive, embryo viability assessment tool that has been designed to meet clinical test criteria and proven to add critical information to the decision-making practices of clinical embryologists. In describing this novel test, we review the criteria for development and validation of a clinical test, assess the scientific underpinning of prediction using time-lapse imaging, and introduce new advances in automation enabled by state-of-the-art computer vision software.

Clinical Testing

The goal of clinical testing is to help clinicians improve assessment or treatment decisions by determining a disease risk probability (in the case of a screening test) or diagnosing a disease (in the case of a diagnostic test) [12]. Typically, a clinical test is developed against a reference standard test that is more invasive, more risky, or prohibitively expensive. A clinical test may also be developed as a first-pass surrogate for a more invasive procedure (e.g., venous ultrasonography serves as a surrogate marker of vein thrombosis and reduces the need for a highly invasive venography procedure [13]; cell-free fetal DNA analysis of maternal blood can detect fetal genetic anomalies without requiring invasive amniocentesis or chorionic villus sampling procedures [14]).

In clinical embryology, several noninvasive candidate technologies have been proposed as surrogates for invasive embryo assessment and predictors of embryo developmental potential, including culture media assessment [15–17], cumulus cell assessment [18, 19], and time-lapse imaging [20–22]. Parallel advances in assay and embryo biopsy techniques have resulted in increased use of preimplantation genetic screening (PGS) and preimplantation genetic diagnostics (PGD) together with blastocyst culture for assessing not only the genetic and chromosomal status of an embryo but also its overall implantation potential [23, 24]. While embryo biopsy is invasive to the embryo and typically relevant for IVF patients indicating a need for PGS or PGD, noninvasive technologies have the potential to be more economical and more broadly applicable. However, most noninvasive technologies are in early development stages; as such, they have not been prospectively validated in independent clinical trials and lack the basic prerequisites for successful clinical translation.

Three major requirements are needed in order to successfully implement a novel embryo assessment technology or test into the IVF laboratory. First, a predictive biomarker based on scientific evidence and validated in clinical studies must be associated with a confirmable and desirable outcome. Second, the detection of the predictive biomarker must be accurate, reliable, and practical to use by clinicians. Finally, the combined test (predictive biomarker + detection method) must be characterized for performance and shown to provide actionable information that improves the standard of care. In addition to these major requirements, scientists have increasingly demanded that new technologies be brought to patients via an evidence-based approach that includes basic research, which provides scientific understanding and clinical confidence in the test [10, 11, 22]. In a recent review, Palmer et al. noted that in reproductive medicine, it is common for only the first milestone—report of a novel biomarker correlation—to be achieved; whereas, successful culmination of all milestones ideally results in content for regulatory submission documents and eventual regulatory approval [11]. In support of this approach, new standards for reporting diagnostic accuracy (STARD) are being required of authors seeking to publish new test results [25].

The Eeva Test

The *Eeva™* Test (Auxogyn; Menlo Park, CA, USA) was designed with clinical test criteria in mind and combines both a highly robust predictive marker of embryo development and a novel detection assay to rapidly obtain quantitative measurements of the biomarker in a clinical setting. Briefly, the Eeva Test consists of: (1) a multi-well dish that provides individual culture for embryos with the same media drop, (2) an imaging system that collects data inside a standard incubator, and (3) intelligent software that analyzes and measures cell division timings. Collectively, Eeva provides quantitative information regarding embryo development by Day 3 (Fig. 22.1). Below we detail the underlying science and technology behind Eeva, and

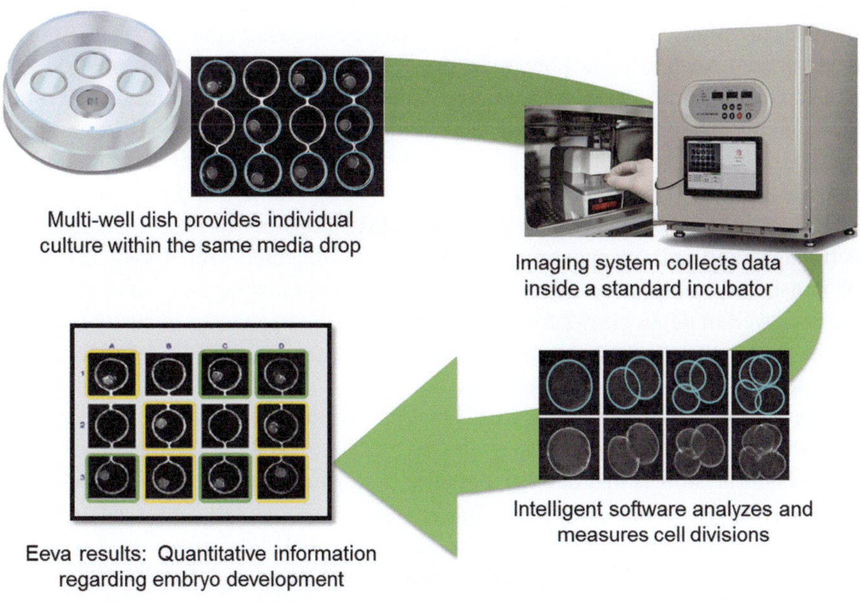

Fig. 22.1 The Eeva™ Test in the IVF laboratory workflow

we further describe clinical results from the first prospective, multicenter study that compares the use of Eeva results combined with morphology (adjunctive grading method) against morphology alone (traditional morphology grading method).

Predictive Information Enabled BY Time-Lapse

The first major requirement of a clinical test is identifying a predictive biomarker with strong correlation to a measureable, clinical outcome. Recently, increasing availability and usage of time-lapse imaging systems—both homemade and commercial variations—have enabled researchers to identify potential image biomarkers during human embryo culture in a safe and noninvasive manner. Time-lapse systems currently vary in a number of ways, harboring variations in format/footprint (e.g., some are enclosed in stand-alone box formats [26, 27], while others integrate seamlessly with conventional incubators [28–31]), embryo culture environment (e.g., some require individual culture of embryos [27], while others enable group culture [28–31]), and mode of illumination (e.g., most offer brightfield imaging while others offer darkfield or multimodal imaging). Importantly, all systems inherently have optical alignment, focusing, image capture, and image storage capabilities and utilize low power illumination that exposes embryos to overall less light than conventional microscopy [27, 29, 31]. As a result of these advances, the clinical embryology field has been able to study the function and consequences of dynamics occurring during human embryo development and explore application to clinical practice.

Time-lapse imaging in clinical embryology has a relatively long history that can be broken into two phases: an observational phase and a predictive phase. Beginning in 1997, time-lapse imaging had been focused on observing new aspects of embryo development, such as polar body extrusion, fertilization, pronuclear formation and abuttal, cytoplasmic flares, and embryo hatching [26, 32–34]. Since 2010, time-lapse imaging has shifted focus to identifying predictive parameters that can help assess developmental outcomes of the embryo, such as blastocyst development, implantation, and most recently ploidy [27, 29, 30]. Numerous publications since 2010 have reported statistically significant correlations between time durations of cell stages and embryo outcomes. These studies, together with studies that have demonstrated safety of time-lapse and continuous monitoring of human embryos, are reviewed in detail elsewhere [20–22]. Overall, the increasing intensity of interest in time-lapse suggests that noninvasive biomarker discovery is feasible, ongoing, and promising for use in the clinic.

Time-lapse biomarkers have great potential as predictive clinical tests, but the reproducibility of their predictive ability is critical to validating clinical utility. An analysis of the studies that defined a precise time window for embryo development prediction showed that the major predictors are biomarkers observed in early embryo development, before the 5-cell stage. In particular, the time from 2-to-3 cell (P2) and the time from 3-to-4 cell (P3) were reported in six out of seven of the studies that investigated which embryos are most likely to become a blastocyst, implant, or be euploid [27, 29, 35–37] (Fig. 22.2) and several following reports [35, 38].

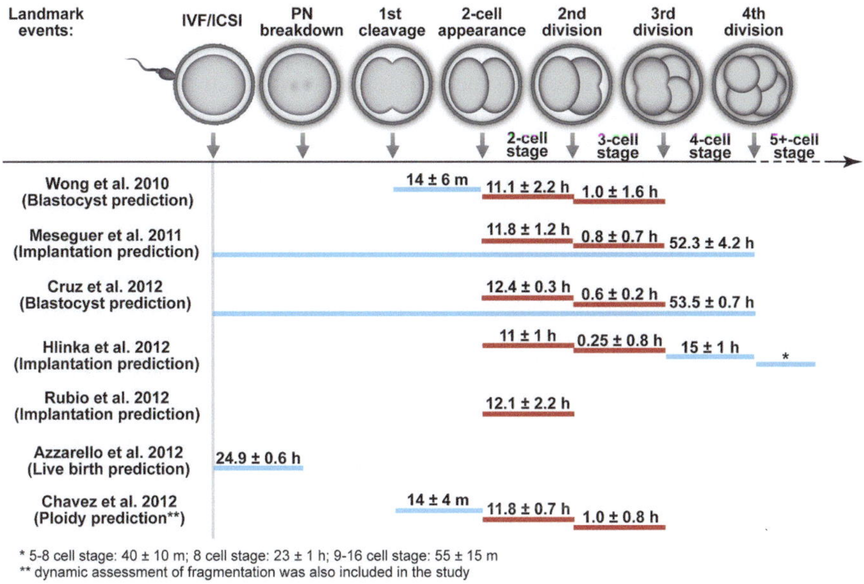

Fig. 22.2 Overview of published time-lapse biomarkers that are predictive of clinical outcomes. Landmark events captured by time-lapse imaging are mapped to the progression of preimplantation embryo development. Time-lapse biomarkers that have been used for prediction in at least three publications—and are implemented in the Eeva Test—are colored dark red while others are *colored light blue*. Average values for embryo outcomes within the optimally predictive windows are labeled above *colored bars* (Adapted with permission from [22])

These P2 and P3 timings were consistent embryo viability predictors even when stimulation protocols [39], fertilization methods [40], culture media [41, 42], and culture environments [43] were varied. In addition to clinical reproducibility, mechanistic studies have also demonstrated that embryos with abnormal P2 and P3 timings exhibit distinct gene expression profiles [29], aneuploidy probabilities [30], and micronuclei patterns [30], compared to embryos with normal P2 and P3 timings. This collection of evidence supports the conclusion that P2 and P3 are reliable across independent datasets, and moreover, are grounded in basic scientific understanding. Development of the Eeva Test, therefore, was based on (1) incorporation of P2 and P3 into a simple classification tree and prediction algorithm and (2) development of intelligent image analysis software that could reliably measure P2 and P3 in a busy clinical laboratory.

Automation Enabled by Intelligent Software

The second major requirement of a clinical test is that it is technically reliable, accurate, and practical for daily laboratory use. Although time-lapse biomarkers may provide great clinical value, extraction of these markers requires manual assessment of hundreds of images per embryo, which would be prohibitively time-consuming and laborious for routine use. In order for predictive time-lapse biomarkers to be clinically realized, novel detection methods are required to automatically extract and quantify image data in a high-throughput fashion.

Computer vision software that can analyze embryo videos in real time is now transforming the time-lapse imaging field and allowing predictive biomarkers to be rapidly quantified in the clinical laboratory. Image analysis software is widespread in many areas of clinical laboratory medicine, such as oncology and pathology. In reproductive medicine, software tools for quantitative and rapid image analysis of sperm quality [44] and for screening cervical cytology samples [45, 46] are also available. Applied to clinical embryology, image analysis software is particularly challenging due to several unique features of the developing human embryo. Blastomeres of the human embryo may divide in multiple dimensions (e.g., in and out of plane) and may include confounding events (e.g., fragmentation, reverse cleavage, abnormal cleavage). In addition, for each patient, multiple embryos developing at variable rates must be surveyed.

In their 2010 report demonstrating the first use of three cell cycle parameters to predict embryo development, Wong et al. also established the first proof-of-concept of cell tracking software used to measure the cell cycle parameters in human embryos [29]. The Wong et al. approach utilized computer vision techniques to simulate images and compare the simulations to observed image data for 14 cryo-preserved embryos. In their study, dark field imaging was employed as it provided strong contrast of blastomere membranes for model estimations. The development of the Eeva Test introduced a data driven probabilistic framework that uses approximate inference to quantify P2 and P3, and validated Eeva's predictive performance for approximately 1,000 fresh human embryos [31]. Eeva software predictions were shown to have good (>90 %) agreement with manual predictions made by human observers [31]. Separate from this technological advance, other groups have performed research to help automate the morphological analysis of static embryo images to the blastocyst stage [47, 48] and the detection of cytoplasmic waves generated post-fertilization [49]. Since the objective in designing the Eeva Test was to provide embryologists with quantitative information about embryo development, the test focused on the clinically and scientifically validated predictive markers P2 and P3 and integrated automated software to quantify these validated parameters.

Clinical Outcomes for Eeva

The final and often most elusive requirement for a novel clinical embryology test is that it is characterized for performance and shown to improve the standard of care. When performing a retrospective study, it is relatively straightforward to extract one or more promising biomarkers from a sampling of time-lapse videos. However, it is challenging and significantly less common to demonstrate comparable performance of the biomarker on an independent set of prospectively collected test data from multiple centers. It is rarer still that new potential selection methods are compared to traditional embryo selection methods based on morphology. Here we describe how Eeva provides actionable information that may improve current embryo selection based on morphology.

Eeva Study Design and Independent Validation

Following the development of the integrated Eeva Test, we conducted a prospective, five-center clinical study that was designed to assess its performance on a diverse and independent clinical dataset and to evaluate the effectiveness and utility of using the test as an adjunct to traditional morphological assessment (ClinicalTrials.gov #NCT01369446) [31]. Specifically, we sought to test Eeva's ability to assist embryologists in selecting embryos that have the greatest potential to develop into usable blastocysts (i.e., blastocysts suitable for transfer or freezing) as well as Eeva's impact on embryologists' embryo selection decisions.

Our initial results demonstrating the predictive power of time-lapse biomarkers P2 and P3 for identifying embryos with high developmental competence were consistent with Wong et al. and other successive studies [29]. Using refined cutoffs of P2: 9.33–11.45 h and P3:0–1.73 h, Eeva automatically differentiated a usable blastocyst from arrested embryo with significantly improved diagnostic specificity (85 %) compared to traditional morphology (57 %, $p<0.0001$) [31]. Specificity, or the ability to correctly predict which embryos will arrest, is highly relevant to embryo selection since traditional morphology is most limited in selecting among "good morphology" embryos. Furthermore, the development and validation of the Eeva Test was performed on clinical data collected from five IVF clinics undergoing their own standard procedures for stimulation, egg retrieval, embryo culture, and insemination, suggesting broad applicability of Eeva in diverse clinical embryology laboratories.

Eeva Improves Embryo Selection

Since clinical embryologists are faced daily with the challenge of selecting among several comparable embryos those which are the top candidates for transfer, it was important to assess the impact of Eeva on embryologists' embryo assessment decisions. Our prospective study design evaluated the embryo assessment of three experienced clinical embryologists for 755 embryos. Two methods of embryo assessment were compared: in the first arm, embryologists made predictions about embryo development using Day 3 morphology only (traditional grading method); in the second arm, the same embryologists made predictions about embryo development using Day 3 morphology plus Eeva results (adjunctive grading method) (Fig. 22.3a). When Eeva was used adjunctively with Day 3 morphology, each embryologist's likelihood of selecting embryos that would develop to blastocysts was significantly improved

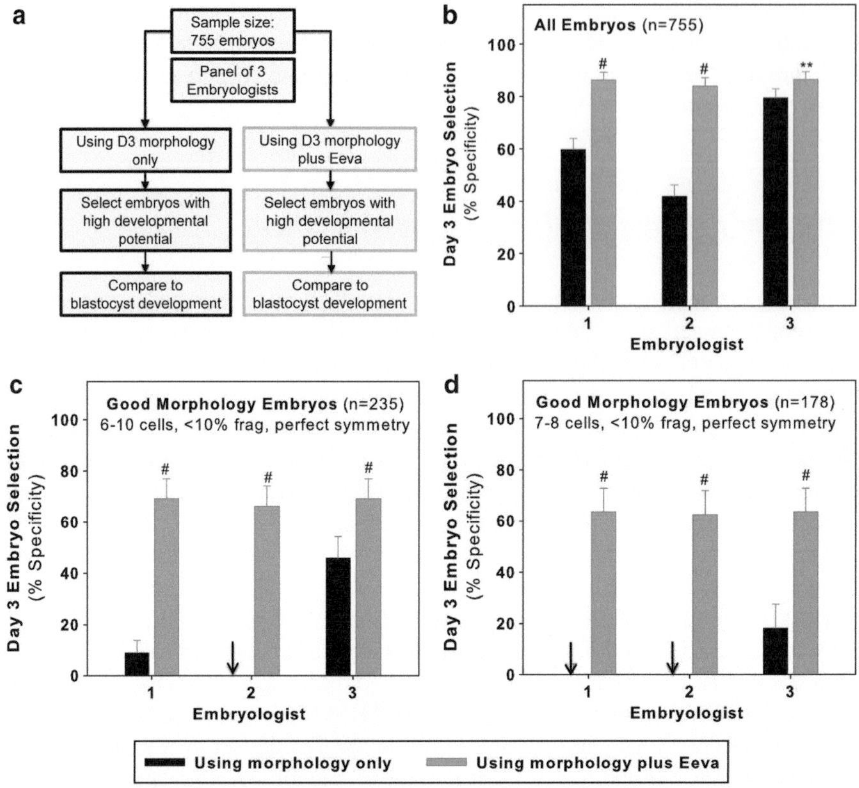

Fig. 22.3 Adjunctive use of D3 morphology plus Eeva results significantly improves the specificity of D3 embryo selection. (**a**) Design for an embryo selection cohort study comparing the use of D3 morphology vs. D3 morphology plus Eeva results. (**b–d**) D3 embryo selection by individual embryologists (1, 2, and 3) using morphology only versus morphology plus Eeva for (**b**) all embryos ($n=755$), (**c**) "good morphology" embryos ($n=235$), defined using a criteria of 6–10 cells, <10 % fragmentation, and perfect symmetry, and (**d**) "good morphology" embryos ($n=178$), defined using a more stringent criteria of 7–8 cells, <10 % fragmentation, and perfect symmetry. Note that embryologists 1 and 2 were very conservative in their morphology assessments and expected that almost all D3 "good morphology" embryos would become usable blastocysts. Error bars represent upper 95 % confidence interval. $^{**}p<0.01$, $\#p<0.0001$ (Adapted with permission from [31])

compared to traditional morphology methods alone (Fig. 22.3b). This improvement was augmented among a subset of $n=235$ embryos that were pre-selected as having "good" morphology (6–10 cells, <10 % fragmentation, perfect symmetry) (Fig. 22.3c) and a subset of $n=178$ embryos where "good" morphology was more stringently defined (7–8 cells, <10 % fragmentation, perfect symmetry) (Fig. 22.3d). As expected, each case demonstrated remarkably high interindividual variability when morphology alone was used for embryo assessment. The ability to predict blastocyst formation by Day 3 has clinical value as it could potentially improve IVF success rates while avoiding the risks associated with extended culture for blastocyst transfer [50–55].

Eeva Reduces Variability

Using Eeva results as an adjunct to morphology, the average of the three embryologists' prediction specificities were significantly improved (68.2 ± 1.7 % for morphology plus Eeva vs. 18.3 ± 23.3 % for morphology alone, $p<0.05$) [31]. The embryologists' performances were also more consistent, as the standard deviation among embryologists was reduced. Since intra- and inter-operator variability in morphological grading has been shown to negatively impact IVF success rates [4, 6], adjunctive use of the Eeva Test may improve the standardization, reproducibility, and ultimate success of Day 3 embryo selection.

Eeva Correlates to Implantation and Pregnancy

While the first critical steps in developing the Eeva Test as a predictive and automated clinical assay have been achieved, further work is needed to confirm the impact of Eeva results on implantation and pregnancy outcomes. Towards this goal, we performed a first analysis examining whether the time-lapse markers used by the Eeva Test correlate with implantation and pregnancy outcomes. We focused our analysis on embryos that were transferred at the blastocyst stage using standard morphological selection criteria (without Eeva results). Of 141 embryos transferred at the blastocyst stage, those embryos denoted by Eeva as having a high probability to develop (Eeva High indicating P2: 9.33–11.45 h and P3:0–1.73 h) had a statistically higher chance of implantation than those embryos denoted by Eeva as having a low probability to develop (Eeva Low indicated by P2 or P3 out of specific timing windows) (49 % vs. 21 %, $p<0.001$) (Fig. 22.4). Similarly, for these 77 blastocyst transfer patients, those with at least one Eeva High embryo transferred were more likely to achieve clinical pregnancy (60 % vs. 40 %, $p=0.09$) and ongoing pregnancy (56 % vs. 37 %, $p=0.11$) than those with only Eeva Low embryos transferred. These results add further evidence to recent retrospective reports showing correlation between P2, P3, and implantation [27] and pregnancy outcomes [56]. Additional prospective studies with implantation and pregnancy outcomes and sufficient sample size to draw statistically significant conclusions are underway.

Conclusion and Future Work

The Eeva Test is the first clinical test that has been validated in a prospective, multicenter study and shown to add value to embryologists' morphological evaluations by improving Day 3 embryo assessment and reducing inter-observer variability. It combines both a highly robust predictive marker of embryo development and a novel automated detection assay to rapidly obtain quantitative measurements of the biomarker in the clinical embryology laboratory. Therefore, the Eeva Test meets several important prerequisites for implementation in clinical practice: it is

Patient Population	# Pts	# Embs	Avg Age (years)	Implantation Rate	Clinical Pregnancy Rate	Ongoing Pregnancy Rate
At least 1 Eeva High transferred	47	89	32.1 ± 5.2	**49%** (44/89) 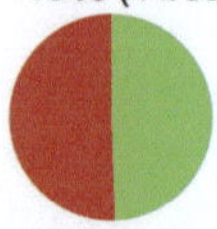	**60%** (28/47) 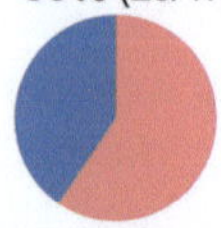	**55%** (26/47) 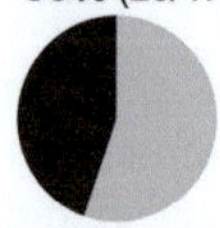
Only Eeva Lows transferred	30	52	32.2 ± 5.1	**21%** (11/52) 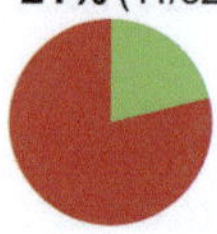	**40%** (12/30) 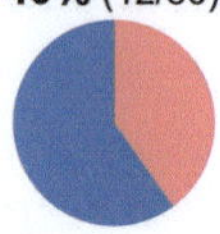	**37%** (11/30) 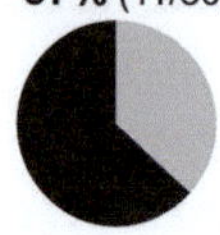
p-value			*p=0.9*	*p<0.001*	*p=0.09*	*p=0.11*

Fig. 22.4 Time-lapse markers used by the Eeva Test are correlated with positive implantation and pregnancy outcomes. A retrospective analysis of implantation and pregnancy rates was performed for two populations of patients with Eeva imaging and blastocyst transfer based on morphology only. The two patient populations included those with at least 1 Eeva High transferred (i.e., one Eeva High embryo could be transferred with another Eeva High or Eeva Low embryo) and those with only Eeva Low transferred (i.e., one or more Eeva Low embryos were transferred). The Eeva High vs. Low denominations are based on whether time-lapse markers P2 and P3 are within defined time windows (P2: 9.33–11.45 h and P3: 0–1.73 h) (Adapted with permission from [22])

scientifically and clinically validated, it considers a practical intended use model, and it has demonstrated clinical utility compared to standard of care.

This first generation platform will be further improved through planned and ongoing studies. Specifically, a prospective study focused on implantation and pregnancy is currently underway and will evaluate the implantation rates for embryos selected using Eeva as an adjunct to Day 3 morphological grading. Studies evaluating the impact to Day 5/6 morphology-based selection are also warranted, as blastocyst culture is an independent strategy for embryo selection that may be circumvented with earlier Eeva information. In parallel, we continue to identify promising time-lapse biomarker candidates, rigorously validate their clinical robustness, and iterate our automation and prediction algorithms. Future versions of the Eeva Test may incorporate complementary morphological features and timings, blastocyst stage milestones, and other prospectively validated parameters. We expect that automated analysis of these more complex morphological and timing features will require increasingly sophisticated approaches and likely a combination of illumination techniques. The introduction of any automated algorithm will be accompanied with the full spectrum of clinical validation steps described here to ensure safety and efficacy for clinical use.

Acknowledgments We gratefully acknowledge the physicians, embryologists, and patients who participated in the development and validation of Eeva, including Dr.'s Susan P. Willman, Kristen Ivani, Philip E. Chenette, Joe Conaghan, Robert Boostanfar, Anh Le, Valerie L. Baker, Mariluz Suarez, Mary E. Abusief, and Marina Gvakharia. We also thank the clinical, scientific, and computer vision groups at Auxogyn, Inc. for their technical contributions and insightful discussion.

References

1. van Montfoort AP, Dumoulin JC, Land JA, Coonen E, Derhaag JG, Evers JL. Elective single embryo transfer (eSET) policy in the first three IVF/ICSI treatment cycles. Hum Reprod. 2005;20(2):433–6.
2. Alpha E. The Istanbul consensus workshop on embryo assessment: proceedings of an expert meeting. Hum Reprod. 2011;26(6):1270–83.
3. Racowsky C, Vernon M, Mayer J, Ball GD, Behr B, Pomeroy KO, et al. Standardization of grading embryo morphology. Fertil Steril. 2010;94(3):1152–3.
4. Baxter Bendus AE, Mayer JF, Shipley SK, Catherino WH. Interobserver and intraobserver variation in day 3 embryo grading. Fertil Steril. 2006;86(6):1608–15.
5. Montag M, Liebenthron J, Koster M. Which morphological scoring system is relevant in human embryo development? Placenta. 2011;32 Suppl 3:S252–6.
6. Paternot G, Devroe J, Debrock S, D'Hooghe TM, Spiessens C. Intra- and inter-observer analysis in the morphological assessment of early-stage embryos. Reprod Biol Endocrinol. 2009;7:105.
7. Munne S, Tomkin G, Cohen J. Selection of embryos by morphology is less effective than by a combination of aneuploidy testing and morphology observations. Fertil Steril. 2009; 91(3):943–5.
8. Kroener L, Ambartsumyan G, Briton-Jones C, Dumesic D, Surrey M, Munne S, et al. The effect of timing of embryonic progression on chromosomal abnormality. Fertil Steril. 2012;98(4):876–80.
9. Alfarawati S, Fragouli E, Colls P, Stevens J, Gutierrez-Mateo C, Schoolcraft WB, et al. The relationship between blastocyst morphology, chromosomal abnormality, and embryo gender. Fertil Steril. 2011;95(2):520–4.
10. Harper J, Cristina Magli M, Lundin K, Barratt CLR, Brison D. When and how should new technology be introduced into the IVF laboratory? Hum Reprod. 2012;27(2):303–13.
11. Palmer SS, Barnhart KT. Biomarkers in reproductive medicine: the promise, and can it be fulfilled? Fertil Steril. 2013;99(4):954–62.
12. Bodurtha J, Strauss 3rd JF. Genomics and perinatal care. N Engl J Med. 2012;366(1):64–73.
13. Kucher N. Clinical practice. Deep-vein thrombosis of the upper extremities. N Engl J Med. 2011;364(9):861–9.
14. Simpson JL. Cell-free fetal DNA and maternal serum analytes for monitoring embryonic and fetal status. Fertil Steril. 2013;99(4):1124–34.
15. Hardarson T, Ahlstrom A, Rogberg L, Botros L, Hillensjo T, Westlander G, et al. Non-invasive metabolomic profiling of Day 2 and 5 embryo culture medium: a prospective randomized trial. Hum Reprod. 2012;27(1):89–96.
16. Vergouw CG, Kieslinger DC, Kostelijk EH, Botros LL, Schats R, Hompes PG, et al. Day 3 embryo selection by metabolomic profiling of culture medium with near-infrared spectroscopy as an adjunct to morphology: a randomized controlled trial. Hum Reprod. 2012;27(8): 2304–11.
17. Seli E, Robert C, Sirard MA. OMICS in assisted reproduction: possibilities and pitfalls. Mol Hum Reprod. 2010;16(8):513–30.
18. Huang Z, Wells D. The human oocyte and cumulus cells relationship: new insights from the cumulus cell transcriptome. Mol Hum Reprod. 2010;16(10):715–25.

19. Wathlet S, Adriaenssens T, Segers I, Verheyen G, Janssens R, Coucke W, et al. New candidate genes to predict pregnancy outcome in single embryo transfer cycles when using cumulus cell gene expression. Fertil Steril. 2012;98(2):432–9.e1-4.
20. Kirkegaard K, Agerholm IE, Ingerslev HJ. Time-lapse monitoring as a tool for clinical embryo assessment. Hum Reprod. 2012;27(5):1277–85.
21. Wong C, Chen A, Behr B, Shen S. Time-lapse microscopy and image analysis in basic and clinical embryo development research. Reprod Biomed Online. 2012;26(2):120–9.
22. Chen AA, Tan L, Suraj V, Reijo Pera R, Shen S. Biomarkers identified with time-lapse imaging: discovery, validation, and practical application. Fertil Steril. 2013;99(4):1035–43.
23. Yang Z, Liu J, Collins GS, Salem SA, Liu X, Lyle SS, et al. Selection of single blastocysts for fresh transfer via standard morphology assessment alone and with array CGH for good prognosis IVF patients: results from a randomized pilot study. Mol Cytogenet. 2012;5(1):24.
24. Forman EJ, Upham KM, Cheng M, Zhao T, Hong KH, Treff NR, et al. Comprehensive chromosome screening alters traditional morphology-based embryo selection: a prospective study of 100 consecutive cycles of planned fresh euploid blastocyst transfer. Fertil Steril. 2013; pii:S0015-0282(13)00557–8.
25. Ochodo EA, Bossuyt PM. reporting the accuracy of diagnostic tests: the STARD initiative 10 years on. Clin Chem. 2013;59(6):917–9.
26. Mio Y, Maeda K. Time-lapse cinematography of dynamic changes occurring during in vitro development of human embryos. Am J Obstet Gynecol. 2008;199(6):660.e1–5.
27. Meseguer M, Herrero J, Tejera A, Hilligsoe KM, Ramsing NB, Remohi J. The use of morphokinetics as a predictor of embryo implantation. Hum Reprod. 2011;26(10):2658–71.
28. Vajta G, Peura TT, Holm P, Paldi A, Greve T, Trounson AO, et al. New method for culture of zona-included or zona-free embryos: the Well of the Well (WOW) system. Mol Reprod Dev. 2000;55(3):256–64.
29. Wong C, Loewke K, Bossert N, Behr B, De Jonge C, Baer T, et al. Non-invasive imaging of human embryos before embryonic genome activation predicts development to the blastocyst stage. Nat Biotechnol. 2010;28(10):1115–21.
30. Chavez SL, Loewke KE, Han J, Moussavi F, Colls P, Munne S, et al. Dynamic blastomere behaviour reflects human embryo ploidy by the four-cell stage. Nat Commun. 2012;3:1251.
31. Conaghan J, Chen AA, Willman SP, Ivani K, Chenette PE, Boostanfar R, et al. Improving embryo selection using computer-automated time-lapse imaging plus day 3 morphology: results from a prospective multi-center trial. Fertil Steril. 2013;100(2):412–9.e5.
32. Martini E, Flaherty SP, Swann NJ, Payne D, Matthews CD. Analysis of unfertilized oocytes subjected to intracytoplasmic sperm injection using two rounds of fluorescence in-situ hybridization and probes to five chromosomes. Hum Reprod. 1997;12(9):2011–8.
33. Hardarson T, Lofman C, Coull G, Sjogren A, Hamberger L, Edwards RG. Internalization of cellular fragments in a human embryo: time-lapse recordings. Reprod Biomed Online. 2002;5(1):36–8.
34. Pribenszky C, Matyas S, Kovacs P, Losonczi E, Zadori J, Vajta G. Pregnancy achieved by transfer of a single blastocyst selected by time-lapse monitoring. Reprod Biomed Online. 2010;21(4):533–6.
35. Cruz M, Garrido N, Herrero J, Perez-Cano I, Munoz M, Meseguer M. Timing of cell division in human cleavage-stage embryos is linked with blastocyst formation and quality. Reprod Biomed Online. 2012;25(4):371–81.
36. Hlinka D, Kalatova B, Uhrinova I, Dolinska S, Rutarova J, Rezacova J, et al. Time-lapse cleavage rating predicts human embryo viability. Physiol Res. 2012;61(5):513–25.
37. Rubio I, Kuhlmann R, Agerholm I, Kirk J, Herrero J, Escribá M-J, et al. Limited implantation success of direct-cleaved human zygotes: a time-lapse study. Fertil Steril. 2012;98(6):1458–63.
38. Hashimoto S, Kato N, Saeki K, Morimoto Y. Selection of high-potential embryos by culture in poly(dimethylsiloxane) microwells and time-lapse imaging. Fertil Steril. 2012;97(2):332–7.
39. Munoz M, Cruz M, Humaidan P, Garrido N, Perez-Cano I, Meseguer M. Dose of recombinant FSH and oestradiol concentration on day of HCG affect embryo development kinetics. Reprod Biomed Online. 2012;25(4):382–9.

40. Dal Canto M, Coticchio G, Mignini Renzini M, De Ponti E, Novara PV, Brambillasca F, et al. Cleavage kinetics analysis of human embryos predicts development to blastocyst and implantation. Reprod Biomed Online. 2012;25(5):474–80.
41. Ciray HN, Aksoy T, Goktas C, Ozturk B, Bahceci M. Time-lapse evaluation of human embryo development in single versus sequential culture media—a sibling oocyte study. J Assist Reprod Genet. 2012;29(9):891–900.
42. Basile N, Morbeck D, Garcia-Velasco J, Bronet F, Meseguer M. Type of culture media does not affect embryo kinetics: a time-lapse analysis of sibling oocytes. Hum Reprod. 2013; 28(3):634–41.
43. Kirkegaard K, Hindkjaer JJ, Ingerslev HJ. Effect of oxygen concentration on human embryo development evaluated by time-lapse monitoring. Fertil Steril. 2013;99(3):738–44.e4.
44. Krause W, Viethen G. Quality assessment of computer-assisted semen analysis (CASA) in the andrology laboratory. Andrologia. 1999;31(3):125–9 [Review].
45. Dziura B, Quinn S, Richard K. Performance of an imaging system vs. manual screening in the detection of squamous intraepithelial lesions of the uterine cervix. Acta Cytol. 2006;50(3):309–11 [Comparative Study].
46. Lozano R. Comparison of computer-assisted and manual screening of cervical cytology. Gynecol Oncol. 2007;104(1):134–8 [Clinical Trial Comparative Study].
47. Filho ES, Noble JA, Wells D. A review on automatic analysis of human embryo microscope images. Open Biomed Eng J. 2010;4:170–7.
48. Filho ES, Noble JA, Poli M, Griffiths T, Emerson G, Wells D. A method for semi-automatic grading of human blastocyst microscope images. Hum Reprod. 2012;27(9):2641–8.
49. Swann K, Windsor S, Campbell K, Elgmati K, Nomikos M, Zernicka-Goetz M, et al. Phospholipase C-zeta-induced Ca^{2+} oscillations cause coincident cytoplasmic movements in human oocytes that failed to fertilize after intracytoplasmic sperm injection. Fertil Steril. 2012;97(3):742–7.
50. Papanikolaou EG, D'Haeseleer E, Verheyen G, Van de Velde H, Camus M, Van Steirteghem A, et al. Live birth rate is significantly higher after blastocyst transfer than after cleavage-stage embryo transfer when at least four embryos are available on day 3 of embryo culture. A randomized prospective study. Hum Reprod. 2005;20(11):3198–203.
51. Papanikolaou EG, Camus M, Kolibianakis EM, Van Landuyt L, Van Steirteghem A, Devroey P. In vitro fertilization with single blastocyst-stage versus single cleavage-stage embryos. N Engl J Med. 2006;354(11):1139–46.
52. Blake DA, Farquhar CM, Johnson N, Proctor M. Cleavage stage versus blastocyst stage embryo transfer in assisted conception. Cochrane Database Syst Rev. 2007;4, CD002118.
53. Kallen B, Finnstrom O, Lindam A, Nilsson E, Nygren KG, Olausson PO. Blastocyst versus cleavage stage transfer in in vitro fertilization: differences in neonatal outcome? Fertil Steril. 2010;94(5):1680–3.
54. Kalra SK, Ratcliffe SJ, Barnhart KT, Coutifaris C. Extended Embryo Culture and an Increased Risk of Preterm Delivery. Obstet Gynecol. 2012;120(1):69–75. doi:10.1097/AOG.0b013e31825b88fc.
55. Diamond MP, Willman S, Chenette P, Cedars MI. The clinical need for a method of identification of embryos destined to become a blastocyst in assisted reproductive technology cycles. J Assist Reprod Genet. 2012;29(5):391–6.
56. Meseguer M, Rubio I, Cruz M, Basile N, Marcos J, Requena A. Embryo incubation and selection in a time-lapse monitoring system improves pregnancy outcome compared with a standard incubator: a retrospective cohort study. Fertil Steril. 2012;98(6):1481–9.e10.

Chapter 23
Predicting Embryo Implantation Potential Using Video Monitoring by the EmbryoScope™ Time-Lapse System

Belén Aparicio, Alberto Tejera IVI, Laura Romany, Arancha Galán, and Marcos Meseguer

Introduction

Standard methods of embryo assessment in an IVF laboratory are based on subjective morphology evaluations. These evaluations are done at discrete time points because of the negative effects that manipulation and interrupted incubation has on embryo development, but information for selecting the best embryos is limited. The efforts aimed at improving pregnancy rates have focused on the search for additional markers of viability and new methods of retrieving more information for embryo evaluation to supplement current criteria for embryo selection.

Time-lapse technology represents a powerful tool in assisted reproduction techniques. It is based on specially designed instruments which take images of the embryos at set time intervals during incubation for minimized manipulation. This technique provides additional information to the embryologist by enabling evaluation of embryos from a dynamic point of view to study exact timings of important events during embryo development.

The aim of time-lapse technology is to improve IVF success rates by having extra information to describe embryos with higher developmental potential. The embryologist therefore has a wider range of variables to rely on for the selection of viable embryos, which—all other things being equal—should result in a better embryo selection.

B. Aparicio • A.T. IVI • L. Romany • A. Galán • M. Meseguer (✉)
In Vitro Fertilization Laboratory, IVI Valencia, Valencia, Spain
e-mail: marcos.meseguer@ivi.es

Z.P. Nagy et al. (eds.), *Clinical Embryology: A Practical Guide*,
DOI 10.1007/978-1-4614-8376-2_23,

EmbryoScope™ Time-Lapse Technology

The EmbryoScope™ time-lapse system (ES) (Unisense FertiliTech A/S, Aarhus, Denmark) is a tri-gas oocyte/embryo incubator with a built-in microscope and camera to automatically acquire images of up to 72 individual embryos from six patients during development (Fig. 23.1).

Culture conditions can be set as for conventional incubators. Temperature and gas concentrations are registered and logged by an embedded PC which automatically generates a graph for easy monitoring of the incubator conditions over time.

EmbryoScope® time-lapse instruments are designed to optimize culture environment. The system has a non-humidified incubation chamber with a very short recovery time of O_2 and CO_2 concentrations, a direct heat transfer system for stable culture temperature even at door openings, and active carbon and HEPA filters to remove VOCs and other particles. Furthermore, all system components potentially in contact with embryos or embryo environment are toxicity tested prior release from the manufacturer.

The Microscope Imaging System

The imaging system in the ES uses low intensity red light (635 nm) from a single LED with short illumination times for image acquisition to minimize embryo exposure to light and to avoid damaging short wavelength light [1, 2].

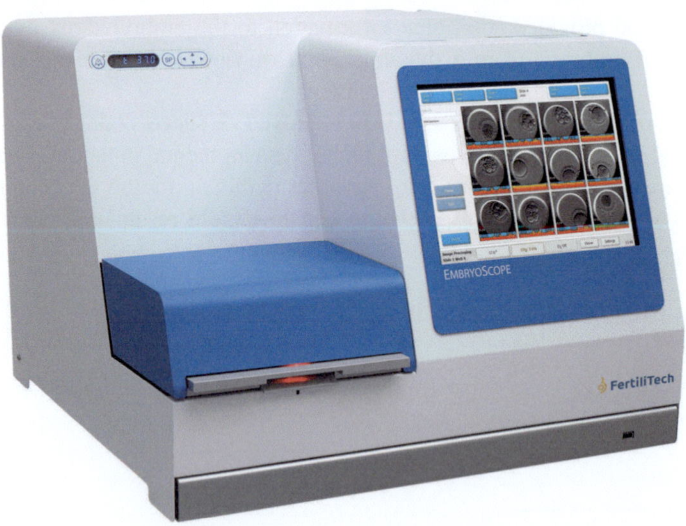

Fig. 23.1 EmbryoScope™ instrument (Unisense FertiliTech A/S, Aarhus, Denmark), where the embryos can be seen in the screen on the right while the incubator itself is on the left

Optics employed to perform the imaging of oocytes/embryos closely resemble those of an inverted microscope with Hoffman modulation contrast. However, as the microscope unit is fully automated and the images are recorded as in a digital microscope. The design is much more compact than in a conventional laboratory microscope. The 20× objective lens is custom build (Leica) and optimized at relevant wavelengths.

Digital images are recorded by a highly sensitive CCD camera (1,280×1,024 pixels) with a resolution of 3 pixels/μm and image stacks are acquired at equidistant focal planes during embryo culture. The number of planes acquired can be selected by the embryologist (up to 17 planes).

Although recording several thousand images during embryo culture, the total exposure time in the EmbryoScope® time-lapse system during culture and acquisition of images is significantly lower than the microscope light exposure time reported for a standard IVF treatment [1].

Description of EmbryoSlide® Culture Dishes

The EmbryoSlide® (EmbryoSlide®, UnisenseFertilitech, Aarhus, Denmark) holds up to 12 embryos each in individual wells with a design patented one-to-one identification system for easy identification under the microscope (Fig. 23.2). The well numbers are equivalent to the embryo identifier associated to time-lapse recordings in the system. Embryos settle in a central depression at the bottom of each well (micro-well) and are normally cultured in 25 μL droplets each under a common oil overlay.

EmbryoSlide® culture dishes are packed in sterile pouches and are recommended to be prepared in a sterile, non-heated environment.

Upon media and oil loading and appropriate temperature and gas equilibration, EmbryoSlide® culture dishes can be loaded with embryos before transfer to the EmbryoScope® time-lapse system for culture and monitoring.

Working Procedure/Methodology

The text below describes the working procedures as performed at IVI clinics.

Oocytes are placed in the micro-well just after microinjection (day 0). Therefore, the exact timing for each embryo division is calculated in hours after microinjection.

For placing embryos safely in the micro-well we use Stripper® pipettes (MXL3-275 de MidAtlantic Diagnostics, Inc.) and ensure embryo settlement at well bottom by microscope inspection.

When culturing embryos in the EmbryoScope® time-lapse system, EmbryoSlide® culture dishes containing the individually cultured embryos must be loaded in the EmbryoScope® time-lapse system both physically and electronically. Physical load

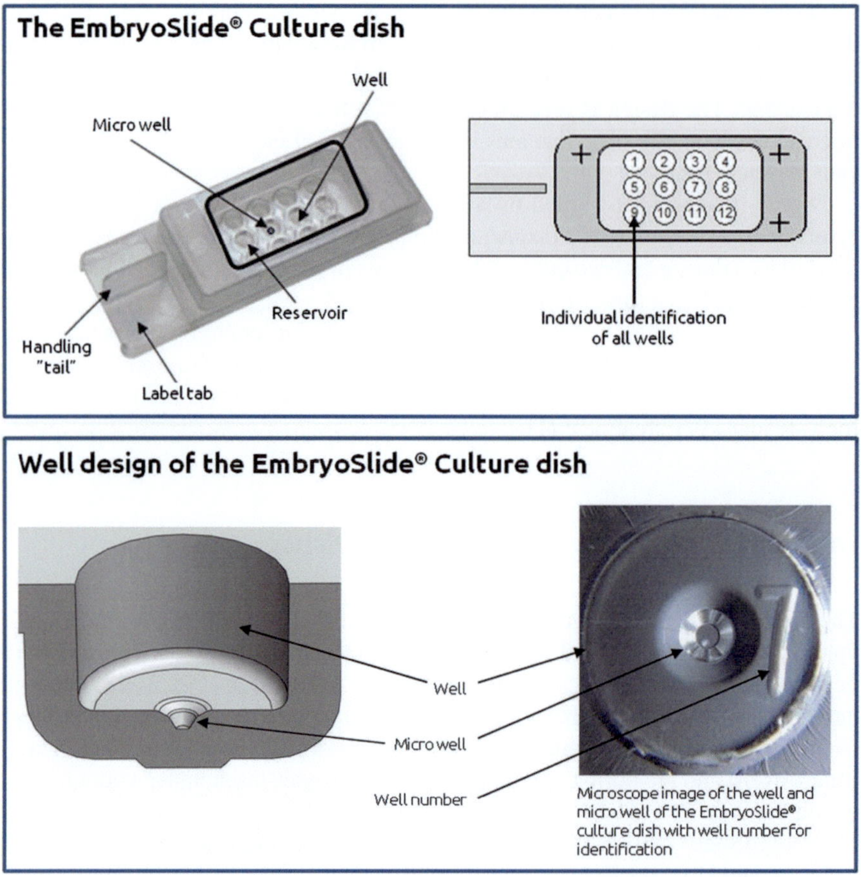

Fig. 23.2 On the *top* of the image we can see the EmbryoSlide culture dish and a diagram where the wells are numbered. The *bottom* of the figure is focused on one well of the slide

is easily done by inserting into the specially designed dish holder of the embryo chamber. Electronic load is equally easily achieved at the touch of a single button on the EmbryoScope® Home screen ("Add Slide," Fig. 23.3).

Introduction of an EmbryoSlide® in the EmbryoScope® time-lapse system prompts information to be added about the patient (Patient identification, date and time of fertilization) and a check for association with time-lapse images (Fig. 23.4).

It is very important to introduce at the correct time at which the microinjection has been performed, as all recorded events will be defined taking that time as starting point.

In the table that appears in the right-hand side (Fig. 23.4) we add any information related to each particular embryo.

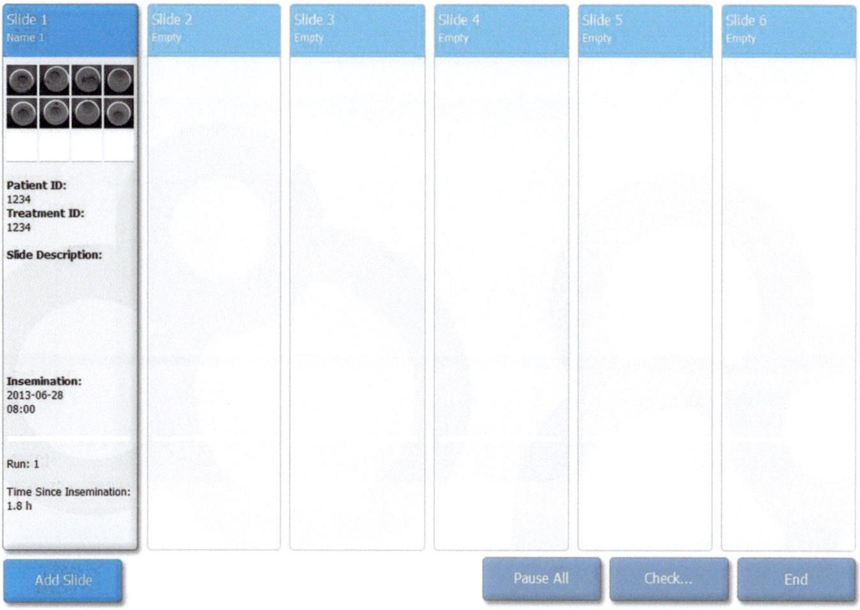

Fig. 23.3 EmbryoScope® Home screen where we can see how many empty gaps available before electronic load of a new slide

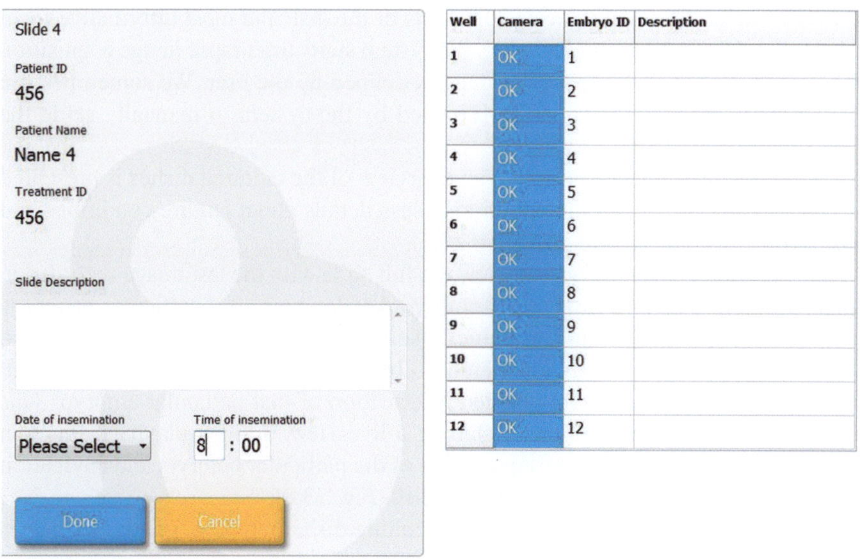

Fig. 23.4 Screen shown in the EmbryoScope™ once a new EmbryoSlide is introduced to add information of that particular patient

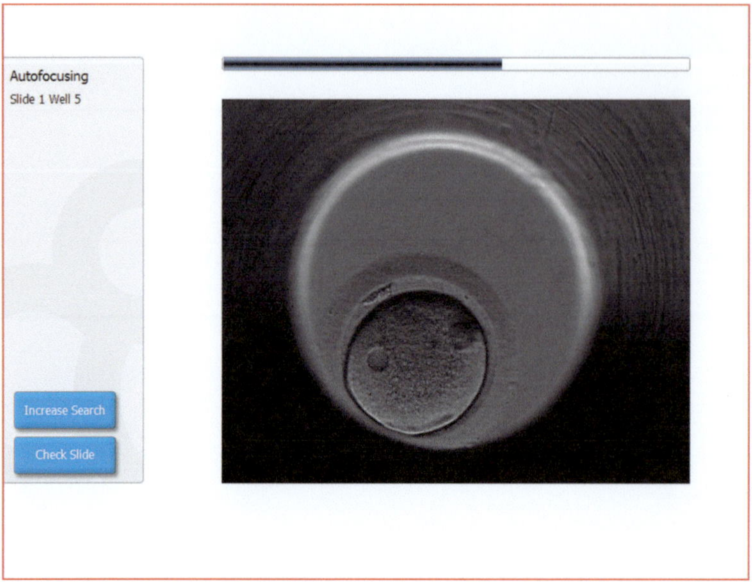

Fig. 23.5 Screen shown in the EmbryoScope™ while automatic autofocusing of the wells and the oocytes introduced is being developed by the software

Once the EmbryoSlide® culture dish has been placed inside the embryo chamber the software automatically locates the wells of the dish and most informative focal plane (Fig. 23.5). After autofocusing, the system starts time-lapse image acquisition from each well in multiple focal planes as defined by the user. We sometimes use the refocus option ("New Focus") provided by the system to manually settle the focus plane (Fig. 23.6).

While the instrument is running, an overview of the cultured dishes is presented on the Home screen with the option to access details about culture conditions and each EmbryoSlide® culture dish (Fig. 23.7).

By pressing a Slide tab we can view the full slide with the last image recorded in each well. Such an overview of the embryo development of a particular patient is very informative and useful for a quick overview of instrument content. It is also possible to focus on an individual embryo by a single touch on the screen which retrieves last image and more detailed information of that particular embryo. This feature includes several options including a live view, a video playback function which will play the entire time-lapse video of the particular embryo, and navigation within the current EmbryoSlide® culture dish (Fig. 23.8).

All data related to each EmbryoSlide® culture dish, including time-lapse images and incubation summaries, are saved in an integrated PC and on the appertaining EmbryoViewer™ workstation (EV).

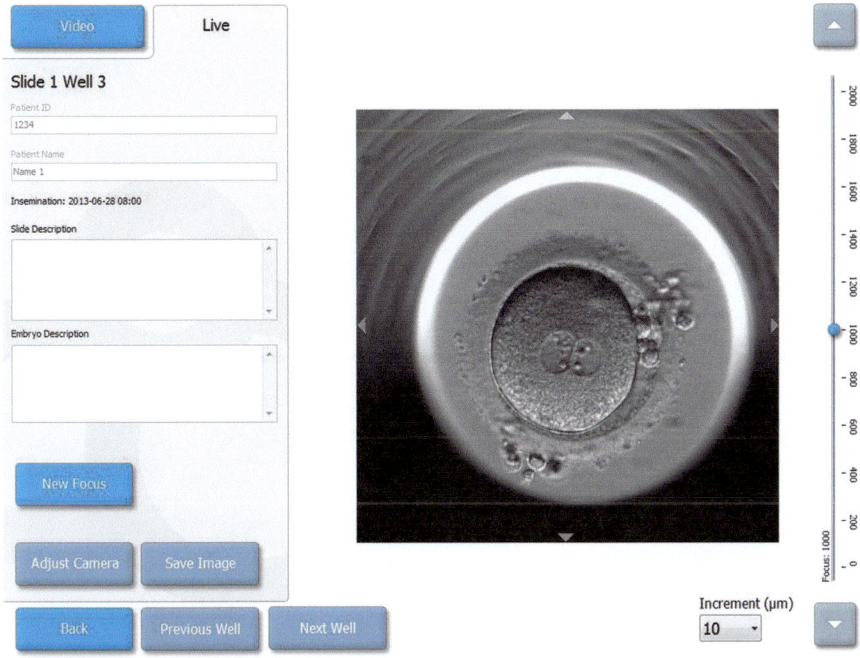

Fig. 23.6 Manual focus to improve the automatic focus provided by the software in order to have the most informative focal planes

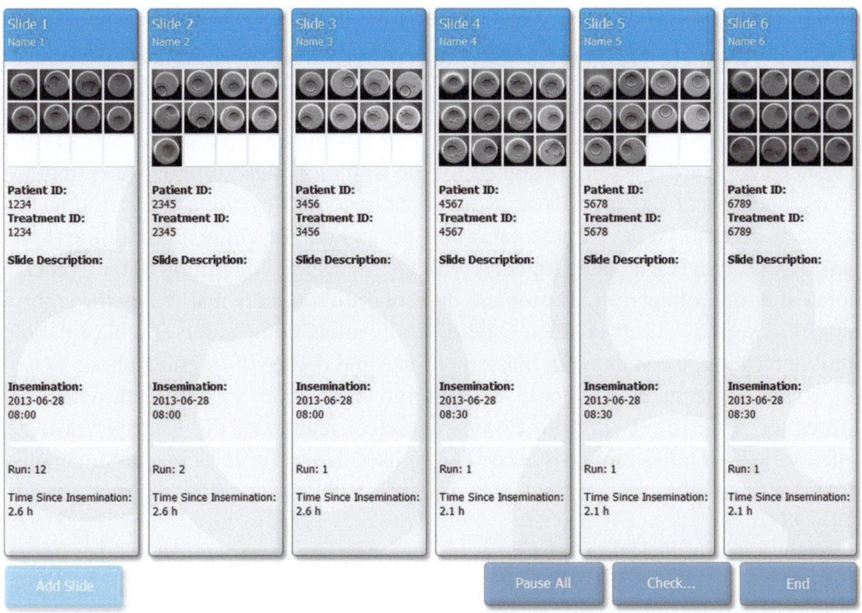

Fig. 23.7 Home screen shown in the instrument while running. It is possible to enter in each particular slide for further information

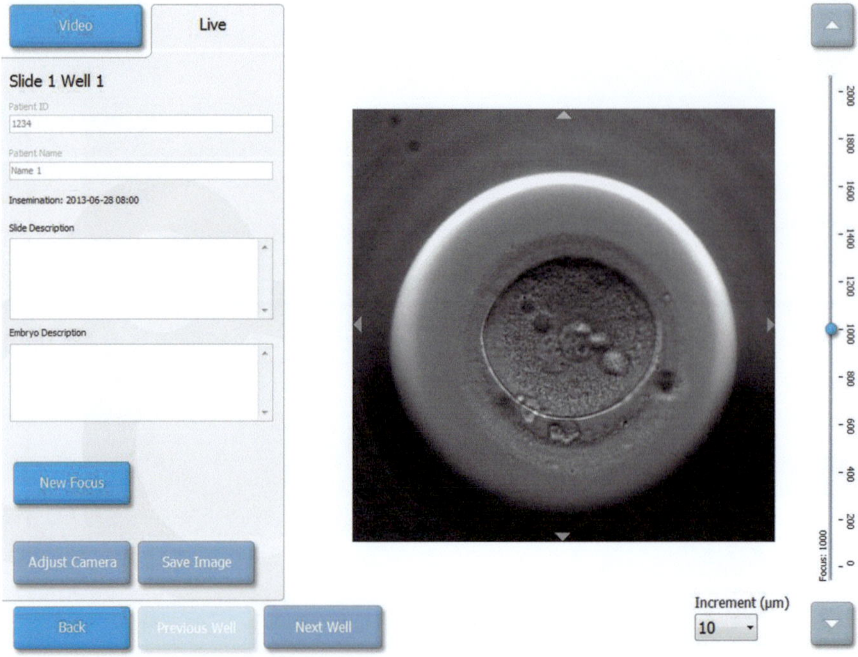

Fig. 23.8 This is the screen shown once entering in a particular well from the Home screen where the video recorded up to that moment can be visualized

Image Analysis Using the EmbryoViewer™ Software

The EmbryoViewer™ software (Unisense FertiliTech A/S, Aarhus, Denmark) is an advanced software specially designed for the EmbryoScope® time-lapse system for image analysis of the time-lapse acquisitions recorded by the system. Using this software, all embryo developmental events throughout the entire culture time (up to blastocyst stage) is annotated together with the corresponding timing of the events in hours after microinjection. Blastomere divisions are routinely marked by the embryologist as well as events characteristic of fertilization, compaction and blastulation, multinucleation, unevenness in blastomere size and degree of fragmentation.

At all our centers we apply the embryo evaluation algorithm designed by Meseguer et al. [5] Using the Compare&Select feature of the EmbryoViewer™ software which ranks embryos according to user-defined criteria this automatically provides the quality grade or category for each embryo according to the algorithm (Fig. 23.9).

The EmbryoViewer™ workstation provides the user with decision tools to mark embryo images once the selection of which embryos to be used for transfer, freezing, or kept in the laboratory for further observation is performed (green for transfer, blue for freezing, red for not viable, and yellow for observation) (Fig. 23.10).

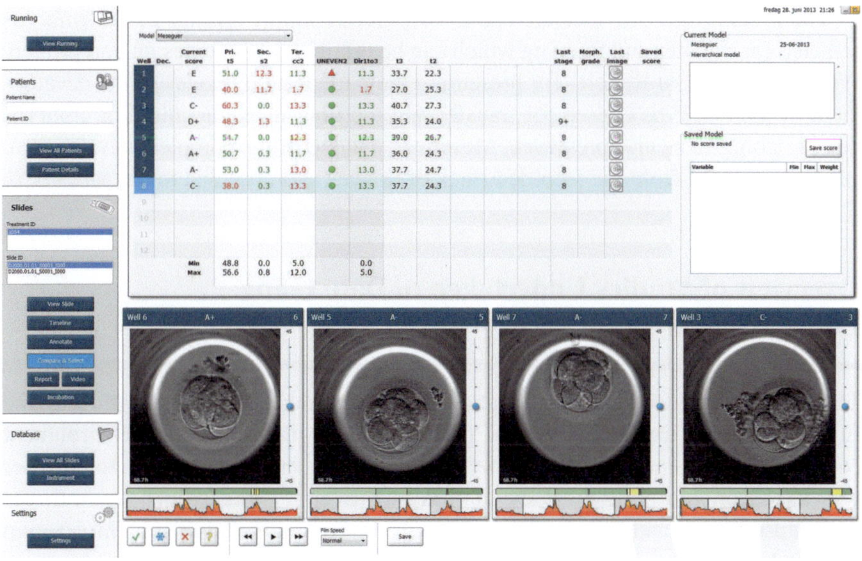

Fig. 23.9 Image shown when embryos are categorized using the algorithm designed by Meseguer. We can see the category assigned for each embryo. It is also shown if timings of the most relevant parameters are inside the optimal ranges and the exclusion criteria

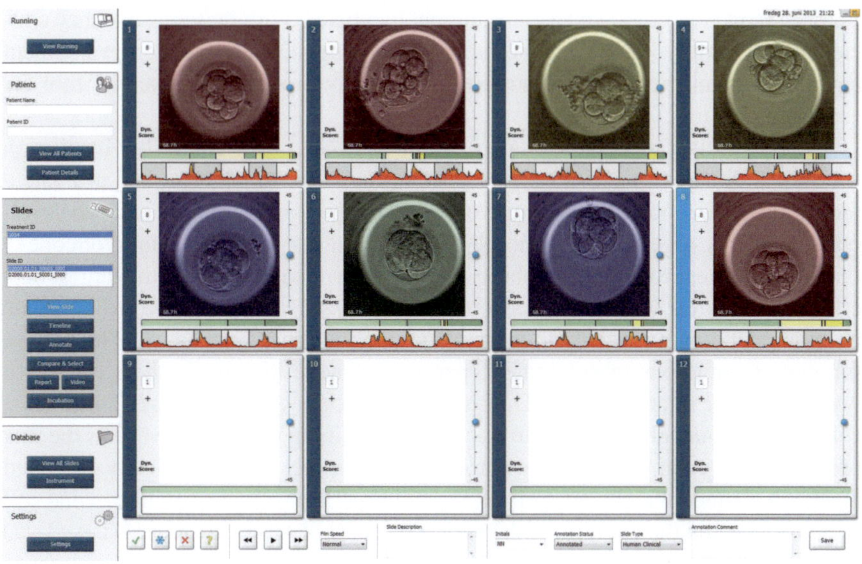

Fig. 23.10 Screen shown in the EmbryoViewer™ with wells marked with different colors according to final decision (transfer, vitrification, or further observation)

The system also provides the option to generate report formats of the embryos selected for transfer and freezing which can be tailored to clinic design and printed. We use the "Patient Report" for presenting the patient with images of the development of the embryos chosen for transfer and the final image acquired of embryos that are going to be cryopreserved. Moreover, a video of the complete development can be generated from the recorded stack of images and provided to the patients.

Overview of Studies Undertaken to Date Using EmbryoScope™

The study presented by Cruz et al. was the first step to evaluate whether the EmbryoScope™ time-lapse system provides a safe and controlled environment compared to conventional incubators [3]. In this study, embryo selection for transfer was based on morphological evaluation at the same time points for both the time-lapse system and the conventional incubator groups, the additional information provided by the time-lapse system not being taken into account.

Results obtained showed no significant variation between the two incubator groups when comparing embryo quality, development, and ongoing pregnancy rates which confirmed the safety of the system for clinical use.

Kirkegaard et al. also developed a randomized clinical trial to evaluate the safety of the EmbryoScope™ time-lapse system before introducing the instrument in a clinical setting. Results obtained in this study confirm no differences on development, clinical pregnancy, or implantation rates between incubation in the EmbryoScope™ system and a conventional incubator. With these results, they concluded that EmbryoScope™ time-lapse system supports embryonic development equally and can therefore be introduced clinically providing a potential tool for embryo evaluation [4].

Upon demonstration of the safety as an incubator with controlled incubation conditions, the next purpose of Meseguer's group was to generate and evaluate a tool for the selection of viable embryos based on the exact timing of embryo development events together with morphological patterns by using EmbryoScope™ time-lapse system to monitor embryo development. They presented the largest data set on transferred ICSI-generated embryos analyzed by time-lapse, to correlate morphokinetic parameters with implantation and pregnancy rates [5]. The precise timings of numerous morphokinetic parameters were identified where time zero was the time of microinjection. Division into two cells was defined as t2, into three cells t3, into four cells t4, and into five cells t5, defining time of cleavage as the first observed time point when the newly formed blastomeres were completely separated by clearly defined membrane. Cell cycle duration was also evaluated, the second cell cycle (cc2) being the duration of the period as a two-blastomere embryo (i.e., t3–t2) and the second synchrony (s2), synchrony in division from two-blastomere embryo to four-blastomere embryo (i.e., t4–t3). The four quartiles for the timing of each of these parameters were compared with the percentage of successfully implanting embryos in each of the quartiles. Optimal ranges were established considering the

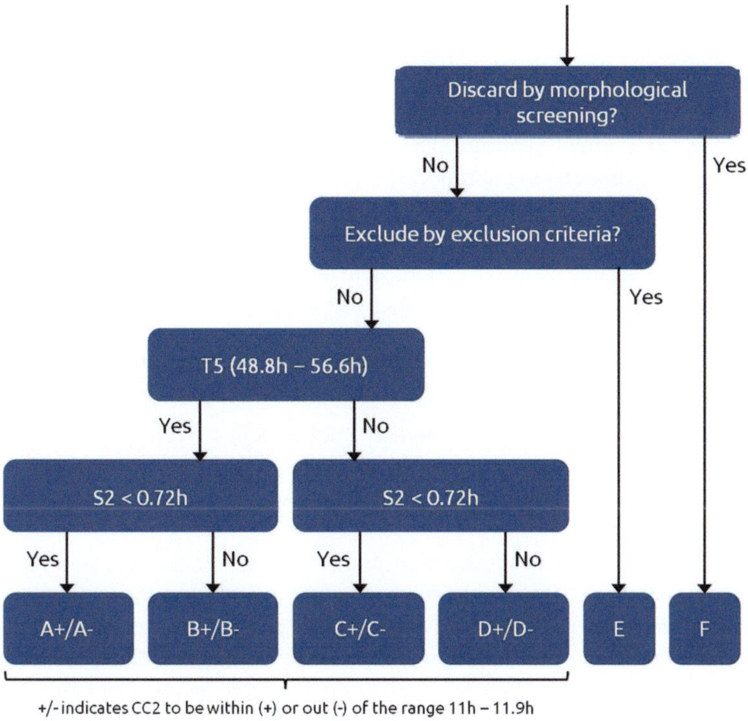

Fig. 23.11 Diagram of the algorithm including the most relevant timings to select the best embryos

two consecutive quartiles with the highest implantation probabilities in each category. Statistical analysis defined the most relevant parameters for embryo evaluation. The results obtained were then used to design a hierarchical classification algorithm for the selection of embryos with the highest implantation potential. The timing of the cleavage to five cells turned out to have the best correlation with implantation success and was superior to the timing of the first cell division used in earlier studies of early cleavage [5].

The algorithm starts with a morphological screening of the embryos to discard the embryos that are clearly not viable and which are consequently classified as category F. The next step in the algorithm is to exclude embryos fulfilling at least one of the following exclusion criteria: (1) uneven blastomere size after the first cleavage (when the embryo has two cells). Blastomeres were considered uneven if the average diameter of the large blastomere was 25 % larger than the average diameter of the small blastomere; (2) abrupt division from one to three cells or (3) multinucleation at the four-cell stage (category E). After evaluation for these criteria, the remaining levels of the hierarchy are defined according to the defined ranges of some of the variables (t5, s2). Once the embryo is classified with a specific grade, the timing of cc2 is taken into account, adding a plus (+) if it is inside the range established as optimal or minus (–) if it is outside this optimal range. In this way, embryos are graded A^+–D^-, E, or F using the algorithm (Fig. 23.11).

One of the exclusion criteria defined in Meseguer's algorithm was studied in detail by Rubio et al. [6]. By using the EmbryoScope™ time-lapse system they precisely identified each cell cycle and observed abnormal lengths of the cell cycle, such as the abrupt cleavage of human embryos from two to three cells in less than 5 h, defined as a direct cleavage (DC 2–3). Clinical pregnancy and implantation rates of embryos undergoing abrupt cell division from two to three cells were studied to evaluate the clinical applicability of this morphokinetic parameter. The known implantation rate of DC2–3 embryos was statistically significantly lower than for embryos with a normal cleavage pattern. The incidence of direct cleavage was about 14 % in the total embryonic cohort which, combined with the markedly decreased implantation rate of direct cleavage, suggests this to be a strong morphokinetic parameter for clinical use.

Using this algorithm and the EmbryoScope™ time-lapse system, Basile et al. compared different culture media, demonstrating identical timings and proportion of optimal embryos for the two media analyzed [7]. These results validate the algorithm for embryo selection developed by Meseguer et al. [5] in diverse culture conditions.

The further use of the described algorithm by Meseguer et al. [5] is in the largest retrospective study to date on pregnancy outcomes comparing conventional incubation with time-lapse technology [8]. Even though prospective studies are obviously preferable, this was a first approximation where all the available data from ten different IVI clinics were analyzed, adding up to a large quantity of heterogeneous information. A key limitation of this study, because of its retrospective design, was that patients were not evenly or randomly distributed between the two different incubators, which can affect and distort final conclusions. Because of this, it was essential to analyze for any confounding factors that may significantly influence pregnancy rates and their uneven distribution between incubators. Oocyte source, maternal age, day of transfer, and number of retrieved oocytes were identified as significant confounding factors and included in a logistic regression model. The results obtained suggested a relative 20 % improvement in pregnancy rates in the time-lapse incubator system compared with the conventional incubator, which implies a larger impact than the improvement associated with blastocyst culture [8]. For treatments with conventional incubators, the average clinical pregnancy rate per initiated cycle with oocyte retrieval was 44.9 %. If they had been incubated using time-lapse, a relative improvement of 20 % would imply an expected clinical pregnancy rate for the same cycles of 53.9 %, an absolute improvement of 9 %. These results need to be confirmed with prospective studies which have already been started.

Using the algorithm described above, Cruz et al. [9] developed the largest time-lapse analysis of human blastocysts to date to demonstrate associations between various cleavage stage kinetic parameters and the ability of the embryos to reach the blastocyst stage [9]. This study compared the blastocyst rate and morphological features for cleavage stage embryos, which were graded according to their morphokinetic development. The blastocyst rate and morphology were highest for embryos from the best morphokinetic grade A and gradually decreased to the lowest rates and qualities for the lowest grade D. From their results, Cruz et al. concluded that time-lapse-based evaluation of the exact timing of early events in embryo development is a promising tool for the prediction of blastocyst formation and quality.

In a recent study, Dal Canto et al. [10] studied EmbryoScope® acquired time-lapse images and found human embryo cleavage rates to be suggestive of their ability to develop to the blastocyst stage and to implant. They showed similar cleavage patterns up to the six-cell stage of embryos that later developed into blastocyst and those that did not, but highlighted the importance of timings of cleavage to the seven- and eight-cell stages for predicting blastocyst potential. In this study implanting embryos developed to the eight-cell stage in a significantly shorter period than those unable to implant. With these results, they concluded that cleavage from the two- to the eight-cell stage occurs progressively earlier in embryos with the ability to develop to expanding blastocysts and to implant [10].

Very recently, the EmbryoScope® time-lapse system has been demonstrated of great value in assisting more resource consuming laboratory procedures due to the precise and continuous recordings of embryonic development.

Preimplantation genetic diagnosis encourages further investigations using time-lapse systems such as the impact of blastomere removal and correlation of morphokinetic parameters with aneuploidy risk.

Kirkegaard et al. presented the first study to evaluate the effect of blastomere biopsy on early human embryonic development using time-lapse analysis. Using the EmbryoScope™ time-lapse they demonstrated that although cleavage stage embryo biopsy prolongs the cell stage at which the biopsy is performed, the cleavage rate after this initial delay seems unaffected [11]. Biopsied and non-biopsied embryos started hatching at the same time, which caused duration of the blastocyst stage to be shorter in the biopsied group, due to a shorter time from reaching the full blastocyst stage until hatching. Moreover, the study confirms previous findings from studies on assisted hatching, showing the embryo to hatch through the artificial breach in zona pellucida. The study hereby contributes to the understanding of the effect of blastomere biopsy and the early development of the human embryo.

To evaluate the difference in morphokinetics between aneuploid and euploid embryos [12], Campbell et al. compared morphokinetic variables of these two groups of embryos using EmbryoScope® time-lapse images. Their results showed that multiple aneuploid embryos were delayed at the initiation of compaction (t_{sc}) and the time to reach full blastocyst stage (t_B). Embryos having single or multiple aneuploidy also presented a delay in initiation of blastulation (t_{SB}) compared with euploid embryos [12].

Morphokinetic variables found to differ between euploid and aneuploid embryos were used to build a risk classification model by classifying the embryos into groups depending on the value of the variables t_{SB} and t_B and finally developed the following algorithm: low risk, $t_B < 122.9$ h and $t_{SB} < 96.2$ h; medium risk, $t_B < 122.9$ h and $t_{SB} \geq 96.2$ h; high risk, $t_B \geq 122.9$ h (Table 23.1).

This same group also developed a retrospective analysis to evaluate the effectiveness and potential impact of this classification model for unselected IVF patients without biopsy and preimplantation genetic screening (PGS) [13].

Table 23.1 Classification of ploidy with associated incidence rates and probability of aneuploidy

Risk class	No. of embryos	Incidence of aneuploid embryos	Probability of an embryo being aneuploid
Low, $t_B < 122.9$ h and $t_{SB} < 96.2$ h	36	0.36	0.37
Medium, $t_B < 122.9$ h and $t_{SB} \geq 96.2$ h	49	0.69	0.69
High, $t_B \geq 122.9$ h	12	1.00	0.97

Table 23.2 Known implantation data rate for fetal heart beat and live birth for each aneuploidy risk class

Risk class	Fetal heart beat in known implantation data	Live birth in known implantation data
Low, $t_B < 122.9$ h and $t_{SB} < 96.2$ h	72.7[a] ($n = 33$)	61.1[b] ($n = 18$)
Medium, $t_B < 122.9$ h and $t_{SB} \geq 96.2$ h	25.5[a] ($n = 51$)	19.2[b] ($n = 26$)
High, $t_B \geq 122.9$ h	0 ($n = 4$)	0 ($n = 2$)

[a] $p < 0.0001$
[b] $p < 0.01$

When the aneuploidy risk classification model was applied, the medium- and low-risk classes for aneuploidy were significantly different from each other with respect to known implantation rates (Table 23.2). Of the few embryos classified as high risk subsequent to transfer, none implanted. The aneuploidy risk classification model, therefore, indicated the predictive power of this algorithm to identify and avoid selecting embryos at high risk of implantation failure using noninvasive objective criteria.

In summary, time-lapse systems improve our knowledge of the real-time distribution of the main events of embryo development making possible to establish, with accuracy and objectivity, the basis of the embryo development timing. The EmbryoScope® technology provides flexibility in working routines and evaluation protocols due to the platform design. This technology might also improve effectiveness of IVF cycles increasing the ability to identify embryos with higher implantation potential, in order to perform elective single embryo transfer reducing multiple pregnancy rates.

References

1. Ottosen LDM, Hindkjær J, Ingerslev J. Light exposure of the ovum and preimplantation embryo during ART procedures. J Assist Reprod Genet. 2007;24(2):99–103.
2. Takenaka M, Horiuchi T, Yanagimachi R. Effects of light on development of mammalian zygotes. Proc Natl Acad Sci USA. 2007;104(36):14289–93.
3. Cruz M, Gadea B, Garrido N, Pedersen KS, Martínez M, Pérez-Cano I, et al. Embryo quality, blastocyst and ongoing pregnancy rates in oocyte donation patients whose embryos were monitored by time-lapse imaging. J Assist Reprod Genet. 2011;28(7):569–73.

4. Kirkegaard K, Hindkjaer JJ, Grøndahl ML, Kesmodel US, Ingerslev HJ. A randomized clinical trial comparing embryo culture in a conventional incubator with a time-lapse incubator. J Assist Reprod Genet. 2012;29(6):565–72.
5. Meseguer M, Herrero J, Tejera A, Hilligsøe KM, Ramsing NB, Remohí J. The use of morphokinetics as a predictor of embryo implantation. Hum Reprod. 2011;26(10):2658–71.
6. Rubio I, Kuhlmann R, Agerholm I, Kirk J, Herrero J, Escriba MJ, et al. Limited implantation success of direct-cleaved human zygotes: a time-lapse study. Fertil Steril. 2012 Dec;98(6):1458–63.
7. Basile N, Morbeck D, García-Velasco J, Bronet F, Meseguer M. Type of culture media does not affect embryo kinetics: a time-lapse analysis of sibling oocytes. Hum Reprod. 2013;28(3):634–41.
8. Meseguer M, Rubio I, Cruz M, Basile N, Marcos J, Requena A. Embryo incubation and selection in a time-lapse monitoring system improves pregnancy outcome compared with a standard incubator: a retrospective cohort study. Fertil Steril. 2012;98(6):1481–9.e10.
9. Cruz M, Garrido N, Herrero J, Perez-Cano I, Munoz M, Meseguer M. Timing of cell division in human cleavage-stage embryos is linked with blastocyst formation and quality. Reprod Biomed Online. 2012;25(4):371–81.
10. Dal Canto M, Coticchio G, Mignini Renzini M, De Ponti E, Novara PV, Brambillasca F, et al. Cleavage kinetics analysis of human embryos predicts development to blastocyst and implantation. Reprod Biomed Online. 2012 Nov;25(5):474–80.
11. Kirkegaard K, Hindkjaer JJ, Ingerslev HJ. Human embryonic development after blastomere removal: a time-lapse analysis. Human Reprod. 2012;27(1):97–105.
12. Campbell A, Fishel S, Bowman N, Duffy S, Sedler M, Hickman CFL. Modelling a risk classification of aneuploidy in human embryos using non-invasive morphokinetics. Reprod Biomed Online. 2013;26(5):477–85.
13. Campbell A, Fishel S, Bowman N, Duffy S, Sedler M, Thornton S. Retrospective analysis of outcomes after IVF using an aneuploidy risk model derived from time-lapse imaging without PGS. Reprod Biomed Online. 2013;27(2):140–6.

Part V
Genetic Testing of Embryos

Chapter 24
Embryo Biopsy for PGD: Current Perspective

Steven J. McArthur, Don Leigh, Maria Traversa, James Marshall, and Robert P.S. Jansen

This chapter sets out to examine the major recent advances in embryo biopsy, specifically blastocyst-stage biopsy and preimplantation genetic testing and diagnosis (together *PGD*) which are transforming singleton live birth rates in families at risk of passing on monogenic diseases or chromosomal translocations.

The Development of Embryo Biopsy

Embryo biopsies for clinical PGD generally were performed at day 3, when the embryo typically was at the 6- to 8-cell stage, and involved the removal of one or two blastomeres. The zona was breached by dissolving the protein with acid Tyrode's solution. The embryo was incubated in a calcium-/magnesium-free medium to reduce cell–cell interactions and make the removal of cells easier. There has been debate about the impact of removing multiple cells, and in general it was considered that two-cell removal was more detrimental than removing just a single cell and should not be performed—although the reliability of amplification of two cells was considered less prone to allele dropout. An alternative biopsy approach involved the removal of either the first and second polar bodies—either sequentially on day 0 and day 1, or both at day 1. PCR analysis of blastomeres or polar bodies involves amplification of a single allelic copy of the target. Similarly, analysis by FISH is a single-cell test. Biopsy at the blastocyst stage, when embryos typically comprise upward of 100 cells, enables the removal of 3–5 trophectoderm cells without significant cell mass depletion. Putting several cells into a PCR reaction should decrease the likelihood of amplification failure (allele dropout, or ADO) and, with FISH analyses, should provide an opportunity to confirm signal patterns.

S.J. McArthur, BSc (✉) • D. Leigh, PhD (UNSW) • M. Traversa, BSc, Msc, (Med)
J. Marshall, BAppSc (UTS) • R.P.S. Jansen, MD CREI
Sydney IVF, Sydney, Australia
e-mail: Steve.mcarthur@sydneyivf.com

Z.P. Nagy et al. (eds.), *Clinical Embryology: A Practical Guide*,
DOI 10.1007/978-1-4614-8376-2_24, © Springer Science+Business Media New York 2013

Table 24.1 Embryos available for testing for monogenic disease mutations by biopsy on day 3[a] and on day 5–6

	Egg retrievals	Embryos biopsied	Inconclusive test result	Conclusive, favorable test	Embryos transferred fresh	Tested embryos cryostored
Day 3 biopsy + day 5–6 transfera	91	595 av. 6.5 embryos	61 (10.3%)	261 (43.8%)	103	158 (60.5%)
Day 5–6 biopsy + day 5–6 transfer	177	655 av. 3.7 embryos	46 (7.0%)	305 (46.5%)	121	184 (60.3%)

See McArthur et al. [7] for more detailed interpretation of the data
[a] All embryos were developed to blastocysts before transfer

During the early 2000s, Genea (formerly Sydney IVF)moved comprehensively to blastocyst culture and blastocyst-stage transfers and cryostorage and experienced a corresponding increase in take-home baby rates, substantial reductions in multiple pregnancies, and reduced rates of miscarriage [1–7]. In 2004, we described the first clinical application of blastocyst biopsy to routine PGD practice [1]. Embryos were "hatched" on day 3 using a Hamilton Thorne Zilos Tk near-infrared laser and were then incubated for another 2 days to enable blastocoel expansion and herniation of trophectoderm cells through the opened zona for biopsy [1, 6]. Suitable embryos were placed in 5 μL drops of standard medium under oil. A holding pipette, the same as used in ICSI practice, was employed to immobilize the embryo, while a 30-μL biopsy pipette was used to collapse the blastocyst cavity and hold the tissue sample. Several pulses with the laser set at low level loosened cell–cell interactions 3–5, permitting a small piece of tissue to be teased off the exposed trophectoderm. The embryo was then removed and placed into fresh medium for further incubation (until the results were known and the embryo was transferred, cryostored, or disposed of). The tissue piece was washed and placed into PCR tubes or fixed to glass slides for analysis using FISH.

The advantage of moving from cleavage-stage to blastocyst-stage PGD was demonstrated by comparison of embryo biopsies performed (a) at the day 3 cleavage stage and followed by the transfer of embryos that went on to blastulate successfully, with (b) embryo biopsies taken *at* the blastocyst stage (day 5–6) and followed by almost immediate transfer [7]. This study, in other words, *examined the efficacy of day 3 biopsy vs. day 5 or 6 on the embryo, while controlling for the embryo's ability to blastulate*; patients in this trial had PGD not for infertility or miscarriages but to prevent further propagation of a serious monogenic family disease. The outcome (Table 24.1) implies that, in comparison with the biopsy of blastocysts, day 3 cleavage-stage PGD reduces the implantation potential of at least some embryos. (The same could still also be true of blastocyst biopsy, but appears to be to a much lesser extent.)

Table 24.1 shows the technical outcome data for the embryos biopsied (595 for day 3; 656 for days 5–6), with an average of 6.5 embryos biopsied and tested per retrieval at cleavage, compared with an average of 3.7 embryos biopsied and tested per retrieval when the blastocyst stage was awaited before performing PGD. The proportion of embryos with a conclusive test and with a normal result, thus suitable for transfer, was still approximately 50% in each series, which means that taking the biopsy later in embryo development conferred appreciable laboratory and clinical efficiency through not having to test embryos whose development was compromised. The late-biopsied blastocysts had almost twice the chance of implanting than did the blastocysts that had been biopsied on day 3.

Table 24.2 shows the outcomes of the embryo transfer procedures. In spite of a lower average number of embryos transferred (1.1 vs. 1.5 per transfer procedure), and without taking into account later further pregnancies from cryostored biopsied embryos, the day 5–6 biopsy transfers resulted in fewer miscarriages and a higher absolute ongoing pregnancy rate, as well as the expected lower rate of multiple pregnancy. There was one obvious monozygotic twinning event, involving an embryo biopsied on day 3. In about 60% of cases in each series, additional embryos that had tested normally were cryostored for further attempts at pregnancy.

Preimplantation Screening for Aneuploidy

It has been known for more than 15 years that IVF embryos show a high rate of chromosome aneuploidy [8]. It has also been understood for many more years that a chance acquisition of an abnormal number of chromosomes is a frequent event in human conception and, in particular, is the commonest cause for pregnancies to miscarry. It might therefore be expected that screening IVF embryos for aneuploidies before selecting an embryo to transfer should materially improve the chance of pregnancy, reduce the risk of miscarriage, and (by enabling embryos to be transferred efficiently and efficaciously one at a time) greatly reduce the multiple pregnancy rate, thus lessening perinatal morbidity and mortality. The target—improved live birth rates from IVF and less costs for community—is worthy and logical.

Aneuploidy Risk

Several authors have reported that the age of the woman undergoing IVF has a significant bearing on the extent of aneuploidy in the resulting embryos. Studies on the origin of the nondisjunction chromosome anomalies have suggested that most of the abnormalities originate predominantly from female meiosis, especially meiosis I, although analysis of preimplantation embryo polar bodies with FISH has indicated that meiosis II errors could be similar in number [9]. Analysis of later-stage embryos would therefore be able to identify both meiosis I and meiosis II errors (as well as revealing aneuploidies brought by the fertilizing sperm). Generally, a predisposition to aneuploidy beyond maternal age effect has been hampered by the fact that few

Table 24.2 Clinical outcomes following biopsy at the cleavage-stage vs. biopsy at the stage of blastocyst, each with transfer of embryos fresh on day 5 or 6

	Embryos transferred *n*	Transfer procedures *n*	Pregnancy per retrieval	Implantation per embryo[a]	Miscarriage	Live birth or ongoing pregnancy	Multiple at confinement		
							Single	Twin	Triple
Day 3 biopsy + day 5–6 transferred	1	38	11	11	4	7	7		
	2	28	12	15	1	10	7	2	1
$n = 91$ retrievals	3	3	1	1	0	1	1		
	All av. 1.5	69 (75.8%)	24/91 (26.4%)	27/103 (26.2%)	5/91 (20.1%)	18/91 (19.8%)	15	3 Multiples (16.7%)	
Day 5–6	1	105	54	54	8	46	46		
biopsy + day 5–6	2	8	4	5	1	3	2	1	
transferred	3	0							
$n = 177$ retrievals	All av. 1.1	113 (63.8%)	58/177 (32.8%)	59/121 (48.8%)	9/58 (15.5%)	49/177 (27.7%)	48	1 Multiple (2%)	

Data from McArthur et al. [7]

[a] The implantation rate for blastocysts biopsied from the trophectoderm as blastocysts (48.8%) was highly significantly better than the implantation rate for blastocysts biopsied using a single cell removed at the day 3 cleavage stage (26.2%, $P < 0.01$)

studies have looked for or been able to identify genetic causes; rare recessive genetic states that interfere with meiosis have been described [10]. While not extensive, there have been a number of reports suggesting that among women undergoing IVF and experiencing subsequent implantation failure, the chromosome abnormality rate in their embryos is quite high compared to the other IVF cohorts [11–13]. Screening embryos for aneuploidy could reduce the number of embryos subsequently needed to initiate a successful and continuing pregnancy [14]. The efficacy of the screening process must obviously take into account any detrimental aspects of the biopsy and culture processes to be considered truly beneficial for the patient's progress.

Aneuploidy Screening in IVF Programs

Examination of a restricted number of chromosomes using FISH for aneuploidy screening as a routine may not be helpful in all cases and in fact can be harmful if biopsy procedures are not efficient. Mastenbroek et al. showed that biopsy of day 3 (cleavage-stage) embryos for limited PGS—screening for aneuploidy of chromosomes 13, 16, 17, 18, 21, X, and Y—can reduce the chance of an ongoing pregnancy in women aged 35–41 having in vitro fertilization (IVF) [15]. Our considerations above (Tables 24.1 and 24.2) suggest that interfering with an early embryo might lie behind this detrimental result, but other factors could also be important. For the Mastenbroek study, these included such straightforward concerns as the time the embryos spent being manipulated in potentially altered culture conditions across the variety of IVF clinics where the biopsies were performed. They also include more complex issues, such as the inadvertent exclusion from transfer of mosaic embryos in which the biopsied cell happened to be the only cell with the trisomy (a situation that can follow a mitotic nondisjunction event) [9].

Between August 2004 and November 2006, we studied the impact of screening for aneuploidy in younger infertile women (<38 years, median 33.5 years), employing biopsies of blastocysts [5]. All women were in their first or second attempt at IVF. Agreement to have one embryo transferred (eSET) was a precondition for entry. Patients were withdrawn from the study if there were fewer than eight ovarian follicles over 1 cm diameter at 8–10 days of stimulation, fewer than four embryos with seven or more cells on day 3 of culture, or fewer than three blastocysts for biopsy on day 5 or 6; no women had cycles canceled because of a poor response. The biopsies consisted of 2–9 trophectoderm cells and were tested by at least 5-color fluorescent in situ hybridization for, at minimum, chromosomes 13, 18, 21, X, and Y. We compared outcomes between the screened group (Group A, normal ≥5-color pattern in all the removed trophectoderm cells for the transferred embryo) and the principal control group (Group B, with zona opening but no biopsy); we also made comparisons with the women who were withdrawn from the study before randomization because of suboptimal responses to stimulation (Group C) and with women who were eligible but elected not to take part in the study (Group D). Table 24.3 gives the results up to the time the trial was suspended. Pregnancies are clinical pregnancies with a normal fetal heart rate on ultrasound scanning in the first trimester.

Table 24.3 Pregnancy rates after preimplantation genetic screening for aneuploidy from biopsy of blastocysts on day 5 or 6 of development using 5- or 7-color FISH

Group A. Biopsy				Group B. No biopsy (control)			
n	P	NP	%P	*n*	P	NP	%P
56	25	30	45.5%	48	26	20	56.5%
Group C. Poor response, withdrawn				Group D. Eligible, nonparticipating			
n	P	NP	%P	*n*	P	NP	%P
107	36	71	33.6%	1,194	564	630	47.2%

From Jansen et al. [5], with permission
P pregnant; *NP* not pregnant

The clinical pregnancy rate (pregnancies with a normal fetal heart rate at 6 weeks' gestation) was high (46.4% of egg retrieval procedures overall), irrespective of whether PGS was performed or not, and is consistent with results we [2, 6] and others [16] have reported previously for elective single blastocyst transfers.

Among the women who underwent biopsy for aneuploidy screening (Group A), the pregnancy rate at 45.5% was insignificantly less than among women who were eligible for the trial but did not take part (Group D, 47.2%) and was trending to be higher than among women who were withdrawn from the trial prior to randomization because of a suboptimal response (Group C, 33.6%; $c^2 = 1.7$, $P < 0.1$, 1-tailed). We could thus find no evidence of clinically important detriment from blastocyst biopsy in women of normal reproductive age. The pregnancy rate compares favorably, with the 25% clinical pregnancy rate reported by Mastenbroek et al.

Unexpectedly, Group B, the embryos subjected to zona opening by near-infrared laser, a standard preparatory step for biopsy and performed on day 3 or 4 (see above), produced the highest clinical pregnancy rate of the groups (56.5%), which while not statistically significantly different from either the biopsied embryos (Group A, $c^2 = 0.8$) or the eligible but nonparticipant women's embryos (Group D, $c^2 = 1.2$), the trend was opposite to that required to disprove the null hypothesis, and the clinical trial was stopped.

The reason for the strong performance of the embryos in the principal control group, if it is true, is not clear. Assisted hatching by opening of the zona, while advocated from time to time for the embryos of older women to facilitate hatching and implantation, has not been shown to be beneficial among women under 40 or with good blastocyst development. More likely, a too strict set of criteria for assumed meiotic nondisjunction led to overinterpretation and rejection of some blastocysts that would, if left unscreened, have developed normally and contributed to the total number of embryos suitable for transfer.

Testing for Chromosomal Translocations

Reciprocal translocations occur in about 1 in 625 newborns and usually result from the exchange of two terminal segments from different chromosomes, ordinarily resulting in a genome that is balanced. Exchanges can also take place close to the centromeres of two acrocentric chromosomes; these Robertsonian translocations, which occur in about 1 in 900 newborns, also ordinarily provide a balanced genome and bring the overall prevalence of balanced translocations among newborns to about 1:380 [17]. When diploid germ cells with these karyotypes eventually undergo meiosis, however, the chromosomes involved segregate abnormally and yield a varying but significantly high level of unbalanced haploid states among oocytes and spermatozoa—an unbalanced state that is continued into the embryo and which results in implantation failure, miscarriage, stillbirth, or abnormalities at birth. Balanced translocations are ten times more common among couples presenting for treatment with IVF [18].

With *reciprocal translocations*, homologous pairing during meiosis 1 produces a tetravalent structure instead of the usual bivalent. Subsequent segregation to respective daughter cell spindles takes one of three modes: *2:2 alternate segregation* (producing alternately a normal or a balanced abnormal complement, the latter perpetuating the familial condition but both with a balanced genome); *adjacent 1 and 2 segregations* (producing segmental monosomies and trisomies); and comparatively rarely, 3:1 *segregations* (involving nondisjunction of a whole chromosome and producing more complete monosomies and trisomies) [19]. Overall, 75% of embryos from a parent with a balanced reciprocal translocation show partially or fully aneuploid chromosome complements (14 different unbalanced combinations compared to two balanced combinations), considerably reducing the number of otherwise healthy appearing embryos available for transfer after PGD.

In *Robertsonian translocations*, a trivalent structure is formed during meiosis 1, with three main segregation modes possible (and nine different chromosome combinations), namely, *alternate* (which returns dosage to its balanced state), *2:1 segregations* (producing complementary monosomies and trisomies), and *3:0 segregation* (produce double trisomy or double monosomy).

Traditional PGD for translocations involves FISH, utilizing either breakpoint-spanning probes (which require access to extensive probe libraries and complicated workups) or (much more simply) combinations of commercially available, quality-controlled centromeric, locus-specific, and subtelomeric probes attached to standard fluorochromes. The use of PGD to screen balanced from unbalanced chromosome sets in the embryos then significantly reduces the failure rate for implantation and should result in fewer miscarriages among the embryos available for transfer [13, 20]. Again, to be truly beneficial, the process of biopsy must do the least amount of harm to the embryo's continued development and to its ability to implant. Table 24.4 shows our experience with cleavage- and blastocyst-stage biopsies among couples with recurrent miscarriage attributable to a balanced reciprocal translocation in one of them. The live baby results have been lower compared to those we obtain after testing for monogenic disease (Table 24.2), possibly reflecting the large decrement in transferable embryos seen with reciprocal translocations following the demonstration of unbalanced cells by FISH-based PGD. These apparent unbalanced outcomes can be of biological origin but can also be false, due to inherent error rates observed with FISH-based protocols [21] or reflective of a benign mosaic state, but in either case contributing to false positive interpretation of FISH signals and leading to the exclusion of otherwise normal embryos.

Table 24.4 Clinical outcomes of PGD for balanced translocation using FISH and from using STR-based PCR

	Reciprocal translocations		Robertsonian translocations	
	FISH	STR-PCR	FISH	STR-PCR
Patients	54	22	17	7
Mean age	35.2	33.1	36.0	33.3
Cycles with egg retrieval	112	22	51	6
Cycles with embryo biopsy	73	22	31	6
Biopsied embryos	320	61	142	17
Actionable PGD result	304	60	136	17
Embryos for transfer	74 (23%)	20 (33%)	44 (31%)	13 (76%)
Embryo transfer cycles	54	13	27	5
Embryos transferred	1.2	1	1.2	1
Total embryos transferred	62	13	32	5
Positive pregnancy test	20	7	14	3
Implantation rate/embryo (%)	32	54	44	60
FH-positive pregnancy rate per transfer	15 (24%)	6 (46%)	12 (38%)	2 (40%)
FH-positive pregnancy rate per egg retrieval (%)	13	27	24	33

Data from McArthur et al. [7] and Traversa et al. [22]

All embryos were biopsied and transferred at the blastocyst stage. Results do not include pregnancies from the embryos cryostored

In our published series for translocations using FISH [7], 95 egg retrievals were performed and led to biopsy and testing among couples with a *balanced reciprocal translocation*; there were 10 pregnancies among 26 patients who had day 3 biopsies, seven of which went to term—a miscarriage rate of 33%. Of the 12 pregnancies among 21 couples for whom biopsy was performed on day 5–6, eight miscarried (38%). Twenty-three egg retrievals among 15 couples with a *Robertsonian translocation* led to biopsies and testing; there were 3 pregnancies among 7 couples with day 3 biopsies, each of which went to term, and 8 pregnancies among 7 couples with day 5–6 biopsies, one of which miscarried and one of which was an ongoing monozygotic twin pregnancy. Combining day 3 with day 5–6 biopsies, the miscarriage rate after PGD for Robertsonian translocation exclusion was 18%, whereas PGD for excluding unbalanced reciprocal translocations was followed by a miscarriage rate of 45%.

Monogenic Diseases

Monogenic diseases considered appropriate for PGD are those uncommon or rare, fatal, or chronically disabling familial conditions that occur as a result of mutations in a single gene. The location of the mutation can be in an exon, a splice point, or within the control regions and affects the functioning of the specific gene.

Inheritance is Mendelian, and classically there are three major classes of phenotypic expression:

1. *Dominant inheritance*, where every individual who inherits the single gene change is likely to be affected by the disorder and will carry a 50% chance of passing on the affected gene to offspring. An example is Huntington's disease. PGD analysis for such mutations must be reliable in detecting a mutation change in a background of normal DNA sequence.
2. *Recessive inheritance*, where carriers of mutations themselves are not affected by the disorder but who partner with another carrier for a mutation in the same gene then produce a reproductive risk for their offspring of 25% for an affected child and 50% for a carrier child. An example is cystic fibrosis. Mutation analysis for these conditions needs to address the ability to analyze for a mutation in a homozygote state or often in a compound heterozygous state.
3. *X-linked inheritance* where, essentially, mutations on the X chromosome typically result in female carriers who have a 25% risk of producing affected male offspring and a 25% risk of reproducing the carrier state in female offspring. An example of a recessive X-linked gene disorder is hemophilia A. An example of an incompletely dominant X-linked disorder is fragile-X syndrome, which causes severe mental retardation in males but which also has a heterozygous female phenotype that includes premature ovarian failure. Analysis must be reliable but, unlike other recessive diseases, or the dominant diseases, there is no normal background DNA sequence for males. Female carriers contribute a non-mutated X chromosome, so confidence with the analysis must be the same as for the autosome mutations.

The starting point for PCR in the case of a single cell from a day 3 biopsy is usually just a single copy of DNA (there is obviously more DNA available with multicellular trophectoderm biopsies). In principle—and regrettably sometimes also in practice—failure of the mutated DNA to amplify (ADO) produces a false-negative result, leading to an incorrect conclusion of a normal state. Any biopsy testing process must be as reliable as possible to avoid any miscalls.

The Near Future for Translocation Testing

STR-Based Molecular Strategies

Our experience, above, revealed no obvious advantage for blastocyst-stage biopsies compared with day 3 cleavage-stage biopsies when FISH is used to infer balanced chromosomal patterns for either reciprocal or Robertsonian translocations. In each case, miscarriage rates remain particularly high for apparently balanced reciprocal translations. We have since reported a molecular strategy utilizing PCR for PGD in translocation carriers that examines highly polymorphic short tandem repeat sequences (STRs), application of which has significantly improved outcomes after biopsies at the blastocyst stage [22].

Using STR profiling to identify chromosomal segments on either side of the known breakpoints, in conjunction with standard cytogenetic segregation tables to predict each unbalanced state, we directly identify the monoallelic and triallelic states that are the direct cause of the phenotypic abnormality and reproductive loss which results from these malsegregants and, in turn, is the immediate pathogenic mechanism behind the reason PGD is offered to translocation carriers. The method requires extensive screening of chromosome-specific STRs to define those markers for which the carrier is heterozygous and where alleles are not shared with the partner. To make this PCR-based test efficient, chosen markers are multiplexed to obtain results within primary or secondary amplifications. The method also lends itself to other PCR-based PGD objectives conducted simultaneously, such as monogenic disease exclusion. Verification of the method has come from the rebiopsy of embryos diagnosed as unbalanced: in each of six cases in which samples were assessed for segmental chromosomal gains and losses using conventional CGH (see below), the predicted malsegregations were confirmed.

Conclusive results in our hands rose to 99% using STR profiling, compared with 93% with blastocyst-based FISH. Any apparent mosaicism seen in the trophectoderm sample has the potential to complicate the interpretation of the translocation state, especially when using FISH, where any visible abnormality tends to disqualify the embryo for transfer, on the subjective basis that failure of a chromosome to hybridize or to hybridize ambiguously is always possible. STR profiling, on the other hand, encompasses multiple loci on each side of the translocation point, reducing ADO-based errors (false monoallelic states from diploid alleles, false biallelic states for trisomic alleles).

Table 24.4 compares our FISH-based blastocyst biopsy experience with our STR-PCR experience. Patients with reciprocal translocations still show the expected predominantly unbalanced segregation patterns predicted by theory, but fewer embryos are falsely disqualified from transfer. Patients with Robertsonian translocations also fare better. Robertsonian translocation carriers can be prone to uniparental disomy, especially when chromosomes 14 and 15 are involved (see [22]); STR-PCR, unlike FISH, enables biparental inheritance to be looked for and to be confirmed or excluded. Finally, the time needed for actionable results with STR-PCR is just 4–5 h, compared with the 6–16 h required for FISH hybridization and interpretation.

The Near Future for Aneuploidy Screening

The majority of aneuploidies arise during female meiosis. The minority are brought to the embryonic genome by the fertilizing sperm and are equally pathogenic. A small number take origin in the first few cleavage divisions through mitotic nondisjunction. The latter lead to mosaic states in the embryo: clearly, the later this happens, the smaller the proportion of triploid cells and the more patchy the distribution among inner cell mass and trophectoderm derivatives. There is a large body of published knowledge on the recognized outcomes, such as confined placental mosaicism. In the embryo proper, trisomic cells will be at a disadvantage compared with their euploid neighbors as tissues and organs develop. Our experience with karyotyping 82 cell lines derived from inner cell masses of slow and stalled embryos, assumed to disproportionally display aneuploidies, provides an indication of this process (Bradley et al., manuscript under review). Sixty-nine (84%) displayed only a normal, diploid karyotype, indicating likely self-correction of mitotic nondisjunction-based mosaic states; a limited number tested showed no cases of loss of heterozygosity, which would indicate uniparental disomy as a consequence of self-correction of meiotic errors. The 13 cellular outgrowths that were cytogenetically abnormal included six single trisomies, a double trisomy, a monosomy, three triploidies, a triploidy with an additional chromosome 22, and a balanced reciprocal translocation. In each of the trisomies, meiotic nondisjunction was confirmed by demonstrating triallelic states for STRs on the affected chromosome. There were no mosaic cell lines.

Thus, for reasons of both relative numbers (mitotic trisomies are from the start mosaic states, whereas meiotic trisomies are pure) and, possibly, a qualitative difference between independent aneuploid states compared with diploid states, the key objective of screening for aneuploidy should be less to count chromosomes than it is to recognize dominant original parent of origin states for any of the 24 chromosomes.

Fluorescent In Situ Hybridization

Specific staining of embryo chromosomes with FISH has been the preferred method to identify the chromosome copy number in a fixed cell preparation. The probes bind to defined regions on the usually interphase cell chromosomes immobilized on a standard microscope slide, usually at interphase. Generally, the probes are purified cloned regions of the specific chromosome, subtracted for repetitive sequences. These probes are labeled with a unique fluorophore which can be visualized with fluorescence microscopy. The preparation and quality control of such material generally means that a commercial supply of the probes is the preferred choice for routine clinical use.

There are limitations to commercially available probe sets. The number of fluorophore colors falls far short of the minimum of 24 required. The fluor needs to be chemically active to attach to the DNA probe and also stable enough to remain attached during the hybridization process. Once hybridized, the color must be able to be visualized using, typically, UV excitation and filtered emission. High-energy wavelength excitation can result in rapid photo bleaching of the fluorophore and hence insufficient time to enumerate the hybridization pattern. The number of fluorophore colors falls far short of the minimum of 24 required. The commercial suppliers have limited their probe labels to a very small set that meet manufacturing standards and the exacting requirements for clinical use. These fluors must be spectrally separable using specific but simple microscope filters. In practice, this means that only 5–7 or so chromosomes can be checked in one hybridization event. Consequently, the number of chromosomes that are there to be counted using FISH means that multiple cycles of hybridization, enumeration, probe stripping, and rehybridization are needed. Each cycle runs the risk of target loss and/or degraded target sites, either of which can result in incorrect chromosome enumeration and thus a misreading of chromosome number—technical considerations that preclude more than 2 or 3 rounds of hybridization. Temporally, adding more than a very few hybridizations would take too much time to permit the transfer of IVF embryos fresh.

Single blastomere biopsy from day 3 embryos gives a single, simple answer: a normal chromosome complement or an abnormal complement. The problems of mosaicism and technical difficulties discussed above, however, still lead to embryos being incorrectly classified and then being excluded from transfer. Biopsy at the blastocyst stage does not resolve these problems but does offer an opportunity to see multiple hybridization signals for a set of cells. Nonetheless, a conservative reading of those signals has meant that observation of mosaic states in multicell biopsies has resulted in the exclusion of embryos that are likely to be substantially normal and suitable for transfer. The policy of disqualifying an embryo for transfer on the basis of 1 or 2 aberrant cells might need to be reexamined.

All other current karyotyping methods applicable to extremely low copy numbers of chromosomes, including analyses of single cells with day 3 embryo biopsies and of typically fewer than ten cells with blastocyst trophectoderm biopsies requires preliminary amplification of DNA copy number.

The first way to satisfy this challenge is to greatly increase the number of chromosome targets to be amplified, enabling any genomic shortcomings in genome-wide amplifications to be overcome by averaging. Over the last few (very few) years, advances in whole genome amplification has advanced the place of the technique of *comparative genomic hybridization* (CGH) by increasing its resolving power within chromosomes as well as improving its quantitative reliability in estimating preamplification DNA copy number.

Comparative Genomic Hybridization

Developed as a chromosomal screen to analyze genomic changes in cancers almost 20 years ago [23], CGH reveals copy amounts of all 22 autosomes and the two sex chromosomes to a resolution of ten million base pairs or so. The technique uses a combination of molecular and cytogenetic approaches to evaluate chromosome complements. Testing cancers with CGH is simpler than testing embryos, however, because generally with cancer samples there is no shortage of extracted DNA to be tested, whereas embryo biopsy specimens are much more limited.

Wells and Delhanty reported CGH analysis of individual cells from human day 3 embryos a decade ago [24]. Wilton and others reported the first reported successful clinical preimplantation use of CGH technique a year later [25]. While the use of CGH promised to deliver a total chromosome aneuploidy screen and the possibility of identifying any chromosome imbalance in an embryo, its labor intensity and its time-consuming nature (which required the embryos to be frozen while testing proceeded over periods of many days) precluded transfer of embryos during the biopsy cycle. There were only a few further reports over the ensuing 6 years [26–28]. Often, what was observed were relatively complex chromosome combinations; these then were given causal roles to explain implantation failure, but screening out aneuploid embryos did not improve embryo implantation rates. In spite of its promise, CGH has not been reported to be in routine use by any group. Recently, however, a report from Wells et al. has reported high implantation rates for blastocysts biopsied and analyzed with CGH after improved whole genome amplification [29]. The embryos were transferred after vitrification and later thawing, and produced an impressive thawed blastocyst implantation rate of 67%—which would warrant routine use, at least in selected patients.

The use of classical CGH on metaphase chromosomes demands high levels of skill, many days of analysis, and the freezing of biopsied embryos until the karyotype is known. One approach to minimizing labor requirements and shortening the testing time has been to employ DNA microarrays [30]. On the one hand, the timing suits polar body analyses and day 3 cleavage-stage biopsies, but both of these sample types offer only a single-cell genome for amplification and analysis, whereas blastocyst biopsy offers several cells to average out the amplification biases more effectively. On the other hand, the additional expense of CGH, however performed, is coming to be more generally appreciated as another reason for identifying embryos that can blastulate before biopsy and testing, in effect providing a self-screening process that reduces the costs of the testing for the individual patient. A pilot study looking at the analysis of polar bodies for aneuploid detection of female origin has been commenced by a consortium from the European Society for Human Reproduction. Implantation rates and pregnancy outcome data are still to be collected. Recent advances combining blastocyst-stage biopsy, micro-array CGH and vitrification have produced high embryo implantation rates and clinical pregnancy outcomes allowing a viable clinical service to be offered [31].

To date, therefore, it is blastocyst-stage biopsy that has given valuable improvement in implantation rates, and it waits to be seen whether the still prevalent day 3 biopsies and day 0–1 biopsies of polar bodies can achieve the same outcomes. With the use of a DNA amplification-based approach, the interpretation problems associated with low-level somatic mosaicism common in embryos and seen with FISH are partially overcome. The tissue sample, typically consisting of 3–5 cells, is analyzed as a whole (and is taken to represent the embryo as a whole), thus producing an averaging effect for the constitutional chromosomes under investigation.

References

1. de Boer KA, Catt JW, Jansen RPS, Leigh D, McArthur S. Moving to blastocyst biopsy for preimplantation genetic diagnosis and single embryo transfer at Sydney IVF. Fertil Steril. 2004;82(2):295–8.
2. Henman M, Catt JW, Wood T, Bowman MC, de Boer KA, Jansen RPS. Elective transfer of single fresh blastocysts and later transfer of cryostored blastocysts reduces the twin pregnancy rate and can improve the in vitro fertilization live birth rate in younger women. Fertil Steril. 2005;84(6):1620–7.
3. Jansen RPS. Female age and the chance of a baby from one in-vitro fertilisation treatment. Med J Aust. 2003;178:258–61.
4. Jansen RPS. Benefits and challenges brought by improved results from in vitro fertilization. Intern Med J. 2005;35(2):108–17.
5. Jansen RPS, Bowman MC, de Boer KA, Leigh DA, Lieberman DB, McArthur SJ. What next for preimplantation genetic screening (PGS)? Experience with blastocyst biopsy and testing for aneuploidy. Hum Reprod. 2008;23(7):1476–8.
6. McArthur SJ, Leigh D, Marshall JT, de Boer KA, Jansen RPS. Pregnancies and live births after trophectoderm biopsy and preimplantation genetic testing of human blastocysts. Fertil Steril. 2005;84(6):1628–36.
7. McArthur SJ, Leigh D, Marshall JT, Gee AT, de Boer KA, Jansen RPS. Blastocyst trophectoderm biopsy and preimplantation genetic diagnosis for familial monogenic disorders and chromosomal translocations. Prenat Diagn. 2008;28(5):434–42.
8. Munné S, Lee A, Rosenwaks Z, Grifo J, Cohen J. Diagnosis of major chromosome aneuploidies in human preimplantation embryos. Hum Reprod. 1993;8(12):2185–91.
9. Kuliev A, Verlinsky Y. Meiotic and mitotic nondisjunction: lessons from preimplantation genetic diagnosis. Hum Reprod Update. 2004;10:401–7.
10. Bolor H, Mori T, Nishiyama S, et al. Mutations of the SYCP3 gene in women with recurrent pregnancy loss. Am J Hum Genet. 2009;84(1):14–20.
11. Landwehr C, Montag M, Van der Ven K, Weber RG. Rapid comparative genomic hybridization protocol for prenatal diagnosis and its application to aneuploidy screening of human polar bodies. Fertil Steril. 2008;90(3):488–96.
12. Vialard F, Hammoud I, Molina-Gomes D, et al. Gamete cytogenetic study in couples with implantation failure: aneuploidy rate is increased in both couple members. J Assist Reprod Genet. 2008;25(11–12):539–45.
13. Voullaire L, Collins V, Callaghan T, McBain J, Williamson R, Wilton L. High incidence of complex chromosome abnormality in cleavage embryos from patients with repeated implantation failure. Fertil Steril. 2007;87(5):1053–8.
14. Schoolcraft WB, Katz-Jaffe MG, Stevens J, Rawlins M, Munne S. Preimplantation aneuploidy testing for infertile patients of advanced maternal age: a randomized prospective trial. Fertil Steril. 2009;92(1):157–62.
15. Mastenbroek S, Twisk M, van Echten-Arends J, et al. In vitro fertilization with preimplantation genetic screening. N Engl J Med. 2007;357(1):9–17.
16. Milki AA, Hinckley MD, Westphal LM, Behr B. Elective single blastocyst transfer. Fertil Steril. 2004;81(6):1697–8.
17. Van Dyke DL, Weiss L, Robertson JR, Babu VR. The frequency and mutation rate of balanced autosomal rearrangements in man estimated from prenatal genetic studies for advanced maternal age. Am J Hum Genet. 1983;35:301–8.
18. Stern C, Pertile M, Norris H, Hale L, Baker H. Chromosome translocations in couples with in-vitro fertilization implantation failure. Hum Reprod. 1999;14:2097–101.
19. Wilton L. Preimplantation genetic diagnosis for aneuploidy screening in early human embryos: a review. Prenat Diagn. 2002;22(6):512–8.
20. Otani T, Roche M, Mizuike M, Colls P, Escudero T, Munne S. Preimplantation genetic diagnosis significantly improves the pregnancy outcome of translocation carriers with a history of

recurrent miscarriage and unsuccessful pregnancies. Reprod Biomed Online. 2006;13(6): 869–74.
21. Munné S, Sandalinas M, Escudero T, Fung J, Gianaroli L, Cohen J. Outcome of preimplantation genetic diagnosis of translocations. Fertil Steril. 2000;73:1209–18.
22. Traversa MV, Carey L, Leigh D. A molecular strategy for routine preimplantation genetic diagnosis in both reciprocal and Robertsonian translocation carriers. Mol Hum Reprod. 2010;16(5):329–37.
23. Kallioniemi A, Kallioniemi OP, Sudar D, et al. Comparative genomic hybridization for molecular cytogenetic analysis of solid tumors. Science. 1992;258(5083):818–21.
24. Wells D, Escudero T, Levy B, Hirschhorn K, Delhanty JD, Munné S. First clinical application of comparative genomic hybridization and polar body testing for preimplantation genetic diagnosis of aneuploidy. Fertil Steril. 2002;78(3):543–9.
25. Wilton L, Williamson R, McBain J, Edgar D, Voullaire L. Birth of a healthy infant after preimplantation confirmation of euploidy by comparative genomic hybridization. N Engl J Med. 2001;345(21):1537–41.
26. Gutiérrez-Mateo C, Gadea L, Benet J, Wells D, Munné S, Navarro J. Aneuploidy 12 in a Robertsonian (13;14) carrier: case report. Hum Reprod. 2005;20(5):1256–60.
27. Obradors A, Fernandez E, Oliver-Bonet M, et al. Birth of a healthy boy after a double factor PGD in a couple carrying a genetic disease and at risk for aneuploidy: case report. Hum Reprod. 2008;23(8):1949–56.
28. Peng W, Takabayashi H, Ikawa K. Whole genome amplification from single cells in preimplantation genetic diagnosis and prenatal diagnosis. Eur J Obstet Gynecol Reprod Biol. 2007;131(1):13–20.
29. Wells D, Fragouli E, Stevens J, Munné S, Schoolcraft WB, Katz-Jaffe MG. Fertil Steril. 2010; 90:s80.
30. Hu DG, Webb G, Hussey N. Aneuploidy detection in single cells using DNA array-based comparative genomic hybridization. Mol Hum Reprod. 2004;10(4):283–9.
31. Traversa MV, Marshall J, McArthur S, Leigh D. The genetic screening of preimplantation embryos by comparative geneome hybridisation. Reprod Biol. 2011;10 (Supp 3):51–60.

Chapter 25
Microarrays and CGH for PGD of Chromosome Abnormalities and Gene Defects

Gary Harton and Santiago Munné

Fish and Array-Based Testing

More than 50% of cleavage-stage embryos produced in vitro are chromosomally abnormal, increasing to up to 80% in women over 42 years of age [1–4]. Although some abnormal embryos arrest during extended culture, most do not, and even at the blastocyst stage, more than half of all embryos are abnormal (mean maternal age 38 years) [5]. The majority of numerical chromosome abnormalities detected in embryos are not compatible with implantation or birth which negatively affects the success of assisted reproductive treatments. The detrimental effect of aneuploidy is illustrated by the high prevalence of chromosome abnormalities detected in spontaneous abortions, exceeding 70% in some studies [6–11]. It has been hypothesized that selection of embryos for transfer based on chromosome normalcy (euploidy) could improve success rates in assisted reproductive procedures [12]. This process is known as preimplantation genetic diagnosis (PGD) of aneuploidy or preimplantation genetic screening (PGS). For a glossary of terms (see Glossary).

Shortcomings of Pre-Array Technologies

The first PGD strategies to be described employed fluorescence in situ hybridization (FISH) analysis of cells biopsied from day-3 embryos [12–16], trophectoderm cells biopsied from blastocyst-stage embryos [17], or polar bodies biopsied from oocytes or zygotes [18–21]. The FISH methods allowed analysis of 5–12 chromosomes in each oocyte or embryo but were unable to provide a full evaluation of the

G. Harton, BS, TS (ABB) • S. Munné, PhD (✉)
Department of Molecular Genetics, Reprogenetics, LLC, 3 Regent Street, Suite 301, Livingston, NJ 07039, USA
e-mail: munne@reprogenetics.com

Z.P. Nagy et al. (eds.), *Clinical Embryology: A Practical Guide*,
DOI 10.1007/978-1-4614-8376-2_25, © Springer Science+Business Media New York 2013

chromosome complement. Nevertheless, that was enough to detect more than 80% of chromosomally abnormal embryos detected by array technology [22].

Some studies utilizing FISH-based strategies reported an improvement in implantation rates, reduction in spontaneous abortions, and/or an increase in take-home-baby rates [15, 21, 23–32]. However, these studies were not randomized. Other studies, some performed in a randomized fashion, did not produce significant improvements or showed a detrimental effect of PGD for aneuploidy [33–36]. Several reasons for these conflicting results have been advanced.

The biological argument, which does not explain differences in reports, but attempts to understand why some studies observed a negative effect on outcome, argues that cleavage-stage embryos have such high rates of chromosomal mosaicism that any analysis based upon a single cell is unreliable. Although it is true that mosaicism is common in cleavage-stage embryos (about 30% according to FISH analyses) [1–4], the majority of these embryos display chromosome abnormalities in every cell. In such cases, the biopsied cell may not be chromosomally identical to the remaining cells of the embryo, they may contain errors affecting different chromosomes, but the clinical diagnosis of "abnormal" is still valid. Large follow-up studies of preimplantation embryos diagnosed using FISH estimate only a 5–7% error caused by mosaicism [15, 37] when embryos are reanalyzed in all their cells by FISH. Even less, only 2% when analyzed by array CGH [38], thus mosaicism is unlikely to be the primary cause of poor outcomes following PGD.

The most probable cause of intercenter differences in PGD results are variations in the biopsy and genetic technologies employed. These encompass all aspects of the process and have been previously reviewed [39]. Here we will discuss briefly only a few of the key factors. Probably the most important variable in PGD is the embryo biopsy itself. One of the studies showing no difference in IVF outcome following PGD involved biopsy of two cells from each cleavage-stage embryo [33]. However, the same group later reported that two-cell biopsy, in contrast to single-cell biopsy, is detrimental to embryo development [40].

Even biopsying one cell in suboptimal conditions could be extremely damaging to embryo potential. A study conducted by Mastenbroek et al. [35] reported an astonishingly high rate of diagnostic failure (20%), resulting in many embryos being transferred without a diagnosis. The implantation rate of these undiagnosed embryos was 59% lower than the control. In this case, the only difference between the control and test groups appears to have been the biopsy, suggesting that embryo viability was drastically reduced by the biopsy procedures used in the clinics involved.

The second most important factor in obtaining good results can be summarized in the "error rate." The steps after biopsy involve fixation, FISH with a variety of potentially different protocols and probes, and cell scoring. However, the overall accuracy of these steps can be summarized in a single number, which is the error rate of a PGD laboratory. This error rate can be obtained by reanalyzing all the cells of nonreplaced embryos (abnormal embryos and arrested normal embryos) and determining if the original diagnosis was correct. Unfortunately, error rates vary widely, ranging from 2–7% [2, 15, 38] to 40–50% [22, 41] depending on the PGD laboratory. As shown in a recent review, error rates around 50% will in fact decrease implantation rates [39].

When performed using appropriate, well-validated methods, FISH can detect 90% of the chromosome abnormalities detected by CGH [16, 42], and some PGD laboratories do appear to obtain consistently good results with FISH and cleavage-stage embryo biopsy. Regardless, the field of PGD is evolving away from biopsying at this stage of embryo development and is increasingly focusing on biopsy of polar bodies from oocytes or zygotes or removal of trophectoderm cells from blastocysts. These embryonic stages may be more resilient to technical manipulation. Additionally, the limited chromosomal screening conveyed by FISH is increasingly being replaced by comprehensive methods of DNA analysis, which detect close to 100% of chromosomal abnormalities. The new wave of aneuploidy testing technologies is extremely redundant (each chromosome tested multiple times at different sites), readily automated, less subjective, and theoretically less prone to errors.

Comprehensive DNA Analysis Techniques

Here we will cover three techniques that are currently being used for PGD of chromosome abnormalities. Comparative genome hybridization (CGH) was first applied to day-3 embryo biopsies [43–47]. However, CGH is time consuming and is incompatible with day-3 biopsy and transfer by day 5, necessitating cryopreservation of embryos while testing is carried out. At the time that it was first applied, embryo freezing was a relatively inefficient technique and the low survival rate of thawed embryos likely neutralized any beneficial effects of CGH. For these reasons, CGH was temporarily abandoned and not applied again until the development of vitrification [48]. In conjunction with vitrification, CGH has been clinically applied to polar bodies [49–51] and blastocyst biopsies [5, 52]. The combination of CGH, blastocyst biopsy, and vitrification significantly improved implantation rates in a recent study, from 46.5% in controls to 72.2% in cycles with screening, with nearly 100% of blastocysts surviving biopsy [5]. However, many clinics are not yet proficient at blastocyst culture and vitrification. Furthermore, freezing adds extra cost to the cycle, and a majority of patients prefer to have a fresh cycle. Thus, for the time being, day-3 biopsy combined with comprehensive chromosome analysis remains the choice for most physicians and patients.

Two other techniques, microarray CGH (array CGH or aCGH) [53–57] and single-nucleotide polymorphism (SNP) microarrays [58–60], can be used for comprehensive chromosome analysis of single cells from day-3 biopsy and yield results in 24 h. The rapid turnaround time for these methods eliminates the need to cryopreserve embryos while testing is carried out.

Array CGH (aCGH) is already widely used for the cytogenetic analysis of prenatal and postnatal samples [61–66] since it is rapid and cost-effective and allows chromosomal regions to be screened at high resolution. Several types of aCGH platform are available for the purposes of aneuploidy screening. The variety most commonly used for the purpose of PGD utilizes bacterial artificial chromosome (BAC) probes, about 150,000 bp in length, covering all chromosome bands and giving a 4 MB or lower resolution. Even higher resolutions are achievable but not generally recommended since at that level, the difference between clinically significant duplications/deletions and normally occurring copy number variations is less clear. A microarray recently validated for PGD had 4,000 probes and thus covered ~25% of the genome sequence [58]. Microarray CGH has a similar accuracy rate to conventional CGH and should therefore be capable of producing similar results to those obtained in the promising CGH study performed by Schoolcraft et al. [5].

CGH and aCGH provide a quantitative analysis based on comparing the relative amount of DNA from two different sources, one from the clinical sample (e.g., a cell from an embryo) and another from a chromosomally normal individual. DNA samples from the two sources are differentially labeled and hybridized to either metaphase chromosomes (CGH) or probes on a microarray (aCGH). In the case of aCGH, each probe reveals the relative amounts of these two DNAs at a single chromosomal site. Since multiple copies of each probe are placed on the microarray and each chromosome is tested at many distinct loci, the diagnosis is very accurate.

Chromosome imbalances (aneuploidies, unbalanced translocations, deletions, and duplications) are easily detected using CGH and aCGH, but a limitation of these approaches is that diploidy cannot be distinguished from changes involving loss or gain of an entire set of chromosomes (e.g., haploidy, triploidy, tetraploidy, etc.). How important is this? In a recently submitted paper by Munne et al. (personal communication), about 7.7% (n = 91,073) of the supposedly 2PN embryos tested were polyploid or haploid but the majority of them had additional abnormalities detectable by CGH or array CGH and only 1.8% of all embryos were homogeneously polyploid or haploid. Furthermore, of those, the majority arrested by day 4, leaving only 0.2% of developing embryos uniformly polyploid or haploid. This suggests that failure to detect polyploid embryos may rarely lead to a misdiagnosis but is unlikely to have a significant impact on the clinical efficacy of the screening using aCGH or CGH.

Single nucleotide polymorphisms are areas of the genome where a single nucleotide in the DNA sequence varies within the population. Most SNPs are biallelic, existing in one of two forms, and are found scattered throughout the genome. By determining the genotype of multiple SNPs along the length of each chromosome, a haplotype (a contiguous series of polymorphisms on the same chromosome) can be assembled. This ultimately allows the inheritance of individual chromosomes or pieces of chromosomes to be tracked from parents to embryos. Current SNP microarrays simultaneously assay hundreds of thousands of SNPs, while utilizing powerful software to distinguish how many copies of each chromosome was inherited by an embryo [58, 60, 67].

All of the new generation of chromosome screening methods (CGH, aCGH, and SNP microarrays) rely on whole genome amplification (WGA) to amplify DNA from the single cell or small number of cells removed from a developing embryo [68]. CGH can be performed in combination with a variety of WGA methods; however, SNP microarrays are more sensitive to the type of amplification technique used and are not compatible with all methods. Currently, WGA methods like multiple displacement amplification (MDA), GenomePlex, and PicoPlex are most commonly used for SNP microarrays. These amplification methods allow for better overall coverage of the genome compared with earlier WGA methods (e.g., degenerate oligonucleotide primed PCR) and are less inclined to preferentially amplify some parts of the genome while leaving others unamplified or under amplified.

Currently, a few PGD groups around the world are validating SNP microarrays and analysis software for clinical use in PGD for aneuploidy screening. It is expected that data from the clinical use of SNP microarrays will closely match the data from CGH and aCGH testing. While the technologies differ greatly, both types of arrays (CGH-based and SNP-based) are trying to answer the same question; how many copies of each chromosome is present in a sample?

The small size of the SNP array probes can lead to poor hybridization efficiencies and low signal intensities for individual probes. This factor, coupled with the failure of WGA methods to amplify the entirety of the genome, can lead to many probes yielding no result (i.e., a low "call rate"). Also, allele dropout (ADO) and/or preferential amplification (PA) of one SNP allele versus another can lead to a great deal of "noise" in the system, which requires sophisticated interpretation. Several methods for the cleaning up of data from SNP microarrays have been developed: qualitative methods, looking only at the inheritance of specific SNPs and requiring comparison with parental DNA samples; quantitative approaches, assessing only the intensity of SNP calls; and techniques combining qualitative and quantitative methods, using both SNP intensity calls and inheritance patterns.

For qualitative approaches, it is necessary to assess parental DNA prior to clinical embryo testing. The key requirement is the deduction of the four parental haplotypes for each chromosome. Embryo testing is then focused on detecting the individual parental haplotypes, revealing how many chromosomes were inherited from each parent, i.e., karyomapping [58]. This approach has the disadvantage that mitotic abnormalities, in which only two haplotypes are present in a trisomy (i.e., caused by duplication of one of the two chromosomes in the embryo after fertilization), will not be detected. This can misdiagnose a substantial amount of embryos since 30% of aneuploid embryos contain mitotic abnormalities (mosaics) [15]. A quantitative approach compares the intensity of each SNP against the other SNPs. A purely quantitative approach for aneuploidy screening may not require parental testing ahead of the cycle; however, this approach would not be compatible with combination testing of single gene defects with aneuploidy screening (discussed below). This approach is currently the least developed. A qualitative/quantitative approach has also been applied clinically, and probably can obviate the issues mentioned above for purely qualitative or quantitative approaches [60, 67]. All of the analysis approaches still share one limitation and that is the diagnosis of tetraploidies. In a tetraploid cell, only two haplotypes are present (i.e., a postmeiotic duplication of a euploid cell); therefore, all SNPs will have the same intensity.

SNP-based microarrays offer some advantages over aCGH: (a) if qualitative analysis is employed, SNP-based microarrays can also detect the parental origin of any chromosome abnormalities. This may be valuable in rare instances of young couples producing many chromosome abnormalities but of little relevance to cases of advanced maternal age where at least 90% of the aneuploidies will be maternal in origin, and those of paternal origin are most likely mitotic error where the paternal chromosome was randomly recruited as the extra chromosome. These errors offer no predictive value for other embryos in the cohort or for future cycles; (b) SNP microarrays applied to PGD for chromosome rearrangements can differentiate between normal and balanced (carrier) embryos. However, because the rate of abnormalities in translocation cases is generally very high (>80%) [69], the great majority of PGD cycles do not have a surplus of embryos with a balanced chromosome constitution. In most cases, whatever balanced embryos are available are needed for transfer; (c) SNP arrays can directly produce a fingerprint of the embryo, allowing for assessment of which of the transferred embryos led to a pregnancy. However, if a laboratory is using aCGH, a similar test can be performed by utilizing a small aliquot of the DNA produced by WGA to perform conventional DNA fingerprinting; (d) finally, qualitative SNP arrays can also detect uniparental disomy (UDP), although this is a very rare event (e.g., UDP 15 occurs in 0.001% of newborns (OMIM)).

A major disadvantage of a qualitative or combination approach to SNP array analysis is the need to assess parental DNA ahead of the PGD cycle. This complicates patient management, adds substantially to the cost of the test, and precludes ad hoc decisions on biopsy for PGD. Approximately 20% of IVF cycles with planned PGD are canceled on day 3 due to low embryo numbers. Thus, these patients would have spent money on precycle parental testing that was ultimately unnecessary.

Validation of aCGH and SNP Arrays

Due to the intrinsic and often unforeseen problems with every new technology, a novel method should always be validated against other, more established methods [70]. Assessing a new approach against itself may preclude the detection of technique-related flaws. Thus, validation by inadequate methods such as the analysis of cell lines with defined chromosome abnormalities which cannot mimic mosaicism and other peculiarities of the cell being tested; analysis of eggs or embryos by one technique with analysis of polar bodies or the remainder of the embryo by the same technique which will preclude identifying abnormalities not detectable by that technique; blindly replacing undiagnosed embryos (either by single embryo transfer or fingerprinting the embryo) and following pregnancies and clinical losses to determine the fate of each tested embryo which does not account for the status of nonimplanted embryos; or using the SNP calls in one chromosome as internal controls for other SNPs in that same chromosome [60] may lead to false assumptions. In addition, the use of analysis tools that are qualitative in nature will miss the presence of two chromosomes of the same grandparental origin, and the errors caused by mosaicism will not be taken into account in this validation mode, resulting in bogus 99.9% confidence results.

In our opinion, the optimal method for validating a new technique is to reanalyze those embryos that were not transferred to the patient, either because they underwent arrest or because they were diagnosed chromosomally abnormal. The reanalysis of these embryos should be done with another well-established technique, the "gold standard." This would discern shortcomings of the new method under evaluation and account for issues related to embryo biology, such as mosaicism. The only problem with this approach is that euploid arresting embryos may become abnormal (karyokinesis without cytokinesis) from day 3 to day 5 before reanalysis [71, 72] and there is a scarcity of nonreplaced normal embryos.

To simplify comparison between studies, an error should be classified as diagnosing an embryo as euploid when reanalysis shows that it was abnormal or vice versa. Due to the extent of mosaicism, an error rate per chromosome has questionable relevance and no clinical importance compared to an error rate per embryo.

SNP microarrays have undergone a variety of validation experiments, such as comparison of PGD results and analysis of babies born [67, 73], SNP microarray reanalysis of embryos previously analyzed by SNP arrays [59], and using data from one set of SNPs as internal controls for another set of SNPs. To date, no studies have confirmed the original diagnosis by reanalyzing the remaining embryonic cells with a different technique.

Microarray CGH for PGD has been validated by analysis of single cells from known cell lines (Dagan Wells, personal communication) and by analyzing eggs with aCGH and comparing them to the results obtained using aCGH of the corresponding PBs (Montag and Gianaroli, personal communication). In a recent study, day-3 embryos analyzed by PGD with aCGH that were not replaced because of chromosome or morphological abnormalities were reanalyzed in most of their remaining cells by FISH using 12 probes for the most common chromosome abnormalities plus probes for any chromosomes found abnormal according to aCGH. Only 1.9% of embryos were found to be incorrectly diagnosed [58]. This is even lower than the 7% error rate expected solely from mosaicism as calculated in FISH studies [15]. Most likely, analyzing all of the chromosomes leads to the ascertainment of more chaotic embryos, further lowering the overall error rate.

Clinical Results

Of the techniques discussed, CGH is the one for which the greatest quantity of clinical data is available [5, 49, 50, 52]. Sher et al. [49] detected a 74% ongoing pregnancy rate per transfer and 63% per retrieval in women with an average age of 37.5 years. For patients of a similar age, receiving blastocyst transfer, Schoolcraft et al. [5] detected a significant increase in implantation rates, from 46.5 to 72.2% ($p < 0.001$) following embryo selection using CGH. Interestingly, both studies showed high implantation rates and both avoided cleavage-stage embryo biopsy and transferred embryos that had previously been cryopreserved in a later cycle. In addition to the potential benefits of transferring euploid embryos, there may be additional advantages associated with transfer in a nonstimulated cycle [74]. Loss of blastocyst-stage embryos after devitrification in the study by Schoolcraft et al. was minimal (0.7%) [5].

Regarding day-3 biopsy followed by aCGH and day-5 replacement, our most recent data [75] showed that only 118/151 PGD cycles had normal embryos for transfer in a population 38 years of age. The pregnancy rate was 59% per transfer compared with 38% in controls with a transfer ($p < 0.001$). The ongoing pregnancy rate for the PGD group was 54% per transfer, compared with 31.1% in controls with a transfer ($p < 0.001$). These results are encouraging but not as impressive as the day-5 (blastocyst) biopsy results. It is probable that the difference between clinical results obtained using CGH and aCGH is related to the stage at which biopsy was carried out rather than to differences in the method of chromosome screening. It is very likely that aCGH will replicate the results obtained by CGH when applied in conjunction with blastocyst biopsy. In summary, although data on the clinical application of comprehensive chromosome analysis techniques is preliminary, all studies suggest a significant improvement in ART results.

Less clinical data is available from SNP-based microarrays. In presentations at ASRM, Schlenker et al. [76] reported that CGH and SNP microarrays provided the same high implantation rates after blastocyst biopsy and vitrification. Also, in an ongoing RCT using 24-chromosome analysis by qPCR, higher pregnancies rates were obtained when biopsy was performed on day 5 than in controls with no intervention [77].

Microarrays for PGD of Gene Defects

Neither CGH microarrays nor the SNP microarrays in current use can directly detect gene defect mutations. However, SNP microarrays can be used to indirectly infer the presence or absence of a chromosome segment containing a mutant gene (i.e., identification of the same SNP haplotype as the parental chromosome carrying the mutation). A diagnosis can be performed based upon this sort of information [59]; indeed, this approach has recently been applied clinically for the simultaneous detection of gene defects and chromosome abnormalities [78].

In the case of aCGH, although gene defects cannot be detected directly, enough DNA is produced during the WGA step of the procedure that an aliquot can be used for aCGH analysis of chromosome abnormalities and another taken for PCR-based analysis of gene defects.

The high levels of ADO recorded after WGA mean that direct detection of a mutation using a microarray is likely to be less reliable than existing forms of PGD. Microarray-based diagnosis will be safer using approaches such as karyomapping, where conclusions are based upon the results from multiple linked SNPs, rather than a single mutation site. While the sort of microarrays used for preconception screening are not currently suitable for PGD, it is anticipated that their use will significantly increase the identification of high-risk couples and therefore lead to an increase in the usage of genetic testing modalities such as prenatal testing and PGD.

Glossary

Allele dropout (ADO) The failure to detect an allele in a sample or the failure to amplify an allele during PCR.

Aneuploidy The condition of a cell or of an organism that has additions or deletions of a small number of whole chromosomes from the expected balanced diploid number of chromosomes.

Array comparative genomic hybridization (aCGH) A technique to detect genomic copy number variations at a high resolution level using differentially labeled DNA samples (one of unknown karyotype, one known normal karyotype) after hybridization to specific parts of the genome printed on a glass slide.

Bacterial artificial chromosome (BAC) Artificial chromosome vector derived from bacteria used for cloning relatively large DNA fragments.

Chromosome translocation A chromosomal configuration in which (usually) the ends of two nonhomologous chromosomes have become exchanged.

DNA fingerprint The derivation of unique patterns of DNA fragments obtained using a number of short repeats following polymerase chain reaction allowing discrimination between the genetic makeup of one person from another or one embryo from another.

Comparative genomic hybridization (CGH) A technique that is used to detect chromosome gain or loss by hybridizing DNA from a target cell and a normal cell that are differentially labeled with unique fluorescent dyes to a normal karyotype.

Euploidy The condition of a cell or organism that has one or more complete sets of chromosomes.

Fluorescence in situ hybridization (FISH) A cytogenetic technique that is used to detect and localize the presence or absence of specific DNA sequences on chromosomes.

Haplotype A set of closely linked genetic markers present on one chromosome that tend to be inherited together (not easily separable by recombination).

Karyotype Cytogenetic chromosome analysis with direct visualization of the chromosomes to determine chromosome number and structure/content.

Meiotic error A chromosome error arising during meiosis (reduction division) in an egg or sperm.

Microarray Sometimes called a gene chip or a DNA chip. Microarrays consist of large numbers of molecules (often, but not always, DNA) distributed in rows in a very small space. Microarrays permit scientists to study inheritance of chromosomes and gene expression by providing a snapshot of all the genes that are active in a cell at a particular time.

Mitotic error A chromosome error arising during mitosis (division) of an embryo.

Mosaicism Two or more distinct chromosomal or genetic lineages within an individual embryo.

Polyploidy A cell or an organism having three or more chromosome sets.

Preferential amplification (PA) Phenomenon that occurs during amplification from small amounts of starting DNA where one allele preferentially amplifies more than the other allele.

Preimplantation genetic diagnosis (PGD) Diagnosis of a cell from a preimplantation embryo for a specific genetic disease before embryo transfer.

Preimplantation genetic screening (PGS) Screening of a cell from a preimplantation embryo for the detection chromosomal disorders before embryo transfer.

Single nucleotide polymorphism (SNP) A variation of a single nucleotide of DNA useful in understanding and identifying a higher risk of a disease in particular people.

Whole genome amplification (WGA) The in vitro amplification of a full genome sequence, ideally with even representation of the genome in the amplified product.

References

1. Munné S, Alikani M, Tomkin G, Grifo J, Cohen J. Embryo morphology, developmental rates and maternal age are correlated with chromosome abnormalities. Fertil Steril. 1995;64:382–91.
2. Magli MC, Gianaroli L, Ferrareti AP, Lappi M, Ruberti A, Farfalli V. Embryo morphology and development are dependent on the chromosome complement. Fertil Steril. 2007;87:534–41.
3. Bielanska M, Tan SL, Ao A. Chromosomal mosaicism throughout human preimplantation development in vitro: incidence, type, and relevance to embryo outcome. Hum Reprod. 2002;17:413–9.
4. Munné S, Serena C, Colls P, Garrisi J, Zheng X, Cekleniak N, Lenzi M, Hughes P, Fischer J, Garrisi M, Tomkin G, Cohen J. Maternal age, morphology, development and chromosome abnormalities in over 6000 cleavage-stage embryos. Reprod Biomed Online. 2007; 14:628–34.
5. Schoolcraft WB, Fragouli E, Stevens J, Munné S, Katz-Jaffe MG, Wells D. Clinical application of comprehensive chromosomal screening at the blastocyst stage. Fertil Steril. 2010;94(5):1700–6.
6. Hassold T, Chen N, Funkhouser J, Jooss T, Manuel B, Matsuura J, Matsuyama A, Wilson C, Yamane JA, Jacobs PA. A cytogenetic study of 1000 spontaneous abortions. Ann Hum Genet. 1980;44:151–78.
7. Daniely M, Aviram-Goldring A, Barkai G, Goldman B. Detection of chromosomal aberrations in fetuses arising from recurrent spontaneous abortions by comparitive genome hybridization. Hum Reprod. 1998;13:805–9.
8. Fritz B, Hallermann C, Olert J, Fucs B, Bruns M, Aslan M, Schmidt S, Coerdt W, Muntefering H, Rehder H. Cytogenetic analyses of culture failures by comparative genome hybridization. Re-evaluation of chromosome aberration rates in early spontaneous abortions. Eur J Hum Genet. 2001;9:539–47.
9. Qumsiyeh MB, Kim KR, Ahmed MN, Bradford W. Cytogenetics and mechanisms of spontaneous abortions: increased apoptosis and decreased cell proliferation in chromosomally abnormal villi. Cytogenet Cell Genet. 2000;88:230–5.
10. Carp H, Toder V, Aviram A, Daniely M, Mashiach S, Barkai G. Karyotype of the abortus in recurrent miscarriages. Fertil Steril. 2001;75:678–82.
11. Menasha J, Levy B, Hirschhorn K, Kardon NB. Incidence and spectrum of chromosome abnormalities in spontaneous abortions: new insights from a 12-year study. Genet Med. 2005;7(4):251–63.

12. Munné S, Lee A, Rosenwaks Z, Grifo J, Cohen J. Diagnosis of major chromosome aneuploidies in human preimplantation embryos. Hum Reprod. 1993;8:2185–91.
13. Munné S, Magli C, Bahçe M, Fung J, Legator M, Morrison L, Cohen J, Gianaroli L. Preimplantation diagnosis of the aneuploidies most commonly found in spontaneous abortions and live births: XY, 13, 14, 15, 16, 18, 21, 22. Prenatal Diagn. 1998;18:1459–66.
14. Magli MC, Sandalinas M, Escudero T, Morrison L, Ferrareti AP, Gianaroli L, Munné S. Double locus analysis of chromosome 21 for preimplantation genetic diagnosis of aneuploidy. Prenat Diagn. 2001;12:1080–5.
15. Colls P, Escudero T, Zheng X, Lenzi M, Cinnioglu C, Cohen J, Munné S. Increased efficiency of preimplantation genetic diagnosis for infertility through reanalysis of dubious signals. Fertil Steril. 2007;88:53–61.
16. Colls P, Goodall N, Zheng X, Munné S. Increased efficiency of preimplantation genetic diagnosis for aneuploidy by testing 12 chromosomes. Reprod Biomed Online. 2009;19:532–8.
17. Jansen RPS, Bowman MC, De Boer KA, Leigh DA, Lieberman DB, McArthur SJ. What next for preimplantation genetic screening (PGD)? Experience with blastocyst biopsy and testing for aneuploidy. Hum Reprod. 2008;23:1476–8.
18. Verlinsky Y, Cieslak J, Frieidine M, Ivakhnenko V, Wolf G, Kovalinskaya L, White M, Lifchez A, Kaplan B, Moise J, Valle J, Ginsberg N, Strom C, Kuliev A. Pregnancies following pre-conception diagnosis of common aneuploidies by fluorescence in-situ hybridization. Hum Reprod. 1995;10:1923–7.
19. Verlinsky Y, Kuliev A. Preimplantation diagnosis of common aneuploidies in fertile couples of advanced maternal age. Hum Reprod. 1996;11:2076–7.
20. Kuliev A, Cieslak J, Ilkevitch Y, Verlinsky Y. Chromosomal abnormalities in a series of 6733 human oocytes in preimplantation diagnosis for age-related aneuploidies. Reprod Biomed Online. 2002;6:54–9.
21. Verlinsky Y, Tur-Kaspa I, Cieslak J, Bernal A, Morris R, Taranissi M, Kaplan B, Kuliev A. Preimplantation testing for chromosomal disorders improves reproductive outcome of poor prognosis patients. Reprod Biomed Online. 2005;11:219–25.
22. Coulam CB, Jeyendram RS, Fiddler M, Pergament E. Discordance among blastomeres renders preimplantation genetic diagnosis for aneuploidy ineffective. J Assist Reprod Genet. 2007;24:37–41.
23. Gianaroli L, Magli C, Ferraretti AP, Munné S. Preimplantation diagnosis for aneuploidies in patients undergoing in-vitro fertilization with a poor prognosis: identification of the categories for which it should be proposed. Fertil Steril. 1999;72:837–44.
24. Munné S, Magli C, Cohen J, Morton P, Sadowy S, Gianaroli L, Tucker M, Márquez C, Sable D, Ferraretti AP, Massey JB, Scott R. Positive outcome after preimplantation diagnosis of aneuploidy in human embryos. Hum Reprod. 1999;14:2191–9.
25. Gianaroli L, Magli MC, Ferraretti AP. The in vivo and in vitro efficiency and efficacy of PGD for aneuploidy. Mol Cell Endocrinol. 2001;183:S13–8.
26. Gianaroli L, Magli MC, Ferraretti AP, Tabanelli C, Trombetta C, Boudjema E. The role of preimplantation diagnosis for aneuploidy. Reprod Biomed Online. 2001;4:31–6.
27. Munné S, Sandalinas M, Escudero T, Velilla E, Walmsley R, Sadowy S, Cohen J, Sable D. Improved implantation after preimplantation genetic diagnosis of aneuploidy. Reprod Biomed Online. 2003;7:91–7.
28. Gianaroli L, Magli C, Ferraretti AP, Tabanelli C, Trengia V, Farfalli V, et al. The beneficial effects of PGD for aneuploidy support extensive clinical application. Reprod Biomed Online. 2004;10:633–40.
29. Munné S, Chen S, Fischer J, Colls P, Zheng X, Stevens J, et al. Preimplantation genetic diagnosis reduces pregnancy loss in women 35 and older with a history of recurrent miscarriages. Fertil Steril. 2005;84:331–5.
30. Munné S, Fischer J, Warner A, Chen S, Zouves C, Cohen J. Referring centers PGD group. Preimplantation genetic diagnosis significantly reduces pregnancy loss in infertile couples: a multi-center study. Fertil Steril. 2006;85:326–32.

31. Garrisi GJ, Colls P, Ferry KM, Zheng X, Garrisi MG, Munné S. Effect of infertility, maternal age and number of previous miscarriages on the outcome of preimplantation genetic diagnosis for idiopathic recurrent pregnancy loss. Fertil Steril. 2009;92:288–95.
32. Rubio C, Buendía P, Rodrigo L, Mercader A, Mateu E, Peinado V, Delgado A, Milán M, Mir P, Simón C, Remohí J, Pellicer A. prognostic factors for preimplantation genetic screening in repeated pregnancy loss. Reprod Biomed Online. 2009;18(5):687–93.
33. Staessen C, Platteau P, Van Assche E, Michiels A, Tournaye H, Camus M, et al. Comparison of blastocyst transfer with or without preimplantation genetic diagnosis for aneuploidy screening in couples with advanced maternal age: a prospective randomized controlled trial. Hum Reprod. 2004;19:2849–58.
34. Platteau P, Staessen C, Michiels A, Van Steirteghem A, Liebaers I, Devroey P. Preimplantation genetic diagnosis for aneuploidy screening in patients with unexplained recurrent miscarriages. Fertil Steril. 2005;83:393–7.
35. Mastenbroek S, Twisk M, Van Echten-Arends J, Sikkema-Raddatz B, Korevaar JC, Verhoeve HR, et al. Preimplantation Genetic Screening in Women of Advanced Maternal Age. New Engl J Med. 2007;357:9–17.
36. Hardarson T, Hanson C, Lundin K, Hillensjo T, Nilsson L, Stevic J, Reismer E, Borg K, Wikland M, Bergh C. Preimplantation genetic screening in women of advanced maternal age caused a decrease in clinical pregnancy rate: a randomized controlled trial. Hum Reprod. 2008;23:2806–12.
37. Munné S, Sandalinas M, Escudero T, Marquez C, Cohen J. Chromosome mosaicism in cleavage stage human embryos: evidence of a maternal age effect. Reprod Biomed Online. 2002;4: 223–32.
38. Gutiérrez-Mateo C, Colls P, Sánchez-García J, Escudero T, Prates R, Ketterson K, Wells D, Munné S. Validation of microarray comparative genomic hybridization for comprehensive chromosome analysis of embryos. Fertil Steril. 2011;95(3):953–8.
39. Munné S, Wells D, Cohen J. Technology requirements for preimplantation genetic diagnosis to improve art outcome. Fertil Steril. 2010;94(2):408–30.
40. De Vos A, Staessen C, De Rycke M, Verpoest W, Haentjens P, Devroey P, Liebaers I, Van de Velde H. Impact of cleavage-stage embryo biopsy in view of PGD on human blastocyst implantation: a prospective cohort of single embryo transfers. Hum Reprod. 2009;12:2988–96.
41. Baart E, Van Opstal D, Los FJ, Fauser BCJM, Martini E. Fluorescence in-situ hybridization analysis of two blastomeres from day-3 frozen-thawed embryos followed by analysis of the remaining embryo on day-5. Hum Reprod. 2004;19:685–93.
42. Munné S, Fragouli E, Colls P, Katz M, Schoocraft W, Wells D. An improved 12-chromosome FISH test could detect 91% of aneuploid blastocysts. Reprod Biomed Online. 2010;20:92–7.
43. Wells D, Sherlock JK, Handyside AH, Delhanty DA. Detailed chromosomal and molecular genetic analysis of single cells by whole genome amplification and comparative genome hybridization. Nucleic Acids Res. 1999;27:1214–8.
44. Voullaire L, Wilton L, Slater H, Williamson R. Detection of aneuploidy in single cells using comparative genome hybridization. Prenat Diagn. 1999;19:846–51.
45. Wells D, Delhanty JDA. Comprehensive chromosomal analysis of human preimplantation embryos using whole genome amplification and single cell comparative genomic hybridization. Mol Human Reprod. 2000;6:1055–62.
46. Wilton L, Williamson R, McBain J, Edgar D, Voullaire L. Birth of a healthy infant after preimplantation confirmation of euploidy by comparative genomic hybridization. N Engl J Med. 2001;345: 1537–41.
47. Wells D, Escudero T, Levy B, Hirschhorn K, Delhanty JDA, Munné S. First clinical application of comparative genome hybridization (CGH) and polar body testing for Preimplantation genetic diagnosis (PGD) of aneuploidy. Fertil Steril. 2002;78:543–9.
48. Kuwayama M. Highly efficient vitrification for cryopreservation of human oocytes and embryos: the Cryotop method. Theriogenology. 2007;67:73–80.
49. Sher G, Keskintepe L, Keskintepe M, Ginsburg M, Maassarani G, Yakut T, Baltaci V, Kotze D, Unsal E. Oocyte karyotyping by comparative genome hybridization provides a highly reliable

method for selecting "competent" embryos, markedly improving in vitro fertilization outcome: a multiphase study. Fertil Steril. 2007;87:1033–40.
50. Fragouli E, Escalona A, Gutierrez-Mateo C, Tormasi S, Alfarawati S, Sepulveda S, Noriega L, Garcia J, Wells D, Munné S. Comparative genomic hybridization of oocytes and first polar bodies from young donors. Reprod Biomed Online. 2009;18:228–37.
51. Fragouli E, Escalona A, Gutierrez-Mateo C, Tormasi S, Alfarawati S, Sepulveda S, Noriega L, Garcia J, Wells D, Munné S. Comparative genomic hybridization of oocytes and first polar bodies from young donors. Reprod Biomed Online. 2009;18:228–37.
52. Fragouli E, Alfarawati S, Katz-Jaffe M, Stevens J, Colls P, Goodall N, Tormasi S, Gutierrez-Mateo C, Prates R, Schoolcraft WB, Munné M, Wells D. Comprehensive chromosome screening of polar bodies and blastocysts from couples experiencing repeated implantation failure. Fertil Steril. 2010;94(3):875–87.
53. Hu DG, Webb G, Hussey N. Aneuploidy detection in single cells using DNA array-based comparative genomic hybridization. Mol Hum Reprod. 2004;10:283–9.
54. Le Caignec C, Spits C, Sermon K, De Rycke M, Thienpont B, Debrock S, Staessen C, Moreau Y, Fryns JP, Van Steirteghem A, Liebaers I, Vermeesch JR. Single-cell chromosomal imbalances detection by array CGH. Nucleic Acids Res. 2006;34:e68.
55. Hellani A, Abu-Amero K, Azouri J, El-Akoum S. Successful pregnancies after application of array-comparative genomic hybridization in PGS-aneuploidy screening. Reprod Biomed Online. 2008;17:841–7.
56. Fishel S, GordonA LC, et al. Birth after polar body array CGH prediction of embryo ploidy following IVF—the future of IVF? Fertil Steril. 2009;93(3):1006–7.
57. Munné S, Gutierrez-Mateo C, Sanchez-Garcia JF, Ketterson K, Prates R, Keningsberg D (2009) Validation of microarray CGH for PGD by FISH reanalysis. Fertil Steril. 2009;92(3) Suppl S2.
58. Handyside AH, Harton GL, Mariani B, Thornhill AR, Affara NA, Shaw MA, Griffin DK. Karyomapping: a universal method for genome wide analysis of genetic disease based on mapping crossovers between parental haplotypes. J Med Genet. 2009;47(10): 651–8.
59. Treff N, Su J, Tao X, Miller KA, Levy B, Scott RT. A novel single-cell DNA fingerprinting method successfully distinguishes sibling human embryos. Fertil Steril. 2010;94(2): 477–84.
60. Johnson DS, Gemelos G, Baner J, Ryan A, Cinnioglu C, Banjevic M, Ross R, Alper M, Barrett B, Frederick J, Potter D, Behr B, Rabinowitz M. Preclinical validation of a microarray method for full molecular karyotyping of blastomeres in a 24-h protocol. Hum Reprod. 2010;25(4):1066–75.
61. Sismani C, Kitsiou-Tzeli S, Ioannides M, et al. Cryptic genomic imbalances in patients with de novo or familial apparently balanced translocations and abnormal phenotype. Mol Cytogenet. 2008;1(1):15.
62. Goobie S, Knijnenburg J, Fitzpatrick D, et al. Molecular and clinical characterization of de novo and familial cases with microduplication 3q29: guidelines for copy number variation case reporting. Cytogenet Genome Res. 2008;123(1–4):65–78.
63. Dimova I, et al. Whole genome analysis by array-based comparative genomic hybridization in patients with congenital malformations. Balkan J Med Genet. 2008;11(1):33–40.
64. Beaudet al, Belmont JW. Array-based DNA diagnostics: let the revolution begin. Annu Rev Med. 2008;59:113–29.
65. Heinrich U, et al. Array comparative genomic hybridisation in clinical diagnostics: principles and applications. J Lab Med. 2009;33(5):255–66.
66. Stejskalová E, et al. Cytogenetic and array comparative genomic hybridization analysis of a series of hepatoblastomas. Cancer Genet Cytogenet. 2009;194(2):82–7.
67. Treff NR, Su J, Kasabwala N, Tao X, Miller KA, Scott Jr RT. Robust embryo identification using first polar body single nucleotide polymorphism microarray-based DNA fingerprinting. Fertil Steril. 2009;90(Suppl):S82–3.
68. Vanneste E, Voet T, Le Caignec C, et al. Chromosome instability is common in human cleavage-stage embryos. Nat Med. 2009;15(5):577–83.

69. Munné S, Sandalinas M, Escudero T, Fung J, Gianaroli L, Cohen J. Outcome of preimplantation genetic diagnosis of translocations. Fertil Steril. 2000;73:1209–18.
70. Scott R, Treff N. Assessing the reproductive competence of individual embryos: a proposal for the validation of new "-omics" technologies. Fertil Steril. 2010;94(3):791–4.
71. Munné S, Alikani M, Grifo J, Cohen J. Monospermic polyploidy and atypical embryo morphology. Human Reprod. 1994;9:506–10.
72. Márquez C, Sandalinas M, Bahçe M, Alikani M, Munné S. Chromosome abnormalities in 1255 cleavage-stage human embryos. Reprod Biomed Online. 2000;1:17–27.
73. Scott TR (2010) Choosing the best embryo for transfer. In: 2010 Syllabus, Pacific Coast Reproductive Society, Rancho Mirage, CA, p. 51–63.
74. Shapiro BS, Daneshmand ST, Garner FC, Aguirre M, Hudson C, Thomas S. High ongoing pregnancy rates after deferred transfer through bipronuclear oocyte cryopreservation and post-thaw extended culture. Fertil Steril. 2009;92:1594–9.
75. Munné S, Surrey M, Grifo J, et al. Preimplantation Genetic Diagnosis using array CGH significantly increases ongoing pregnancy rates per transfer. Fertil Steril. 2010;94:(4)Suppl S81.
76. Schlenker T, Stevens J, Rawlins M, McCormick S, Katz-Jaffe MG, Schoolcraft WB. Clinical success with vitrification following trophectoderm biopsy for comprehensive chromosomal screening. Fertil Steril. 2009;92(Suppl):S-71.
77. Scott RT, Tao X, Taylor D, Ferry KM, Treff NR. A prospective randomized controlled trial demonstrating significantly increased clinical pregnancy rates following 24 chromosome aneuploidy screening: biopsy and analysis on day 5 with fresh transfer. Fertil Steril. 2010; 94:Suppl S2(O-65).
78. Handyside A, Grifo J, Gabriel A, Thornhill A, Griffin D, Ketterson K, Prates R, Tormasi S, Fischer J, Munné S. First clinical application of karyomapping for PGD of Gaucher disease combined with 24 chromosome screening. Reprod Biomed Online. 2010;20 Suppl 1:S16.

Part VI
Cryopreservation

Chapter 26
Sperm Cryopreservation

Fabio Firmbach Pasqualotto, Eleonora Bedin Pasqualotto, Edson Borges Jr., and Ashok Agarwal

The first reported observations of the effects of low temperatures on spermatozoa were performed by Lazaro Spallanzani in 1776, and the first to discuss the possible uses of sperm banks was the Italian Paolo Mantegazza, who wrote the following sentence in 1866: "It might even be that a husband who has died on a battle-field can fecundate his own wife after he has been reduced to a corpse and produce legitimate children after his death" [1]. However, sperm cryopreservation did not become a realistic proposition until the discovery in 1949 of the potent cryoprotective properties of glycerol [2]. The first human births resulting from artificial insemination of cryopreserved semen were reported by Bunge and Sherman in 1953 [3]. Since that time, many children have been born as a result of this rather simple procedure of assisted reproduction. Theoretical considerations suggested that long-term cryostorage would require the use of temperatures lower than −130°C, the glassy-transition temperature, below which ice-crystal growth is inhibited [4]. Consequently, liquid nitrogen (−196°C) storage became the standard very early in the history of sperm banking [5].

Nowadays, human semen cryopreservation is an extensively performed routine technique in fertility clinics and hospitals worldwide. Sperm cryopreservation may provide the opportunity for future fertility in a variety of situations. Although semen cryopreservation has proven to be very valuable, the quality of frozen sperm is highly affected during the process.

F.F. Pasqualotto, MD, PhD (✉)
Department of Urology, University of Caxias do Sul, Bairro Sao Pelgrino, RS, Brazil
e-mail: fabio@conception-rs.com.br

E.B. Pasqualotto, MD, PhD
Department of Gynecology, University of Caxias do Sul, Caxias do Sul, RS, Brazil
e-mail: eleonora@conception-rs.com.br

E. Borges Jr., MD
Fertility—Center for Assisted Fertilization, São Paulo, Brazil

A. Agarwal, PhD, HCLD (ABB), EMB (ACE)
Director, Center for Reproductive Medicine, Cleveland Clinic, Euclid Avenue 9500, Cleveland, OH 44195, USA

Z.P. Nagy et al. (eds.), *Clinical Embryology: A Practical Guide*,
DOI 10.1007/978-1-4614-8376-2_26,

General Aspects of Sperm Cryopreservation

It is generally accepted that the motility and fertilizing ability of frozen sperm do not correlate each other, and sublethal damages occurring within the sperm cell are thought to be responsible for this difference [6]. Generally, living cells undergoing cryopreservation are subjected to two major factors that are responsible for cryoinjury in a sequential manner (low temperature and crystallization of intracellular and extracellular water). These factors have deleterious effects on the sperm plasma membrane as changes in lipid composition and location [7–9]. These insults to the sperm membrane are in turn responsible for cell leakage of many intracellular components resulting in reduced sperm metabolic activities. Therefore, cytoplasmic and membrane-bound proteins and enzymes, as well as other components, are eliminated from the sperm cell [10–13]. These cryoinjuries include loss of membrane fluidity and integrity [14–16], oxidative stress leading to lipid peroxidation [17, 18], DNA fragmentation [19–21], and cytoskeleton modifications [22]. Also, freezing process causes disruption of cold-sensitive microtubule containing structures such as the meiotic spindle [23–27]. However, Donnely et al. demonstrated that sperm frozen unprepared from seminal fluid appears to be more resistant to freezing damage than frozen prepared sperm either by Percoll density centrifugation or a direct swim-up procedure and frozen in seminal plasma. In fact, although progressive motility is significantly greater in fresh prepared sperm compared with fresh unprocessed semen, prepared sperm suffer a greater decrease in progressive motility than raw semen after freezing. In addition, progressive motility is significantly improved by preparation of thawed semen, although the sperm velocity does not change. Progressive motility may be significantly improved by freezing prepared sperm in seminal plasma, although values are still significantly lower than that of the fresh samples. This is again due to the presence of seminal plasma because human sperm are particularly sensitive to free-radical assault due to their high content of polyunsaturated fatty acids and lack of repair mechanisms [28]. Further improvements can be achieved by selecting out the subpopulation of sperm with best motility and DNA integrity and freezing these sperm in seminal plasma, making this the optimal procedure. Therefore, freezing sperm in seminal plasma improves motility and DNA integrity after thawn [28]

Anyway, cryopreservation of human sperm remains an essential tool for the preservation of male fertility. Freezing of sperm before initiation of treatment provides to patients a type of "fertility insurance" and may allow them to father their own children through the use of in vitro fertilization (IVF) or intracytoplasmic sperm injection (ICSI). On the other hand, human spermatozoa have unusual cryobiological behavior, and improvements in their survival have not been achieved by the standard approaches of cryobiology. In fact, despite continuous methodological optimization, the process of cryopreservation and thawing leads to an activation of apoptosis signal transduction in a certain amount of the cryopreserved spermatozoa probably contributing to the reduction of the fertilizing capacity [29–31]. In fact, the mitochondria are preferentially susceptible to apoptotic stimuli due to their compartmentation within the midpiece region [32, 33].

As far as sperm membrane damage is concern, the susceptibility of the sperm of other mammal species to cryodamage during the freezing process appears to be related to a high ratio of saturated vs. unsaturated fatty acids, together with low cholesterol content [34]. Interestingly, human sperm membranes have unusually high cholesterol contents, and these high levels are known to stabilize membranes during cooling [35]. Recently, a study showed that higher cholesterol contents do not appear to protect sperm against cryodamage. Conversely, calcium equilibrium appears to be essential for a good postthaw recovery. On the other hand, mitochondrial activity is not reflecting the possibilities of sperm survival and is probably not a good indicator of the sperm metabolism. Although further experiments are needed to improve postthaw recovery, some calcium chelators (i.e., EDTA) or determinate phospholipids, which would prevent calcium flux into the sperm, may be added to the sperm freezing medium. Although ICSI may be used for men with severe sperm pathologies and the generation of poor results after the thawing of sperm, there are some specific cases where an improvement in the freezing methods are essential, such as in management of sperm donor samples [36].

Sperm membrane integrity becomes impaired with translocation of phosphatidylserine from the inner to the outer leaflet of the sperm plasma membrane [37, 38]. This translocation is considered one of the early signs of terminal phase of apoptosis [39]. The specific binding of annexin V to phosphatidylserine can be used for detection [40] and magnetic separation of spermatozoa with disturbed plasma membrane [41].

According to Paasch, sperm freezing showed a significant overall activation of caspases with a decrease in mitochondrial membrane potential. Both mature and immature fractions had significant activation of caspases followed by a decreased number of sperm with intact mitochondrial membrane potential after cryopreservation. In addition, cryopreservation and thawing induce caspase activation in mature annexin V1 in ejaculated human spermatozoa as well as in immature annexin V1 and annexin V2 sperm. Cells without susceptibility to apoptosis activation can thus be separated by magnetic field by magnetic cell sorting (MACS) technique, which may prove to be of clinical relevance [42]. In fact, the separation of a distinctive population of nonapoptotic spermatozoa with intact membranes may optimize the cryopreservation–thawing outcome. Magnetic-activated cell sorting using annexin V microbeads enhances sperm motility and cryosurvival rates following cryopreservation [43]. However, MACS using annexin V microbeads enhances the percentage of spermatozoa with intact transmembrane mitochondrial potential and mitochondrial integrity survival rates following cryopreservation [33].

The change in the plasma membrane selective permeability caused by cold shock induces the loss of many components from the sperm cell resulting in reduced metabolic activities. During this process, cytoplasmic and membrane-bound proteins are lost [44–46]. Recently, a decrease in P25b and P34H (fertility markers according to Syllivan) after human sperm cryopreservation has been shown. However, this decrease in P34H detection is most likely a consequence of cryopreservation-induced damage to the sperm plasma membrane rather than total cell damage. Due to the fact that sperm deficient in P34H are unable to bind to the egg's zona pellucida (ZP) [47], lower levels of P34H observed in cryopreserved semen may correlate with the loss of fertility after freezing–thawing of human sperm.

According to Morris et al., viability on thawing does not appear to correlate with conventional theories of cellular freezing injury, suggesting that, for human spermatozoa, other factors determine viability following freezing and thawing. Improved methods of cryopreservation may be developed by specifically manipulating the manner in which cells experience physical changes instead of imposing a linear temperature reduction. Treatments which followed a chosen nonlinear concentration profile, referred to as "controlled concentration," allowed recovery of almost all the cells which were motile before freezing [48].

Effect of Storage Temperature on Sperm Cryopreservation

The standard method for preservation of human sperm is storage in liquid nitrogen at a temperature of −196°C [2]. A number of studies have documented that improvements in cooling technique and the use of improved cryopreservatives, as well as thawing at 37°C in a water bath, improve postthaw sperm quality [3]. It appears, however, that the loss of sperm motility with the cryopreservation process does not increase with prolonged periods of cryopreservation, making long-term storage feasible. In fact, it has been reported that the semen of six donors was stored for 28 years suggesting that it may be possible to store human sperm virtually indefinitely if it is kept under liquid nitrogen. This is a pertinent information for clinicians to refer pubescent boys and young men for sperm banking before chemotherapy. Some of these young men may require sperm storage for long periods (years) [49–52].

Sperm cryopreservation in liquid nitrogen at −196°C has become standard protocol in most andrology facilities. Because this technique is pretty much acceptable everywhere, little consideration has been given to the potential effectiveness of short- or long-term storage of sperm at higher temperatures. Unfortunately, not every place has consistent access to liquid nitrogen cryopreservation facilities. Trummer et al. showed that sperm storage at −70°C is linked with a greater loss of sperm motility than is storage at −196°C. The reduction in motility noted at 1 week, however, was fairly modest. Unfortunately, the loss of sperm motility increased dramatically after 3 months of storage. These results indicate that short-term storage of sperm at −70°C may be a viable option if liquid nitrogen storage facilities are not available. Long-term storage at this temperature (70°C), however, appears to be linked with an unacceptable reduction in sperm motility [53].

Even though the standard protocol of sperm storage at −196°C is widely used in almost every center, the technical aspects of freezing and thawing sperm and preparing cryopreservation media have been refined over the years [54–57]. Various methods of cryopreservation have been evaluated for their effects on sperm motility [58–60]. However, the methods for freezing and thawing semen that optimize motility recovery have not been firmly established. In addition, the optimum rate of temperature drop during freezing remains controversial [54, 58, 59]. The flash-freezing technique in which the sample is plunged directly into liquid nitrogen produces sperm recovery rates that are comparable to those seen with computer-controlled, slow-staged freezing [60]. In addition, a variety of cryoprotectants are available to protect sperm from the negative effects of the cryopreservation process. Many andrology laboratories use TES and Tris yolk buffer (TYB; Irvine Scientific, Santa Ana, CA), but some of the other media commonly used are the following: Sperm Freezing Medium (Medi-Cult, Copenhagen, Denmark) and Enhance Sperm Freeze (Conception Technologies, San Diego, CA). However, a recent study by Nallella et al. showed that Irvine Scientific method is associated with more flash freezing compared with the Cleveland Clinic Foundation method and results in better preservation of sperm motility and a higher cryosurvival rate. According to their study, TES and TYB is most effective at protecting sperm from the negative effects of the cryopreservation process [61]. This may be due to the presence of egg yolk along with glycerol.

The advantages of the fast-freezing and slow-staged cooling methods have long been debated. Studies have reported results in favor of both the fast-freezing method [62] and the slow-staged cooling method [63–65]. A recent study showed that there was no difference in sperm quality preservation when semen samples is frozen by fast-freezing technique or by slow, controlled freezing method, either in liquid nitrogen or vapor-phase nitrogen [66].

Another study has showed that freezing spermatozoa in alginic acid microcapsules resulted in an increase of immobilized spermatozoa by 18.3%, compared with the standard protocol. The method of cryopreservation of small amounts of spermatozoa is a feasible and easy method that does not demand special laboratory equipment. Because microcapsules are dissolved under microscopic control, a 100% recovery rate of spermatozoa is estimated. Furthermore, microencapsulation of spermatozoa excludes the possibility of contamination with foreign material, either spermatozoa or genetic material. With microcapsules, the recovered spermatozoa can be divided into samples and cryopreserved separately for consecutive ICSI procedures. This gives the opportunity to collect spermatozoa, independently from oocyte recovery and ICSI, and assures the availability of spermatozoa on the day of ICSI [67].

Cryopreservation of Human Spermatozoa Within Oocyte Empty Zona

Men who have azoospermia can now be treated through the surgical isolation of spermatozoa using microsurgical epididymal sperm aspiration (MESA) or testicular sperm extraction (TESE) [68]. However, multiple testicular operations are not only costly but may lead to adverse physiologic effects and possible testicular failure [69]. The need to repeat these procedures can be avoided by the use of sperm cryopreservation [70]. Cohen et al. were the first to demonstrate that the ZP is an ideal vehicle for sperm cryopreservation [71]. After removal of the cellular material from oocytes or embryos, the empty ZP provides a suitable vehicle for preserving the few spermatozoa that can be obtained from patients with severe male infertility [71]. Cryopreservation in ZP avoids the loss of sperm that occurs with the dilution and washing of sperm during conventional cryopreservation procedures [72]. The rate of recovery of motile sperm after cryopreservation in ZP is higher than after conventional cryopreservation with cryoseeds and dithiothreitol [72–74]. With cryopreservation in ZP, TESE or MESA could be performed without regard to the timing of egg retrieval [75].

Sperm Cryopreservation in Specific Situations

Obstructive Azoospermia

Obstructive azoospermia is caused by several different etiologic processes. Ejaculatory duct obstruction, vasectomy, postinfection obstruction, and congenital bilateral absence of the vas deferens are some of the major causes of obstruction. An important approach in management of patients with obstructive azoospermia is retrieval of sperm for various assisted reproductive technology (ART) procedures through MESA, TESE, and percutaneous epididymal sperm aspiration (PESA).

In general, spermatozoa from epididymis are considered more mature than the testicular spermatozoa and provide a higher pregnancy rate [76]. Often, it is not possible to retrieve spermatozoa from the epididymis. In some cases, there might be a complete absence of epididymis. TESE is the modality of choice in the management of nonreconstructable obstruction of the excurrent duct system, when epididymal sperm aspiration is not available or unsuccessful. It is possible to extract a large number of spermatozoa from the epididymis or testicular tissues of patients with azoospermia of obstructive etiology. In fact, pregnancy outcome in obstructive azoospermia using these spermatozoa is higher than in nonobstructive azoospermia [77]. Only a small portion of these spermatozoa are needed for IVF/ICSI techniques, and the remaining tissue can be divided into several aliquots and cryopreserved for subsequent use. After carrying out a TESE procedure, the testicular tissue can be divided into several aliquots and cryopreserved. This would favor multiple ICSI cycles [78], thereby avoiding further surgical biopsies to retrieve spermatozoa in the future [79]. Generally, the time from biopsy to processing and freezing is within 1 and 1.5 h; however, a recent case report showed pregnancy even with the interval between the biopsy and the testicular tissue cryopreservation up to 15 h. Therefore, for many programs, the use of cryopreserved testicular tissue avoids the need for fresh testicular tissue at the time of ICSI [51].

Nonobstructive Azoospermia

In contrast to obstructive azoospermia, where viable sperm can easily be retrieved from the frozen specimens, the impaired quality of the testicular tissue present in nonobstructive azoospermic (NOA) patients does not allow for cryopreservation and later use for ICSI in all cases. As has been demonstrated for ejaculated sperm, a significant decrease in sperm motility and viability by freezing and thawing also occurred for testicular sperm [80]. This implies that cases with extremely low numbers of sperm retrieved can hardly be considered candidates for cryopreservation.

Even in a program with low-restrictive criteria for patient allocation and cryopreservation of testicular sperm, diagnostic testicular sperm retrieval followed by cryopreservation may be the procedure of choice. In order to counteract the reasonable risk of not finding sperm or only immotile sperm, scheduling fresh surgery as backup or counseling the couple for donor sperm as backup is recommended. The use of totally immotile sperm after thawing should be discouraged on the basis of the present data [81].

Patients with Cancer

Recent advances in the diagnosis and treatment of malignant diseases has brought into focus certain quality-of-life issues, such as the problem of infertility [82]. The impact of these problems is magnified in malignant diseases that predominantly affect patients in the reproductive age group. An increasing number of people are being successfully treated for cancer, and for those with an expectation of long-term survival, the late effects of treatment are of concern. In fact, in the past, cancer survivors tended to be most concerned about disease recurrence and treatment side effects. As survival rates have increased, however, patients are now also concerned about quality-of-life issues such as preserving fertility potential [83].

Depending on the underlying disease, the age of the oncological patient, the type of therapeutic agent used to treat the cancer, the cumulative doses used, and the duration of the treatment, 10–100% of surviving cancer patients will show reduced semen parameters after their cure. An average of 15–30% of cured cancer patients remain sterile in the long term [84].

The degree of testicular damage is drug specific and dose related. Ninety-seven percent of men with Hodgkin's disease (HD) who were treated with MOPP (mechlorethamine, vincristine, procarbazine, and prednisone) became azoospermic compared with 54% of those treated with ABVD (adriamycin, bleomycin, vinblastine, and dacarbazine). Only 14% of those in the MOPP group recovered spermatogenesis compared with 100% in the ABVD group [85]. Men with testicular germ cell cancer can expect irreversible impairment of the gonadal function at cumulative cisplatin doses 400 mg/m^2 [86]. In the case of irradiation to the adult male testis, permanent azoospermia can be induced by doses in excess of 400 cGy, whereas recovery of spermatogenesis is seen at doses of 300 cGy or below [87].

According to a study by Spermon et al., before the cancer being diagnosed, 79 (66%) of 120 couples who attempted to conceive succeeded within 1 year. After treatment, 38 (43%) of 88 couples conceived within 1 year. Seven couples used cryopreserved sperm to conceive a child after treatment. The different treatment modalities do not significantly influence the outcome of patients' wish for children.

Congenital malformations were recorded in approximately 4% of the children born before or after treatment. Therefore, although the majority of the patients with testicular cancer have a fulfilled wish with regard to children, it seems to be more difficult to father a child after treatment compared with the case in the general population. Because it is not possible to predict which patient will have fertility problems after treatment, cryopreservation should be offered to every testicular cancer patient. In addition, an increased risk for congenital malformations is not observed [88].

It is recommended that all male cancer patients up to age 55 (at least or according to institutional criteria) be referred for sperm cryopreservation. The age of 55 years is the maximum recommended age for freezing sperm according to the Human Fertilisation & Embryology Authority (HFEA) regulations [89]. Further deterioration have been observed following cancer treatment, and this is of a major importance to young patients. Sperm quality following cancer treatment depends on many factors: initial sperm characteristics, type of cancer, and therapeutic approach. Unfortunately, it is impossible to predict who will have normal spermatogenesis and who will become azoospermic.

In many cancer subjects, sperm quality is already reduced before receiving any treatment. Studies have been shown that semen quality in adolescent male patients with cancer found that semen parameters may be diminished, and sperm cryopreservation during potentially sterilizing treatment should be considered [90–92]. At present, sperm banking remains the only proven method, although hormonal manipulation to enhance recovery of spermatogenesis and cryopreservation of testicular germ cells are possibilities for the future [5, 93–95]. According to Hallak et al., patients with testicular cancer, leukemia, and lymphoma had the worst seminal quality compared to other cancer groups [96, 97]. Patients with malignant diseases in general have lower total motile sperm count and motility compared to normal semen donors. Furthermore, and of utmost importance, the authors concluded that prefreeze or postthaw semen quality in cancer patients is not affected by the type of disease. According to Gandini et al., the recovery of spermatogenesis after chemotherapy or radiotherapy in their group of testicular cancer patients studied was not a function of pretherapy sperm parameter quality [93]. Therefore, cryopreservation of semen should be offered to cancer patients irrespective of the type of the disease [5, 98–100].

The intersection of cancer and reproduction raises ethical issues for both cancer and fertility specialists, including issues of experimental vs. established therapies, the ability of minors to give consent, the welfare of expected children, and posthumous reproduction. In some respects, cancer-related infertility is not markedly different than other kinds of infertility. In other way, however, the context of cancer gives rise to issues of patient and offspring welfare that do not arise in other infertility settings. Reproductive physicians play important roles in helping to preserve the reproductive capacities of young cancer patients. First, they are involved in developing and using procedures to preserve gametes, embryos, and gonadal tissue before treatment. Second, fertility specialists will assist cancer survivors in using preserved gametes and tissue or in providing other assistance in reproduction [101].

Men who once had little or no chance of establishing a pregnancy through assisted techniques now have fertility rates approaching that of a couple undergoing standard IVF when there is no male infertility involved. However, according to

Zapzalka et al., most of the oncologists (74%) are unaware of recent advances in reproductive technology in which only a few sperm are needed for successful IVF with ICSI [102]. This lack of awareness may be contributing to underutilization of sperm cryopreservation by male cancer patients. Coincidentally, the number of patients that the oncologists estimated to actually cryopreserve sperm is also very small (27%). This leads to speculation that if more oncologists knew of the existence of ICSI, the percentage of patients who cryopreserve sperm might increase.

According to Schover et al., 19% of the 283 survivors of cancer from the Cleveland Clinic Foundation tumor registry had significant anxiety that their cancer treatment could affect negatively their children's future, and only 57% received information from their healthcare providers about infertility after cancer [103].

Other reproductive concerns are discussed even less often. For instance, patients with cancer may have chromosomal abnormalities in the malignant cell of origin and an increased frequency of human sperm chromosomal abnormalities after radiotherapy has been reported. However, reassuringly, studies have shown that children born after completion of cancer treatment have no increased risk for chromosomal abnormalities or birth defects before or after treatment.

Intraoperative Sperm Harvesting During a Vasectomy Reversal and Cryopreservation

The availability of ICSI technique has encouraged some surgeons to offer cryopreservation of sperm that may be harvested during vasectomy reversals. Cryopreservation of sperm during vasoepididymostomy is especially important because of a reported 35% rate of azoospermia after microsurgical vasoepididymostomy [104]. Other investigators have reported that motile sperm were present in the intraoperative vasal and epididymal fluid in 35% of 603 vasectomy reversals [105]. However, performance of a vasal or epididymal anastomosis should be prioritized over sperm harvesting during vasectomy reversals. The surgeon should perform the reversal at the location farthest from the testicle where intact sperm, regardless of their motility, are present, rather than closer to the testicle in order to harvest motile sperm. Before sperm harvesting and cryopreservation are performed, the patient and his partner should assess the cost effectiveness of, and their ability to afford, IVF/ICSI. When harvesting sperm during vasectomy reversals, surgeons must alert laboratory personnel to cryopreserve small aliquots of sperm that are appropriate for later use with ICSI rather than larger aliquots for either vaginal or intrauterine insemination (IUI) or IVF without ICSI [106, 107].

Prior to the Absence of the Partner

If it is anticipated that the male partner will be unavailable during the optimal time for the procedure, it is possible to cryopreserve a semen sample prior to his departure as a backup in the event he is prevented from providing a sample at the time of the procedure. While this may not be optimal, it can often keep the time and finances invested in a procedure from being wasted due to unforeseen circumstances [108].

Assisted Reproduction

Since the introduction of a method for freezing human semen, the indications for sperm cryobanking have been greatly expanded by recent breakthroughs in assisted reproduction, for one's own future use and donor banking [5]. However, it has been shown that the process of freezing and thawing is related with a variable loss of sperm quality [109].

Although the adverse effect of freezing and thawing upon sperm quality is even more pronounced in cases of poor semen quality, with the advent of ICSI, only a small number of motile spermatozoa are required for a successful fertilization [110, 111]. In fact, ICSI can be performed with fresh and cryopreserved spermatozoa from ejaculated semen from patients with oligoasthenoteratozoospermia (OAT) or from spermatozoa extracted from the epididymis or testis in cases of obstructive or nonobstructive azoospermia [112].

It is well known that IUI with cryopreserved sperm results in a lower pregnancy rate compared to fresh sperm, but many studies have been showing that fertilization and pregnancy rates of ICSI using cryopreserved spermatozoa are similar of freshly obtained sperm [113–117].

Even though there is no doubt that cryopreserved spermatozoa can be used to fertilize oocytes by ICSI, more studies comparing the efficacy of ICSI with either fresh or cryopreserved ejaculated spermatozoa from infertile patients should be performed. Also, the majority of studies comparing fresh and cryopreserved sperm have shown results from sperm surgically retrieved [114–117]. Borges et al. demonstrated that when the semen sample had motility decreased, the fertilization rate is higher with fresh sperm than with cryopreserved sperm. However, the implantation and pregnancy rates miscarriage rates are similar. This finding corroborates the idea that the cryopreservation process may cause more damage to patients with asthenozoospermia than patients with normal semen analysis or oligozoospermia. In fact, it is postulated by the authors that the worst normal fertilization rate detected in men with asthenozoospermia compared to normozoospermic or oligozoospermic men could be because the semen with low motility may have abnormalities in the sperm even before the cryopreservation, and the damage caused by the cryopreservation could be much higher than detected in other sperm characteristics [112].

According to a study published by Schmidt et al., following antineoplastic treatment, 43% of the men had motile spermatozoa in the ejaculate, but 57% were azoospermic. A total of 151 ART cycles were performed [55 IUI, 82 ICSI, and 14 ICSI–frozen embryo replacement (FER)]. Their clinical pregnancy rate per cycle was 14.8% after IUI, 38.6% after ICSI, and 25% after ICSI–FER. The corresponding delivery rates were 11.1, 30.5, and 21%. Cryopreserved semen was used in 58%

of the pregnancies. The delivery rate per cycle was similar after using fresh or cryopreserved spermatozoa. Therefore, male cancer survivors have a good chance of fathering a child by using either fresh ejaculated sperm or cryopreserved sperm [118]. Recently, Agarwal et al. [94] reported the outcome of ART in 29 male cancer survivors all using cryopreserved semen. A total of 87 cycles were performed with a mean pregnancy rate of 18.3% per cycle (7% after IUI, 23% after IVF, and 37% after ICSI).

Male cancer patients should be encouraged to freeze numerous sperm samples even when sperm count and motility are poor [119]. In these cases, ICSI is a powerful technique compared with intrauterine injection since thawed sperm samples with poor parameters can produce relatively high fertilization rates resulting in normal pregnancies and deliveries. The possibility to repeat treatments even in face of a limited number of sperm samples appears to be of utmost importance.

There are concerns that men with cancer who initiate a pregnancy either before or after treatment may have children who are at an increased risk for congenital anomalies. However, Hansen et al. studied the rate of congenital abnormalities in children born to fathers with cancer before treatment and observed a congenital malformation rate of 3.8%, which is comparable to the general population [120]. Redman et al. found no congenital abnormalities in three children who were born using cryopreserved semen from patients with Hodgkin's disease [121]. Moreover, Spermon et al. reported a 4% rate of congenital malformations in children born before or after treatment of testicular cancer, compared with 2.2% in the general population [89]. Thus, cancer patients should be informed that, currently, there is no available evidence for increased incidence of congenital abnormalities in children.

In recent years, some physicians have raised doubts regarding the justification and necessity of providing the facilities for banking spermatozoa before cancer treatment because of the relatively small number of men who used it following completion of treatment and consequently the small number of children born as a result of cryopreserved spermatozoa. Indeed, it seems that 5–15% of the patients who banked their semen before treatment return for fertility purposes. The reasons for that are: short period of original disease, anxiety about potential risks for the children, and uncertainty about their long-term health and recovery or waiting for possible recovery of gonadal function. Hallak et al. surveyed 56 patients at the Cleveland Clinic who requested to discontinue storing of spermatozoa, and they concluded that most patients decided to discontinue sperm banking because they either regained fertility or had improved semen quality [122]. Even if properly counseled, not all patients will eventually bank semen before their treatment. One study reported that only 42% of appropriately counseled patients did bank their semen to counter sterility [123], while another recent study reported a value of 54% [124].

The Cleveland Clinic survey revealed that, of those currently childless, 76% wanted children in the future [125]. Moreover, approximately 80% of the patients viewed themselves positively as actual or potential parents. Addressing this issues immediately upon diagnosis helps young cancer patients and their families to face the disease and cope with treatment in a more optimistic light. Currently, all male cancer patients of reproductive age who will have treatment that may affect testicular function and who may desire children in the future should cryopreserve sperm before the initiation of therapy. It is vital therefore to keep records of patients having postcancer infertility treatment and to monitor the children born as a consequence of these treatments.

While many oncologists now tend to use less gonadotoxic treatments, semen cryopreservation should always be offered to each cancer patient since recovery of spermatogenesis cannot be guaranteed for the individual patient, because of important interindividual variances or because a therapeutic regimen may be started with limited gonadotoxicity, but eventually a more gonadotoxic therapy may be indicated because of treatment failure.

Sperm Cryopreservation in Boys

Another point of interest is the prepubertal boys with malignant disease. Spermatozoa can be obtained by masturbation from about the age of the 14 years. To preserve fertility, it is necessary to determine the risk of fertility impairment before instituting cancer therapy. Predicting the impact of treatment on reproductive function in individual children based on expected exposures is notoriously unreliable. Current tools, both biochemical and biophysical, are unsuitable for assessing actual reproductive impacts in prepubertal and peripubertal children. Even when pubertal onset and progression is apparently normal, the integrity of gametes may have been compromised.

Cryopreservation of semen and subsequent IVF is the only standard option for postpubertal males, and spermarche is the watershed around which options for boys are defined. Spermarche typically is an early to midpubertal event and occurs before the ability to achieve ejaculation [126]. In the mature adolescent, semen is usually obtained by masturbation, with electrostimulation or vibratory stimulation as alternatives (the latter two may be applicable in peripubertal boys). However, the rate at which viable samples are obtained is highly variable. These adolescents are often sick as well as embarrassed and uncomfortable. One study of 62 attempts by adolescents to bank sperm before therapy resulted in totally normal semen in only four [127]. Adolescents may be more successful if unaccompanied by parents [92, 128].

Testicular tissue cryopreservation would be an important technique for fertility preservation in prepubertal boys, who do not yet have sperm in the ejaculate and who are scheduled to undergo gonadotoxic treatment [129]. If the boy already has spermatozoa in his semen, it is best to freeze sperm [92, 130]. Cryopreservation of testicular cell suspension has been proposed as an alternative method suitable for patients with azoospermia and young patients who are not yet producing sperm [131]. Banking of testicular tissue in prepubertal boys before gonadotoxic treatment is a crucial step in fertility preservation [129]. Testicular biopsies for fertility preservation are therefore ethically justified [132]. However, malignancy recurrence prevention is an important prerequisite for any clinical application of testicular stem cell transplantation. Therefore, the storage of prepubertal testicular tissue is currently emerging as a potential solution [92, 129, 133–135]. After being cured, the frozen–thawed tissue may theoretically be transplanted [133, 135], xenotransplanted [136, 137], or matured in vitro [138, 139]. So far, the testicular stem cell transplantation has provided the most promising results in animal models, mostly murine models. Also, ethically, autologous testicular stem cell transplantation may be more acceptable than xenotransplantation strategies.

Anyway, for pubertal boys, who are too young to ejaculate, cryopreservation of testicular biopsy and TESE after cryopreservation might be an option for fertility preservation [140]. For prepubertal boys, when full spermatogenesis is not yet ongoing, it is essential to store the spermatogonia and the neighboring cells as undamaged integrated tissue [141]. Preservation of Sertoli cells and cell-to-cell contacts in testicular tissue have proved to be important for subsequent maturation of spermatogonia [142].

A study by Kliesch et al. demonstrated that adolescent patients, aged 14–17 years, are good candidates for semen banking [130]. In a large series, Bahadur et al., reported that 86% of 238 boys of postpubertal age up to 19 years old could produce a semen sample for cryostorage [92]. In four out of the remaining 33 boys, eventually, sperm recovered from a urine sample was cryopreserved [92]. A study involving 45 male adolescents showed that for 20 of them (44.5%), semen cryopreservation was not performed because they were not judged as being mature enough to deliver a semen sample by masturbation. Another four boys failed to deliver a semen sample because of masturbation problems and finally, for two boys, semen was collected by alternative methods such as penile vibrostimulation or electroejaculation, both performed under general anesthesia [143]. Electroejaculation in adolescents may be an alternative to masturbation in order to obtain semen for cryostorage [144, 145].

Concluding, the safety and effectiveness of the ART are essential issues. It is important to have ethics approval and strong motivation for all procedures included in programs for fertility preservation in young patients [100, 132, 146, 147]. Children and their parents should be informed about the experimental stage of the study. However, it is important to inform all patients facing infertility as a side effect of gonadotoxic chemo- and radiotherapies about the options available to preserve their future fertility [148–150].

Another interesting situation about cryopreservation is the one involving boys with cryptorchidism. Boys with cryptorchidism often face fertility problems in adult life despite having orchiopexy performed at a very young age. During this operation, a biopsy of the testis is normally taken in order to evaluate their infertility potential and the presence of malignant cells. Evaluating biopsies from 11 testes (eight boys), one fresh and two cryopreserved pieces were cultured for 2 weeks and prepared for histology. The morphology of the fresh and frozen–thawed samples were similar, with well-preserved seminiferous tubules and interstitial cells. A similar picture appeared after 2 weeks of culture, but a few of the cultured biopsies contained small necrotic areas. The presence of spermatogonia was verified by c-kit-positive immunostaining. Production of testosterone and inhibin B (ng/mm^3 testis tissue) in the frozen–thawed pieces is on average similar to that of the fresh samples [151]. Therefore, Kvist et al. concluded that intact testicular tissue from young boys with nondescended testes tolerates cryopreservation with surviving spermatogonia and without significant loss of the ability to produce testis-specific hormones in vitro. It may be an option to freeze part of the testis biopsy, which is routinely removed during the operation for cryptorchidism, for fertility preservation in adult life.

Sperm DNA Damage and Cryopreservation

An intact chromatin structure is extremely important for the fertilizing ability of the sperm, and it has been shown that defective spermiogenesis is associated with abnormal remodeling of sperm chromatin and membrane components, which in turn results in morphologically abnormal spermatozoa. Sperm chromatin structure, once believed to be stable during the cryopreservation process, is now found to be altered during freezing–thawing of spermatozoa. In addition, cryopreservation appears to reduce the ability of sperm chromatin to decondense during fertilization, suggesting the detrimental effect of freezing–thawing on sperm chromatin.

Recently, several groups have reported the effect of cryopreservation on sperm DNA integrity [152–158]. Although in some reports there appears to be an increase in sperm DNA fragmentation after thawing, in other studies, no such effect was found [152–158]. It has been demonstrated by Toro et al. that processing of semen for ART, including incubation and cryopreservation of semen, may result in increased sperm DNA fragmentation. Therefore, unnecessary incubation of semen in the laboratory should be avoided. In fact, cryopreservation has deleterious effects on sperm DNA by inducing DNA fragmentation and oxidation, but the mechanisms underlying such damages need to be elucidated by further investigations. Cryopreservation induces apoptotic sperm DNA fragmentation in men, regardless of sperm concentration. Men with oligospermia present with higher precryopreservation and postcryopreservation apoptotic sperm DNA fragmentation [155]. In fact, they noticed the same increase in DNA fragmentation in normospermic as well in oligospermic infertile patients [155]. Interestingly, in a very elegant study, Adiga et al. found a strong correlation between the amount of initial sperm DNA damage and postthaw survival [156]. However, no significant enhancement in DNA damage was observed by the cryopreservation of spermatozoa with several amounts of DNA damage. Neither the presence nor the type of cryoprotectant affects the DNA integrity of spermatozoa after cryopreservation and separation using density gradient centrifugation [158]. Individuals with lower prefreeze fragmentation in separation using density gradient centrifugation have larger increases in fragmentation and are less likely to exhibit lower levels of fragmentation postthaw [158].

Step by Step Protocol of Laboratory Procedures

Equipment and Reagents

- Microcell counting chamber from Conception Technologies
- 5-μL Eppendorf pipette
- Aliquot mixer
- Vortex
- –20°C Freezer
- LN2 container with racks
- Sterile specimen container
- Sterile 15-mL centrifuge tubes with caps
- Sterile serological pipettes (1, 2, and 5 mL capacity)
- Sterile Nunc cryovials (1 and 2 mL capacity)
- Colored cryomarkers
- Test tube racks (for 15-mL test tubes)
- Cryovial racks
- Stainless steel canes for cryovials
- Plastic cryosleeves
- Cryogloves
- Latex gloves
- 37°C Incubator
- LN2 from supplier
- Eosin–nigrosin stain
- Microslide
- Coverslips
- Sperm washing media
- Makler chamber
- Freezing medium (Test yolk buffer with glycerol; TYB-G) from Irvine Scientific, Sabta Ana, CA
- Sperm washing media (HTF): Enhance-W from Conception Technologies, La Jolla, CA

Procedure (Aspiration from Surgery)

Technical note: Sterile techniques should be used throughout specimen processing. Gloves are mandatory for all procedures dealing with body fluids. Latex, however, may be toxic to sperm. Therefore, care should be taken to prevent contamination of the specimen with latex or talc. Vinyl gloves are an available alternative.

1. Cryopreservation worksheet labeled with the patient name, diagnosis, and LN2 container and rack. If there is more than one specimen, then have a worksheet for each specimen.

2. Every time a laboratory receives the notice that an aspirate is ready, take one bottle of frozen test yolk media and put into the 37°C incubator to thaw.
3. A technologist will go to the surgery room to retrieve the specimen(s). Keep the vials warm in your hands.
4. Normally, two to three specimen will arrive from surgery. Make sure the name of the patient as well as the specimen number.
5. Using sterile technique, measure the volume of each specimen and record on the appropriate cryopreservation worksheet.
6. Centrifuge the specimen in the original container for 5 min at 1,600 rpm.
7. Label three sterile 15-mL conical centrifuge tubes with the patient's name and specimen number.
8. Transfer the supernatant of specimen 1 and specimen 2, and if there is specimen 3 also in the "supernatant" tube. Both supernatants are now combined into one tube.
9. Add 0.5 mL HTF (sperm washing media) to each pellet to resuspend. Mix gently.
10. Transfer a drop of each specimen into a prelabeled conical cup for semen analysis.
11. Perform the following on each specimen aspirate: regular manual semen analysis, Endtz test (leukocytospermia test), eosin–nigrosin stain procedure, Tygerberg's strict criteria form morphology evaluation.
12. Always notify if the surgeon found no motile sperm on the wet prep.
13. Within 1 h of specimen collection, add an aliquot of freezing medium equal to 25% of the resuspended aspirate volume to the centrifuge tube with a sterile pipette.

    Note: Since the resuspended volume for each aspirate is 0.5 mL, then divide 0.5 by 4 to obtain 0.13. Therefore, add 0.13 mL of freeze media four times to the specimen.
14. Gently rock the specimen(s) with the freezing media for 5 min on an aliquot mixer.
15. Repeat steps 13 and 14 three times or until the volume of freezing media added is equal to the specimen volume in step 9.
16. Centrifuge the tube labeled "supernatant" for 5 min at 1,600 rpm.
17. Remove the supernatant from the "supernatant" tube. Resuspend the pellet with 0.5 mL of HTF (sperm washing media). Mix gently. Remove one drop for a semen analysis.

    Note: If no motile sperm is found in the "supernatant" tube, then do not start freezing. If motile sperm is found, then freeze as in steps 13–15.

    During the mixing steps above, use appropriately colored cryomarkers to label 2-mL cryovials and canes. The volume added to the vial should not exceed 1.8 mL per vial.
18. Label an additional 1.0-mL cryovial as in for each specimen. This will contain a leftover aliquot of the cryodiluted specimen to be assessed of cryosurvival 24 h after freezing in LN2.
19. A visual inspection should therefore be made of the cryodiluted specimen for motility. A manual motility can be done using a Microcell chamber or a Makler chamber and a Nikon 2-phase microscope. The percent motility should be documented on the cryopreservation worksheet under cryodilution motility.

20. Distribute the well-mixed, cryodiluted semen into prelabeled vials using a 1- or 2-mL sterile serological pipette. Add at least 0.2 mL to the smaller 1.0-mL cryovial.
21. Place labeled vials into a plastic freezing rack along with canes and cryosleeves and put into a –20°C freezer for 8 min. Do not open the freezer in any circumstance during this incubation.

    Note: Exposure to freezing conditions should occur within 1.5 h of specimen collection.
22. After the 8-min incubation, remove the rack and canes from the 20°C freezer. Place a maximum of two cryovials into bottom slots of canes upside down. Put into cryosleeves.
23. After a minimum 2-h incubation in liquid nitrogen vapors, turn cases upside down, immerging them into liquid nitrogen.
24. After a minimum of 24 h in liquid nitrogen, thaw the aliquot in the 1.0-mL cryovial.
25. Using cryogloves, remove cane containing the vial and snap it out. Loosen the cap and place in the 37°C incubator for 20 min.
26. Mix the vial well and analyze manually.
27. Record the cryosurvival area of the cryopreservation worksheet.
28. Assess cryosurvival in the formal:

$$\frac{\%\text{motility of postthaw specimen}}{\%\text{motility of prefreeze specimen}}$$

Procedure (Semen from Ejaculate)

Technical note: Sterile techniques should be used throughout specimen processing. Gloves are mandatory for all procedures dealing with body fluids. Latex, however, may be toxic to sperm. Therefore, care should be taken to prevent contamination of the specimen with latex or talc. Vinyl gloves are an available alternative.

1. Cryopreservation worksheet labeled with the patient name, diagnosis, and LN2 container and rack. If there is more than one specimen, then have a worksheet for each specimen.
2. Using sterile technique, measure the volume of each specimen and record on the appropriate cryopreservation worksheet.
3. Perform the following on the semen sample: regular manual semen analysis, Endtz test (leukocytospermia test), eosin–nigrosin stain procedure, Tygerberg's strict criteria form morphology evaluation.
4. Within 1 h of specimen collection, add an aliquot of freezing medium equal to 25% of the resuspended aspirate volume to the centrifuge tube with a sterile pipette.
5. Note: Since the resuspended volume for each aspirate is 0.5 mL, then divide 0.5 by 4 to obtain 0.13. Therefore, add 0.13 mL of freeze media four times to the specimen.

6. Gently rock the specimen(s) with the freezing media for 5 min on an aliquot mixer.
7. Repeat step 4 three times or until the volume of freezing media added is equal to the specimen volume in step 2.
8. During the mixing steps above, use appropriately colored cryomarkers to label 2-mL cryovials and canes. The volume added to the vial should not exceed 1.8 mL per vial.
9. Label an additional 1.0-mL cryovial as in for each specimen. This will contain a leftover aliquot of the cryodiluted specimen to be assessed of cryosurvival 24 h after freezing in LN2.
10. A visual inspection should therefore be made of the cryodiluted specimen for motility. A manual motility can be done using a Microcell chamber or a Makler chamber and a Nikon 2-phase microscope. The percent motility should be documented on the cryopreservation worksheet under cryodilution motility.
11. Distribute the well-mixed, cryodiluted semen into prelabeled vials using a 1- or 2-mL sterile serological pipette. Add at least 0.2 mL to the smaller 1.0-mL cryovial.
12. Place labeled vials into a plastic freezing rack along with canes and cryosleeves and put into a −20°C freezer for 8 min. Do not open the freezer in any circumstance during this incubation.
13. Note: Exposure to freezing conditions should occur within 1.5 h of specimen collection.
14. After the 8-min incubation, remove the rack and canes from the 20°C freezer. Place a maximum of two cryovials into bottom slots of canes upside down. Put into cryosleeves.
15. After a minimum 2-h incubation in liquid nitrogen vapors, turn cases upside down, immerging them into liquid nitrogen.
16. After a minimum of 24 h in liquid nitrogen, thaw the aliquot in the 1.0-mL cryovial.
17. Using cryogloves, remove cane containing the vial and snap it out. Loosen the cap and place in the 37°C incubator for 20 min.
18. Mix the vial well and analyze manually.
19. Record the cryosurvival area of the cryopreservation worksheet.
20. Assess cryosurvival in the formal:

$$\frac{\%\text{motility of postthaw specimen}}{\%\text{motility of prefreeze specimen}}$$

Perspectives

Although still purely experimental at this stage, testicular stem cell transplantation may provide an adequate solution to preserve the progenitive capacity of prepubertal boys. Also, even though still surrounded by complex ethical issues, cryobanking of testicular tissue from prepubertal boys may now be considered an acceptable strategy, analogous to cryobanking of ovarian cortex in young girls. However, in contrast to girls, in boys, stem cells are the target of storage, which represents an important difference in terms of potential future applications for preserving fertility.

Conclusions

Reproductive physicians play important roles in helping to preserve the reproductive capacities of young cancer patients. First of all, the reproductive physicians are involved in developing and using procedures to preserve sperm and gonadal tissue before treatment. Secondly, fertility specialists will assist cancer survivors in using preserved gametes and tissue or in providing other assistance in reproduction. The fact that the patient has just been diagnosed with cancer or survived the acute or extended phase of coping with cancer distinguishes the cancer patient from other fertility patients. Variations in type of cancer, time available to onset of treatment, age, partner status, type and dosage of chemotherapy, and risk of sterility with a given treatment regimen require that each case has its own treatment strategy. Consultation with the patient's oncologist often is essential. A key issue at the time of treatment of the cancer is whether it is medically feasible to obtain gametes or gonadal tissue for storage and later use. Questions about the patient's health and prognosis will also arise when the patient is deciding later whether to reproduce.

References

1. Bunge RG, Keettel WC, Sherman JK. Clinical use of frozen semen. Fertli Steril. 1954;5: 520–9.
2. Hammond J. The effect of temperature on the survival in vitro of rabbit spermatozoa from the vagina. J Exp Biol. 1930;7:175–91.
3. Walton J. The effect of temperature on the survival in vitro of rabbit spermatozoa obtained from the vas deferens. J Exp Biol. 1930;7:201–19.
4. Shettles LB. The respiration of human spermatozoa and their response to various gases and low temperatures. Am J Physiol. 1940;128:408–15.
5. Picton HM, Kim SS, Gosden RG. Cryopreservation of gonadal tissue and cells. Br Med Bull. 2000;56:603–15.
6. Watson PF. Recent developments and concepts in the cryopreservation of spermatozoa and the assessment of their post-thawing function. Reprod Fertil Dev. 1995;7:871–91.
7. Schiller J, Arnhold J, Glander HJ, Arnold K. Lipid analysis of human spermatozoa and seminal plasma by MALDI-TOF mass spectrometry and NMR spectroscopy—effects of freezing and thawing. Chem Phys Lipids. 2000;106:145–56.
8. Schuffner A, Morshedi M, Oehninger S. Cryopreservation of fractionated, highly motile human spermatozoa: effect on membrane phosphatidylserine externalization and lipid peroxidation. Hum Reprod. 2001;16:2148–53.
9. Duru NK, Morshedi MS, Schuffner A, Oehninger S. Cryopreservation—thawing of fractionated human spermatozoa is associated with membrane phosphatidylserine externalization and not DNA fragmentation. J Androl. 2001;22:646–51.

10. Lasso JL, Noiles EE, Alvarez JG, Storey BT. Mechanism of superoxide dismutase loss from human sperm cells during cryopreservation. J Androl. 1994;15:255–65.
11. Zilli L, Schiavone R, Zonno V, Rossano R, Storelli C, Vilella S. Effect of cryopreservation on sea bass sperm proteins. Biol Reprod. 2005;72:1262–7.
12. Gadea J, Selles E, Marco MA, Coy P, Matas C, Romar R, et al. Decrease in glutathione content in boar sperm after cryopreservation. Effect of the addition of reduced glutathione to the freezing and thawing extenders. Theriogenology. 2004;62:690–701.
13. Ollero M, Bescos O, Cebrian-Perez JA, Muino-Blanco T. Loss of plasma membrane proteins of bull spermatozoa through the freezing–thawing process. Theriogenology. 1998;49:547–55.
14. Hazel JR. Thermal adaptation in biological membranes: is homeoviscous adaptation the explanation? Annu Rev Physiol. 1995;57:19–42.
15. Holt WV, North RD. Effects of temperature and restoration of osmotic equilibrium during thawing on the induction of plasma membrane damage in cryopreserved ram spermatozoa. Biol Reprod. 1994;5:414–24.
16. Quinn PJ. Effects of temperature on cell membranes. Symp Soc Exp Biol. 1988;42:237–58.
17. Chatterjee S, Gagnon C. Production of reactive oxygen species by spermatozoa undergoing cooling, freezing, and thawing. Mol Reprod Dev. 2001;59:451–8.
18. Mazzilli F, Rossi T, Sabatini L, Pulcinelli FM, Rapone S, Dondero F, et al. Human sperm cryopreservation and reactive oxygen species (ROS) production. Acta Eur Fertil. 1995;26:145–8.
19. Chohan KR, Griffin JT, Carrell DT. Evaluation of chromatin integrity in human sperm using acridine orange staining with different fixatives and after cryopreservation. Andrologia. 2004;36:321–6.
20. Peris SI, Morrier A, Dufour M, Bailey JL. Cryopreservation of ram semen facilitates sperm DNA damage: relationship between sperm andrological parameters and the sperm chromatin structure assay. J Androl. 2004;25:224–33.
21. Linfor JJ, Meyers SA. Detection of DNA damage in response to cooling injury in equine spermatozoa using single-cell gel electrophoresis. J Androl. 2002;23:107–13.
22. Holt WV, North RD. Cryopreservation, actin localization and thermotropic phase transitions in ram spermatozoa. J Reprod Fertil. 1991;91:451–61.
23. Boiso I, Marti M, Santalo J, Ponsa M, Barri PN, Veiga A. A confocal microscopy analysis of the spindle and chromosome configurations of human oocytes cryopreserved at the germinal vesicle and metaphase II stage. Hum Reprod. 2002;17:1885–91.
24. Songsasen N, Yu IJ, Ratterree MS, VandeVoort CA, Leibo SP. Effect of chilling on the organization of tubulin and chromosomes in rhesus monkey oocytes. Fertil Steril. 2002;77:818–25.
25. Park SE, Son WY, Lee SH, Lee KA, Ko JJ, Cha KY. Chromosome and spindle configurations of human oocytes matured in vitro after cryopreservation at the germinal vesicle stage. Fertil Steril. 1997;68:920–6.
26. Zenzes MT, Bielecki R, Casper RF, Leibo SP. Effects of chilling to 0 degrees C on the morphology of meiotic spindles in human metaphase II oocytes. Fertil Steril. 2001;75:769–77.
27. Pickering SJ, Johnson MH. The influence of cooling on the organization of the meiotic spindle of the mouse oocyte. Hum Reprod. 1987;2:207–16.
28. Donnelly ET, McClure N, Lewis SEM. Cryopreservation of human semen and prepared sperm: effects on motility parameters and DNA integrity. Fertil Steril. 2001;76:892–900.
29. Paasch U, Sharma RK, Gupta AK, Grunewald S, Mascha EJ, Thomas Jr AJ, Glander HJ, Agarwal A. Cryopreservation and thawing is associated with varying extend of activation of apoptotic machinery in subsets of ejaculated human spermatozoa. Biol Reprod. 2004; 71:1828–37.
30. Peris SI, Morrier A, Dufour M, Bailey JL. Cryopreservation of ram semen facilitates sperm DNA damage: relationship between sperm andrological parameters and the sperm chromatin structure assay. J Androl. 2004;25:224–33.
31. Sakkas D, Urner F, Bizzaro D, Manicardi G, Bianchi PG, Shoukir Y, Campana A. Sperm nuclear DNA damage and altered chromatin structure: effect on fertilization and embryo development. Hum Reprod. 1998;13(Suppl):11–9.

32. Grunewald S, Paasch U, Said TM, Sharma RK, Glander HJ, Agarwal A. Caspase activation in human spermatozoa in response to physiological and pathological stimuli. Fertil Steril. 2005;83 Suppl 1:1106–12.
33. Grunewald S, Paasch U, Said TM, Rasch M, Agarwal A, Glander H-J. Magnetic-activated cell sorting before cryopreservation preserves mitochondrial integrity in human spermatozoa. Cell Tissue Bank. 2006;7:99–104.
34. White IG. Lipids and Ca^{+2} uptakes of sperm in relation to cold shock and preservation: a review. Reprod Fertil Dev. 1993;5(6):639–58.
35. Drobnis EZ, Crowe LM, Berger T, Anchordoguy TJ, Overstreet JW, Crowe JH. Cold shock damage is due to lipid phase transitions in cell membranes: a demonstration using sperm as a model. J Exp Zool. 1993;265(4):432–7.
36. Meseguer M, Garrido N, Martinez-Conejero JA, Simon C, Pellicer A, Remohi J. Role of cholesterol, calcium, and mitochondrial activity in the susceptibility for cryodamage after a cycle of freezing and thawing. Fertil Steril. 2004;81:588–94.
37. Glander HJ, Schaller J. Binding of annexin-V to plasma membranes of human spermatozoa: a rapid assay for detection of membrane changes after cryostorage. Mol Hum Reprod. 1999;5:109–15.
38. Hinkovska-Galcheva V, Petkova D, Koumanov K. Changes in the phospholipid composition and phospholipids asymmetry of ram sperm plasma membranes after cryopreservation. Cryobiology. 1989;26:70–5.
39. Martin SJ, Reutelingsperger CP, McGahon AJ, Rader JA, van Schie RC, LaFace DM, Green DR. Early redistribution of plasma membrane phosphatidylserine is a general feature of apoptosis regardless of the initiating stimulus: inhibition by overexpression of Bcl-2 and Abl. J Exp Med. 1995;182:1545–56.
40. Paasch U, Grunewald S, Fitzl G, Glander HJ. Deterioration of plasma membrane is associated with activation of caspases in human spermatozoa. J Androl. 2003;24:246–52.
41. Shen HM, Dai J, Chia SE, Lim A, Ong CN. Detection of apoptotic alterations in sperm in subfertile patients and their correlations with sperm quality. Hum Reprod. 2002;17:1266–73.
42. Paasch U, Sharma RK, Gupta AK, Grunewald S, Mascha E, Thomas Jr AJ, Glander H-J, Agarwal A. Cryopreservation and thawing is associated with varying extent of activation of apoptotic machinery in subsets of ejaculated human spermatozoa. Biol Reprod. 2004;71:1828–37.
43. Said TM, Grunewald S, Paasch U, Rasch M, Agarwal A, Glander H-J. Effects of magnetic-activated cell sorting on sperm motility and cryosurvival rates. Fertil Steril. 2005;83:1442–6.
44. Lasso JL, Noiles EE, Alvarez JG, Storey BT. Mechanism of superoxide dismutase loss from human sperm cells during cryopreservation. J Androl. 1994;15:255–65.
45. Zilli L, Schiavone R, Zonno V, Rossano R, Storelli C, Vilella S. Effect of cryopreservation on sea bass sperm proteins. Biol Reprod. 2005;72:1262–7.
46. Lessard C, Parent S, Leclerc P, Bailey JL, Sullivan R. Cryopreservation alters the levels of the bull sperm surface protein P25b. J Androl. 2000;21:700–7.
47. Boue F, Sullivan R. Cases of human infertility are associated with the absence of P34H an epididymal sperm antigen. Biol Reprod. 1996;54:1018–24.
48. Morris GJ, Acton E, Avery S. A novel approach to sperm cryopreservation. Hum Reprod. 1999;14:1013–21.
49. Schuffner A, Stockler S, Costa S, Centa L. Long-term cryopreserved semen results in a live birth 12 years later. J Urol. 2004;171:358.
50. Sergerie M, Mieusset R, Daudin M, Thonneau P, Bujan L. Ten-year variation in semen parameters and sperm deoxyribonucleic acid integrity in a healthy fertile man. Fertil Steril. 2006;86:1513–8.
51. Bhakoo HS, Vaccaro P, Crickard K, Sullivan MW. Live birth following intracytoplasmic sperm injection after a 15-hour weather-related delay in cryopreservation of testicular sperm. Fertil Steril. 2005;83:464–5.

52. Clarke GN, de Liu Y, Baker HW. Recovery of human sperm motility and ability to interact with the human zona pellucida after more than 28 years of storage in liquid nitrogen. Fertil Steril. 2006;86:721–2.
53. Trummer H, Tucker K, Young C, Kaula N, Meacham RB. Effect of storage temperature on sperm cryopreservation. Fertil Steril. 1998;70:1162–4.
54. Punyatanasakchai P, Sophonristsuk A, Weerakiet S, Wansumrit S, Chompurat D. Comparison of cryopreserved human sperm in vapor and liquid phases of liquid nitrogen, effect on motility parameters, morphology, and sperm function. Fertil Steril. 2008;90:1978–82.
55. Calamera JC, Buffone MG, Doncel GF, Brugo-Olmedo S, de Vicentiis S, Calamera MM, Storey BT, Alvarez JG. Effect of thawing temperature on the motility recovery of cryopreserved human spermatozoa. Fertil Steril. 2010;93:789–94.
56. Vutyavanich T, Piromlertamorn W, Nunta S. Rapid freezing versus slow programmable freezing of human spermatozoa. Fertil Steril. 2009;93:1921–8.
57. Sherman JK. Improved methods of preservation of human spermatozoa by freezing and freeze-drying. Fertil Steril. 1963;14:49–64.
58. Kruger TF, Menkveld R, Standerl FS, Lombard CJ, Van der Merwe JP, Van Zyll JA, et al. Sperm morphologic features as a prognostic factor in vitro fertilization. Fertil Steril. 1986;46: 1118–23.
59. Fjallbrant B, Ackerman DR. Cervical mucus penetration in vitro by fresh and frozen-preserved human semen specimen. J Reprod Fertil. 1969;20:515–7.
60. Pironcheva GL, Miteva K, Vaisberg C, Russev G. Influence of freezing at different temperatures on the transcription activity of buffalo sperm chromatin. Cytobios. 1995;83:207–10.
61. Nallella KP, Sharma RK, Allamaneni SSR, Aziz N, Agarwal A. Cryopreservation of human spermatozoa: comparison of two cryopreservation methods and three cryoprotectants. Fertil Steril. 2004;82:913–8.
62. Verheyen G, Pletincx I, Van Steirtegham A. Effect of freezing methods, thawing temperature, and post-thaw dilution/washing on motility (CASA) and morphology characteristics of high-quality human sperm. Hum Reprod. 1993;8:1672–84.
63. Ragni G, Caccamo AM, Serra AD, Guercilena S. Computerized slow-staged freezing of semen from men with testicular tumors or Hodgkin's disease preserves sperm better than standard vapor freezing. Fertil Steril. 1990;53:1072–5.
64. Stanic P, Tandara M, Sonicki Z, Simunic V, Radakovic B, Suchanek E. Comparison of protective media and freezing techniques for cryopreservation of human semen. Eur J Obstet Gynecol Reprod Biol. 2000;91:65–70.
65. Serafini P, Marrs RP. Computerized staged-freezing technique improves sperm survival and preserves penetration of zona-free hamster ova. Fertil Steril. 1986;45:854–8.
66. Amesse LS, Srivastava G, Uddin D, Pfaff-Amesse T. Comparison of cryopreserved sperm in vaporous and liquid nitrogen. J Reprod Med. 2003;48:319–24.
67. Herrier A, Eisner S, Bach V, Weissenbom U, Beier HM. Cryopreservation of spermatozoa in alginic acid capsules. Fertil Steril. 2006;85:208–13.
68. Schoysman R, Vanderzwalmen P, Segal-Bertin G, van de Casseye M. Successful fertilization by testicular spermatozoa in an in-vitro fertilization programme. Hum Reprod. 1993;8: 1339–40.
69. Schlegel PR, Su LM. Physiological consequences of testicular sperm extraction. Hum Reprod. 1997;12:1688–92.
70. Silber SJ, Van Steirteghem AC, Liu J, Nagy Z, Tournaye H, Devroey P. High fertilization and pregnancy rate after intracytoplasmic sperm injection with spermatozoa from testicular biopsy. Hum Reprod. 1995;10:148–52.
71. Cohen J, Garrisi GJ, Congedo-Ferrara TA, Kieck KA, Schimmel TW, Scott RT. Cryopreservation of single human spermatozoa. Hum Reprod. 1997;12:994–1001.
72. Ye Y, Xu C, Qian Y, Jin F, Huang H. Evaluation of human sperm function after being cryopreserved within the zona pellucida. Fertil Steril. 2009;92:1002–8.
73. Bongso A, Jarina AK, Ho J, Ng SC, Ratnam SS. Comparative evaluation of three sperm-washing methods to improve sperm concentration and motility in frozen-thawed oligozoospermic and normozoospermic samples. Arch Androl. 1993;31:223–30.

74. Sawetawan C, Bruns ES, Gail SP. Improvement of post-thaw motility in poor quality human semen. Fertil Steril. 1993;60:706–10.
75. Hsiek Y, Tsai H-D, Chang CC, Lo H-Y. Cryopreservation of human spermatozoa within human or mouse empty zona Pellucidae. Fertil Steril. 2000;73:694–8.
76. Pasqualotto FF, Rossi-Ferragut LM, Rocha CC, Iaconelli Jr A, Borges Jr E. Outcome of in vitro fertilization and intracytoplasmic injection of epididymal and testicular sperm obtained from patients with obstructive and nonobstructive azoospermia. J Urol. 2002;167:1753–6.
77. Pasqualotto FF, Rossi LM, Guilherme P, Ortiz V, Iaconelli Jr A, Borges Jr E. Etiology-specific outcomes of intracytoplasmic sperm injection in azoospermic patients. Fertil Steril. 2005;83:606–11.
78. Park YS, Lee SH, Song SJ, Jun JH, Koong MK, Seo JT. Influence of motility on the outcome of in vitro fertilization/intracytoplasmic sperm injection with fresh vs. frozen testicular sperm from men with obstructive azoospermia. Fertil Steril. 2003;80:526–30.
79. Prabakaran SA, Agarwal A, Sundaram A, Thomas Jr AJ, Sikka S. Cryosurvival of testicular spermatozoa from obstructive azoospermic patients: The Cleveland Clinic experience. Fertil Steril. 2006;86:1789–91.
80. Verheyen G, Nagy Z, Joris H, De Croo I, Tournaye H, Van Steirteghem A. Quality of frozen–thawed testicular sperm and its preclinical use for intracytoplasmic sperm injection into in vitro-matured germinal-vesicle stage oocytes. Fertil Steril. 1997;67:74–80.
81. Verheyen G, Vernaeve V, Van Landuyt L, Tournaye H, Devroey P, Van Steirteghem A. Should diagnostic testicular sperm retrieval followed by cryopreservation for later ICSI be the procedure of choice for all patients with non-obstructive azoospermia? Hum Reprod. 2004; 19:2822–30.
82. Pasqualotto FF, Agarwal A. Should we offer semen cryopreservation to men with testicular cancer? Cleve Clin J Med. 2001;68:101–2.
83. Agarwal A, Allamaneni SSR. Disruption of spermatogenesis by the cancer disease process. J Natl Cancer Inst Monogr. 2005;34:9–12.
84. Schrader M, Muller M, Straub B, Miller K. The impact of chemotherapy on male fertility: a survey of the biologic basis and clinical aspects. Reprod Toxicol. 2001;15:611–7.
85. Viviani S, Ragni G, Santoro A, Perotti L, Caccamo E, Negretti E, Valagussa P, Bonadonna G. Testicular dysfunction in Hodgkin's disease before and after treatment. Eur J Cancer. 1991;27:1389–92.
86. Pont J, Albrecht W. Fertility after chemotherapy for testicular germ cell cancer. Fertil Steril. 1997;68:1–5.
87. Apperley JF, Reddy N. Mechanism and management of treatment related gonadal failure in recipients of high dose chemoradiotherapy. Blood Rev. 1995;9:93–116.
88. Spermon JR, Kiemeney LALM, Meuleman EJH, Ramos L, Wetzels AMM, Witjes JA. Fertility in men with testicular germ cell tumors. Fertil Steril. 2003;79:1543–9.
89. Laguna MP, Pizzocaro G, Klepp O, Algaba F, Kisbenedek L, Leiva O. European Association of Urology guidelines on testicular cancer. Eur Urol. 2001;40:102–10.
90. Aubier F, Flamant F, Brauner R, Caillaud JM, Chaussain JM, Lemerle J. Male gonadal function after chemotherapy for solid tumors in childhood. J Clin Oncol. 1989;7:304–9.
91. Bahadur G, Chatterjee R, Ralph D. Testicular tissue cryopreservation in boys. Ethical and legal issues. Hum Reprod. 2000;15:1416–20.
92. Bahadur G, Ling KL, Hart R, Ralph D, Wafa R, Ashraf A, Jaman N, Mahmud S, Oyede AW. Semen quality and cryopreservation in adolescent cancer patients. Hum Reprod. 2002;17: 3157–61.
93. Gandini L, Lombardo F, Salacone P, Paoli D, Anselmo AP, Culasso F, Dondero F, Lenzi A. Testicular cancer and Hodgkin's disease: evaluation of semen quality. Hum Reprod. 2003; 18:796–801.
94. Agarwal A, Ranganathan P, Kattal N, Pasqualotto FF, Hallak J, Khayal S. Fertility after cancer: a prospective review of assisted reproductive outcome with banked semen specimens. Fertil Steril. 2004;81:342–8.
95. Anger JT, Gilbert BR, Goldstein M. Cryopreservation of sperm: indications, methods and results. J Urol. 2003;170:1079–84.

96. Hallak J, Pasqualotto FF, Sharma RK, Thomas AJ, Jr., Agarwal A. Prefreeze and postthaw semen quality in men with cancer. Poster presented in American Urological Association annual meeting, Anaheim, USA; 2–7 June 2001.
97. Hallak J, Kolettis P, Sekhon V, Thomas Jr AJ, Agarwal A. Sperm cryopreservation in patients with testicular cancer. Urology. 1999;54:894–9.
98. Bahadur G. Fertility issues for cancer patients. Mol Cell Endocrinol. 2000;27:117–22.
99. Agarwal A. Semen banking in patients with cancer: 20 years experience. Int J Androl. 2000;23:16–9.
100. Bahadur G, Ozturk O, Muneers A, Wafa R, Ashraf A, Jaman N, Patel S, Oyede AW, Ralph DJ. Semen quality before and after gonadotoxic treatment. Hum Reprod. 2005;20:774–81.
101. The Ethics Committee of the American Society for Reproductive Medicine. Fertility preservation and reproduction in cancer patients. Fertil Steril. 2005;83:1622–8.
102. Zapzalka DM, Redmon HB, Pryor JL. A survey of oncologists regarding sperm cryopreservation and assisted reproductive techniques for male cancer patients. Cancer. 1999;86:1812–7.
103. Schover LR, Rybicki LA, Martin BA, Bringeisen KA. Having children after cancer. A pilot survey of survivors' attitudes and experiences. Cancer. 1999;86:697–709.
104. Matthews GJ, Schlegel PN, Goldstein M. Patency following microsurgical vasoepididymostomy and vasovasostomy: temporal considerations. J Urol. 1995;154:2070–3.
105. Belker AM, Bergamini D. The feasibility of cryopreservation of sperm harvested intraoperatively during vasectomy reversals. J Urol. 1997;157:1292–4.
106. Hoekstra T, Witt M. The success, yield and outcome of microscopic aspiration at the time of vasal reconstruction. J Urol. 1996;155:364A.
107. The practice committee of the American Society for Reproductive Medicine. Vasectomy reversal. Fertil Steril. 2006;86(S4):S268–71.
108. Pasqualotto FF, Pasqualotto EB. Banco de sêmen e reprodução assistida para casais após tratamento do câncer no homem. Reprod Hum. 2005;1:21–30.
109. Mortimer D. Current and future concepts and practices in human sperm cryobanking. Reprod Biomed Online. 2004;9:134–51.
110. Marcus-Braun N, Braun G, Potashnik G, Har-Vardi I. Effect of cryopreservation on quality and fertilization capacity of human sperm. Eur J Obstet Gynecol Reprod Biol. 2004;116:63–6.
111. Kuczynski W, Dhont M, Grygoruk C, Grochowski D, Wolczynski S, Szamatowicz M. The outcome of intracytoplasmic injection of fresh and cryopreserved ejaculated spermatozoa—a prospective randomized study. Hum Reprod. 2001;16:2109–13.
112. Borges Jr E, Rossi LM, Freitas CVL, Guilherme P, Bonetti TCS, Iaconelli Jr A, Pasqualotto FF. Fertilization and pregnancy outcome after intracytoplasmic injection using fresh or cryopreserved ejaculated spermatozoa. Fertil Steril. 2007;87:316–20.
113. Van Steirteghem A, Nagy P, Joris H, Janssenswillen C, Staessen C, Verheyen G, et al. Results of intracytoplasmic sperm injection with ejaculated, fresh and frozen-thawed epididymal and testicular spermatozoa. Hum Reprod. 1998;13:134–42.
114. Schlegel PN. Debate: is ICSI a genetic time bomb? No: ICSI is safe and effective. J Androl. 1999;20:18–22.
115. Perraguim-Jayot S, Audebert A, Emperaire JC, Parneix I. Ongoing pregnancies after intracytoplasmic injection using cryopreserved testicular spermatozoa. Hum Reprod. 1997;12: 2706–9.
116. Gil-Salom M, Romero J, Mínguez Y, Molero MD, Remohí J, Pellicer A. Testicular sperm extraction and intracytoplasmic sperm injection: a chance of fertility in nonobstructive azoospermia. J Urol. 1998;160:2072–3.
117. De Croo I, Van der Elst J, Everaert K, De Sutter P, Dhont M. Fertilization, pregnancy and embryo implantation rates after ICSI with fresh or frozen-thawed testicular spermatozoa. Hum Reprod. 1998;13:1893–7.
118. Schmidt KLT, Larsen E, Bangsbøll S, Meinertz H, Carlsen E, Andersen EN. Assisted reproduction in male cancer survivors: fertility treatment and outcome in 67 couples. Hum Reprod. 2004;19:2806–10.

119. Revel A, Haimov-Kochman R, Porat A, Lewin A, Simon A, Laufer N, Gino H, Meirow D. In vitro fertilization–intracytoplasmic sperm injection success rates with cryopreserved sperm from patients with malignant disease. Fertil Steril. 2005;84:118–22.
120. Redman JR, Bajorunas DR, Goldstein MC, Evenson DP, Gralla RJ, Lacher MJ, et al. Semen cryopreservation and artificial insemination for Hodgkin's disease. J Clin Oncol. 1987; 5:233–8.
121. Hansen PV, Glavind K, Panduro J, Pedersen M. Paternity in patients with testicular germ cell cancer: pretreatment and post-treatment findings. Eur J Cancer. 1991;27:1385–9.
122. Hallak J, Sharma RK, Thomas Jr AJ, Agarwal A. Why cancer patients request disposal of cryopreserved semen specimens posttherapy: a retrospective study. Fertil Steril. 1998;69:889–93.
123. Kliesch S, Kamischke A, Nieschlag E. Cryopreservation of human sperm. In: Nieschlag E, Behre H, editors. Andrology. Male reproductive health and dysfunction. Berlin: Springer; 1997. p. 347–55.
124. Rousillon E, Pariene JL, Hostyn B, Merian G, Ferriere JM, Le Guillou M. Fertilité masculine après chimiothérapie: à propos d'une série de 26 patients traités pour cancer du testicule stade 1. Andrologie. 1888;9:42–7.
125. Agarwal A. Semen banking in patients with cancer: 20 years experience. Int J Androl. 2000;23:16–9.
126. Kulin HE, Frontera MA, Demers LM, et al. The onset of sperm production in pubertal boys. Am J Dis Child. 1989;143:190–3.
127. Postovsky S, Lightman A, Aminpour D, et al. Sperm cryopreservation in adolescents with newly diagnosed cancer. Med Pediatr Oncol. 2003;40:355–9.
128. Greenberg ML, Urbach SL. Preserving the fertility of children with cancer. Med J Aust. 2006;185:532–3.
129. Hovatta O. Cryopreservation of testicular tissue in young cancer patients. Hum Reprod Update. 2001;7:378–83.
130. Kliesch S, Behre H, Jurgens H, Nieschlag E. Cryopreservation of semen from adolescent patients with malignancies. Med Pediatr Oncol. 1996;26:20–7.
131. Brook PF, Radford JA, Shalet SM, Joyce AD, Gosden RG. Isolation of germ cells from human testicular tissue for low temperature storage and autotransplantation. Fertil Steril. 2001;75:269–74.
132. Tournaye H, Goossens E, Verheyen G, Frederickx V, De Block G, Devroey P, Van Steirteghem A. Preserving the reproductive potential of men and boys with cancer: current concepts and future prospects. Hum Reprod Update. 2004;10:525–32.
133. Schlatt S. Prospects and problems for germ cell transplantation in the male. Int J Androl. 1999;22:13–8.
134. Aslam I, Fishel S, Moore H, Dowell KK, Thornton S. Fertility preservation of boys undergoing anti-cancer therapy: a review of the existing situation and prospects for the future. Hum Reprod. 2000;15:2154–9.
135. Schlatt S, von Schonfeldt V, Schepers AG. Male germ cell transplantation: an experimental approach with a clinical perspective. Br Med Bull. 2000;56:824–36.
136. Schlatt S, Honaramooz A, Boiani M, Scholer HR, Dobrinski I. Progeny from sperm obtained after ectopic grafting of neonatal mouse testes. Biol Reprod. 2003;68:2331–5.
137. Honaramooz A, Snedaker A, Boiani M, Scholer H, Dobrinski I, Schlatt S. Sperm from neonatal mammalian testes grafted in mice. Nature. 2002;418:778–81.
138. Nagano M, Patrizio P, Brinster RL. Long-term survival of human spermatogonial stem cells in mouse testes. Fertil Steril. 2002;78:1225–31.
139. Feng LX, Chen Y, Dettin L, Pera RA, Herr JC, Goldberg E, Dym M. Generation and in vitro differentiation of a spermatogonial cell line. Science. 2002;297:392–5.
140. Hovatta O, Foudila T, Siegberg R, Johansson K, von Smitten K, Reima I. Pregnancy resulting from intracytoplasmic injection of spermatozoa from a frozen–thawed testicular biopsy specimen. Hum Reprod. 1996;11:2472–3.
141. Ehmcke J, Hubner K, Scholer HR, Schlatt S. Spermatogonia: origin, physiology and prospects for conservation and manipulation of the male germ line. Reprod Fertil Dev. 2006;18:7–12.

142. Ogawa T, Ohmura M, Ohbo K. The niche for spermatogonial stem cells in the mammalian testis. Int J Hematol. 2005;82:381–8.
143. Muller J, Sonksen J, Sommer P, Schmiegelow M, Petersen PM, Heilman C, Schmiegelow K. Cryopreservation of semen from pubertal boys with cancer. Med Pediatr Oncol. 2000; 34:191–4.
144. Schmiegelow ML, Sommer P, Carlsen E, Sonksen JO, Schmiegelow K, Muller JR. Penile vibratory stimulation and electroejaculation before anticancer therapy in two pubertal boys. J Pediatr Hematol Oncol. 1998;20:429–30.
145. Hovav Y, Dan-Goor M, Yaffe H, Almagor M. Electroejaculation before chemotherapy in adolescents and young men with cancer. Fertil Steril. 2001;75:811–3.
146. Tournaye H. Recovery, survival and functional evaluation by transplantation of frozen-thawed mouse germ cells. Hum Reprod. 2004;19:948–53.
147. Jahnukainen K, Hou M, Petersen C, Setchell B, Soder O. Intratesticular transplantation of testicular cells from leukemic rats causes transmission of leukemia. Cancer Res. 2001; 61:706–10.
148. Robertson JA. Cancer and fertility: ethical and legal challenges. J Natl Cancer Inst Monogr. 2005;34:104–6.
149. Wallace WH, Anderson RA, Irvine DS. Fertility preservation for young patients with cancer: who is at risk and what can be offered? Lancet Oncol. 2005;6:209–18.
150. Keros V, Hultenby K, Borgstro B, Fridstro M, Jahnukainen K, Hovatta O. Methods of cryopreservation of testicular tissue with viable spermatogonia in pre-pubertal boys undergoing gonadotoxic cancer treatment. Hum Reprod. 2007;22:1384–95.
151. Kvist K, Thorup J, Byskov J, Hoyer PE, Mollgard K, Yding Andersen C. Cryopreservation of intact testicular tissue from boys with cryptorchidism. Hum Reprod. 2006;21:484–91.
152. Kalthur G, Adiga SK, Upadhya D, Rao S, Kumar P. Effect of cryopreservation on sperm DNA integrity in patients with teratospermia. Fertil Steril. 2008;89:1723–7.
153. Toro E, Fernandez S, Colomar A, Casanovas A, Alvarez JG, Lopez-Teijon M, Velilla E. Processing of semen can result in increased sperm DNA fragmentation. Fertil Steril. 2009;92:2109–12.
154. Zribi N, Chakroun NF, El Euch H, Gargouri J, Bahloul A, Keskes LA. Effects of cryopreserved on human sperm deoxyribonucleic acid integrity. Fertil Steril. 2010;93:159–66.
155. De Paula TS, Bertolla RP, Spaine DM, Cunha MA, Schor N, Cedenho AP. Effect of cryopreservation on sperm apoptotic deoxyribonucleic acid fragmentation in patients with oligospermia. Fertil Steril. 2006;86:597–600.
156. Adiga SK, Khan Z, Upadhya D, Kalthur G, Kumar P. Ability of deoxyribonucleic acid-damaged sperm to withstand freeze-thaw-induced damage during cryopreservation. Fertil Steril. 2009;92:959–63.
157. Thomson LK, Fleming SD, Barone K, Zieschang JA, Clark AM. The effect of repeated freezing and thawing on human sperm DNA fragmentation. Fertil Steril. 2010;93:1147–56.
158. Thomson LK, Flemming SD, Schulke L, Barone K, Zieschang J-A, Clark AM. The DNA integrity of cryopreserved spermatozoa separated for use in assisted reproductive technology is unaffected by the type of cryoprotectant used but is related to the DNA integrity of the fresh separated preparation. Fertil Steril. 2009;92:991–1001.

Chapter 27
Slow Freezing of Oocytes

Giovanni Coticchio and Lucia De Santis

Introduction

Assisted reproduction technology (ART) is becoming an increasingly important strategy to preserve female fertility. Until a decade ago, in an ART context, the only option available to preserve fertility for a woman at risk of loss of ovarian function was embryo cryopreservation. The storage of embryos is a sound, well established, and safe procedure, but it entails major downsides, such as ethical objections to the generation of conceptuses that might never be used, the need of single women to resort to donor sperm, and legal complications in case of separation of the couple. More recently, new avenues have been opened to preserve female fertility through ART. Ovarian tissue cryopreservation and orthotopic re-implantation have shown the potential to restore ovarian function for a period of time and offer a chance for natural conception. However, so far, only very few full-term pregnancies have been achieved. Therefore, the efficacy of this approach remains to be established. Oocyte cryopreservation is powerfully emerging as an efficient ART procedure able to preserve female fertility without the implications which afflict embryo cryopreservation. Historically, control rate slow cooling (CRSC) has been the technological standard of human embryo cryopreservation. This has marked the early history of oocyte cryopreservation. Consistent advances of CRSC protocols have given oocyte cryopreservation the dignity of a routine procedure in many human IVF laboratories. Progress in the last few years has been also driven by the development of the vitrification approach.

G. Coticchio, BSc, MSc, MMedSc, PhD (✉)
Biogenesi, Reproductive Medicine Centre, Istituti Clinici Zucchi,
Via Zucchi 24, Monza, 20052, Italy
e-mail: coticchio.biogenesi@grupposandonato.it

L. De Santis, BSc, MSc
IVF Unit, Department of Obstetrics and Gynecology,
H S. Raffaele, Universita Vita-Salute, Milan, Italy
e-mail: desantis.lucia@hsr.it

Z.P. Nagy et al. (eds.), *Clinical Embryology: A Practical Guide*,
DOI 10.1007/978-1-4614-8376-2_27, © Springer Science+Business Media New York 2013

Methodological Aspects of Oocyte Cryopreservation

Oocyte cryopreservation, irrespective of whether CRSC or vitrification is applied, requires a rigorous system of management to control technical (type of protocol, cryopreservation media) and procedural (time of oocyte culture before and after cryopreservation, oocyte manipulation, operator experience) factors that could affect the viability of the stored material. In terms of operative times and mobilization of resources, cryopreservation can represent a conspicuous part of the activity of an IVF laboratory. Therefore, cryopreservation and long-term storage in liquid nitrogen necessitate of specific work areas. These areas should be adjacent to the core of the laboratory, accessible only by authorized staff, and equipped with systems to ensure sufficient air changes to prevent accumulation of liquid nitrogen vapours and monitor oxygen levels. The choice of a CRSC system should be supported by the use to two cryofreezers, to ensure safe backup and give the opportunity to run separate cycles of freezing at appropriate times, if required. Cryofreezers produce temperature graphs of the freezing process that represent an important document of quality control for each cryopreservation cycle. Liquid nitrogen levels in dewars used for medium-/long-term storage should be monitored at regular intervals and reported in a dedicated logbook. Dewars may be equipped with electronic monitoring systems able to send information to remote terminals, such as PC and mobile phones. Laboratory staff should be properly instructed on safety measures on the use of liquid nitrogen and have access to devices for personal protection. Quality-control and quality-assurance programmes require monitoring and recording of the procedures adopted for the cryopreservation of oocytes. These data may be used at later stages for various purposes, for example, assessments of efficacy and reproducibility. Each laboratory should have operative instructions describing the cryopreservation protocols and flow charts showing the path that oocytes follow from recovery to their use after cryopreservation. All aspects pertaining cryopreservation procedure (information for the identification of the couple, cryopreservation protocols, storage details) should be fully described and reported in a logbook and an electronic database backed up at regular intervals.

Possible Effect of Slow Freezing on Human Oocytes

Fully grown oocytes from antral follicles may be cryopreserved at the immature—germinal vesicle (GV)—or mature stage. Although immature oocyte cryopreservation has been recently suggested to represent a possible route for fertility preservation especially in women facing the prospect of gonadotoxic therapies [1], the storage of mature oocytes has gained a far larger interest as an alternative to embryo cryopreservation. The pre-ovulatory mature oocyte is an individual entity, ready for fertilization and relatively autonomous from cumulus cells which have accompanied and supported its development throughout oogenesis. Its cryopreservation, therefore, is not complicated by the need to maintain unaltered a sophisticated tissue and intricate cell contacts, as in the case of the preservation of ovarian tissue. Nevertheless, the cellular and biochemical integrity of the single oocyte is exposed to a risk of irreversible damage during the process of cryopreservation. Rupture of the oolemma and widespread cell disruption is a relatively common event. This occurs in 20–30% of cases even with the most efficient CRSC protocols [2, 3], a frequency that has become less acceptable following the recently reported successes of the vitrification approach by which survival rates in excess of 90% can be achieved. Overt oocyte death may be observed immediately after thawing and release from the storage device (usually a 250-mL straw) or during exposure to thawing solutions. Clearly, this may represent an effect of physical damage caused by intracellular ice formation or osmotic stress dictated by dehydration and rehydration events taking place during replacement of intracellular water with cryoprotective agents (CPAs) and/or vice versa. Cell death may occur even hours after the completion of the process of thawing and rehydration. Gook et al. [4] reported a decrease in survival rate of oocytes over the 24 h following thawing. Clearly, oocyte cryopreservation by CRSC requires further development in order to improve survival rates.

Survival after thawing is obviously crucial, but does not necessarily ensure or coincide with cell integrity. Sublethal damage may affect different cell organelles and structures and/or biochemical pathways. Transmission electron microscopy (TEM) is an investigative tool often believed either obsolete or out of fashion by many, but in fact, it is extremely valuable for the study of cell damage that may be generated by cryopreservation. In human oocytes stored by a CRSC protocol developed for human embryos, about 30 years ago, Sathananthan observed fractures in the zona pellucida, oolemma irregularities, and widespread disorganization of the ooplasm. After exposure to dimethyl sulfoxide (DMSO) at 0°C, he also found that parts of the endoplasmic reticulum, Golgi, mitochondria, and the cytosol were damaged to some extent [5]. A subsequent study showed how sometimes TEM fails to detect structural anomalies that may have significant implications for the oocyte physiology. Van Blerkom and Davies [6] described cytokinesis anomalies and cleavage arrest in embryos developed from cryopreserved human oocytes, despite electron microscopy analysis carried out after thawing had not shown gross cytoplasmic alterations. Afterwards, electron microscopy studies on cryopreserved human oocytes were interrupted for over a decade, as a consequence of the inadequacy of the cryopreservation methodology available in the nineties to ensure high survival rates. With the development of improved protocols [3, 7, 8], ultrastructural studies again attracted a significant interest. By comparing fresh and frozen–thawed oocytes, Ghetler et al. [9] reported substantial decrease in the number of cortical granules (CG) as an effect of cryopreservation. This supports the inference that stored oocytes should be microinjected by intracytoplasmic sperm injection (ICSI) rather than inseminated by standard IVF to prevent possible fertilization failure caused by hardening of the zona pellucida. In effect, a few years after it became available, ICSI was chosen as the elective route to achieve fertilization in cryopreserved oocytes [10] and is now recognized as a standard of treatments involving cryopreserved oocytes [11–14]. Despite that, the question of a non-physiological release of CG in cryopreserved oocytes remains open. By using epifluorescence microscopy, Gook et al. [4] showed that, in comparison to fresh material, the staining specific for CG was unaffected in cryopreserved material. They also showed that in frozen oocytes, fertilization could be achieved through standard IVF [15]. The possibility to use standard IVF has been reported by other authors [16]. However, further ultrastructural analysis has confirmed that a partial loss of CG occurs following cryopreservation. This has been observed qualitatively in oocytes cryopreserved with CRSC protocols involving the use of 0.1 or 0.3 mol/L sucrose as a constituent of the freezing solution [17]. Similar findings were described by Gualtieri et al. [18]. Consistent with this, oocytes stored by a CRSC protocol including ethylene glycol (EG) as an intracellular CPA [19] or by vitrification [20] appear to be affected by a loss of CG. Recent observations provide quantitative data suggesting that about two thirds of the original population of CG is lost and presumably their contents released in the perivitelline space, as a result of cryopreservation. This phenomenon appears therefore rather ubiquitous in cryopreserved oocytes, irrespective of the cryopreservation approach (CRSC or vitrification) or specific protocol. Whether CG release is always sufficient to cause zona hardening in frozen oocytes is not clear, although the detection of thickening and change in texture of the inner surface of the ZP is in line with this hypothesis [17].

Another recurrent characteristic found in cryopreserved oocytes is the increased presence of vacuolar structures. The nature of these formations has not been well characterized. They may be found in fully grown immature oocytes, but in metaphase II (MII) oocytes, they are rare and have been interpreted as a sign of cytoplasmic immaturity or, vice versa, ageing. Because vacuoles may also derive from a general response to injury [21], in the case of oocyte cryopreservation, they may represent a manifestation of cell stress. Rather consistently, the presence of vacuoles was described in association with a variety of CRSC protocols [9, 17, 19]. It is tempting to hypothesize that vacuoles located peripherally may evolve from crypt-like invaginations and clusters of endocytic vesicles which form in the oocyte cortex following simple exposure to CPA [22]. However, if this assumption is correct, it remains to be explained why oocytes vitrified through the cryoleaf method, which are exposed to high concentrations of CPAs, do not exhibit an increase in the number of vacuoles, as recently reported [20]. Regardless their origin, it is possible that vacuoles may be adopted as a specific indicator of cryodamage and reduced developmental potential in cryopreserved oocyte, considering that an increased number of vacuoles [17] and a reduced developmental ability [11, 23] are concomitantly associated to certain CRSC protocols, although this has not been confirmed through a prospective randomized control trial. Preliminary evidence suggest that vitrification protocols may be associated with high implantation ability [14] and a normal or low occurrence of vacuoles [20].

Mitochondria and elements of the smooth endoplasmic reticulum (SER) may also be affected by cryopreservation. Individually, these two types of organelles play well-characterized roles in all cells. In particular in oocytes, not only are mitochondria central to the energy generation process but also can produce intermediates of the tricarboxylic acid cycle and reducing equivalents that may be employed in antioxidant defence. The SER complex is instead well characterized as an organelle system competent to the translation, modification, packaging, and delivery of proteins destined to the plasmalemma or exocytotic compartments. In the oocyte, the association between mitochondria and SER elements contributes to the generation of the typical oscillations in cytosolic free calcium which are triggered by the fertilizing spermatozoon and are interpreted by the oocyte biochemical machinery as a start signal for fertilization [24]. Magnitude and frequency of calcium oscillation have also been found to influence much later events of development, such as organogenesis and fetal growth [25]. For such reasons, mitochondria-SER aggregates are particularly important for the physiology of the oocyte. Mitochondria and SER elements, separately or in close association with each other, are often found unaltered in oocytes cryopreserved with CRSC protocols relying on propane-1,2-diol (PrOH) as a intracellular CPA [17] and used in the clinical practice [11, 23]. This is a reassuring evidence in the light of the role of mitochondria-SER associations in the mechanism of intracellular calcium signalling, as discussed above. Conversely, other cryopreservation conditions may be in fact deleterious to mitochondria-SER aggregates. In particular, in oocytes cryopreserved by a CRSC protocol including EG as an intracellular CPA, pronounced disorganization of these aggregates may be noticed [19]. Why some cryopreservation conditions can generate damage to the mitochondria-SER aggregates is still to be understood. It may be relevant to this question the fact that, so far, mitochondria-SER aggregate disarrangements have been reported only in association with the use of EG, but not PrOH. Perceptible, although moderate, underdeveloped mitochondria-SER aggregates were also observed in oocytes vitrified with a solution containing EG [20]. However, such findings are largely insufficient to conclude that EG can specifically and directly affect the constitution of mitochondria-SER aggregates. Overall, these studies confirm the usefulness of TEM to investigate oocyte quality after cryopreservation.

One of the factors that could cause a partial loss of oocyte viability after cryopreservation is the phenomenon of in vitro ageing. In fact, only for a limited period of time the mature oocyte is able to maintain a particular condition that is essential for successful fertilization and development. Such a condition corresponds biochemically to relatively high levels of maturation-promoting factor (MPF) and microtubule-activated protein kinase (MAPK), two key regulators of the meiotic and mitotic cell cycles, and from a cellular standpoint to the arrest of the meiotic process at the MII stage. The MPF and MAPK activities can decrease either as an effect of a spontaneous biochemical decay occurring within a few hours after PBI extrusion or secondarily to extrinsic factors, such as inappropriate manipulation in vitro. Cryopreservation could interfere with the mechanism of meiotic control of the oocyte, either directly, through the stresses generated by the process of freezing-thawing (or vitrification-warming), or indirectly, because of an excessively protracted maintenance in culture before and/or after cryopreservation. Recent evidence suggests that biochemical cryodamage is not purely hypothetical. In fact, in sheep oocytes, cumulus removal and vitrification can affect the MPF and MAPK levels after in vitro maturation [26]. A similar phenomenon may occur in human oocytes after cryopreservation. In coincidence with the use of a protocol involving 0.3 mol/L sucrose as non-penetrating CPA [3], over a period of 2 h after thawing, MAPK is unaffected in comparison to fresh controls. Conversely, during the same interval, MPF activity is initially maintained unaltered but undergoes a significant decrease thereafter [27]. It is striking that the observed decrease in MPF mirrors a progressive loss in the organization of the MII spindle that is known to occur with a similar dynamics in frozen–thawed oocytes [28]. Because high levels of MPF are critical to maintain the integrity of the MII spindle, it is tempting to speculate that after thawing, a decrease in the activity of the former may cause a loss in the organization of the latter.

These findings may have significant implications for the clinical use of frozen–thawed oocytes. In particular, considering the observed delayed reduction in MPF activity, it might be appropriate to limit to 1 h the period of post-thaw culture that is implemented in preparation for ICSI, thereby preventing possible losses in spindle and chromosome configuration, or premature exit from the MII arrest. The importance of the time factor in oocyte cryopreservation seems to be suggested also by data that indicate that the oocyte ability to give rise to a viable pregnancy tends to decrease if the overall time spent in culture before and after cryopreservation exceeds a certain number of hours (Borini et al., unpublished observations). Other recent studies appear to confirm that an excessively protracted period of culture between retrieval and cryopreservation may have a negative impact on the developmental ability of human oocytes [29, 30].

Clinical Outcome of Oocyte Cryopreservation

Cryopreservation strategies can profoundly affect the clinical outcome of oocyte cryopreservation and make difficult the comparison among different studies. In certain contexts, constrains of religious, ethical, or legal nature limit the number of embryos that may be produced and transferred during each cycle of treatment. In frozen–thawed oocyte (or vitrified-warmed) cycles, these restrictions can be met by thawing only a small proportion of the stored material at a time to the end of having 2–3 viable oocytes suitable for insemination, avoiding wastage of material [11]. As an effect of a legal restriction implemented in Italy from March 2004 to April 2009, the practice established by law to thaw a limited number of oocytes for treatment cycle has been adopted systematically and described in various studies conducted [12, 23, 29, 31]. In other studies, no limit was imposed on the number of oocytes that could be thawed and, consequently, the number of embryos that could be cultured and transferred [32, 33]. The different implications of these two strategies are rather obvious. The thawing of only a few oocytes per cycle involves a higher risk of cycle drop out as an effect of high rates of fertilization or cleavage failure [11]. Furthermore, with only a few oocytes available, embryo selection is not applicable, and in some cases, the number of embryos available for transfer may be insufficient. This scenario, which is unlikely to occur when several oocytes are thawed at the same time, affects the clinical outcome in terms of implantation and pregnancy rates. For this reason, the comparison of implantation rates achieved in studies in which the mean number of transferred embryos was different appears rather arbitrary and non-informative [11, 34]. An example of the inadequacy of pregnancy rate per transfer as a measure of efficacy is offered by a study [31] in which by using a freezing protocol specific from cleavage stage embryos, a success rate of 16.7% was achieved. In fact, in the same study, the pregnancy rate per thawing cycle was 7.7%, as a consequence of a high incidence (50%) of cycles cancelled for failed survival or fertilization. Gook and Edgar [35, 36] have proposed a more objective standard to assess the efficacy of treatments involving frozen oocytes or embryos. By considering that during an IVF treatment the initial amount of biological material (oocytes) undergoes a decrease at different stage of the process (fertilization, cleavage, selection for freezing, and thawing), they estimated that from an original pool of 100 fresh oocytes, about 5 implantations from frozen embryo can be achieved. Gook and Edgar suggests that the same kind of analysis should be adopted also for the assessment of the clinical efficacy of oocyte cryopreservation, including in the calculation all the events of pre- and post-storage loss of the original material. Only under those conditions the relative values of the diverse cryopreservation methods can emerge. For example, it is well know that a considerable increase (35–40% to 70–75%) in the survival rate oocytes cryopreserved by CRSC may be obtained by augmenting from 0.1 to 0.3 mol/L the concentration of sucrose in the freezing solution [3]. A higher sucrose concentration is also beneficial to the fertilization rate [12, 23, 31]. However, the reduced loss of material during the thawing and fertilization phases is accompanied by a decreased implantation rate in comparison to the outcome derived by the use of the protocol based on 0.1 mol/L sucrose [11, 31]. Therefore, in final analysis, the two protocols result equivalent if assessed on the number of implantations (approximately 2.4–2.6 in both cases) that can be obtained from 100 thawed oocytes. By using other protocols, implantation rates per thawed oocyte of about 5% can be achieved, a result that make oocyte freezing rather comparable to embryo freezing. By adopting a freezing protocol based on sodium-free media, Boldt et al. [33] reported an implantation rate per thawed oocyte of 5.3%. In that study, however, only 23 patients were included, and the initial rate of success has not been confirmed by the treatment of larger series of patients. A comparable implantation rate per thawed oocyte has been reported in another study [2] in which oocytes were cryopreserved with a protocol based on different sucrose concentrations in freezing and thawing solutions (0.2 and 0.3 mol/L, respectively). Parmegiani et al. [29] have also achieved a result of a similar magnitude. However, in general, these studies are rather numerically smaller in comparison to those involving frozen embryos. For example, Edgar et al. [37] reported an experience based on more than 5,000 frozen–thawed embryos.

Safety of Oocyte Cryopreservation

Oocyte cryopreservation has raised health concerns derived from the possibility that oocyte cell damage secondary to freezing-thawing is a frequent event that may expose the conceptus to an increased risk of developmental anomalies. The number of babies born from cryopreserved oocytes is steadily increasing. In 2004, Borini et al. [11] described 11 births from cryopreserved oocytes. These children had an average weight of 3.2 kg, normal karyotype, and no malformations. Shortly afterwards, Chen et al. [32] reported the birth of 5 children from cryopreserved oocytes with normal karyotypes. Other authors [2, 12, 23, 31, 33, 38, 39] documented 65 births from frozen oocytes but did not describe details on their genotype in a systematic fashion. In the 18 births of Levi Setti et al. [12], a mean gestational age of 37.1 weeks and weight of 2,807 g were observed. So far, the largest group of children from cryopreserved oocytes has been described in a preliminary study of Borini et al. [40] where 4 cases of developmental anomalies were found (Rubinstein–Taybi syndrome, 47XXX, chromosome 19 hypomethylation, and choanal atresia) in 146 births. Tur Kaspa et al. [41] analysed more than 37 studies on children from cryopreserved oocytes. In 555 live births, 5 developmental anomalies were identified. This corresponds to a frequency of congenital abnormality comparable to the one that affects spontaneous conceptions. The criteria adopted for this analysis have been questioned. In particular, it has been objected that the overall number of births was overestimated as a result of duplication of sets of original data [42]. However, the absence of an association between oocyte cryopreservation and congenital anomalies is confirmed by a different analysis including over 900 births [43]. Eight children were found affected of various anomalies at birth, a result that, again, is comparable to the frequency occurring in spontaneous births.

The debate on the safety of oocyte cryopreservation remains open. For example, data on the frequency of spontaneous abortion are lacking. Nevertheless, current evidence does not seem to support the existence of specific health risks and legitimate the use of oocyte cryopreservation as a treatment for women requiring an assisted reproduction technology treatment.

Conclusions

Oocyte cryopreservation by CRSC has become a well-established procedure able to compete with embryo freezing, especially after recent progress in the development of novel protocols and conditions. Safety concerns have not been confirmed, although further and more rigorous studies are needed. Future development of oocyte CRSC will depend on the application novel theoretical models which can predict better cryopreservation conditions and thereby improve oocyte quality after freezing–thawing.

References

1. Oktay K, Demirtas E, Son WY, Lostritto K, Chian RC, Tan SL. In vitro maturation of germinal vesicle oocytes recovered after premature luteinizing hormone surge: description of a novel approach to fertility preservation. Fertil Steril. 2008;89:228.e19–22.

2. Bianchi V, Coticchio G, Distratis V, Di Giusto N, Flamigni C, Borini A. Differential sucrose concentration during dehydration (0.2 mol/l) and rehydration (0.3 mol/l) increases the implantation rate of frozen human oocytes. Reprod Biomed Online. 2007;14: 64–71.
3. Fabbri R, Porcu E, Marsella T, Rocchetta G, Venturoli S, Flamigni C. Human oocyte cryopreservation: new perspectives regarding oocyte survival. Hum Reprod. 2001;16:411–6.
4. Gook DA, Osborn SM, Johnston WI. Cryopreservation of mouse and human oocytes using 1,2-propanediol and the configuration of the meiotic spindle. Hum Reprod. 1993;8:1101–9.
5. Sathananthan AH, Trounson A, Freemann L, Brady T. The effects of cooling human oocytes. Hum Reprod. 1988;3:968–77.
6. Van Blerkom J, Davis PW. Cytogenetic, cellular, and developmental consequences of cryopreservation of immature and mature mouse and human oocytes. Microsc Res Tech. 1994; 27:165–93.
7. Stachecki JJ, Cohen J, Willadsen SM. Cryopreservation of unfertilized mouse oocytes: the effect of replacing sodium with choline in the freezing medium. Cryobiology. 1998;37:346–54.
8. Quintans CJ, Donaldson MJ, Bertolino MV, Pasqualini RS. Birth of two babies using oocytes that were cryopreserved in a choline-based freezing medium. Hum Reprod. 2002;17:3149–52.
9. Ghetler Y, Skutelsky E, Ben Nun I, Ben Dor L, Amihai D, Shalgi R. Human oocyte cryopreservation and the fate of cortical granules. Fertil Steril. 2006;86:210–6.
10. Porcu E, Fabbri R, Seracchioli R, Ciotti PM, Magrini O, Flamigni C. Birth of a healthy female after intracytoplasmic sperm injection of cryopreserved human oocytes. Fertil Steril. 1997;68:724–6.
11. Borini A, Bonu MA, Coticchio G, Bianchi V, Cattoli M, Flamigni C. Pregnancies and births after oocyte cryopreservation. Fertil Steril. 2004;82:601–5.
12. Levi Setti PE, Albani E, Novara PV, Cesana A, Morreale G. Cryopreservation of supernumerary oocytes in IVF/ICSI cycles. Hum Reprod. 2006;21:370–5.
13. Kuwayama M, Vajta G, Kato O, Leibo SP. Highly efficient vitrification method for cryopreservation of human oocytes. Reprod Biomed Online. 2005;11:300–8.
14. Cobo A, Kuwayama M, Perez S, Ruiz A, Pellicer A, Remohi J. Comparison of concomitant outcome achieved with fresh and cryopreserved donor oocytes vitrified by the Cryotop method. Fertil Steril. 2008;89:1657–64.
15. Gook DA, Schiewe MC, Osborn SM, Asch RH, Jansen RP, Johnston WI. Intracytoplasmic sperm injection and embryo development of human oocytes cryopreserved using 1,2-propanediol. Hum Reprod. 1995;10:2637–41.
16. Li XH, Chen SU, Zhang X, Tang M, Kui YR, Wu X, et al. Cryopreserved oocytes of infertile couples undergoing assisted reproductive technology could be an important source of oocyte donation: a clinical report of successful pregnancies. Hum Reprod. 2005;20:3390–4.
17. Nottola SA, Macchiarelli G, Coticchio G, Bianchi S, Cecconi S, De Santis L, et al. Ultrastructure of human mature oocytes after slow cooling cryopreservation using different sucrose concentrations. Hum Reprod. 2007;22:1123–33.
18. Gualtieri R, Iaccarino M, Mollo V, Prisco M, Iaccarino S, Talevi R. Slow cooling of human oocytes: ultrastructural injuries and apoptotic status. Fertil Steril. 2009;91:1023–34.
19. Nottola SA, Coticchio G, De Santis L, Macchiarelli G, Maione M, Bianchi S, et al. Ultrastructure of human mature oocytes after slow cooling cryopreservation with ethylene glycol. Reprod Biomed Online. 2008;17:368–77.
20. Nottola SA, Coticchio G, Sciajno R, Gambardella A, Maione M, Macchiarelli G, et al. Ultrastructural changes in human metaphase II oocytes cryopreserved by vitrification Reproductive biomedicine online. Reprod Biomed Online. 2009;19 Suppl 3:17–27.
21. Ghadially FN. Ultrastructural Pathology of the Cell and Matrix. 2nd ed. London, UK: Butterworths; 1982.
22. Schalkoff ME, Oskowitz SP, Powers RD. Ultrastructural observations of human and mouse oocytes treated with cryopreservatives. Biol Reprod. 1989;40:379–93.
23. Borini A, Sciajno R, Bianchi V, Sereni E, Flamigni C, Coticchio G. Clinical outcome of oocyte cryopreservation after slow cooling with a protocol utilizing a high sucrose concentration. Hum Reprod. 2006;21:512–7.

24. Fissore RA, Kurokawa M, Knott J, Zhang M, Smyth J. Mechanisms underlying oocyte activation and postovulatory ageing. Reproduction. 2002;124:745–54.
25. Ozil JP, Huneau D. Activation of rabbit oocytes: the impact of the Ca2+ signal regime on development. Development. 2001;128: 917–28.
26. Bogliolo L, Ariu F, Fois S, Rosati I, Zedda MT, Leoni G, et al. Morphological and biochemical analysis of immature ovine oocytes vitrified with or without cumulus cells. Theriogenology. 2007;68: 1138–49.
27. Borini A, Bogliolo L, Coticchio G, Bianchi V, Nicoli A, Valli B, et al. Activity of maturation promoting factor (MPF), but not microtubule-activated protein kinase (MAPK) decreases over time in frozen thawed human oocytes. Hum Reprod. 2009;24:i88.
28. Bromfield JJ, Coticchio G, Hutt K, Sciajno R, Borini A, Albertini DF. Meiotic spindle dynamics in human oocytes following slow-cooling cryopreservation. Hum Reprod. 2009;24: 2114–23.
29. Parmegiani L, Cognigni GE, Bernardi S, Ciampaglia W, Infante F, Pocognoli P, et al. Freezing within 2 h from oocyte retrieval increases the efficiency of human oocyte cryopreservation when using a slow freezing/rapid thawing protocol with high sucrose concentration. Hum Reprod. 2008;23:1771–7.
30. Parmegiani L, Bertocci F, Garello C, Salvarani MC, Tambuscio G, Fabbri R. Efficiency of human oocyte slow freezing: results from five assisted reproduction centres. Reprod Biomed Online. 2009; 18:352–9.
31. De Santis L, Cino I, Rabellotti E, Papaleo E, Calzi F, Fusi FM, et al. Oocyte cryopreservation: clinical outcome of slow-cooling protocols differing in sucrose concentration. Reprod Biomed Online. 2007;14:57–63.
32. Chen SU, Lien YR, Chen HF, Chang LJ, Tsai YY, Yang YS. Observational clinical follow-up of oocyte cryopreservation using a slow-freezing method with 1,2-propanediol plus sucrose followed by ICSI. Hum Reprod. 2005;20:1975–80.
33. Boldt J, Tidswell N, Sayers A, Kilani R, Cline D. Human oocyte cryopreservation: 5-year experience with a sodium-depleted slow freezing method. Reprod Biomed Online. 2006;13: 96–100.
34. Lucena E, Bernal DP, Lucena C, Rojas A, Moran A, Lucena A. Successful ongoing pregnancies after vitrification of oocytes. Fertil Steril. 2006;85:108–11.
35. Gook DA, Edgar DH. Cryopreservation of the human female gamete: current and future issues. Hum Reprod. 1999;14:2938–40.
36. Edgar DH, Gook DA. How should the clinical efficiency of oocyte cryopreservation be measured? Reprod Biomed Online. 2007; 14:430–5.
37. Edgar DH, Archer J, McBain J, Bourne H. Embryonic factors affecting outcome from single cryopreserved embryo transfer. Reprod Biomed Online. 2007;14:718–23.
38. Porcu E, Fabbri R, Damiano G, Giunchi S, Fratto R, Ciotti PM, et al. Clinical experience and applications of oocyte cryopreservation. Mol Cell Endocrinol. 2000;169:33–7.
39. Parmegiani L, Cognigni GE, Bernardi S, Ciampaglia W, Infante F, Pocognoli P, et al. Freezing within 2 h from oocyte retrieval increases the efficiency of human oocyte cryopreservation when using a slow freezing/rapid thawing protocol with high sucrose concentration. Hum Reprod. 2008;23(8):1771–7.
40. Borini A, Cattoli M, Mazzone S, Trevisi MR, Nalon M, Iadarola I. Survey of 105 babies born after slow-cooling oocyte cryopreservation. Fertil Steril. 2007;88:S13–4.
41. Tur-Kaspa I, Gal M, Horwitz A. Genetics and health of children born from cryopreserved oocytes. Fertil Steril. 2007;88:S14.
42. Maher B. Little consensus on egg freezing. Nature. 2007;449:958.
43. Noyes N, Porcu E, Borini A. Over 900 oocyte cryopreservation babies born with no apparent increase in congenital anomalies. Reprod Biomed Online. 2009;18:769–76.

Chapter 28
Vitrification: Research in Animal Models

Gábor Vajta

Cryopreservation of Mammalian Oocytes: The Ultimate Challenge in Mammalian Cryobiology

During the past 50 years, impressive success has been achieved in cryopreservation of male gametes and preimplantation stage embryos of mammals. Techniques were established mostly in domestic animals, predominantly in cattle, because of the high demand of the breeding industry. Artificial insemination with frozen-thawed semen in cattle is now the most frequently used assisted reproductive technique in mammals. Transfer of frozen-thawed morulae and blastocysts is also a routine technology, although the numbers of transferred embryos are stagnating worldwide since years for reasons not closely related to the efficiency of the technology. To a lesser extent, the same techniques are also applied in sheep, goats, horses, and pigs. These techniques are also successful in experimental animals, especially in the most widely used species, mouse.

However, the advancement in cryopreservation of female gametes was slow, and the efficiency was—and still is—frustratingly low. The only exception is mouse, where traditional freezing of oocytes has resulted in high survival and developmental rates [1]. Curiously, this fact had a controversial effect on the development of a successful cryopreservation technique for humans, as methods successfully used in mouse were inappropriate for human oocyte cryopreservation. In this regard, experiences obtained from oocyte cryopreservation of some domestic species provided much more important information for establishing a successful human oocyte cryopreservation method, although none of the tested domestic species have exactly the same oocyte type of cryosensitivity as humans.

In general, the problems related to oocyte cryopreservation are attributed to several physical and biological factors [2] including the size and shape of oocytes.

G. Vajta, MD, PhD, DSc (✉)
Vajta Embryology Consulting, Rakosi and Vajta Trust, Brinsmead, QLD, Australia
e-mail: gabor.vajta@hotmail.com

Z.P. Nagy et al. (eds.), *Clinical Embryology: A Practical Guide*,
DOI 10.1007/978-1-4614-8376-2_28,

The extremely large size—oocytes are close to be detectable with naked eyes—and almost perfect round shape make equal distribution of potentially harmful cryoprotectant solutions within the cells difficult, accordingly toxic damage may develop at the periphery while the center is still not protected by the cryoprotectants. Additionally, oocytes in most mammalian species including humans are very sensitive to chilling injuries, that is, damages between +15 and −5°C. This sensitivity is generally attributed to the injury of the meiotic spindle, lipid-containing membranes, and lipid droplets. The damage of the spindle may be reversible; however, the injury of lipid structures, especially the lipid droplets, seems to be fatal, although the specific function of these droplets is still unclear [3–7]. The premature release of cortical granules caused by the cryopreservation process may also cause zona hardening and hampering sperm penetration.

On the other hand, parallel investigations with other developmental stages suggest the role of other, still unknown factors contributing in this sensitivity, as zygotes with the same size are much more tolerant toward cryoinjuries; the absence of the meiotic spindle of immature oocytes would suggest less cryosensitivity, but in fact, the contrary is true; and data regarding cryopreservation-induced cortical granule exocytosis and zona hardening are controversial; besides, this problem can be easily eliminated by the application of intracytoplasmic sperm injection. Moreover, oocytes of different mammalian species seem to suffer different types of injuries, for example, morphological survival of bovine oocytes is easy to achieve, but the seemingly intact oocytes may fail to get fertilized and activated, while in humans, the signs of cryodamage are easy to recognize minutes after warming; on the other hand, a light microscopically intact MII phase human oocyte after warming has almost or entirely the same developmental competence as its noncryopreserved counterpart.

In spite of these controversies and differences, research in domestic animals has contributed considerably in the establishment of a successful human oocyte cryopreservation system that is now acknowledged worldwide and may be regarded as the greatest achievement in reproductive cryobiology in the first decade of our century.

Research in Domestic Animals Promoting Human Embryology

As mentioned above, the initial embryo cryopreservation techniques based on traditional freezing were successfully adopted for mouse oocytes, but—apart from some exceptional achievements—the human application resulted in very low efficiency that hampered to achieve any practical goals. Accordingly, embryologists had to follow to ways for improvement: to find an entirely new approach or to make stepwise efforts to increase the efficiency of traditional freezing. During the past 2 decades, serious efforts were made in both direction, and eventually, the outcome of both ways has justified the invested energy. Experiments in domestic animals contributed mostly in the former way—to find a radically different solution for the problem—and the latest comparative experiments seem to prove the superiority of this approach.

Except for some sporadic reports in several species, traditional freezing of oocytes of domestic animals was proved to be a dead end. Accordingly, the alternative of traditional slow-rate freezing, vitrification, was applied for the purpose.

Unfortunately, oocyte cryopreservation did not and still does not belong to the priorities in domestic animal embryology. This research area is almost entirely motivated by commercial factors, to increase quantity and quality of livestock. While sperm and embryo preservation is a strategic goal, only very few reasons and very special situations justify the cryostorage of oocytes. Although the benefits of conservation of maternal genome may be considerable in some elite animals, or endangered breed, in practice, this possibility is almost entirely disregarded. Accordingly, achievements in this field were the results of enthusiasm of a few devoted groups, and their efforts were never rewarded. In contrast, research in this direction was financially unsupported, rarely tolerated, and most of offspring derived from cryopreserved oocytes as the result of painstakingly long efforts ended up with early slaughter. Paradoxically, this very limited and unsupported research has eventually led to the establishment of the most successful technology of human oocyte cryopreservation.

General Features of Techniques Used for Oocyte Cryopreservation

All cryopreservation methods attempt to reduce damages during the procedure and—to a lesser extent—to support the regeneration of biological samples from the unavoidable injuries. Most damages develop during the cooling and warming process—some of them at seemingly harmless high temperatures above or around 0°C, while the storage itself below −150°C, most commonly at −196°C, is a relatively harmless part of the procedure. The commonly accepted two major cryopreservation techniques that have emerged over the past decades for oocytes and embryos use different approaches to achieve these goals. Traditional slow-rate freezing attempts to establish a balance between various sources of injuries (ice crystal formation, toxic injury, osmotic and fracture damage, etc. [8]; reviewed in detail recently [9, 10]) by minimizing all of them to a tolerable level. As indicated by the name, the cooling rate is relatively slow; accordingly, samples are held for a relatively long period of time under physiological temperature close to 0°C and accordingly may suffer chilling injury [7, 11–13].

The principle of vitrification is the total elimination of ice crystal formation. In practical work, there are several ways to achieve this goal: to increase the concentration of cryoprotectants, to increase both cooling and warming rates, and to minimize the volume of the solution containing the sample to reduce the chance of ice nucleation. The initial vitrification methods were based on the traditional tools of cryobiology (standard insemination straws or cryovials); accordingly, the achievable cooling and warming rates were limited, and the benefits compared to traditional slow-rate freezing were moderate. Later, special tools were applied or developed for the purpose including electron microscopic grids, narrow plastic or glass capillaries, loops, and thin plastic filmstrips (reviewed by Vajta et al. [14]), allowing the increase of cooling and warming rates with an order of magnitude. This approach offered two benefits: a considerable reduction in the required concentration of cryoprotectants and the dramatic decrease in chilling damage, as samples passed extremely quickly through the dangerous temperature zones (+15 to −5°C) and reached the safe higher or lower degrees at cooling and warming, respectively; accordingly, the time was restricted for the damage to develop in full extent. This benefit which was initially regarded as a by-product of new vitrification techniques has eventually become the major advantage of the application of vitrification for chilling sensitive samples including the MII phase mammalian oocytes [15, 16].

Unfortunately, the required high cooling and warming rates require a direct contact with the cooling and warming solution, that is, with liquid nitrogen or the rehydrating solution containing the osmotic buffer. This direct contact may result in liquid nitrogen-mediated cross-contamination and disease transmission. Although cryopreservation of samples in mammalian embryology was not proven to be responsible for any disease transmission, the theoretical danger exists, and the possibility has also been proven under experimental conditions [17]. There are several ways to eliminate the possibility of contamination: performing cooling and warming in sterile solutions while storing samples in safe containers or in the vapor of liquid nitrogen, using sterile metal surfaces for cooling, or applying sophisticated closed systems [18–22]. However, in some of these systems, either the overall efficiency seems to be compromised or the security or practicality of the system is compromised. Accordingly, the ultimate solution for establishment of a fully safe and highly efficient vitrification system still requires future research.

Results Achieved in Animal Models

As mentioned earlier, the first success in mammalian oocyte cryopreservation has been achieved in mouse by traditional freezing [1]. Even the birth of the first human baby preceded by 6 years the first achievements in domestic animals ([23, 24], respectively). However, vitrification has become soon the preferred approach for cryopreservation of mammalian oocytes. The first mouse pups achieved from vitrified oocytes were reported by Nakagata in 1989 [25]; and in 1992, in parallel with traditional freezing, vitrification has also resulted in the birth of a healthy calf [26]. During the subsequent years, vitrification has become the choice when cryopreservation of domestic animal oocytes was considered.

The introduction of special tools and high-rate cooling and warming techniques had significant impact on the efficiency [14, 27]. Refinement of these techniques has also permitted the birth of calves after vitrification of immature oocytes [28], even with a subsequent round of blastocyst vitrification [29]. Cattle cytoplasts (enucleated oocytes) were also successfully used after vitrification for embryonic or somatic cell nuclear transfer [30, 31].

The extreme chilling sensitivity—due to the high cytoplasmic lipid content—has hampered cryopreservation of porcine embryos and oocytes for long. Eventually, physical removal of these lipid droplets [32] has improved outcomes, but the required micromanipulation has made the procedure too complicated for routine application. A modification of this technique including partial zona digestion and high-speed centrifugation to separate lipids from the remaining components of the cytoplasm [33] opened the way for obtaining live piglets after somatic cell nuclear transfer by using either zona-included or zona-free oocytes [34, 35].

In other domestic species, only sporadic attempts were reported, including horse [36] and buffalo [37]. No reports are available about full-term development in sheep and goat after oocyte cryopreservation, although late-stage fetuses have been achieved (Ledda, personal communication).

Future Perspectives

Although a very limited number of offspring were born after oocyte cryopreservation in domestic animals, the achievements have paved the road for establishment of a highly successful method in humans. Accordingly, innovative approaches applied in domestic species may open new possibilities for future human application, too.

One possibility is the application of cytoskeleton relaxants. The initial approach with cytochalasin B was reported to be successful in pigs [38–40]; however, the benefits were questioned by others [20, 41]. Results achieved with Taxol seem to be more equivocal and promising [40, 42–45], but the human use of this potent anticancer agent to promote cryosurvival of healthy oocytes may not be justified [46].

The other, more recent possibility to improve cryosurvival of oocytes is the pretreatment with carefully selected and strictly controlled sublethal stress effect to increase the stress tolerance. The first and so far the most significant approach toward this direction was the application of high hydrostatic pressure (HHP). In porcine oocytes, the treatment does not result in light microscopic alterations, but induced higher resistance and developmental competence after various interventions including cryopreservation [47, 48]. As an analogue, osmotic pressure was also applied successfully before cryopreservation to increase survival and developmental rates [49, 50]. These achievements may only mean the start of a promising new approach, which may eventually help to increase the efficiency of cryopreservation of oocytes in many other mammalian species including humans.

References

1. Whittingham DG. Fertilization in vitro and development to term of unfertilized mouse oocytes previously stored at –196 degrees C. J Reprod Fertil. 1977;49:89–94.
2. Stachecki JJ, Cohen J. An overview of oocyte cryopreservation. Reprod Biomed Online. 2004;9:152–63.
3. Martino A, Pollard JA, Leibo SP. Effect of chilling bovine oocytes on their developmental competence. Mol Reprod Dev. 1996;45:503–12.
4. Pickering S, Braude P, Hohnson M, et al. Transient cooling to room temperature can cause irreversible disruption of the meiotic spindle in the human oocyte. Fertil Steril. 1990;54:102–8.
5. Santhananthan AH, Ng SC, Trounson A, et al. The effects of ultrarapid freezing on meiotic and mitotic spindles of oocytes and embryos. Gamete Res. 1998;21:385–401.
6. Rienzi L, Martinez F, Ubaldi F, et al. Polscope analysis of meiotic spindle changes in living metaphase II human oocytes during the freezing and thawing procedures. Hum Reprod. 2004;19:655–9.
7. Ghetler Y, Yavin S, Shalgi R, et al. The effect of chilling on membrane lipid phase transition in human oocytes and zygotes. Hum Reprod. 2005;20:3385–9.
8. Mazur P. Cryobiology: the freezing of biological systems. Science. 1970;168(934):939–49.
9. Coticchio G, Bonu MA, Sciajno R, Sereni E, Bianchi V, Borini A. Truths and myths of oocyte sensitivity to controlled rate freezing. Reprod Biomed Online. 2007;15:24–30.
10. Leibo SP. Cryopreservation of oocytes and embryos: optimization by theoretical versus empirical analysis. Theriogenology. 2008;69:2–47.
11. Aman RR, Parks JE. Effects of cooling and rewarming of the meiotic spindle and chromosomes of in vitro matured bovine oocytes. Biol Reprod. 1994;50:103–10.
12. Leibo SP, Martino A, Kobayashi S, Pollard JW. Stage-dependent sensitivity of oocytes and embryos to low temperatures. Anim Reprod Sci. 1996;42:45–53.
13. Isachenko V, Soler C, Isachenko E, Perez-Sanchez F, Grishchenko V. Vitrification of immature porcine oocytes: effects of lipid droplets, temperature, cytoskeleton, and addition and removal of cryoprotectant. Cryobiology. 1998;36:250–3.
14. Vajta G, Kuwayama M, Holm P, et al. Open pulled straw vitrification: a new way to reduce cryoinjuries of bovine ova and embryos. Mol Reprod Dev. 1998;51:53–8.
15. Shaw JM, Jones GM. Terminology associated with vitrification and other cryopreservation procedures for oocytes and embryos. Hum Reprod Update. 2003;9:583–605.
16. Vajta G, Nagy ZP. Are traditional freezers still needed in the embryo laboratory? Review on vitrification. Reprod Biomed Online. 2006;12:779–96.
17. Bielanski A, Nadin-Davis S, Sapp T, Lutze-Wallace C. Viral contamination of embryos cryopreserved in liquid nitrogen. Cryobiology. 2000;40:110–6.
18. Bielanski A, Hanniman A. Non-cross contamination of bovine embryos with microbes using the OPS vitrification system. Reprod Fertil Dev. 2007;29:232 [Abstr].
19. Bielanski A, Vajta G. Risk of contamination of germplasm during cryopreservation and cryobanking in IVF units. Hum Reprod. 2009;24:2457–67.
20. Gupta MK, Uhm SJ, Lee HT. Cryopreservation of immature and in vitro matured porcine oocytes by solid surface vitrification. Theriogenology. 2007;67:238–48.
21. Han X, Ma H, Jiao A, Critser JK. Investigations on the heat transport capability of a cryogenic oscillating heat pipe and its application in achieving ultra-fast cooling rates for cell vitrification cryopreservation. Cryobiology. 2008;56:195–203.
22. Lee HJ, Elmoazzen H, Wright D, Biggers J, Rueda BR, Heo YS, Toner M, Toth TL. Ultra-rapid vitrification of mouse oocytes in low cryoprotectant concentrations. Reprod Biomed Online. 2010;20: 201–8.
23. Chen C. Pregnancy after human oocyte cryopreservation. Lancet. 1986;1(8486):884–6.
24. Fuku E, Kojima T, Shioya Y, Marcus GJ, Downey BR. In vitro fertilization and development of frozen-thawed bovine oocytes. Cryobiology. 1992;29:485–92.

25. Nakagata N. High survival rate of unfertilized mouse oocytes after vitrification. J Reprod Fertil. 1989;87:479–83.
26. Hamano S, Koikeda A, Kuwayama M, Nagai T. Full-term development of in vitro-matured, vitrified and fertilized bovine oocytes. Theriogenology. 1992;38(1):085–90.
27. Martino A, Songsasen N, Leibo SP. Development into blastocysts of bovine oocytes cryopreserved by ultra-rapid cooling. Biol Reprod. 1996;54:1059–69.
28. Vieria AD, Mezzalira A, Barieri DP, et al. Calves born after open pulled straw vitrification of immature bovine oocytes. Cryobiology. 2002;45:91–4.
29. Vieria AD, Forell F, Feltrin C, Rodrigues JL. Calves born after direct transfer of vitrified bovine in vitro-produced blastocysts derived from vitrified immature oocytes. Reprod Domest Anim. 2008;43:314–8.
30. Booth PJ, Vajta G, Høj A, Holm P, Jacobsen H, Greve T, Callesen H. Full-term development of nuclear transfer calves produced from open pulled straw (OPS) vitrified cytoplasts. Theriogenology. 1999;51:99–1006.
31. Hou YP, Dai YP, Zhu SE, Zhu HB, Wu TY, Gong GC, Wang HP, Wang LL, Liu Y, Li R, Wan R, Li N. Bovine oocytes vitrified by the open pulled straw method and used for somatic cell cloning supported development to term. Theriogenology. 2005;64: 1389–91.
32. Nagashima H, Kashiwazaki N, Ashman RJ, Grupen CG, Seamark RF, Nottle MB. Removal of cytoplasmic lipid enhances the tolerance of porcine embryos to chilling. Biol Reprod. 1994;51: 618–22.
33. Esaki R, Ueda H, Kurome M, et al. Cryopreservation of porcine embryos derived from in vitro-matured oocytes. Biol Reprod. 2004;71:432–7.
34. Li R, Lai L, Wax D, et al. Cloned transgenic swine via in vitro production and cryopreservation. Biol Reprod. 2006;75:226–30.
35. Du Y, Li J, Kragh PM, Zhan Y, Schmidt M, Boegh IB, Zhang X, Purup S, Kuwayama M, Jorgensen AL, Pedersen AM, Villemoes K, Yang H, Bolund L, Vajta G. Piglets born from vitrified cloned blastocysts produced with a simplified method of delipation and nuclear transfer. Cloning Stem Cells. 2007;9:470–6.
36. Maclellan LJ, Carnevale EM, Coutinho da Silva MA, et al. Pregnancies from vitrified equine oocytes collected from super-stimulated and non-stimulated mares. Theriogenology. 2002;58: 911–9.
37. Neglia G, Gasparrini B, Caracciolo di Brienza V, Di Palo R, Zicarelli L. First pregnancies to term after transfer of buffalo vitrified embryos entirely produced in vitro. Vete Res Commun. 2004;28:233–6.
38. Dobrinsky JR, Pursel VG, Long CR, Johnson LA. Birth of piglets after transfer of embryos cryopreserved by cytoskeletal stabilization and vitrification. Biol Reprod. 2000;62: 546–70.
39. Somfai T, Dinnyés A, Sage D, Marosán M, Carnwath JW, Ozawa M, Kikuchi K, Niemann H. Development to the blastocyst stage of parthenogenetically activated in vitro matured porcine oocytes after solid surface vitrification. Theriogenology. 2006;66:415–22.
40. Zhang J, Nedambale TL, Yang M, Li J. Improved development of ovine matured oocytes following solid surface vitrification (SSV). Effect of cumulus cells and cytoskeleton stabilizer. Anim Reprod Sci. 2008;110:46–55.
41. Fujihira T, Kobayashi M, Hochi S, Hirabayashi M, Ishikawa H, Ohsumi S, Fukui Y. Developmental capacity of Antarctic minke whale (*Balaenoptera bonaerensis*) vitrified oocytes following in vitro maturation, and parthenogenetic activation or intracytoplasmic sperm injection. Zygote. 2006;14:89–95.
42. Park SE, Chung HM, Cha KY, Hwang WS, Lee ES, Lim JM. Cryopreservation of ICR mouse oocytes: improved post-thawed preimplantation development after vitrification using taxol, a cytoskeleton stabilizer. Fertil Steril. 2001;75:1177–84.
43. Shi WQ, Zhu SE, Zhang D, Wang WH, Tang GL, Hou YP, Tian SJ. Improved development by taxol pre-treatment after vitrification of in vitro matured porcine oocytes. Reproduction. 2006;131:795–804.

44. Morató R, Izquierdo D, Albarracín JL, Anguita B, Palomo MJ, Jiménez-Macedo AR, Paramio MT, Mogas T. Effects of pre-treating in vitro matured bovine oocytes with the cytoskeleton stabilizing agent taxol prior to vitrification. Mol Reprod Dev. 2008;75: 191–201.
45. Morató R, Mogas T, Maddox-Hyttel P. Ultrastructure of bovine oocytes exposed to Taxol prior to OPS vitrification. Mol Reprod Dev. 2008;75:1318–26.
46. Jordan MA, Kamath K. How do microtubule-targeted drugs work? An overview. Curr Cancer Drug Targets. 2007;7:730–42.
47. Pribenszky C, Du Y, Molnár M, Harnos A, Vajta G. Increased stress tolerance of matured pig oocytes after high hydrostatic pressure treatment. Anim Reprod Sci. 2008;106:200–7.
48. Du Y, Pribenszky C, Molnár M, Zhang X, Yang H, Kuwayama M, Pedersen AM, Villemoes K, Bolund L, Vajta G. High hydrostatic pressure (HHP): a new way to improve in vitro developmental competence of porcine matured oocytes after vitrification. Reproduction. 2008;135:13–7.
49. Lin L, Du Y, Liu Y, Kragh PM, Li J, Purup S, Kuwayama M, Zhang X, Yang H, Bolund L, Vajta G. Elevated NaCl concentration improves cryotolerance and developmental competence of porcine oocytes. Reprod Biomed Online. 2009;18:360–6.
50. Lin L, Kragh PM, Purup S, Kuwayama M, Du Y, Zhang X, Yang H, Bolund L, Callesen H, Vajta G. Osmotic stress induced by sodium chloride, sucrose or trehalose improves cryotolerance and developmental competence of porcine oocytes. Reprod Fertil Dev. 2008;21:338–44.

Chapter 29
Oocyte Vitrification

Ana Cobo

The essential role of cryopreservation in ART has become obvious since the commencement of the infertility treatment, becoming a more flexible and efficient practice. Semen and embryo cryopreservation has been a successful strategy, routinely applied in IVF procedure for a long time. However, in spite of numerous studies conducted over the last 20 years, the reliability of oocyte cryopreservation is just being confirmed currently. All of the efforts that have been made are clearly justified, mostly because an efficient oocyte cryopreservation program would be quite welcome and widely applied in ART, since there are many other indications for oocytes cryopreservation different of the abovementioned egg banking for ovum donation. Potential beneficiaries of this technology would be cancer patients who need an option for fertility preservation before undergoing the potential sterilizing treatment [1], or women who wish to delay their motherhood due to a variety of reasons [2], government restrictions on IVF [3, 4], ethical reasons against embryo cryopreservation, and practical reasons such us unavailability of the male gamete the day of pick up, due to a variety of reasons [5, 6].

Despite all of this wide diversity of potential applications, egg banking has not been a routine procedure until very recently; in fact, there are still very few centers worldwide that routinely apply oocyte cryopreservation in their clinical routine. This fact can be explained because the methodology to cryopreserve human oocytes has been disappointing, with results that have not always been reproducible. Lately, vitrification has proven to be a very efficient method for successful oocyte cryostorage. Some fundamental principles of cryobiology would be helpful to understand why it has been extremely difficult to reach the goal of safely cryopreserved human oocytes.

A. Cobo, PhD (✉)
IVI Valencia (Sede Central), Plaza de la Policía local, 3, 46015 Valencia, Spain
e-mail: acobo@ivi.es

Z.P. Nagy et al. (eds.), *Clinical Embryology: A Practical Guide*,
DOI 10.1007/978-1-4614-8376-2_29,

Cryobiology Background

There are some reasons that could explain the low rate of successes that has been traditionally observed. Some of them include the size, shape, and cell number regarding oocytes. These gametes are the largest cells of the human body, and this could explain, at least in part, the great differences in cryotolerance between them and, for example, the spermatozoa. In addition, the spherical shape of the oocyte could disturb the uniform distribution of cryoprotectants (CPAs). Finally, considering the oocytes as a unique cell, they have only one chance of success, and there are few possibilities to restore from a serious damage; this situation is completely different from the one observed in tissues composed by millions of cells, in which the damage could be compensated in different proportions.

Other major factors responsible for the high oocyte sensitivity to cryopreservation include chilling injury and intracellular ice crystal formation. These factors are related to the cryopreservation method. There are two main strategies in cryobiology: slow cooling and vitrification. During the former, the cells are gradually dehydrated in the presence of CPAs, and the temperature is lowered at a very slow cooling rate (−0.3°C) [7]. In this way, the cells are exposed to low temperatures during an extended period of time, which can lead to what is known as chilling injury [8]. At the final stage, water solidifies into ice crystals. Chilling injury can be defined as the irreversible damage following exposure of cells to low temperatures, from +15 to −5°C before the nucleation of ice [9]. This detrimental event affects mainly the cytoskeleton [10] and cell membranes [11]. The ice crystal formation within the cytoplasm must be avoided at all cost in order to guarantee the survival and integrity of the cells when they are later thawed. Chilling injury can be minimized during vitrification by use of high cooling rates. Moreover, as the sample vitrifies, ice crystal formation is avoided [12].

Vitrification, in particular by means of methodologies that use a minimum volume, is altering this situation by producing results that have not been achieved with other approaches [5]. The physical phenomenon of vitrification takes place when the solidification of the solution occurs not by ice crystallization but by extreme elevation in viscosity, which is achieved by using high cooling rates from −15,000 to −30,000°C per minute, therefore avoiding the risk of chilling injury [12]. This ice-free cryopreservation method has undergone modifications in order to optimize results. One such modification has been to reduce the volume of the vitrification solution containing oocytes, which allows the CPA concentration and, consequently, the cytotoxicity to be decreased [13, 14]. As abovementioned, this procedure circumvents the two major limiting factors for achieving optimal cryopreservation: chilling injury [13] and ice formation [15]. Chilling injury can be minimized during vitrification by use of high cooling rates [12]. The velocity of the process is dependent on the volume of the vitrification solution. Thus, the smaller the volume of the sample, the higher the cooling rate. On the other hand, direct contact with liquid nitrogen also contributes to increase the cooling rate. To avoid ice formation, the vitrification technique makes use of high CPA concentrations [12] despite the fact that such high concentrations are considered toxic to cells [16]. Nonetheless, an appropriate, phased composition of CPA could mitigate the toxic and osmotic consequences of highly concentrated CPAs [5]. In this way, a combination of two or three of these agents can decrease the individual specific toxicity. The most common mixture employed for this purpose consists of EG, DMSO, and sucrose [5]. To optimize the results, in addition to an appropriate selection of CPAs, it is also helpful to use these agents at lower concentration while maintaining the necessary concentration to achieve vitrification. By dramatically increasing the cooling rate, the CPA concentration could be reduced. As a result, a high cooling rate avoids chilling injury and allows the reduction of the concentration of CPA, thereby preserving the cells at nontoxic concentrations of CPA. Several approaches fit these conditions. The "minimum drop vitrification" method was proposed by Arav, using a very small volume of vitrification solution placing the samples on a specific device which must be cooled very quickly [17]. High cooling rates are achieved when samples are loaded in minimum volume that are directly immersed in LN. These methods are also known as open systems. Such high rates are impossible to achieve with hermetically closed vials, which are used in closed systems. Nevertheless, it is worth mentioning that the direct contact of samples with LN has raised some concerns due to the theoretical risk of cross-contamination mainly because the LN itself has been considered as a potential source of pathogen agents. Even though, no any case of cross-contamination has ever been reported in ART in many years of practice, highlighting that such eventuality could be extremely unlikely.

On the other hand, the limit imposed by the cooling rate could be restricted to oocytes since satisfactory results have been obtained after the vitrification of embryos at different developmental stages using closed systems. In any case, there are no formal comparative studies which make possible to draw definitive conclusions. A wide variety of open approaches have been reported in the literature [18–23] as well as closed ones [24, 25].

Clinical Outcomes

A review on human oocyte cryostorage based on all reports on vitrification MII oocytes and providing data regarding implantation and pregnancy outcome depicts the situation of the clinical application of human oocyte cryopreservation [26]. It is worth mentioning that nearly all of these studies assessed employed open systems for vitrification, highlighting the advantage of these systems with regard to oocyte cryopreservation and its most wide application for clinical practice in humans. Within this session, we will focus on our clinical experience using the Cryotop method for vitrification [27]. This device consists of a fine transparent polypropylene film attached to a plastic handle and equipped with a cover straw, into which can be loaded very small volumes of oocytes (up to ~0.1 μL), 10 times lower than the capacity of other minimum volume devices [27].

Our first approach with the vitrification of donor oocytes using the Cryotop method was carried out through the simultaneous comparison of the outcome of both vitrified and fresh oocytes from the same ovarian stimulated cycle; we confirmed the potential of vitrification of oocytes using this methodology [28]. We obtained a 96.7% survival rate and detected no significant difference in fertilization rates (76.3 and 82.2%), day 2 (94.2 and 97.8%) or day 3 embryo cleavage rates (77.6 and 84.6%), or blastocyst formation rates (48.7 and 47.5%) for vitrified and fresh oocytes, respectively. In that study, either vitrified or fresh oocytes belonging to the same cohort were simultaneously inseminated using the same semen sample. In this way, we were able to analyze the potential of vitrified and fresh oocytes under exactly the same conditions. The ratios of good quality embryos on day 3 and at blastocyst stage were similar in both groups. Pregnancy, implantation, miscarriage, and ongoing pregnancy rates (OPRs) per transfer were 65.2, 40.8, 20, and 47.8%, respectively. The potential use of this approach for fertility preservation in cancer patients as well as in other clinical situation in ART has also been highlighted [1, 29].

Although these evidences have been encouraging, the need of a controlled clinical trial to test the efficiency of oocyte vitrification was mandatory. A randomized, prospective, triple-blind, single-center, parallel group controlled clinical trial, including 600 recipients from our ovum donation program, aimed to compare the outcome of vitrified-banked oocytes to the gold standard procedure employing fresh oocytes that has been published by our group [30]. The study was designed to establish the superiority of the OPR of fresh oocytes over that of vitrified oocytes. The primary end point, the OPR per intention-to-treat (ITT) population, was 43.7% for vitrified oocytes, over 41.7% for fresh ones. As shown by the OR, we failed to prove the superiority of fresh oocytes over the vitrified oocytes, and moreover, we were able to assume the noninferiority of the vitrification group. Additionally, the proportion of top-quality embryos obtained either by inseminated oocyte (30.8% vs. 30.8% for day 2 and 36.1% vs. 37.7% for day 3, for vitrified and fresh oocytes, respectively) or by cleaved embryos (43.6% vs. 43.8% for day 2 and 58.4% vs. 60.7% for day 3, respectively) was similar between groups.

The outcome achieved in this controlled randomized clinical trial confirmed demonstrates that cryobanking by applying the vitrification technology can provide successful clinical outcome in oocyte donation programs helping to the validation of this strategy. With no doubt, it is of great importance to ovum donation procedures, as it allows traditional drawbacks associated with the use of fresh oocytes to be overcome. Supported by all this evidence, we have established an oocyte bank that currently operates to meet the basic needs of our donation program contributing greatly to improve the logistics of the program and, what is also relevant, allowing us to keep the quarantine period. To date, we have performed 1,856 ovum donation cycles involving 23,000 cryostored oocytes with an overall survival rate over 90%. A mean number of 1.6 ± 0.7 embryos have been replaced, and an OPR of 47.7% has been achieved. A 63.6% of the patients were able to vitrify surplus embryos; therefore, the cumulative OPR after cryotransfers has been over 60%. Additionally to ovum donation, we have applied oocyte cryopreservation in cases of infertile patients with own oocytes due to the risk of suffering ovarian hyperstimulation syndrome (OHSS), no available semen sample the day of ovum pick-up or many other situations in which the embryo transfer was not advisable. In nearly 450 cycles (mean age 47.4 ± 4.5), the overall survival rate was 84% with a clinical pregnancy rate of 41.5% and 32.8% of implantation rate. Oocyte vitrification has been applied for fertility preservation in cancer patients (N = 70; mean age 32.7 ± 5.7) and for social reasons (N = 158; 35.2 ± 5.8), however no warming procedures have been performed to date.

Other authors have confirmed the excellent profile of oocyte vitrification either with autologous or donated oocytes. Rienzi et al. showed in a prospective, randomized sibling study conducted with autologous oocytes that oocyte vitrification procedure is not inferior to fresh insemination procedure achieving comparable ongoing clinical pregnancy rates [31]. A very recent study has prospectively compared an open vs. closed system between fresh and sibling vitrified oocytes [32]. These authors have observed an impairment of embryo quality after employing the closed system. In contrast, the parameters analyzed were similar between fresh and sibling oocytes vitrified using the open system. Other authors have also endorsed the suitability of oocyte vitrification by the Cryotop method in an oocyte donation program [33]. These authors recommend this approach to be applied in infertile patients with different indications within a routine IVF program. All these evidences strongly support the efficiency of oocyte vitrification.

Practical Aspects of Oocyte Vitrification

Laboratory Procedure

- Aspirate the oocytes from the culture dish and keep them at the tip of the capillary or Pasteur pipette and transfer them within minimum drop volume to 20 μL of buffer solution (BS) supplemented with 20% serum substitute into a reproplate well (Kitazato, Biomedical Supply, Tokyo, Japan) (Fig. 29.1).
- Add 20 μL of equilibration solution (ES) containing 7.5% ethylene glycol (EG) and 7.5% dimethyl sulfoxide (DMSO) surrounding the previous drop containing the oocytes (Kitazato, Biomedical Supply, Tokyo, Japan). Wait for 3 min at room temperature (Fig. 29.1).
- Add another drop of 20 μL of ES in the same way as in the previous step and wait for 3 min more.
- Add 240 μL of ES slowly circling the previous drops and wait between 6 and 9 min. At the end of this step, the oocytes should be re-expanded and should recover their original appearance (Fig. 29.1).
- After equilibrium, aspirate the oocytes at the tip of the pipette. Afterward, place them on the surface of the vitrification solution (VS) containing 15% EG plus 15% DMSO in BS solution (Fig. 29.1). Try to carry a minimum volume of ES solution. Note that the oocytes will float due to the high density of the VS media.

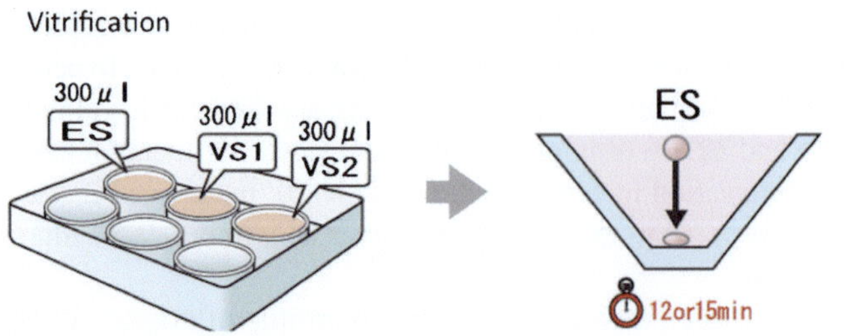

Fig. 29.1 Equilibration procedure

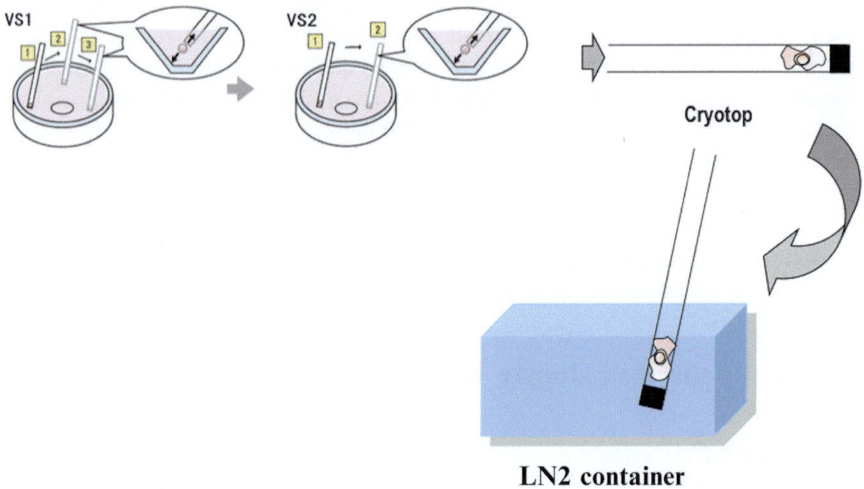

Fig. 29.2 Vitrification procedure

- Dispense 300 μL of VS solution into two well of the reproplate (Kitazato, Medical Supply, Tokyo Japan). Remove the ES medium just placed together with the oocytes (it will be noted clearly due to the difference in density) and wash the pipette outside the VS well. Keep removing continuously and keep on discarding the medium outside the plate. Repeat this operation as many times as possible within 30 s (Fig. 29.2).
- Aspirate the oocytes and bring them to the bottom of the plate (the floating will stop as soon as they start to equilibrate with the medium).
- Repeat the same procedure in the next VS well. Place the oocytes in the bottom of the plate and move them many times around the well, repeating the washing process during 30 more seconds.
- Aspirate the oocytes and maintain them at the tip of the pipette within minimum volume of VS.
- Place the Cryotop under the microscope.
- Proceed to load the oocytes onto the Cryotop within minimum volume.

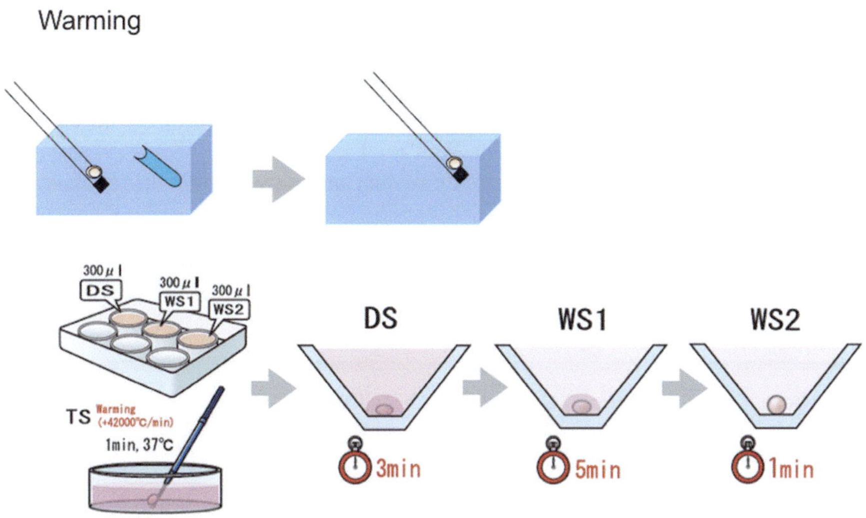

Fig. 29.3 Warming and dilution procedure

- Aspirate excess medium to make sure they are contained within minimum volume.
- Immerse the Cryotop directly into the liquid nitrogen container (Fig. 29.2).
- Place the plastic protector Cryotop.
- Transfer the oocytes to the storage tank.

Warming Procedure

- Remove the Cryotops from the storage tank and handle them submerged into liquid nitrogen. Avoid temperature changes.
- Remove the protective straw maintaining the Cryotops immersed in liquid nitrogen.
- Remove Cryotop from the liquid nitrogen container and submerge it instantly (straight and quick movement) into 1.5 mL of a solution containing 1.0 M sucrose (TS) (Kitazato, Medical Supply, Tokyo, Japan) (Fig. 29.3).
- Visualize the oocytes and immediately start the countdown to 60 s.
- Do not manipulate the oocytes within the first 40 s.
- Retrieve the oocytes from the Cryotop with very gentle manipulations within a minute in TS solution.
- Transfer the oocytes to the DS well in the reproplate (Fig. 29.3). Aspirate the oocytes very gently and continue to aspirate TS until the column reaches approximately 2 mm in length (Fig. 29.3).
- Take the pipette to the DS well and immersed it to the bottom. Dispense the 2-mm column at first. The column of TS within DS will be clear due to the difference in density of both (Fig. 29.3). Leave the oocytes on the "top" of this column. Wait for 3 min.

- Transfer the oocytes to well WS (BS supplemented with 20% SSS) exactly as in the previous step. Wait for 5 min.
- Transfer the oocytes to the next well of WS well. Leave the oocytes on the surface of this media; they will drop down immediately due to the absence of differential density between media. Wait for 1 min.
- Transfer the oocytes to the regular culture dish and place them in the incubator at 37°C Wait for 2 h before ICSI.

References

1. Cobo A, Domingo J, Pérez S, Crespo J, Remohi J, Pellicer A. Vitrification, an effective new approach to oocyte banking in healthy women, could be applied in cancer patients to preserve their fertility. Clin Transl Oncol. 2008;10:268–73.
2. Homburg R, van der Veen F, Silber SJ. Oocyte vitrification—women's emancipation set in stone. Fertil Steril. 2008;91(4 Suppl):1319–20.
3. Boggio A. Italy enacts new law on medically assisted reproduction. Hum Reprod. 2005; 20:1153–7.
4. Borini A, Lagalla C, Bonu MA, Bianchi V, Flamigni C, Coticchio G. Cumulative pregnancy rates resulting from the use of fresh and frozen oocytes: 7 years' experience. Reprod Biomed Online. 2006;12:481–6.
5. Vajta G, Nagy ZP. Are programmable freezers still needed in the embryo laboratory? Review on vitrification Reprod Biomed Online. 2006;12:779–96.
6. Cobo A, Bellver J, Domingo J, Pérez S, Crespo J, Pellicer A, Remohi J. New options in ART: the Cryotop method of oocyte vitrification. Case reports. Introduction. Reprod Biomed Online. 2008;17(1):68–72.
7. Woods EJ, Benson JD, Agca Y, Critser JK. Fundamental cryobiology of reproductive cells and tissues. Cryobiology. 2004;48:146–56.
8. Mazur P. Principles of cryobiology. In: Fuller B, Lane M, Benson E, editors. Life in the Frozen State. New York: CRC Press; 2004. p. 4–55.
9. Watson PF, Morris GJ. Cold shock injury in animal cells. Symp Soc Exp Biol. 1987;41: 311–40.
10. Pickering SJ, Braude PR, Johnson MH, Cant A, Currie J. Transient cooling to room temperature can cause irreversible disruption of the meiotic spindle in the human oocyte. Fertil Steril. 1990;54:102–8.
11. Ghetler Y, Yavin S, Shalgi R, Arav A. The effect of chilling on membrane lipid phase transition in human oocytes and zygotes. Hum Reprod. 2005;20:3385–9.
12. Liebermann J, Dietl J, Vanderzwalmen P, Tucker MJ. Recent developments in human oocyte, embryo and blastocyst vitrification: where are we now? Reprod Biomed Online. 2003;7: 623–33.
13. Vajta G, Kuwayama M. Improving cryopreservation systems Theriogenology. 2006;65:236–44.
14. Kuwayama M, Cobo A, Vajta G. Vitrification of oocytes: general considerations and the use of Cryotop method. In: Liebermann J, Tucker M, editors. Vitrification in assisted reproduction. A user's manual and trouble shooting guide. London: Informa Health Care; 2007.
15. Mazur P. Freezing of living cells: mechanisms and implications. Am J Physiol. 1984; 247:C125–42.
16. Fuller B, Paynter S. Fundamentals of cryobiology in reproductive medicine. Reprod Biomed Online. 2004;9:680–91.
17. Arav A. Vitrification of oocyte and embryos. In: Lauria AGF, Gandolfi F, editors. New trends in embryo transfer. Cambridge: Portland; 1992. p. 255–64.

18. Martino A, Songsasen N, Leibo SP. Development into blastocysts of bovine oocytes cryopreserved by ultra-rapid cooling. Biol Reprod. 1996;54:1059–69.
19. Vajta G, Holm P, Kuwayama M, Booth PJ, Jacobsen H, Greve T, Callesen H. Open Pulled Straw (OPS) vitrification: a new way to reduce cryoinjuries of bovine ova and embryos. Mol Reprod Dev. 1998;51:53–8.
20. Papis K, Shimizu M, Izaike Y. Factors affecting the survivability of bovine oocytes vitrified in droplets. Theriogenology. 2000;54:651–8.
21. Lane M, Gardner DK. Vitrification of mouse oocytes using a nylon loop. Mol Reprod Dev. 2001;58:342–7.
22. Matsumoto H, Jiang JY, Tanaka T, Sasada H, Sato E. Vitrification of large quantities of immature bovine oocytes using nylon mesh. Cryobiology. 2001;42:139–44.
23. Liebermann J, Nawroth F, Isachenko V, Isachenko E, Rahimi G, Tucker MJ. Potential importance of vitrification in reproductive medicine. Biol Reprod. 2002;67:1671–80.
24. Kuwayama M, Ieda S, Zhang J, Kato O. The CryoTip method: Aseptic vitrification of oocytes and embryos. Fertil Steril. 2005;84 Suppl 1:S187.
25. Vanderzwalmen P, Zech N, Prapas Y, Panagiotidis Y, Papatheodorou A, Lejeune B, Jareno D, Vanderzwalmen S, Ectors F. Closed carrier device: a reality to vitrify oocytes and embryos in aseptic conditions. Gynecol Obstet Fertil. 2010;38:541–6.
26. Cobo A, Vajta G, Remohi J. Vitrification of human mature oocytes in clinical practice. Reprod Biomed Online. 2009;19 Suppl 4:4385.
27. Kuwayama M, Vajta G, Kato O, Leibo SP. Highly efficient vitrification method for cryopreservation of human oocytes. Reprod Biomed Online. 2005;11:300–8.
28. Cobo A, Kuwayama M, Perez S, Ruiz A, Pellicer A, Remohi J. Comparison of concomitant outcome achieved with fresh and cryopreserved donor oocytes vitrified by the Cryotop method. Fertil Steril. 2008;89:1657–64.
29. Cobo A, Bellver J, Domingo J, Perez S, Crespo J, Pellicer A, Remohi J. New options in assisted reproduction technology: the Cryotop method of oocyte vitrification. Reprod Biomed Online. 2008;17:68–72.
30. Cobo A, Meseguer M, Remohi J, Pellicer A. Use of cryo-banked oocytes in an ovum donation programme: a prospective, randomized, controlled, clinical trial. Hum Reprod. 2010;25: 2239–46.
31. Rienzi L, Romano S, Albricci L, Maggiulli R, Capalbo A, Baroni E, Colamaria S, Sapienza F, Ubaldi F. Embryo development of fresh 'versus' vitrified metaphase II oocytes after ICSI: a prospective randomized sibling-oocyte study. Hum Reprod. 2010;25(1):66–73.
32. Paffoni A, Guarneri C, Ferrari S, Restelli L, Nicolosi AE, Scarduelli C, Ragni G. Effects of two vitrification protocols on the developmental potential of human mature oocytes. Reprod Biomed Online. 2011;22(3):292–8.
33. Nagy ZP, Chang CC, Shapiro DB, Bernal DP, Elsner CW, Mitchell-Leef D, Toledo AA, Kort HI. Clinical evaluation of the efficiency of an oocyte donation program using egg cryo-banking. Fertil Steril. 2008;92(2):520–6.

Chapter 30
Slow Freezing of Embryos

Liesl Nel-Themaat, Ching-Chien Chang, Thomas Elliott, Patricia Bernal, Graham Wright, and Zsolt Peter Nagy

Historical Overview of Embryo Cryopreservation

Cryobiology (the study of life at low temperature), as we know it today, has come a very long way to where we now have the ability to freeze and thaw living cells while maintaining viability, without any apparent detrimental effects. Currently, cryopreservation plays such a significant role in most biological fields that it is hard to imagine scientific progress without it. Examples range from the use of cryopreserved bacteria for genetic engineering, preservation of frozen tissues for transplantation, and the large number of cell culture studies for disease research to assisted reproduction in humans and animals. To embark on this voyage back in time, one must consider the founding principles that lead to the successes that were ultimately reported during the first half of the twentieth century. Here follows a condensed representation of the history of modern cryopreservation, but a more detailed review can be found in ref. [1].

The start of this exciting journey goes back more than 300 years, to the early experiments by Robert Boyle, who was studying the effects of temperature on the volume of gasses. The foundation laid through his work led to the first Nobel Prize in chemistry, awarded to Jacobus van't Hoff, for groundbreaking work on laws of chemical dynamics and osmotic pressures in solutions. The Boyle-van't Hoff plot still plays a fundamental role in cryobiology, as a means to describe the effect of osmotic pressure on cell volume. The significance of osmotic principles during freezing will be discussed in subsequent sections.

L. Nel-Themaat, PhD • C.-C. Chang, PhD • T. Elliott, BSc • P. Bernal, DVM • G. Wright, BSc
Reproductive Biology Associates, 1100 Johnson Ferry Rd. (Suite 200), Sandy Springs, Atlanta, GA 30342, USA

Z.P. Nagy, MD, PhD, HCLD (ABB), EMB (ACE) (✉)
Scientific and Laboratory Director, Reproductive Biology Associates, Atlanta, GA 30342, USA
e-mail: zsolt.peter.nagy@gmail.com

Z.P. Nagy et al. (eds.), *Clinical Embryology: A Practical Guide*,
DOI 10.1007/978-1-4614-8376-2_30,

During the same era, liquefaction of oxygen, hydrogen, and nitrogen was developed by French physicist, Louis-Paul Cailletet, which later allowed the ultra-cooling of specimens. The importance of this discovery for modern day cryobiology goes without saying.

As interest in life at low temperatures grew, so did the number of publications on the effect of cold on various biological systems. Most noteworthy of these is the work of a Swiss-born Priest named Basile J. Luyet, whose studies are best described by the title of his classic monograph "Life and Death at Low Temperatures." He proceeded to be the founder of the Journal *Biodynamica* and first president of the Society for Cryobiology. Father Luyet is thus generally known as the father of Cryobiology.

The next decades saw major developments in low temperature biology, especially with spermatozoa preservation. In fact, the first observations on cooled spermatozoa occurred in 1866 by Italian military physician, P. Mantegazza, who noted that human spermatozoa became immotile when cooled in snow. He further envisioned the possibility for a deceased soldier to father a child by cooling sperm to maintain viability.

Mutual investigations by John Hammond and Arthur Walton on ejaculated and non-ejaculated sperm, respectively, showed that temperature affects ejaculated and non-ejaculated sperm differently, and that cooling of the latter could preserve it fertilizing capacity. We now know that capacitation is induced by exposure to seminal plasma, which changes membrane properties and renders spermatozoa more susceptible to temperature damage. Interestingly, Hammond predicted that "in these days of rapid aeroplane transport, it might be possible to move entire herds of animals around the world from chilled samples of semen" less than 30 years after the Wright brothers' first flight. So progressive was his thinking, that his vision today is reality with human and animal gametes and embryos that are transported large distances, often across continents and recently even into space!

With the artificial insemination field taking off around 1930, the possible impact that the ability to freeze semen long term became widely recognized, motivating several groups to attempt long term storage of semen by freezing in liquid gas. Success rates varied. It is notable that in 1938, Luyet and Hodapp described an experiment where spermatozoa survived vitrification in liquid air when exposed to a 2 M sucrose solution. Although about 40% initially lost their motility during incubation in the hypertonic solution, all the cells that survived the incubation and were vitrified and warmed survived.

Despite advances, post-thaw survival rates remained typically low, until the accidental breakthrough discovery of the cryoprotective properties of glycerol by Christopher Polge and Audrey Smith under guidance of Alan Parkes in 1947 while working on fowl spermatozoa [2]. (It should be noted that in the previous year, Jean Rostand found that addition of glycerol protected frog spermatozoa from freeze damage. Fertilizing capacity of thawed samples, however, was never confirmed. Furthermore, there are unverified reports of using glycerol as a cryoprotectant for the freezing of mammal and bird semen in Russia.) Polge's discovery was followed by successful freeze-thaw of spermatozoa in various mammalian species [3, 4].

Six years later, Bunge and Sherman reported three human pregnancies resulting from artificial insemination with frozen sperm [5].

The second half of the twentieth century saw great improvements and refinement of the technique, while a wealth of information on freezing principles was produced. This included the necessity of water removal and the addition of cryoprotectants and macromolecules to prevent intercellular ice crystal formation and membrane damage. We will elaborate on these topics in subsequent sections.

The next challenge investigators were facing was that of freezing the female gamete and embryos. At the end of the 1940s, M.C. Chang, who was working under Hammond at the time, started experimenting with cooling embryos and found that while slow-cooled embryos survived, rapidly cooled ones did not [6–8]. He proceeded to produce normal rabbit offspring from zygotes, cleavage- and blastocyst-stage embryos, all stored for at least 24 h at either 10 or 0°C [8, 9]. Chang and Smith both followed these findings by experimenting with rabbit oocytes [10, 11]. Shortly after, Sherman and Lin reported birth of mouse pups from frozen-thawed oocytes that were transferred back into recipient females before being mated. These and other early studies revealed that oocytes are much more sensitive to low temperatures than embryos. During years of subsequent research, the reasons for this difference in sensitivity between oocytes and embryos were investigated, but are beyond the scope of this chapter. For more information on the topic, see ref. [12].

During the late 1950s and early 1960s, Peter Mazur turned his attention toward elucidating mechanisms involved in cell damage during freezing and thawing. Although these fundamental principles will be discussed in the following section, it is noteworthy that his discoveries played a seminal role in the work by Whittingham et al. [13] that led to the first truly successful and repeatable freezing and warming of mouse embryos, as indicated by their high birth rate after transfer. This was followed by more successes in other mammalian species [14, 15], and finally human embryos in the early 1980s [16]. Almost 30 years later, embryo cryopreservation has become an integral part of clinical embryology. The large collection of data available demonstrates that there is no single optimum technique for slow freezing. Instead, numerous different combinations of cryoprotectants, cooling and warming rates can lead to success. One thing that all these techniques do share is that they stem from the principles laid out through the diligent work of the cryobiology pioneers.

Mechanisms of Freeze Damage

Cells are composed 60–85% of water and a mixture of solutes and suspended particles, such as proteins, nucleic acids and lipids. Various studies have shown that about 10% of the water in cells are bound to cellular components, rendering it incapable of freezing (for review, see ref. [17]). As freezing occurs, the *free* water is removed from cells either by crystallization inside the cell, or by moving out of the cell via osmosis through the semi-permeable membrane (due to hypo-osmotic conditions that occurs with extracellular ice crystal formation) to crystallize extracellularly. Intracellular ice formation is the most likely cause of cryodamage, since it can rupture the cell membrane and displace or disrupt organelles. Therefore, it is desirable to dehydrate cells of their *free* water prior to freezing. This outward osmosis can be facilitated by using hypertonic freezing solutions and slow cooling rates, which gives the water time to exit the cell as extracellular ice formation progresses. A direct consequence of dehydration is cell shrinkage, as the cell loses a significant part of its volume. In fact, cells will maintain equal chemical potential of the water inside and outside of the cell, and therefore, the cell volume is (in most cases) inversely proportional to the external osmolality [17].

Another occurrence during osmotic shrinkage is hydrostatic pressure that draws some extracellular solution containing permeating molecules into the cell to replace the water volume that is removed. Thereby, some of the physical stress on the membrane is relieved. Thus, if a cell is inserted into a hypertonic solution, one will witness shrinkage followed by re-expansion to its original volume, as long as the solutes responsible for the high extracellular osmolarity are membrane permeable.

Membrane damage during freezing also occurs when intracellular ice crystals form before complete shrinkage of the cell. As ice forms, solutes in the remainder of the intracellular water cause its freezing temperature to decrease, thereby allowing further dehydration and cell shrinkage. This can be detrimental, since sharp ice crystals can puncture the membrane as the cell volume continues to decrease. It is therefore crucial to not only remove as much water as possible prior to freezing but also allow complete equilibration of the extracellular solution to increase the volume that will remain inside the cell and prevent the membrane from closing in on the ice crystals. This can be accomplished by high concentrations of permeable solutes in the freezing medium combined with a slow freezing rate.

Another proposed source of freeze damage is excessive dehydration that occurs as the osmolarity of extracellular fluid increases when water is removed by ice formation. Some studies suggest that there is a maximum level of shrinkage that a cell can withstand before being damaged, and when this point is superseded during freezing, cell injury occurs [18].

There are indications that cryodamage can also result from the increased concentration of electrolytes that accompanies the *free* water crystallization, independent of the physical damage by ice. Basically, the same mechanisms that cause red blood cells to hemolyze at high salt concentrations apply. A review about this mode of damage and its variants can be found in ref. [19].

Thawing of cells present another set of challenges. In fact, some studies suggest that the majority of cryoinjury occurs during the thawing rather than the cooling process, due to recrystallization of small ice crystals into larger ones [17]. This is especially true with slow rates, which allow enough time for this ice crystal growth.

Much disagreement exists on which is the best method of thawing, which essentially represents the rate of warming. One conclusion that is clear from published works is that the ideal warming rate greatly depends on, and is proportionate to, the cooling rate that was used during freezing. Furthermore, the cell type, cryoprotectants used, and freezing technique also affect which warming method will lead to the highest post-thaw survival rates.

Components of Slow Embryo Freezing

Cryoprotectants

Cryoprotectants are molecules that prevent cryodamage by reducing intracellular ice crystal formation. Their sole purpose in freezing protocols is to protect the cells from cryodamage by preventing the events described above. Two types, permeating and non-permeating cryoprotectants, are normally used in combination to dehydrate (non-permeable) and equilibrate (permeable) cells prior to freezing. Their rate of diffusion into the cell is slower than that of water exiting through osmosis, which necessitates some time for equilibration. Once inside the cell, these agents prevent ice formation by lowering the freezing temperature of the cytoplasm. There are additional theories regarding the mode of protection of cryoprotectants, with strong arguments for all of them.

Some studies suggest that these agents act as replacement diluents to keep relative electrolyte concentrations low when water is removed from the cytoplasm or freezing medium, thereby protecting them from high solute concentrations [20]. Others argue that they substitute the lost water fraction to keep shrinkage to a minimum and increase the unfrozen volume of the cell during freezing and thawing. Yet another school of thought is that cryoprotectants interact with phospholipids in the membrane bilayers to make them more stable. Then there is the fact that cells frozen in media without cryoprotectants are pushed into channels between forming ice crystals, while those that contain cryoprotectants in the media are encapsulated within the ice, with the latter scenario apparently less damaging. Despite the disagreements about the exact modes of protection, it is agreed that these agents are an essential component of freezing solutions. The usability of each ingredient depends on its toxicity to cells, which played a big part in optimization of freezing media for specific cell types.

Today, the most commonly used ingredients for slow-freezing human embryos are permeating 2,1-propanediol and dimethylsulfoxide for cleavage stages and glycerol for blastocysts, whereas sucrose is typically the non-permeating additive. An extensive overview of the various available cryoprotective agents and their use can be found in ref. [21].

Media Formulations and Procedures

As discussed above, numerous different cryoprotectants can assist in protecting embryos from cryodamage when used appropriately. Consequently, there are various medium formulations that can lead to success. Typically, freezing medium consists of a base medium, such as M199, buffered with 4-(2-hydroxyethyl)-1-piperazineethanesulfonic acid (HEPES) and supplemented with either one or a combination of permeating and/or non-permeating cryoprotectants.

Conditions exerted on the embryo by these media can be detrimental if they are not introduced slowly. Therefore, cryoprotectant concentrations are usually increased systematically via a stepwise equilibration technique, allowing water to exit the cell and cryoprotectants to diffuse into the cell gradually. Usually, the first solution will contain permeating cryoprotectants such as propylene glycol and DMSO, while the final freezing medium will contain a higher cryoprotectant concentration (1.0–1.5 M) and sucrose (0.1–0.3 M). Some protocols, however, use a one-step equilibration method with equally successful results, but its effectiveness depends on the species and embryo stage. Equilibrium is reached when the osmotic and chemical gradients caused by water and cryoprotectants inside and outside the cell membrane disappear. Equilibration and loading are then usually performed at room temperature to minimize cytotoxic effects of the cryoprotectants.

Once equilibration is complete, usually after 5–15 min, the embryos are loaded into a cryopreservation carrier. For slow freezing, the most commonly used are plastic straws that can be heat-sealed after loading. They typically accommodate 0.25–0.5 mL of medium in which the embryos are suspended. It is standard procedure to included two small air bubbles before and after the section that will include the embryos, to assist in locating the embryos upon thawing. Cryogenic vials, similar to those used for freezing somatic cells, as well as glass ampoules, have also been used successfully. Each of these has been designed to fit into an automatic, controlled-rate cooling device that carefully regulates the rate of cooling. This, however, can also be achieved by carefully layering the straws/vials at a specific distance above liquid nitrogen vapor. Naturally, the latter is less precise and much more labor intensive.

Initially, the freezing solution containing the embryos are cooled from room temperature, at a rate of 1–3°C/min, to a slightly super-cooled state between −5 and −7°C. Then, seeding is initiated either manually or automatically to start crystallization in a controlled manner and prevent further supercooling. Subsequently, the cooling process is maintained at a reduced rate of 0.3–0.5°C/min to below −30°C. Finally, the embryos are cooled to −180°C at 40°C/min before submersion in liquid nitrogen. Some protocols omit the final cooling phase and require liquid nitrogen submersion once the embryos have reached temperatures below −30°C.

The thawing procedure can be as detrimental to embryo survival as freezing, since recrystallization may occur in the small time window during which the liquid will transition trough the melting temperature. To prevent this, high warming rates are applied. Typically, straws, vials, and ampoules are thawed either in air at room temperature or in a warm water bath at 37°C. Once the freezing solution is completely melted, embryos are removed from the carrier and transferred into a diluent solution. This usually consists of the same medium used for freezing but without the permeating cryoprotectives and the same concentrations of sucrose to remove the permeating cryoprotectants. Rehydration is then achieved by decreasing the sucrose concentration systematically, usually in one or two steps, until all sucrose is removed from the medium. Embryos are subsequently returned to the incubator for conventional embryo culture after the final wash.

Immediate evaluation of survival is achieved visually by assessing the status of the cell membranes. In cases where embryos are cultured after thawing, the developmental competence and blastocyst re-expansion could be indicative of a successful freeze-thaw.

Factors That Determine Success

Embryo Stage

Over the years, research has indicated that embryos at different stages have different tolerance to cryopreservation. The reasons why embryos sometimes survive freeze-thaw better at one stage than another is not clear. Instinctively, from what we know of the affect of surface-volume ration on cryopreservation success (for review, see ref. [17]), we may assume that blastocysts will be most tolerant, followed by morulae, cleavage stage, and lastly, zygotes, based on the size of the individual blastomeres at these respective stages. However, data clearly showed that embryos at the two-pronucleus (2PN) stage are no less tolerant to freezing and thawing than any other stage [22–24]. This becomes more baffling when one considers how challenging oocyte freezing has proven to be. Clearly, the difference in freeze tolerance encompasses more than just the volume of the individual blastomeres. So far, there is no single embryonic stage that is definitely superior in terms of outcome for a frozen embryo transfer (ET) cycle [25]. The parameters associated with assessment of success in embryo freezing are predominantly survival, subsequent development, and implantation. However, results were inconsistent when the survival rates of pronuclear- versus multicellular (days 2 and 3)-stage frozen-thawed embryos were compared [23, 26]. Therefore, there is still no consensus as to which embryonic stage is superior for freezing tolerance, and the decision of freezing stage now primarily depends on the IVF program's management and individual patient cycle parameters. Nonetheless, it is beneficial to know the advantages and disadvantages of all embryonic freezing stages, which will be discussed below.

Pronuclear Stage

Slow freezing at the pronuclear stage has been widely used to cryopreserve human embryos because it gives consistent survival and subsequent development after thawing [22–24]. One major advantage is that the possibility of future embryo biopsy is still reserved when embryo freezing is performed at the pronuclear stage. The pronuclear stage embryo, however, has only one cell, which means embryo survival is either all or nothing. Furthermore, embryo quality cannot be assessed before freezing like what is the case with more advanced embryos since the only measurable quality parameter at this stage is the presence or absence of pronuclei—and zygote scoring may not be as predictable as cleavage- or blastocyst-stage assessment. After thawing, pronuclear stage embryos are typically cultured for at least 1 day—but many times, more days to obtain more data for embryo selection prior to ET. This requires a good number of embryos, enough to obtain the desired number of acceptable blastocysts for ET.

Cleavage Stage

The majority of embryo cryopreservation over the past 2 decades was performed using propanediol and sucrose to slow freeze at the cleavage stage [27]. Survival rates of 60–88% were reported [28–30]. At cleavage stages, the widely accepted criterion for embryo survival in a clinical situation is survival of a minimum of 50% of the original blastomeres. Often, some necrotic blastomeres are present after thawing due to cryodamage. It was therefore suggested to remove those necrotic cells before subsequent culture or ET. We will discuss lysed cell removal (LCR) in subsequent paragraphs. In summary, the main advantages of freezing at the cleavage stage are that embryo cleavage potential has been confirmed before freezing, while cryodamage can be confined to individual blastomeres instead of the entire embryo. Furthermore, it preserves the opportunity to do a day 3 biopsy for genetic screening.

Morula Stage

From all the preimplantation developmental stages, the morula has received the least amount of attention for cryopreservation and ET. However, reports of good outcomes with these procedures at the morula stage exist, and the advantages cited for performing them at this stage include better selection than cleavage stages and safer assisted hatching due to the large perivitelline space [31–33]. The reason for the neglect is not due to poor results, but rather to its intermediate nature. Embryos are typically transferred on day 3 at the cleavage stage or on day 5 at the blastocyst stage. Whether embryos will be transferred on day 3 depends on the number and quality. The advantage of extended culture is the ability to select embryos more extensively based on their developmental and differentiation potential. However, if a patient has too few embryos or they are of suboptimal quality, day 3 transfers are performed. Therefore, should embryos be assigned for day 5 transfer, there are probably enough good quality embryos to culture all the way to the blastocyst stage, which has better selection criteria than the morula stage. It is also beneficial to reduce handling and disturbance of the culture conditions, so quality assessment on day 4 is omitted. Thus, although rarely used, morula-stage cryopreservation is an option for clinics, and its utilization depends on the transfer scheme of the individual clinics.

Blastocyst Stage

Although the early successes in embryo cryopreservation were achieved at the blastocyst stage [34, 35], embryo freezing at this advanced stage was not routinely used until recent years when blastocyst culture systems became optimized. Culturing embryo to the blastocyst stage creates more selection criteria for ET and cryopreservation, due to prolonged monitoring and a more differentiated state. It further allows IVF programs to maintain their pregnancy rates despite transferring fewer embryos [25]. Even though embryos could be selected before freezing, the degree of cryodamage that may occur is hard to predict. Resumption of development is also difficult to assess in cryopreserved blastocysts, since any increase in the number of cells is very difficult to verify and the timeframe of re-expansion for blastocelic activity varies greatly. Also, due to the epithelial-like nature of the trophectoderm and compacted blastomeres of the inner cellular mass, necrotic cells are more difficult to be removed from the blastocyst, which may further impede normal development. Nonetheless, blastocysts have 5–6 days of developmental history that can help to determine, with post-thaw morphology, the overall quality of the thawed embryo.

Embryo Quality

Several studies showed a correlation between embryo quality and freeze tolerance. Typically, cleavage-stage cell divisions are synchronized, resulting in an exponential cell number at any point before the morula stage. Non-exponential blastomere numbers are therefore indicative of asynchronous divisions, fragmentation or degeneration of some of the blastomeres, which are all indicators of inferior embryo quality. Correspondingly, it was shown that embryos with 3, 5, 6, and 7 cells had significantly lower post-thaw survival rates than 2-, 4-, and 8-cell embryos [36–38]. A similar observation was made in the bovine model, where blastocysts of high quality survived freezing better than those of lower quality [39]. Interestingly, Check et al. [40] reported that 4-cell embryos had a similar freezing tolerance to 6–8-cell embryos, suggesting that a slower developmental rate is not included in the quality parameters that affect freeze survival [39]. Although the above-mentioned studies indicate that lower grade embryos are less prone to survive freezing, embryologists may still choose to freeze these inferior embryos to maximize the patient's number of transferable embryos in a given cycle, especially if the other quality parameters are acceptable for transfer before freezing.

Lysed Cell Removal

At the cleavage stage, the widely accepted clinical criterion for embryo survival is a minimum of 50% survival of the original blastomeres. However, necrotic blastomeres resulting from cryodamage are often present after thawing in embryos that are still in the acceptable survival range. These blastomeres can be removed using a technique called LCR, during which the cryodamaged blastomeres are aspirated from the embryo. One study found that after cryopreservation "the percentage of gestational sacs with fetal heartbeat obtained after transfer of fully intact embryos was almost three times higher than that after transfer of partially damaged embryos" [41]. The authors speculated that lysed blastomeres might produce factors as they degrade that are detrimental/toxic to undamaged cells. Additionally, lysed cells could potentially disrupt cell-cell communication between viable blastomeres. Studies in the mouse model demonstrated that LCR can restore developmental potential [42] and promote frozen-thawed embryonic development [43]. LCR has also been used following human embryo cryopreservation at multicellular stages, and results showed that it could significantly improve clinical outcomes [44–46]. It should be noted that in the mentioned experiments, assisted hatching was performed in conjunction with LCR, a practice that was also shown beneficial after vitrification and warming [47] and will be discussed in the next section. In conclusion, removal of degenerated blastomeres is a relatively simple procedure that can significantly impact implantation and pregnancy rates after cryopreservation, especially with slow freezing.

Assisted Hatching

Several reports have claimed that assisted hatching by thinning, breaching, or completely removing the zona pellucida prior to fresh ET significantly improves implantation and chemical pregnancy rates (for recent review, see the publication by The Committee of the Society for Assisted Reproductive technology and the Practice Committee of the American Society for Reproductive Medicine [48]). Various effective techniques have been described, including acid Tyrode's solution drilling/thinning [49], mechanical partial zona dissection [50], laser drilling [51], piezo drilling [52], enzymatic zona digestion [53], and most recently, mechanical zona expansion through hydrostatic pressure [54]. Although the exact alterations that occur in the zona ultra structure as zona hardening occurs remain elusive, oocyte exposure to cryoprotectants and freezing was shown to induce cortical granule exocytosis, zona delamination, and zona fractures [55, 56]. Similar structural changes may occur during embryo freezing, and these alterations in zona structure may prevent zona thinning and subsequent embryo hatching. Studies have demonstrated that assisted hatching following cryopreservation, indeed, improved implantation and pregnancy rates [57, 58]. Therefore, it is common practice to perform assisted hatching in post-thawed embryos. Although conflicting study results and disagreement exist on the benefit for fresh ETs, the most common opinion currently is that the possible advantages of employing it for frozen-thawed ETs exceed its minute risks and thus assisted hatching is typically performed on frozen-thawed embryos.

Additional Considerations

Several other factors may affect embryo survival after freezing, and those discussed below are by no means exclusive.

The technique used during execution of the freezing protocol may severely affect the success rate. One example is performing the step-wise equilibration method in a timely manner with gentle handling of the embryos to prevent mechanical damage during loading. It is thus important that technicians are properly trained to perform all the procedures the correct way.

When embryo biopsy is performed for preimplantation genetic diagnosis, embryos are subjected to crude mechanical disruption, especially in the case of blastocysts. Although the majority of embryos recover from well-executed biopsies, the overall embryo tolerance is affected, thereby decreasing its likelihood to survive freezing and thawing [59]. However, when patients order genetic screening, embryologist may have no choice other than to perform biopsy and subsequent cryopreservation. Therefore, each case should be considered individually based on the total number and quality of embryos, as well as the importance of the genetic diagnosis.

Applications and Impact

Cryopreservation of human embryos was introduced more than 2 decades ago, mainly as an approach to save supernumerary embryos produced after ovarian hyperstimulation [16, 34, 60]. The Society for Assisted Reproduction Technology (SART) and the European Society of Human Reproduction and Embryology (ESHRE) both continuously publish statistics on embryo freezing and birth rates in the United States and Europe, respectively. These are valuable data for seeing the overall impact of cryopreservation on clinical infertility treatment. However, the data does not distinguish between methods of freezing, rendering it impossible to determine the current success rates resulting from slow freezing alone. Since vitrification is becoming more widely used, the weight that slow freezing has in the overall rates is likely decreasing significantly each year, as more clinics are switching over to vitrification for reasons discussed below.

ESHRE reported almost 460,000 in vitro cycles in 2006, of which more than 86,000 (15%) were frozen ETs [61]. Data from SART indicated over 140,000 cycles in the United States, of which about 21,400 (19%) were frozen-thawed ETs. As clinics and patients become more comfortable with the idea of embryo cryopreservation, these percentages should steadily increase. Since we know that at the moment, the large majority of clinics currently still use slow freezing, the impact of this technology on infertility treatment is obvious.

One of the most common reasons a patient may opt for embryo freezing is to preserve excess embryos that were not transferred during the fresh cycle. The advantage of this is that the patient's chances of getting pregnant from a single egg retrieval significantly increase as she can have multiple embryo replacements without having to transfer more than one embryo in a single transfer. This reduces her risk of a multiple pregnancy, and thus various complications.

A major drive toward elective single ET (sET) in the field is further increasing the importance of embryo cryopreservation, allowing the patient additional opportunities for pregnancy should her first eSET not result in one. Furthermore, legislation in some European countries now limits the number of embryos that can be transferred. Embryo freezing provides a way to store the extra embryos and makes it unnecessary for the patient to go through an entire stimulation and retrieval again and again. In Germany, for example, it is illegal to culture more than three embryos from one cycle at a time. Freezing extras at the 2PN stage provides an alternative method to utilize the retrieved eggs to its full potential instead of only continuing with three fertilized eggs.

Another reason why patients may want to freeze embryos is in cases where their ET is canceled due to hyperstimulation. Historically, before freezing became available, this condition required cancellation of the entire treatment cycle and loss of the embryos. Now, with embryo freezing an option, the patient can simply return in subsequent months for frozen embryo replacements without feeling tempted to put herself at risk by having a transfer anyway.

Patients are becoming more interested in genetic screening of embryos. Although day 3 biopsies can be performed for FISH or array CGH analysis to give results in time for a day 5 fresh replacement, the increasing preference is to perform biopsy of blastocysts stage. Without the ability to cryopreserve the biopsied embryos while awaiting results, this would not be possible.

Some patients may have embryos left over after delivering the desired number of babies. Many patients have ethical problems with discarding embryos. A good option for them would be frozen embryo donation, thereby helping couples that could not conceive naturally or by in vitro techniques, and at the same time eliminate the financial burden of storing embryos without feeling guilty. Since the embryos can be thawed out any time, the recipient can be stimulated and scheduled for the ET whenever she is ready.

Open Versus Closed Systems

One issue that has received significant attention in the past few years is that of safety of cryopreservation for the recipient as well as resulting babies born from these embryos. The most cumbersome is transmitted diseases, especially viruses. There are very strict regulations for egg, sperm, and embryo donations, and the donors are screened vigorously before being classified as eligible for donation. Furthermore, there have not been any reports of patients contracting diseases from frozen ETs. However, a growing concern is prompting development of closed systems for storage, where the embryos or cryomedia are never in direct contact with liquid nitrogen. This especially applies to open vitrification techniques. Slow freezing is typically performed in sealed straws, ampoules, or cryovials, which all presumably prevent the exposure to potentially contaminated liquid nitrogen. Therefore, as long as the freezing carriers are used correctly, the risk of contamination of slow-frozen embryos remains dismissible. Thus, one of the most significant advantages of slow-freezing vessels is that they are completely sealed and, if used correctly, exclude any contact with liquid nitrogen (excluding what may condensate from air inside the vessel). Vitrification systems, on the other hand, traditionally require placing the embryo on a carrier device, such as a thin membrane, with minimal amount of medium, followed by direct submersion in liquid nitrogen. These systems are highly criticized for exposing embryos to potentially contaminated fluids and storing them in communal dewars, where the risk of cross-contamination is cumbersome. There are a few companies that are marketing closed-system vitrification equipment, but in our experience success rates are not comparable to that of open vitrification procedures. The caveat of the sealed straws and vials is that the larger volume does not allow vitrification with the current protocols and medium formulations, so slow freezing is the only reliable option when using these closed-system devices.

Slow Freezing Versus Vitrification

Many factors are causing clinics to switch to vitrification instead of traditional slow freezing. Several studies suggest that vitrification results in significantly higher survival and developmental rates than slow freezing [62, 63]. A further driving force for an increased used of vitrification is the practicality of the technique. Apart from being much more cost-effective, the procedure requires significantly less time (typically about 20–30 min total) when compared to the long equilibration methods required by typical slow-freezing protocols (around 1.5–2 h). Thawing following these techniques also differs greatly, with warming a vitrified embryo taking about 20 min versus approximately 45 min for slow-frozen embryos.

Despite these clear advantages of vitrification, many labs still use slow freezing, mainly because of the wealth of clinical data that supports the technique. Switching a well-established, effective method for a new protocol also seems intimidating, thereby preventing implementation of newer technologies. Although currently the vast majority of programs still utilize the slow-freezing method, the number of labs that uses vitrification increases every year and will likely continue to increase. We predict that, in the future, vitrification may become the sole method used for clinical embryo cryopreservation.

Legal and Ethical Considerations

The ability to store embryos for an indefinite amount of time brings up all sorts of ethical and legal issues. First and foremost, ownership of embryos has to be determined before patients that are interested in freezing are admitted to the treatment plan. This becomes very important when couples separate after freezing their embryos. It can also be an issue where family members may want ownership of leftover embryos. Patients should seek legal consult to decide and clearly document what happens to their embryos in any of such circumstances.

Another troublesome issue for patients is that of discarding extra embryos. Often, patients are against destroying embryos, but do not want any more children and also do not feel comfortable donating their embryos. These patients are left with no other option than to continue storing the embryos with the associated costs. Clinics may have difficulty collecting payments from patients after years of storage, and legally, clinics are not authorized to destroy embryos without patient consent. This can be a large burden on IVF programs, especially those with large frozen embryo collections, often from many years ago. The best way for clinics to prevent this situation is to give proper patient guidance on the subject and keep thorough records of patient consent forms before treatment begins.

Future of Slow Freezing in Cryopreservation

Embryo cryopreservation has become such an integral part of infertility treatment that it is hard to imagine that the first successful freezing of a human embryo was less than 30 years ago [16]. Up till now, slow freezing has played the most prominent role. However, because of discussed factors, vitrification is becoming the method of choice for more and more clinics, and it is only reasonable to expect that within the next decade, slow freezing for embryo preservation will be completely replaced by vitrification. Nonetheless, at the moment, many groups still rely on this much older technology for preserving embryos at all different preimplantation stages. Furthermore, slow freezing is routinely used for preservation of spermatozoa, somatic cell lines, and tissue biopsies. Therefore, although embryo cryopreservation may continue without this technology, the vast majority of clinical freezing applications will continue to benefit from slow freezing.

References

1. Leibo SP. The early history of gamete cryobiology. In: Fuller BJ, Lane N, Benson EE, editors. Life in the frozen state. New York: CRC Press; 2004. p. 347–70.
2. Polge C, Smith AU, Parkes AS. Revival of spermatozoa after vitrification and dehydration at low temperatures. Nature. 1949;164:666.
3. Smith AU, Polge C. Survival of spermatozoa at low temperatures. Nature. 1950;166:668–9.
4. Smith AU, Polge C. Storage of bull spermatozoa at low temperatures. Vet Rec. 1950;62:115–16.
5. Bunge RG, Sherman JK. Fertilizing capacity of frozen human spermatozoa. Nature. 1953;172(4382):767–8.
6. Chang MC. Probability of normal development after transplantation of fertilized rabbit ova stored at different temperatures. Proc Soc Exp Biol Med. 1948;68:680–3.
7. Chang MC. The effects of low temperature on fertilized rabbit ova in vitro, and the normal development of ova kept at low temperature for several days. J Gen Physiol. 1948;31:385–410.
8. Chang MC. Transplantation of fertilized rabbit ova; the effect on viability of age, in vitro storage period, and storage temperature. Nature. 1948;161:978.

9. Chang MC. Transplantation of rabbit blastocysts at late stage; probability of normal development and viability at low temperature. Science. 1950;111:544–5.
10. Chang MC. Fertilizability of rabbit ova and the effects of temperature in vitro on their subsequent fertilization and activation in vivo. J Exp Zool. 1952;121:351–81.
11. Smith AU. Behaviour of fertilized rabbit eggs exposed to glycerol and to low temperatures. Nature. 1952;170:374–5.
12. Fuller BJ, Paynter SJ, Watson P. Cryopreservation of human gametes and embryos. In: Fuller BJ, Lane N, Benson EE, editors. Life in the frozen state. New York: CRC Press; 2004. p. 505–39.
13. Whittingham DG, Leibo SP, Mazur P. Survival of mouse embryos frozen to −196 degrees and −269 degrees C. Science. 1972;178: 411–14.
14. Wilmut I, Rowson LE. Experiments on the low-temperature preservation of cow embryos. Vet Rec. 1973;92:686–90.
15. Willadsen SM, Polge C, Rowson LE, Moor RM. Deep freezing of sheep embryos. J Reprod Fertil. 1976;46:151–4.
16. Trounson A, Mohr L. Human pregnancy following cryopreservation, thawing and transfer of an eight-cell embryo. Nature. 1983;305:707–9.
17. Mazur P. Principles of cryobiology. In: Fuller BJ, Lane N, Benson EE, editors. Life in the frozen state. New York: CRC Press; 2004. p. 3–65.
18. Lovelock JE. The haemolysis of human red blood cells by freezing and thawing. Biochim Biophys Acta. 1953;10:28–36.
19. Muldrew K, Acker JP, Elliott JAW, McGann LE. The water to ice transition: implications for living cells. In: Fuller BJ, Lane N, Benson EE, editors. Life in the frozen state. New York: CRC Press; 2004. p. 67–108.
20. Pegg DE. Red cell volume in glycerol/sodium chloride/water mixtures. Cryobiology. 1984;21: 234–9.
21. Swain JE, Smith GD. Cryoprotectants. In: Chian R-C, Quinn P, editors. Fertility cryopreservation. New York: Cambridge University Press; 2010. p. 24–38.
22. Horne G, Critchlow JD, Newman MC, Edozien L, Matson PL, Lieberman BA. A prospective evaluation of cryopreservation strategies in a two-embryo transfer programme. Hum Reprod. 1997;12:542–7.
23. Salumets A, Tuuri T, Makinen S, Vilska S, Husu L, Tainio R, Suikkari AM. Effect of developmental stage of embryo at freezing on pregnancy outcome of frozen-thawed embryo transfer. Hum Reprod. 2003;18:1890–5.
24. Veeck LL. Does the developmental stage at freeze impact on clinical results post-thaw? Reprod Biomed Online. 2003;6:367–74.
25. Noyes N, Reh A, McCaffrey C, Tan O, Krey L. Impact of developmental stage at cryopreservation and transfer on clinical outcome of frozen embryo cycles. Reprod Biomed Online. 2009;19 Suppl 3:9–15.
26. Kattera S, Shrivastav P, Craft I. Comparison of pregnancy outcome of pronuclear- and multicellular-stage frozen-thawed embryo transfers. J Assist Reprod Genet. 1999;16:358–62.
27. Testart J, Lassalle B, Belaisch-Allart J, Hazout A, Forman R, Rainhorn JD, Frydman R. High pregnancy rate after early human embryo freezing. Fertil Steril. 1986;46:268–72.
28. Chi HJ, Koo JJ, Kim MY, Joo JY, Chang SS, Chung KS. Cryopreservation of human embryos using ethylene glycol in controlled slow freezing. Hum Reprod. 2002;17:2146–51.
29. Rama Raju GA, Haranath GB, Krishna KM, Prakash GJ, Madan K. Vitrification of human 8-cell embryos, a modified protocol for better pregnancy rates. Reprod Biomed Online. 2005;11:434–7.
30. Balaban B, Urman B, Ata B, Isiklar A, Larman MG, Hamilton R, Gardner DK. A randomized controlled study of human day 3 embryo cryopreservation by slow freezing or vitrification: vitrification is associated with higher survival, metabolism and blastocyst formation. Hum Reprod. 2008;23:1976–82.
31. Tao J, Tamis R, Fink K. Pregnancies achieved after transferring frozen morula/compact stage embryos. Fertil Steril. 2001;75:629–31.

32. Tao J, Tamis R, Fink K, Williams B, Nelson-White T, Craig R. The neglected morula/compact stage embryo transfer. Hum Reprod. 2002;17:1513–18.
33. Tao J, Craig RH, Johnson M, Williams B, Lewis W, White J, Buehler N. Cryopreservation of human embryos at the morula stage and outcomes after transfer. Fertil Steril. 2004;82:108–18.
34. Cohen J, Simons RF, Edwards RG, Fehilly CB, Fishel SB. Pregnancies following the frozen storage of expanding human blastocysts. J In Vitro Fert Embryo Transf. 1985;2:59–64.
35. Cohen J, Simons RF, Fehilly CB, Fishel SB, Edwards RG, Hewitt J, Rowlant GF, Steptoe PC, Webster JM. Birth after replacement of hatching blastocyst cryopreserved at expanded blastocyst stage. Lancet. 1985;1:647.
36. Lassalle B, Testart J, Renard JP. Human embryo features that influence the success of cryopreservation with the use of 1,2 propanediol. Fertil Steril. 1985;44:645–51.
37. Testart J, Lassalle B, Forman R, Gazengel A, Belaisch-Allart J, Hazout A, Rainhorn JD, Frydman R. Factors influencing the success rate of human embryo freezing in an in vitro fertilization and embryo transfer program. Fertil Steril. 1987;48:107–12.
38. Karlstrom PO, Bergh T, Forsberg AS, Sandkvist U, Wikland M. Prognostic factors for the success rate of embryo freezing. Hum Reprod. 1997;12:1263–6.
39. Han YM, Yamashina H, Koyama N, Lee KK, Fukui Y. Effects of quality and developmental stage on the survival of IVF-derived bovine blastocysts cultured in vitro after freezing and thawing. Theriogenology. 1994;42:645–54.
40. Check JH, Horwath D, Summers-Chase D, Yuan W, Swenson K, Levito C. The effect of blastomere number on embryo survival upon freezing/thawing. Clin Exp Obstet Gynecol. 2009;36(4):209.
41. Van den Abbeel E, Camus M, Van Waesberghe L, Devroey P, Van Steirteghem AC. Viability of partially damaged human embryos after cryopreservation. Hum Reprod. 1997;12:2006–10.
42. Alikani M, Olivennes F, Cohen J. Microsurgical correction of partially degenerate mouse embryos promotes hatching and restores their viability. Hum Reprod. 1993;8:1723–8.
43. Elliott TA, Colturato LF, Taylor TH, Wright G, Kort HI, Nagy ZP. Lysed cell removal promotes frozen-thawed embryo development. Fertil Steril. 2007;87:1444–9.
44. Rienzi L, Nagy ZP, Ubaldi F, Iacobelli M, Anniballo R, Tesarik J, Greco E. Laser-assisted removal of necrotic blastomeres from cryopreserved embryos that were partially damaged. Fertil Steril. 2002;77(6):1196–201.
45. Rienzi L, Ubaldi F, Iacobelli M, Minasi MG, Romano S, Ferrero S, Sapienza F, Baroni E, Tesarik J, Greco E. Developmental potential of fully intact and partially damaged cryopreserved embryos after laser-assisted removal of necrotic blastomeres and post-thaw culture selection. Fertil Steril. 2005;84(4):888–94.
46. Nagy ZP, Taylor T, Elliott T, Massey JB, Kort HI, Shapiro DB. Removal of lysed blastomeres from frozen-thawed embryos improves implantation and pregnancy rates in frozen embryo transfer cycles. Fertil Steril. 2005;84(6):1606–12.
47. Fathi R, Valojerdi MR, Eftekhari-Yazdi P. Effect of laser-assisted hatching and necrotic blastomere removal on the development of vitrified-warmed four-cell mouse embryos. J Assist Reprod Genet. 2008;25:333–9.
48. Practice Committee of Society for Assisted Reproductive Technology, Practice Committee of American Society for Reproductive Medicine. The role of assisted hatching in in vitro fertilization: a review of the literature. A Committee opinion. Fertil Steril. 2008;90:S196–8.
49. Cohen J, Alikani M, Trowbridge J, Rosenwaks Z. Implantation enhancement by selective assisted hatching using zona drilling of human embryos with poor prognosis. Hum Reprod. 1992;7: 685–91.
50. Cohen J, Elsner C, Kort H, Malter H, Massey J, Mayer MP, Wiemer K. Impairment of the hatching process following IVF in the human and improvement of implantation by assisting hatching using micromanipulation. Hum Reprod. 1990;5:7–13.
51. Obruca A, Strohmer H, Sakkas D, Menezo Y, Kogosowski A, Barak Y, Feichtinger W. Use of lasers in assisted fertilization and hatching. Hum Reprod. 1994;9:1723–6.
52. Nakayama T, Fujiwara H, Yamada S, Tastumi K, Honda T, Fujii S. Clinical application of a new assisted hatching method using a piezo-micromanipulator for morphologically low-quality embryos in poor-prognosis infertile patients. Fertil Steril. 1999;71: 1014–18.

53. Fong CY, Bongso A, Ng SC, Anandakumar C, Trounson A, Ratnam S. Ongoing normal pregnancy after transfer of zona-free blastocysts: implications for embryo transfer in the human. Hum Reprod. 1997;12:557–60.
54. Fang C, Li T, Miao BY, Zhuang GL, Zhou C. Mechanically expanding the zona pellucida of human frozen thawed embryos: a new method of assisted hatching. Fertil Steril. 2010; 94:1302–7.
55. Schalkoff ME, Oskowitz SP, Powers RD. Ultrastructural observations of human and mouse oocytes treated with cryopreservatives. Biol Reprod. 1989;40:379–93.
56. Nottola SA, Coticchio G, De Santis L, Macchiarelli G, Maione M, Bianchi S, Iaccarino M, Flamigni C, Borini A. Ultrastructure of human mature oocytes after slow cooling cryopreservation with ethylene glycol. Reprod Biomed Online. 2008;17:368–77.
57. Tucker MJ, Cohen J, Massey JB, Mayer MP, Wiker SR, Wright G. Partial dissection of the zona pellucida of frozen-thawed human embryos may enhance blastocyst hatching, implantation, and pregnancy rates. Am J Obstet Gynecol. 1991;165:341–4; discussion 344–5.
58. Check JH, Hoover L, Nazari A, O'Shaughnessy A, Summers D. The effect of assisted hatching on pregnancy rates after frozen embryo transfer. Fertil Steril. 1996;65:254–7.
59. Joris H, Van den Abbeel E, Vos AD, Van Steirteghem A. Reduced survival after human embryo biopsy and subsequent cryopreservation. Hum Reprod. 1999;14:2833–7.
60. Zeilmaker GH, Alberda AT, van Gent I, Rijkmans CM, Drogendijk AC. Two pregnancies following transfer of intact frozen-thawed embryos. Fertil Steril. 1984;42(2):293–6.
61. de Mouzon J, Goossens V, Bhattacharya S, Castilla JA, Ferraretti AP, Korsak V, Kupka M, Nygren KG, Nyboe Andersen A. Assisted reproductive technology in Europe, 2006: results generated from European registers by ESHRE. Hum Reprod. 2010;25:1851–62.
62. Abdelhafez FF, Desai N, Abou-Setta AM, Falcone T, Goldfarb J. Slow freezing, vitrification and ultra-rapid freezing of human embryos: a systematic review and meta-analysis. Reprod Biomed Online. 2010;20:209–22.
63. Loutradi KE, Kolibianakis EM, Venetis CA, Papanikolaou EG, Pados G, Bontis I, Tarlatzis BC. Cryopreservation of human embryos by vitrification or slow freezing: a systematic review and meta-analysis. Fertil Steril. 2008;90:186–93.

Chapter 31
Vitrification of Embryos

Juergen Liebermann, Joe Conaghan, Zsolt Peter Nagy, and Michael Tucker

Why Cryopreserve Embryos?

Successful cryopreservation of gametes in animal reproduction has a track record of over 60 years. By drawing upon the vast amount of knowledge on gamete and embryo cryopreservation accrued over the years, this led directly to the first pregnancy in humans derived from frozen-thawed embryos in 1983/1984. Since that time, the impact of cryopreservation on the growth and improved efficiency of assisted reproduction in humans has become increasingly appreciated. With approximately one quarter of a million babies born following cryopreservation, this technology has become a well-established and widely used routine procedure that allows important expansion of therapeutic strategies when IVF is used to treat infertility. Currently, controlled ovarian hyperstimulation protocols commonly provide embryos in excess of those needed for fresh transfer. Therefore, techniques have been developed to store these surplus embryos in liquid nitrogen (referred to as cryopreservation) for an indefinite period of time without significant compromise of their quality. Based on data from the Centers for Disease Control and Prevention (CDC) from 2001 to 2004, about 18% of all IVF cycles in the USA used frozen embryos for transfer. In addition, data from the same registry compared live births

J. Liebermann, PhD, HCLD (ABB)
IVF and Embryology Laboratories, Fertility Centers of Illinois,
River North Center, 900 N. Kingsbury, Suite RW6, Chicago, IL 60610, USA

J. Conaghan, PhD
Embryology Laboratories, Pacific Fertility Center, San Francisco, CA, USA

Z.P. Nagy, MD, PhD, HCLD (ABB), EMB (ACE) (✉)
Scientific and Laboratory Director, Reproductive Biology Associates, Atlanta, GA 30342, USA
e-mail: zsolt.peter.nagy@gmail.com

M. Tucker, PhD
IVF and Embryology Laboratories, Shady Grove Fertility, Rockville, MD, USA

Z.P. Nagy et al. (eds.), *Clinical Embryology: A Practical Guide*,
DOI 10.1007/978-1-4614-8376-2_31,

per transfer using frozen and fresh embryos (25% versus 34%, respectively), clearly showing that cryopreservation is an important adjunct to maximize the efficiency of every single patient's oocyte retrieval. The fundamental objectives for successful cryostorage of cells in liquid nitrogen at −196°C can be summarized as follows:

1. Arrest of cellular metabolism with maintenance of structural and genetic integrity.
2. Achieve acceptable cell survival post thaw/warming.
3. Protocol/technique must be consistent and reliable.

Furthermore, all methods and protocols for cryopreservation should be developed such that ice crystal formation and growth inside the cells or tissues must either be eliminated or massively suppressed. One recent hotly debated topic in the area of reproductive cryobiology is whether slow-cooling or rapid-cooling protocols both satisfy the fundamental cryobiological principles for reduction of damage by ice crystal formation during cooling and warming, and which approach is better. It is the case, nonetheless, that both methods of cryopreservation of biological material include six steps:

1. Initial exposure to cryoprotectant
2. Cooling (slow/rapid) to subzero temperatures
3. Low temperature storage
4. Thawing/warming
5. Dilution and removal of the cryoprotective agent
6. Return to a physiological environment

Although initially reported in 1985 as a successful cryopreservation approach for mouse embryos, vitrification has taken a backseat in human assisted reproduction. However, the practical advantages of this cryopreservation method have more recently caught the attention of many ART laboratories as a feasible alternative to traditional slow-freezing methods. Since 1985, 1,500 publications can be found referring to the topic of "vitrification," which is further evidence of the burgeoning growth of interest in this cryopreservation technology. One "drawback" considered by embryologists who are not familiar with the vitrification technique is the use of higher concentration of cryoprotectants, which does potentially mean that the vitrification solutions are more toxic than their counterpart solutions used for conventional slow freezing. However, with better understanding of the physical and biological principles of vitrification, this has led to numerous successful clinical applications of this technique within the field of assisted reproduction. As of today, all developmental stages of human embryos cultured in vitro have been successfully vitrified and warmed, with resulting offspring. Cryopreservation is one of the keystones in the overall picture of comprehensive clinical infertility treatment. These different embryonic stages will continue to be cryopreserved for a variety of different reasons whether practical, political, or personal. Today, slow-freezing technology still has the longest clinical track record and greater "comfort level" among embryologists. Nevertheless, vitrification with its increasing clinical application is showing a trend of greater consistency and better outcomes when compared to slow-freezing technology. Therefore, when (not if) IVF programs overcome the fear of the "unknown," and take on the challenge of the short learning curve with vitrification, then at that point, vitrification will become the clinical standard for human embryo cryopreservation.

Cryopreservation at low temperature slows or totally prevents unwanted physical and chemical change. The major disadvantage to using low temperature cryostorage is that it can lead to the crystallization of water, and thereby, this approach can create new and unwanted physical and chemical events that may injure the cells that are being preserved. Although the results achieved by slow freezing in many cases seem quite successful [1, 2], ice crystal formation still renders traditional slow-freezing programs generally less consistent in their clinical outcomes. Another downside to the slow-freezing approach is the time to complete such freezing procedures for human embryos, which can range from 1.5 to 5 h. This is due to the fact that the slow rate of cooling attempts to maintain a very delicate balance between multiple factors that may result in cellular damage by ice crystallization and osmotic toxicity. Traditionally, slow-freeze embryo cryopreservation has been a positive contributor to cumulative patient pregnancy rates, but ultimately, the limitations of current slow-rate freezing methods in ART have become more evident in the shootout with vitrification-based cryostorage.

Vitrification is one of the more exciting developments in ART in recent years that attempts to avoid ice formation altogether during the cooling process by establishing a glassy or vitreous state rather than an ice crystalline state, wherein molecular translational motions are arrested without structural reorganization of the liquid in which the reproductive cells are suspended. To achieve this glass-like solidification of living cells for cryostorage, high cooling rates in combination with high concentrations of cryoprotectants are used. A primary strategy for vitrifying cells and tissue is to increase the speed of thermal conductivity, while decreasing the concentration of the vitrificants to reduce their potential toxicity. There are two main ways to achieve the vitrification of water inside cells efficiently: firstly, to increase the cooling rate by using special carriers that allow very small volume sizes containing the cells to be very rapidly cooled; and secondly, to find materials with rapid heat transfer. However, one has to take into account that every cell seems to require its own optimal cooling rate, for example, mature unfertilized oocytes are much more sensitive to chilling injury than any of the cell stages of the preimplantation embryo. The earliest attempts using vitrification as an ice-free cryopreservation method for embryos were first reported in 1985 [3]. In 1993, successful vitrification of mouse embryos was demonstrated [4]. Furthermore, bovine oocytes and cleavage stages were vitrified and warmed successfully a few years later [5]. In 1999 and 2000, successful pregnancies and deliveries after vitrification and warming of human oocytes were reported [6, 7]. Since that time, and because it seems to be that both entities appear to be especially chill-sensitive cells in ART, oocytes and blastocysts seem to receive a potentially significant boost in survival rates by avoiding ice crystallization using vitrification [8]. In general, vitrification solutions are aqueous cryoprotectant solutions that do not freeze when cooled at high cooling rates to very low temperature. Interest in vitrification has clearly risen as evinced by the almost exponential growth of scientific publications about vitrification. Vitrification is very simple, requires no expensive programmable freezing equipment, and relies especially on the placement of the embryo in a very small volume of vitrification medium that must be cooled at extreme rates not obtainable in traditional enclosed cryostorage devices such as straws and vials.

During vitrification, by using a cooling rate in the range of 2,500–30,000°c/min or greater, water is transformed directly from the liquid phase to a glassy vitrified state. The physical definition of vitrification is the solidification of a solution at low temperature, not by ice crystallization but by extreme elevation in viscosity during cooling [9, 10]. Vitrification of the aqueous solution inside cells can be achieved by increasing the speed of temperature change and by increasing the concentration of the cryoprotectant used. However, a major potential drawback of vitrification is the use of high concentration of cryoprotectant, and an unintentional negative impact of these cryoprotectants in turn can be their toxicity, which may affect the embryo and subsequent development in utero. It is therefore essential to achieve a fine balance between the speed of cooling and the concentration of the vitrifying cryoprotectants. This is necessitated by the practical limit for the rate of cooling and the biological limit of tolerance of the cells for the concentration of toxic cryoprotectants being used to achieve the cryopreserved state. It is important to note that recently published papers [11–13] have shown that the use of relatively high concentration of cryoprotectants such as 15% (vol/vol) ethylene glycol (EG) used in an equimolar mixture with dimethyl sulfoxide (DMSO) had no negative effect on the perinatal outcomes from blastocyst transfers following vitrification when compared with those from fresh blastocyst transfers.

Vitrification in principle is a simple technology, that is, potentially faster to apply and relatively inexpensive; furthermore, it is becoming clinically established and is seemingly more reliable and consistent than conventional cryopreservation when carried out appropriately [14, 15].

Cryoprotectant agents are essential for the cryopreservation of cells. Basically, two groups of cryoprotectants exist: (1) permeating (*glycerol, ethylene glycol, DMSO*) and (2) nonpermeating (*saccharides, protein, polymers*) agents. The essential component of a vitrification solution is the permeating agent. These compounds are hydrophilic nonelectrolytes with a strong dehydrating effect. Furthermore, these CPAs are able to depress the "freezing point" of the solution. Regarding the high concentration of cryoprotectant used for vitrification, and in view of the known biological and physiochemical effects of cryoprotectants, it is suggested that the toxicity of these agents is a key limiting factor in cryobiology. Not only does this toxicity prevent the use of fully protective levels of these additives, but it may also be manifested in the form of cryoinjury above and beyond that seen occurring due to classical causes of cell damage (osmotic toxicity and ice formation) during cryopreservation. In spite of this, the permeating CPA should be chosen firstly by their permeating property, and secondly on the basis of their potential toxicity. Because the permeating CPA is responsible for the toxicity (*the key limiting factor in cryobiology*), different cryoprotectants have been tested for their relative toxicity, and the results indicate that ethylene glycol (EG; MW 62.02) is the least toxic followed by glycerol. Additionally, these highly permeating cryoprotectants are also more likely to diffuse out of the cells rapidly, and the cells regained their original volume more quickly upon warming, thus preventing osmotic injury. Therefore, the most common and accepted cryoprotectant for vitrification procedures is ethylene glycol (EG). Today, EG is more commonly used in an equimolar mixture with DMSO. Often, additives are added to the vitrification solution such as disaccharides. Disaccharides, for example, sucrose, do not penetrate the cell membrane, but they help to draw out more water from cells by osmosis, and therefore, lessen the exposure time of the cells to the toxic effects of the cryoprotectants. The nonpermeating sucrose also acts as an osmotic buffer to reduce the osmotic shock that might otherwise result from the dilution of the cryoprotectant after cryostorage. In addition, permeating agents are able to compound with intracellular water, and therefore, water is very slowly removed from the cell. Hence, the critical intracellular salt concentration is reached at a lower temperature. Removal of the cryoprotectant agent during warming can present a very real problem in terms of trying to reduce toxicity to the cells. Firstly, because of the toxicity of the vitrification solutions, quick dilution of them after warming is necessary, and secondly, during dilution, water permeates more rapidly in to the cell than the cryoprotective additive diffuses out. As a consequence of the excess water inflow, the cells are threatened by injury from osmotic swelling. In this situation, the nonpermeating sucrose acts as an osmotic buffer to reduce the osmotic shock. During warming, using a high extracellular concentration of sucrose (e.g., 1.0 M) counterbalances the high concentration of the cryoprotectant agents in the cell, as it reduces the difference in osmolarity between the intra- and extracellular compartments. The high sucrose concentration cannot totally prevent the cell from swelling, but it can reduce the speed and magnitude of swelling [16–18].

Pronuclear Stage Embryo Vitrification

Conventional cryopreservation of pronuclear zygotes (2PN) is well established in countries such as Germany where freezing of later stage human embryos is by law or by ethical reasons not allowed. The time to complete the conventional protocol to cryopreserved zygotes is 98 min. In Germany, the clinical pregnancy outcomes arising from the frozen-thawed 2PN cycles are about 18%, with an implantation of around 10% per embryo transferred. The time to complete vitrification of zygotes requires approximately 12 min. Recently, successful vitrification of 2PN embryos with a high survival rate is approximately 90%, cleavage rates on day 2 is greater than 80%, and blastocyst formation of 31%, and pregnancies were reported [19–22] (Table 31.1). Zygote vitrification implemented as a clinical setting can provide a clinical pregnancy rate of close to 30%, with an implantation rate of 17% [22]. The pronuclear stage appears well able to withstand the vitrification and warming conditions, which is probably due to the significant membrane permeability changes that occur postfertilization; such changes to the oolemma may also make it more stable and able to cope with the vagaries of the cold shock and striking osmotic fluctuations that occur during the vitrification process.

Table 31.1 2008/2009 Experience (SG/GRS) with vitrification for zygote cryostorage using EG/DMSO/sucrose protocol and open carrier system

Zygote warming cycles	7
Number of zygotes stored	69
Number warmed	47
Number survived	43 (91.5%)
Cleavage	43 (100%)
Number of ETs (day 3/day 5)	7 (6/1)
Embryos transferred (average)	16 (2.3)
Blastocyst vitrified	3
2PN utilization rate	19/43 (44.2%)
Clinical pregnancies	5 (71.5%)
Implantation rate	6/16 (37.5%)

Cleavage Stage Embryo Vitrification

Reports of human embryo vitrification have been more frequent. Liebermann and Tucker [16] using either the cryoloop or the hemi-straw system (HSS) showed postwarming survival rates (after 2 h of culture of day 3 embryos where more than half of their blastomeres were intact) from 84 to 90% which was dependent on the carrier system used. There was a reasonable further cleavage and compaction rate of 34%. This finding supports previous reports in which high survival rates of eight-cell human embryos using 40% EG were documented [23]. In comparison to traditional slow-rate cryopreservation, a survival rate of cleavage stage embryos of 76% was reported with vitrification [24]. Recently, successful pregnancies and deliveries after vitrification of day 3 human embryos using the OPS have been reported [25, 26]. Their results showed a negative correlation between stage of development and survival, eight-cell embryos showed a higher survival rate (79.2%; 62/78) than did embryos with fewer than six cells (21.1%; 11/53) after vitrification [25]. Despite the fact that Liebermann and Tucker [16] achieved a promising postwarming survival rate, overall only about 34% of the surviving embryos had the developmental potential to reach the compaction stage. Recently, publications on cleavage stage vitrification provided good outcome data. Loutradi et al. [27] were performing a meta-analysis and systematic review by comparing traditional and vitrification protocols for cleavage stage embryos and found a survival rate of 84.0% vs. 97.0%. In addition, clinical pregnancy rates between 35 and 48%, with implantation rates between 15 and 39%, have been reported [28–31]. So, clearly, vitrification appears to have a positive impact on overall embryo utilization. A study on the neonatal outcome of 907 vitrified-warmed cleavage stage embryos found no significant increase in the congenital birth defect rate when compared with pregnancies using fresh cleavage stage embryos [32].

Blastocyst Stage

Both natural and hormone replacement cycles seem to provide comparable levels of receptivity in naturally cycling women, though they differ in level of convenience.

Regardless of the day of cryopreservation of the embryo (whether day 5, 6, or 7), at thawing/warming, blastocysts should be treated as if they had been frozen on the fifth day of development. Vitrification of blastocysts has been undertaken utilizing an "open system" (Cryotop; Kitazato BioPharma Co., Ltd., Fuji-shi, Japan) and a "closed system" (HSV (High Security Vitrification Kit); CryoBio System, L'Aigle, France) after a two-step loading with cryoprotectant agents at 24°C. Briefly, blastocysts were placed in equilibration solution, which is the base medium (HEPES-buffered HTF with 20% synthetic serum substitute (SSS)) containing 7.5% (v/v) ethylene glycol (EG) and 7.5% (v/v) DMSO. After 5–7 min, the blastocysts were washed quickly in vitrification solution, which is the base medium containing 15% (v/v) DMSO, 15% (v/v) EG, and 0.5 M sucrose, for 45–60 s and transferred onto the Cryotop or HSV using a micropipette. Immediately after the loading of not more than two blastocysts in a 1 μL drop on the Cryotop, the carrier was plunged into fresh clean liquid nitrogen (LN2). After loading the embryos, the Cryotop was capped under the LN2 to seal and protect the vitrified material prior to cryostorage. In contrast, after loading the HSV, the straw was heat-sealed and then plunged in LN2, and stored the same way as the Cryotop [12, 13].

To remove the cryoprotectants, blastocysts were warmed and diluted in a two-step process. With the Cryotop or HSV submerged in LN2, the protective cap (Cryotop) or inner straw (HSV) were removed, and then both carriers with the blastocysts were removed from the LN2 and placed directly into a prewarmed (~35–37°C) organ culture dish containing 1 mL of 1.0 M sucrose. Blastocysts were picked up directly from the Cryotop and placed in a fresh drop of 1.0 M sucrose at 24°C. After 5 min, blastocysts were transferred to 0.5 M sucrose solution. After an additional 5 min, blastocysts were washed in the base medium and returned to the culture medium (SAGE Blastocyst Medium, Trumbull, CT, USA) until transfer.

Between January 2004 and December 2009, the *Fertility Centers of Illinois* "IVF Laboratory River North" (Chicago) has vitrified 10,119 blastocysts *without artificial shrinkage* before the cryopreservation procedure (Table 31.2). After 1,737 frozen embryo transfers (FET) including day 5 and day 6 blastocysts with a mean age of the patients of 34.6 ± 5.1 years, to date, we have seen a survival rate, implantation, and clinical pregnancy rate per transfer (cPR) of 96.6, 30.1, and 43.1%, respectively (Table 31.3). In addition, in 482 FET using aseptic vitrification, 927 blastocysts were transferred with a survival, implantation and cPR of 97.5, 33.3, and 47.5%, respectively (Table 31.4). After 6 years of vitrifying blastocysts, the perinatal outcome is as follow: from 464 deliveries with vitrified blastocysts, 576 babies (277 boys and 299 girls) were born (Table 31.3). No abnormalities were recorded.

When the vitrified-warmed blastocysts were divided into day 5 and day 6 groups, the following data were gathered (Table 31.5): In 845 FET transferring day 5 blastocysts, the survival, implantation, and cPR were 96.6, 34.8, and 49.8% compared to 96.5, 25.5, and 36.7% of day 6 blastocysts. As shown in Table 31.5, implantation and cPR occurring in the day 5 blastocysts group were significantly higher than in the day 6 blastocyst group (χ^2; $P < 0.05$; $P < 0.01$, respectively). If we compare day 5 vs. day 6 outcome using a closed system, the following data in terms of survival, implantation, and cPR were observed: 97.7%, 39.6%, and 54.9% vs. 97.2%, 27.2%, and 40.5%, respectively (Table 31.6). As shown in Table 31.6, implantation

Table 31.2 Retrospective data from 2,907 patients (average age 33.6 ± 4.9) with blastocyst cryopreservation by vitrification from January 2004 till December 2009

Day of development	Day 5	Day 6	Day 7	Total
No. of blastocysts vitrified	4,323 (43%)	5,478 (54%)	318 (3%)	10,119

Table 31.3 Retrospective data from the blastocyst cryopreservation program (Fertility Centers of Illinois, Chicago) where vitrification (VIT) technology was applied from January 2004 till December 2009

Technique	VIT
Patient's age (years)	34.6 ± 5.1
No. of warmed cycles	1,754
No. of transfers	1,737
No. of blastocysts warmed	3,465
No. of blastocysts survived (%)	3,346 (96.6)
No. of blastocysts transferred	3,313
Mean no. of blastocysts transferred	1.9
No. of implantations (%)	998 (30.1)
No. of positive pregnancy/warm (%)	860 (49.0)
No. of positive pregnancy/VET (%)	860 (49.5)
No. of clinical pregnancy/warm (%)	748 (42.6)
No. of clinical pregnancy/VET (%)	748 (43.1)
Ongoing pregnancies/VET (%)	631 (36.3)
No. of live births	576 (277 boys and 299 girls)

Values are numbers unless otherwise described
VET vitrified embryo transfer

Table 31.4 Retrospective data from the blastocyst cryopreservation program (*Fertility Centers of Illinois, Chicago*) where aseptic vitrification (aVIT) technology was applied from June 2007 till December 2009

Technique	aVIT
Patient's age (years)	34.2 ± 5.1
No. of warmed cycles	485
No. of transfers	482
No. of blastocysts warmed	959
No. of blastocysts survived (%)	935 (97.5)
No. of blastocysts transferred	927
Mean no. of blastocysts transferred	1.9
No. of implantations (%)	309 (33.3)
No. of positive pregnancy/warm (%)	260 (53.6)
No. of positive pregnancy/VET (%)	260 (53.9)
No. of clinical pregnancy/warm (%)	229 (47.2)
No. of clinical pregnancy/VET (%)	229 (47.5)
Ongoing pregnancies/VET (%)	221 (45.9)
No. of live births	115 (61 boys and 54 girls)

Values are numbers unless otherwise described
VET vitrified embryo transfer

Table 31.5 A comparison of retrospective data from the blastocyst cryopreservation program (*Fertility Centers of Illinois, Chicago*) of vitrified day 5 and day 6 blastocysts from January 2004 till December 2009

Day of development	Day 5	Day 6
Patient's age (years)	34.5 ± 5.3	34.7 ± 4.8
No. of warmed cycles	848	906
No. of transfers	845	892
No. of blastocysts warmed	1,732	1,733
No. of blastocysts survived (%)	1,673 (96.6)	1,673 (96.5)
No. of blastocysts transferred	1,652	1,661
Mean no. of blastocysts transferred	2.0	1.8
No. of implantations (%)	575 (34.8)[a]	423 (25.5)[a]
No. of positive pregnancy/warm (%)	487 (57.4)[b]	373 (41.2)[b]
No. of positive pregnancy/VET (%)	487 (57.6)[b]	373 (41.8)[b]
No. of clinical pregnancy/warm (%)	421 (49.6)[b]	327 (36.1)[b]
No. of clinical pregnancy/VET (%)	421 (49.8)[b]	327 (36.7)[b]
Ongoing/delivered pregnancies (%)	353 (41.8)	278 (31.2)
No. of live births	342	234

Values are numbers unless otherwise described
VET vitrified embryo transfer.
[a]$P < 0.05$
[b]$P < 0.01$

Table 31.6 A comparison of retrospective data from the blastocyst cryopreservation program (*Fertility Centers of Illinois, Chicago*) of aseptic vitrified day 5 and day 6 blastocysts from January 2004 till December 2009

Day of development	Day 5	Day 6
Patient's age (years)	34.2 ± 5.5	34.3 ± 4.4
No. of warmed cycles	235	250
No. of transfers	235	247
No. of blastocysts warmed	472	487
No. of blastocysts survived (%)	461 (97.7)	474 (97.2)
No. of blastocysts transferred	457	470
Mean no. of blastocysts transferred	1.9	1.9
No. of implantations (%)	181 (39.6)[a]	128 (27.2)[a]
No. of positive pregnancy/warm (%)	147 (62.6)[a]	113 (45.2)[a]
No. of positive pregnancy/VET (%)	147 (62.6)[a]	113 (45.7)[a]
No. of clinical pregnancy/warm (%)	129 (54.9)[a]	100 (40.0)[a]
No. of clinical pregnancy/VET (%)	129 (54.9)[a]	100 (40.5)[a]
Ongoing/delivered pregnancies (%)	125 (53.2)	96 (38.9)
No. of live births	78	37

Values are numbers unless otherwise described
VET vitrified embryo transfer
[a]$P < 0.01$

and cPR occurring in the day 5 blastocysts group were significantly higher than transferring day 6 blastocysts (χ^2; $P < 0.01$ for any comparison, respectively). After 3 years of vitrifying blastocysts using a closed system, the perinatal outcome is as follow: 115 babies (61 boys and 54 girls) were born (Table 31.4). No abnormalities were recorded.

Our data have shown that freezing at the blastocyst stage provides excellent survival, implantation, and clinical pregnancy [12, 13]. To achieve this data, the following points should be considered: (a) without a successful blastocyst vitrification storage program, extended culture should never be attempted; (b) the blastocyst is composed of more cells, and therefore, better able to compensate for cryoinjury; (c) the cells are smaller, thus making cryoprotectant penetration faster; and (d) on average, fewer embryos per patient are cryostored, but each one when thawed has a greater potential for implantation, often with an opportunity for an ET with a single blastocyst.

Furthermore, a vitrification solution with a mixture of 7.5% EG/DMSO, followed by a 15% EG/DMSO with 0.5 M sucrose step, is safe for clinical use, giving rise to healthy babies without abnormalities. Vitrification of blastocysts using an open or closed system (Cryotop or HSV) is effective for achieving high implantation and pregnancy rates as seen in fresh embryo transfers.

Although the outcome in terms of implantation and clinical pregnancy is significantly different when comparing day 5 blastocyst to day 6 blastocysts, our data should encourage cryopreservation of day 6 blastocysts as well. Based on the data presented, it is clear that the vitrification of day 6 blastocysts is of clinical value since it can result in live births. This observation is confirmed by Shapiro et al. [33] and Levens et al. [34]; they found that blastocyst development rate impacts outcome in slow cryopreserved blastocyst transfer cycles.

In conclusion, vitrification of human blastocysts is a viable and feasible alternative to traditional slow-freezing methods. The key to this success lies in the more optimal timing of embryo cryopreservation, for example, individual blastocysts may be cryopreserved at their optimal stage of development and expansion. In addition, the repeatedly discussed topic of using open systems (direct contact between cells and LN2) and the possible danger of contamination by bacteria, fungus, or different strains of virus from LN2 can be avoided by moving forward to a closed system providing lower cooling rates, but without a negative impact on the outcome.

Contamination of LN2: Open Versus Closed Systems

There are many potential advantages of vitrification in that it is an easy, cheap, fast, and an apparently successful cryopreservation method; however, there is one issue that is still up for debate. It has been shown that fungi, bacteria, and viruses are able to survive in liquid nitrogen (LN2) [35–40]. Given the direct exposure of the human cells as they are directly plunged into LN2 during the vitrification process, this therefore raises the question as to whether the LN2 has to be sterilized, as it may be a possible source of contamination for those cells. To this point, there has been no fungal, viral, or bacterial contamination that has been described from about 400 publications related to vitrification since the first report in 1985. Bielanski and colleagues [37] demonstrated a viral transmission rate of 21% to human embryos stored in open-freezing containers under experimental conditions of extremely elevated viral presence, while in contrast, all embryos stored in sealed freezing containers were free from contamination. Based on this observation, they proposed that the sealing of freezing containers appears to prevent exposure to potential contaminants. Commercial systems to purify LN2 by filtration have been developed; however, this technology to date has received little practical application in IVF laboratories that have active cryopreservation programs. While it is not totally clear that contamination is a real risk in everyday use of LN2, nevertheless, it may be prudent to consider routine sterilization of LN2 when open carrier systems are used for vitrification, followed by a sealing of that system for cryostorage. Further, there are currently at least three "closed" sealed vitrification systems that are commercially available, with FDA clearance, that represent successful alternatives to open systems for embryo vitrification [13].

Conclusions and Future Directions

Vitrification is a very promising cryopreservation method with many advantages and an ever increasing clinical track record. There exist many variables that can profoundly influence the effectiveness and the survival rates of vitrified cells as shown in Table 31.2. A standardized vitrification protocol applicable to all stages of the preimplantation embryo may not be realistic because of (a) different surface-to-volume ratios; (b) differing cooling rate requirements between oocytes, zygotes, cleavage stage embryos, and blastocysts; and (c) variable chill sensitivity between these different developmental stages. Currently, however, the most widely used protocol applied to any embryo stage is the two-step equilibration in an equimolar combination of the cryoprotectants ethylene glycol and DMSO, at a concentration of 15%, each (v/v) supplemented with 0.5 mol/L sucrose.

An ideal strategy for vitrifying cells and tissue is to increase the speed of thermal conduction and to decrease the concentration of cryoprotectant, thus reducing potential toxicity. There are two main ways to achieve the vitrification of water inside cells efficiently. Firstly to increase the cooling rate by using special carriers that allow very small volume sizes containing the cells to be vitrified, and secondly to find materials with rapid heat transfer. For the adoption of vitrification in ART, as with all new technologies, there has been initial resistance, but as clinical data have been accrued, this technology is becoming more commonly adopted as standard procedure in many IVF programs worldwide. With this increased use in human assisted reproduction will come evolution of the vitrification process as it is fine-tuned to clinical needs, so pushing forward its development to higher levels of clinical efficiency, utilization, and universal acceptance.

Acknowledgments The authors thank the *Fertility Centers of Illinois* (FCI) and the embryologists at the FCI IVF laboratory, River North for their invaluable contributions and support in pushing vitrification to become our standard protocol for cryopreservation of human oocytes and blastocysts within our program.

References

1. Gardner DK, et al. Changing the start temperature and cooling rate in a slow-freezing protocol increases human blastocyst viability. Fertil Steril. 2003;79:407–10.
2. Van den Abbeel E, et al. Slow controlled-rate freezing of sequentially cultured human blastocysts: an evaluation of two freezing strategies. Hum Reprod. 2005;20(10):2939–45.
3. Rall WF, Fahy GM. Ice-free cryopreservation of mouse embryos at –196°C by vitrification. Nature. 1985;313:573–5.
4. Ali J, Shelton JN. Vitrification of preimplantation stages of mouse embryos. J Reprod Fertil. 1993;98:459–65.
5. Vajta G, et al. Open pulled straws (OPS) vitrification: a new way to reduce cryoinjuries of bovine ova and embryos. Mol Reprod Dev. 1998;51:53–8.
6. Kuleshova L, et al. Birth following vitrification of a small number of human oocytes: case report. Hum Reprod. 1999;14:3077–9.
7. Yoon TK, et al. Pregnancy and delivery of healthy infants developed from vitrified oocytes in a stimulated in vitro fertilization-embryo transfer program [letter]. Fertil Steril. 2000;74: 180–1.
8. Walker DL, et al. Vitrification versus programmable rate freezing of late stage murine embryos: a randomized comparison prior to application in clinical IVF. Reprod Biomed Online. 2004;8:558–68.
9. Fahy GM, et al. Vitrification as an approach to cryopreservation. Cryobiology. 1984;21: 407–26.
10. Fahy GM. Vitrification: a new approach to organ cryopreservation. In: Merryman HT, editor. Transplantation: approaches to graft rejection. New York: Alan R Liss; 1986. p. 305–35.
11. Takahashi K, et al. Perinatal outcome of blastocyst transfer with vitrification using cryoloop: a 4-year follow-up study. Fertil Steril. 2005;84:88–92.
12. Liebermann J, Tucker MJ. Comparison of vitrification versus conventional cryopreservation of day 5 and day 6 blastocysts during clinical application. Fertil Steril. 2006;86:20–6.
13. Liebermann J. Vitrification of human blastocysts: an update. Reprod Biomed Online. 2009;19 Suppl 4:4328http://www.rbmonline.com/Article/4328.
14. Tucker MJ, et al. Cryopreservation protocols. In: Patrizio P, Guelman V, Tucker MJ, editors. Color atlas of human assisted reproduction: laboratory and clinical insights. Philadelphia: Lippincott Williams & Wilkins; 2003. p. 257–76.
15. Liebermann J, Tucker MJ. Vitrifying and warming of human oocytes, embryos, and blastocysts: vitrification procedures as an alternative to conventional cryopreservation methods. Mol Biol. 2004;254:345–64.
16. Liebermann J, Tucker MJ. Effect of carrier system on the yield of human oocytes and embryos as assessed by survival and developmental potential after vitrification. Reproduction. 2002;124:483–9.
17. Liebermann J. Potential importance of vitrification in reproductive medicine. Biol Reprod. 2002;67:1671–80.
18. Liebermann J, et al. Recent developments in human oocyte, embryo and blastocyst vitrification: where are we now? Reprod Biomed Online. 2003;7:623–33.
19. Park SP, et al. Ultra-rapid freezing of human multipronuclear zygotes using electron microscope grids. Hum Reprod. 2000;15:1787–90.

20. Jelinkova L, et al. Twin pregnancy after vitrification of 2-pronuclei human embryos. Fertil Steril. 2002;77:412–4.
21. Liebermann J, et al. Blastocyst development after vitrification of multipronucleate zygotes using the flexipet denuding pipette (FDP). Reprod Biomed Online. 2002;4:146–50.
22. Al-Hasani S, Ozmen B, Koutlaki N, Schoepper B, Diedrich K, Schultze-Mosgau A. Three years of routine vitrification of human zygotes: is it still fair to advocate slow-rate freezing? Reprod Biomed Online. 2007;14:288–93.
23. Mukaida T, et al. Vitrification of human embryos based on the assessment of suitable conditions for 8-cell mouse embryos. Hum Reprod. 1998;13:2874–9.
24. Jericho H, Wilton L, Gook DA, Edgar DH. A modified cryopreservation method increases the survival of human biopsied cleavage stage embryos. Hum Reprod. 2003;18(3):568–71.
25. El-Danasouri I, Selman HA. Successful pregnancies and deliveries after a simple vitrification protocol for day 3 human embryos. Fertil Steril. 2001;76:400–2.
26. Selman HA, El-Danasouri I. Pregnancies derived from vitrified human zygotes. Fertil Steril. 2002;77:422–3.
27. Loutradi KE, Kolibianakis EM, Venetis CA, Papanikolaou EG, Pados G, Bontis I, Tarlatzis BC. Cryopreservation of human embryos by vitrification or slow freezing: a systematic review and meta-analysis. Fertil Steril. 2008;90:186–93.
28. Rama Raju GA, Haranath GB, Krishna KM, Prakash GJ, Madan K. Vitrification of human 8-cell embryos, a modified protocol for better pregnancy rates. Reprod Biomed Online. 2005;2005(11):434–7.
29. Desai N, Blackmon H, Szeptycki J, Goldfarb J. Cryoloop vitrification of human day 3 cleavage-stage embryos: post-vitrification development, pregnancy outcomes and live births. Reprod Biomed Online. 2007;14:208–13.
30. Li Y, Chen ZJ, Yang HJ, Zhong WX, Ma SY, Li M. Comparison of vitrification and slow-freezing of human day 3 cleavage stage embryos: post-vitrification development and pregnancy outcomes. Zhonghua Fu Chan Ke Za Zhi. 2007;42:753–5.
31. Balaban B, Urman B, Ata B, Isiklar A, Larman MG, Hamilton R, Gardner DK. A randomized controlled study of human Day 3 embryo cryopreservation by slow freezing or vitrification: vitrification is associated with higher survival, metabolism and blastocyst formation. Hum Reprod. 2008;23:1976–82.
32. Rama Raju GA, Jaya Prakash G, Murali Krishna K, Madan K. Neonatal outcome after vitrified day 3 embryo transfers: a preliminary study. Fertil Steril. 2009;92:143–8.
33. Shapiro B, Richter K, Harris D, Daneshmand S. A comparison of day 5 and 6 blastocysts transfers. Fertil Steril. 2001;75:1126–30.
34. Levens ED, Whitcomb BW, Henessy S, James AN, Yauger BJ, Larsen FW. Blastocyst development rate impacts outcome in cryopreserved\blastocyst transfer cycles. Fertil Steril. 2008;90:2138–43.
35. Tedder RS, Zuckerman MA, Goldstone AH, Hawkins AE, Fielding A, Briggs EM, et al. Hepatitis-B transmission from contaminated cryopreservation tank. Lancet. 1995;346: 137–40.
36. Fountain R, et al. Liquid nitrogen freezer: a potential source of microbial contamination of hematopoietic stem cell components. Transfusion. 1997;37:585–91.
37. Bielanski A, et al. Viral contamination of embryos cryopreserved in liquid nitrogen. Cryobiology. 2000;40:110–6.
38. Bielanski A, et al. Microbial contamination of embryos and semen during long term banking in liquid nitrogen. Cryobiology. 2003;46:146–52.
39. Kyuwa S, et al. Experimental evaluation of cross-contamination between cryotubes containing mouse 2-cell embryos and murine pathogens in liquid nitrogen tanks. Exp Anim. 2003;52: 67–70.
40. Letur-Kornisch H, et al. Safety of cryopreservation straws for human gametes or embryos: a study with human immunodeficiency virus-1 under cryopreservation conditions. Hum Reprod. 2003;18:140–4.

Chapter 32
Directional Freezing of Reproductive Cells, Tissues, and Organs

Amir Arav

The multi thermal gradient (MTG) technique is based on the principles of directional freezing. The directional freezing process is based on controlling the ice crystal propagation through the sample by regulating the velocity of the sample through a predetermined thermal gradient. The directional freezing method permits a very precise and uniform cooling rate [1], which has allowed for successful freezing in the absence of liquid CPAs. Ice formation occurs as the edge of the sample (seeding is initiated), and as the sample is pushed through the thermal gradient, the ice crystals propagate in opposite direction to the sample movement. The ice crystal size and morphology are dependent on this velocity in an inverse proportion; that is, as the ice interface velocity increases, the size of the ice crystals decreases, and vice versa. The result is that the control of the unfrozen fraction size (the area between the ice crystals where the cells and solutes solidify) is controlled by the thermodynamics of the process and not by CPAs such as DMSO, glycerol, and their likes.

This has enabled the successful cryopreservation of what has previously been regarded as impossible such as wild animal's sperm, human cartilage tissue, and large organs (sheep and human ovaries, porcine liver, and rat hearts).

MTG Description

The MTG technique aims to overcome problems related to freezing of large volume of cells, tissue, and organs. The technology is based on a series of heat conductive blocks (usually built of brass or aluminum) arranged in a line, with a straight track running through the blocks. Along the blocks, different temperatures (T1, T2, T3, T4 in Fig. 32.1) can be set, thereby imposing a temperature gradient (G1, G2, G3).

A. Arav, DMV, PhD (✉)
Core Dynamics, 3 Hamazmerah Street, Ness Ziona 70400, Israel
e-mail: arav@agri.huji.ac.il

Z.P. Nagy et al. (eds.), *Clinical Embryology: A Practical Guide*,
DOI 10.1007/978-1-4614-8376-2_32,

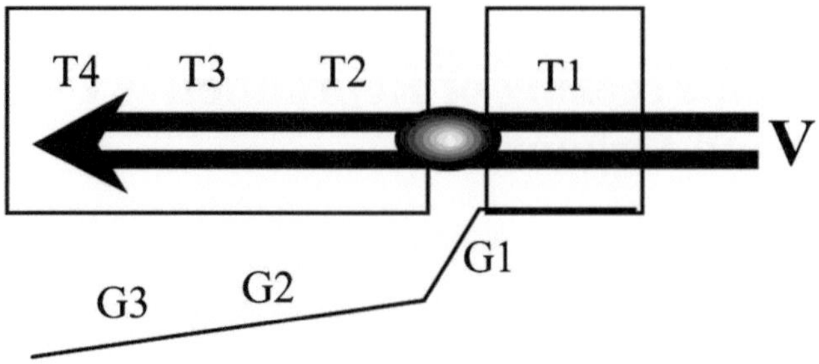

Fig. 32.1 Along the blocks, different temperatures (T1, T2, T3, T4) can be set, thereby imposing a temperature gradient (G1, G2, G3)

The blocks are separated by a gap (D1), and the temperature of the block on one side of the gap (T1) is above the freezing point temperature, whereas the temperature on the other side of the gap (T2) is below the freezing point temperature, thereby imposing a temperature gradient across the gap (G1). Biological samples to be frozen or thawed are placed inside the test tubes and are moved along the track at certain velocities (V). The samples are frozen at rates (cooling rate 1, 2, 3 = G1, 2, 3 × V) according to the specific protocols of the samples.

Sperm Freezing

Several freezing methods are in use for the cryopreservation of spermatozoa. Probably the most widely used one is the vapor freezing method during which the extended semen, packaged into 0.25- or 0.5-mL plastic straws, is held at a predetermined distance above liquid nitrogen for several minutes before being plunged into the liquid nitrogen for storage [2, 3]. Another method is known as the pellet method in which a small volume (usually around 200 μL) of extended semen is placed directly on carbon dioxide ice ("dry ice") and then stored in liquid nitrogen [4]. Other low-tech techniques include the dry-shipper freezing technique [5] or freezing in cold ethanol [6]. In more recent years, controlled rate freezing machines started penetrating the market [7]. In these machines, suitable for freezing extended semen packaged in straws, the rate of both the chilling and the freezing can be programmed and precisely controlled. The drawback of the various conventional freezing methods (vapor, pellet, controlled rate) is that ice crystal growth is uncontrolled in terms of both velocity and morphology, and the crystals may therefore disrupt and kill cells in the sample [8]. The alternative technique, which was described in a recent review as "the only recent significant advancement in semen preservation technology" [9], is the directional freezing technique. This technique uses the Multi Thermal Gradient device (MTG®; IMT Ltd, Ness Ziona, Israel) (Fig. 32.2). After the initial seeding stage, the semen sample is advanced at a constant velocity through a linear temperature gradient. The ice crystal propagation can thus be controlled to

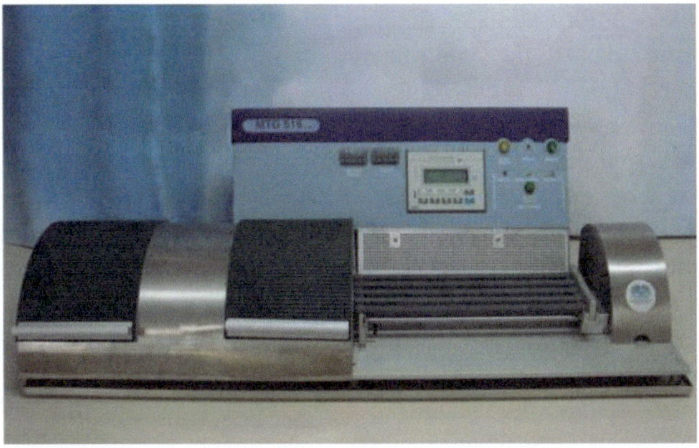

Fig. 32.2 Multi gradient thermal device in which large volume test tubes with samples are advanced at a constant velocity through a predefined temperature gradient to achieve optimal heat transfer and extracellular ice crystallization

optimize crystal morphology and to achieve continual seeding and a homogenous cooling rate throughout the entire freezing process. Damage to the cells, even when freezing in large volumes of 8 mL, is thereby minimized [1, 10–12]. Several studies, conducted by us and others, that used this technology demonstrated the viability and fertilizing ability of frozen–thawed semen from a variety of species [11, 13–23]. The advantages of large volume freezing are apparent when one has to consider the storage space and costs of a large number of samples under liquid nitrogen over extended period of time. In studies conducted on bovine bull semen, we have demonstrated that semen frozen in this way can be thawed, packaged in insemination-dose straws, refrozen and later thawed and used for AI with acceptable fertility results, similar to those achieved in the conventional single-freezing method [11, 24]. Several studies on human sperm showed that some cells preserve their functional capacity even after several freeze–thaw cycles and can be used to fertilize oocytes through ICSI [25–27].

Recently, using the MTG, we have shown that it is possible to freeze cells in the absent of CPS. Freezing only with additives that are dry at room temperatures (such as sugars and proteins) allowing the freeze-drying of cells and storage at a dry state.

Freeze-Drying of Cells

For many years, scientists have been aspiring for the lyophilization of cells for the simplicity it allows in the storage and transportation of dried materials. In a recent publication, we have shown that freeze-dried granulosa cells that were stored for 3 years at room temperature preserved their DNA integrity and were capable to produce normal embryos after nuclear transfer [28, 29]. We have then continued on improving the viability and functionality of the dried cells after rehydration by adding an antioxidant to the lyophilization solution and by changing the freezing and drying parameters. This was done on MNC derived from human umbelical cord blood (UCB) units where we have achieved a viability rate of 85% after rehydration with distilled water. Furthermore, when colony-forming unit assay was done, there was no difference between the numbers of colonies formed before freezing to those formed after freeze-drying and rehydration [30]. This assay has shown that the hematopoietic stem cells have maintained their capability to differentiate into different blood cells following freeze-drying.

Additionally, we have performed freeze-thawing and freeze-drying experiments with MNC derived from mice bone marrow which were transfused into sublethally irradiated mice. We have seen increased survival following injection of freeze-dried and rehydrated cells. The freeze-thawing experiments were done on blood from male mice that were injected into irradiated female mice. One month after the injection of the frozen–thawed cells, blood was taken from the female mice, and PCR was preformed showing the presence of Y chromosome. These preliminary findings suggest that the cells were capable to incorporate into the bone marrow and to form new white blood cells.

We have been able to lyophilize sheep leukocytes and show that their DNA is remained intact and can direct embryonic development after 3 years of storage at room temperature followed by rehydration with pure water. Human hematopoietic stem cells that were lyophilized and rehydrated with water were viable and have maintained their clonogenic capacity, showing that they were able to develop into all blood lineages. This was the first report to show cells that have undergone complete lyophilization and following rehydration have maintained not only their viability but also their functionality.

Whole Ovary Freezing

For many years, attempts to cryopreserve large organs have been ineffective due to problems associated with heat transfer [31] and the nonhomogeneous rate of cooling between the core and the periphery of the organ. To overcome these challenges, two methodologies have been proposed: the first is the MTG freezing technique [13, 17, 20] and the second is the vitrification methodology [32, 33]. Vitrification as a methodology for preserving large biological samples such as vascularized organs has many drawbacks: chemical toxicity and osmotic shock following exposure to very high (>50%) concentrations of cryoprotectant solutions, fractures caused to the vitrified organ by the vitrification procedure [34], and devitrification if the storage temperature is above the glass transition temperature [35].

The novel MTG methodology as shown by the experiments reported here and in other works [36] has solved this problem by maintaining a uniform cooling rate through the entire organ, by using two thermocouples, one in the ovarian cortex and the other in the center part of the medulla, that cooling rate is uniform throughout the periphery and the core of the ovary. Maintaining this uniform cooling rate was made possible by building our freezing devices based on two principles: (a) large mass of conductive material which enables rapid evacuation of latent heat being released due to crystallization in the freezing front, and (b) since the sample is moving through the temperature gradient at a controlled speed, we are able to create a very precise and uniform freezing front (the interface), which allows efficient removal of the latent heat.

The alternative to whole ovary is the cryopreservation of cortical strips. However, this method has major technical limitations since upon thawing and grafting of the cortical tissue, there is a vast loss of follicles during the period of ischemia and before the tissue becomes revascularized [37, 38], compromising ovarian function.

The successful demonstration of long survival—6 years—after whole ovary freezing and retransplant in a large animal does well for ongoing studies on whole human ovary cryopreservation and transplantation [39]. The information gathered from these animal experiments is very relevant to the human application since the sheep ovaries have strong similarities with young women ovaries displaying a high cortical primordial follicle density. There is hardly any data available on aged sheep ovaries since animals are normally culled long before 6 years of age [40]. However, it is the first time that long-term follow-up of whole ovary freezing and transplantation demonstrate a large number of follicles, as shown in the present study [41]. Cryopreservation of intact human ovary with its vascular pedicle is not associated with any signs of apoptosis or ultrastructural alterations in any cell types, confirming that whole-organ vascular transplantation may thus be a viable option in the future [42].

Summary

In summary, directional freezing is a promising technology which enables the freezing of large volume samples including large tissue and whole organs [36, 43, 44].

Concerning organ cryopreservation, with the advances in whole ovary, heart, and liver transplantation surgeries, the availability of an effective cryopreservation methodology is paramount.

References

1. Arav A, Assignee. Device and methods for multigradient directional cooling and warming of biological samples. 1999; US Patent, Patent 5, 873, 254.
2. Roussel JD, Kellgren HC, Patrick TE. Bovine semen frozen in liquid nitrogen vapor. J Dairy Sci. 1964;47(12):1403–6.
3. Sherman JK. Improved methods of preservation of human spermatozoa by freezing and freeze-drying. Fertil Steril. 1963;14:49–64.
4. Gibson CD, Graham EF. The relationship between fertility and post-freeze motility of bull spermatozoa (by pellet freezing) without glycerol. J Reprod Fertil. 1969;20(1):155–7.

5. Roth TL, Bush LM, Wildt DE, Weiss RB. Scimitar-horned oryx (*Oryx dammah*) spermatozoa are functionally competent in a heterologous bovine in vitro fertilization system after cryopreservation on dry ice, in a dry shipper, or over liquid nitrogen vapor. Biol Reprod. 1999; 60(2):493–8.
6. Saroff J, Mixner JP. The relationship of egg yolk and glycerol content of diluters and glycerol equilibration time to survival of bull spermatozoa after low temperature freezing. J Dairy Sci. 1955;38(3):292–7.
7. Landa CA, Almquist JO. Effect of freezing large numbers of straws of bovine spermatozoa in an automatic freezer on post-thaw motility and acrosomal retention. J Anim Sci. 1979;49(5): 1190–4.
8. Watson PF. The causes of reduced fertility with cryopreserved semen. Anim Reprod Sci. 2000;60–61:481–92.
9. Gillan L, Maxwell WMC, Evans G. Preservation and evaluation of semen for artificial insemination. Reprod Fertil Dev. 2004;16: 447–54.
10. Arav A, Zeron Y, Ocheretny A. A new device and method for vitrification increases the cooling rate and allows successful cryopreservation of bovine oocytes. Theriogenology. 2000;53(1):248 [abstract].
11. Arav A, Zeron Y, Shturman H, Gacitua H. Successful pregnancies in cows following double freezing of a large volume of semen. Reprod Nutr Dev. 2002;42(6):583–6.
12. Saragusty J, Gacitua H, Rozenboim I, Arav A. Do physical forces contribute to cryodamage? Biotechnol Bioeng. 2009;104(4): 719–28.
13. Arav A, Revel A, Nathan Y, et al. Oocyte recovery embryo development and ovarian function after cryopreservation and transplantation of whole sheep ovary. Hum Reprod. 2005;20: 3554–9.
14. Gacitua H, Arav A. Successful pregnancies with directional freezing of large volume buck semen. Theriogenology. 2005;63(3):931–8.
15. Hayakawa H, Yamazaki T, Oshi M, Hoshino M, Dochi O, Koyama H. Cryopreservation of conventional and sex-sorted bull sperm using a directional freezing method. Reprod Fertil Dev. 2007;19(1):176–7 [abstract].
16. Hermes R, Arav A, Saragusty J, Göritz F, Pettit M, Blottner S, Flach E, Eshkar G, Boardman W, Hildebrandt TB. Cryopreservation of Asian elephant spermatozoa using directional freezing; 2003 Apr 10–Oct 10. Minneapolis, MN, USA. p. 264 [abstract].
17. O'Brien JK, Robeck TR. Development of sperm sexing and associated assisted reproductive technology for sex preselection of captive bottlenose dolphins (*Tursiops truncatus*). Reprod Fertil Dev. 2006;18(3):319–29.
18. Reid CE, Hermes R, Blottner S, Goeritz F, Wibbelt G, Walzer C, Bryant BR, Portas TJ, Streich WJ, Hildebrandt TB. Split-sample comparison of directional and liquid nitrogen vapour freezing method on post-thaw semen quality in white rhinoceroses (Ceratotherium simum simum and Ceratotherium simum cottoni). Theriogenology. 2009;71(2):275–91.
19. Saragusty J, Gacitua H, King R, Arav A. Post-mortem semen cryopreservation and characterization in two different endangered gazelle species (*Gazella gazella and Gazella dorcas*) and one subspecies (*Gazella gazelle acaiae*). Theriogenology. 2006;66(4): 775–84.
20. Saragusty J, Gacitua H, Pettit MT, Arav A. Directional freezing of equine semen in large volumes. Reprod Domest Anim. 2007;42(6):610–5.
21. Saragusty J, Hildebrandt TB, Behr B, Knieriem A, Kruse J, Hermes R. Successful cryopreservation of Asian elephant (*Elephas maximus*) spermatozoa. Anim Reprod Sci. 2009;115(1–4): 255–66.
22. Si W, Hildebrandt TB, Reid C, Krieg R, Ji W, Fassbender M, Hermes R. The successful double cryopreservation of rabbit (*Oryctolagus cuniculus*) semen in large volume using the directional freezing technique with reduced concentration of cryoprotectant. Theriogenology. 2006;65(4):788–98.
23. Si W, Lu Y, He X, Ji S, Niu Y, Tan T, Ji W. Improved survival by cryopreservation rhesus macaque (*Macaca mulatta*) spermatozoa with directional freezing technique. Reprod Fertil Dev 2009;22(1): 217 [abstract].

24. Saragusty J, Gacitua H, Zeron Y, Rozenboim I, Arav A. Double freezing of bovine semen. Anim Reprod Sci. 2009;115(1–4):10–7.
25. Bandularatne E, Bongso A. Evaluation of human sperm function after repeated freezing and thawing. J Androl. 2002;23(2):242–9.
26. Polcz TE, Stronk J, Xiong C, Jones EE, Olive DL, Huszar G. Optimal utilization of cryopreserved human semen for assisted reproduction: recovery and maintenance of sperm motility and viability. J Assist Reprod Genet. 1998;15(8):504–12.
27. Rofeim O, Brown TA, Gilbert BR. Effects of serial thaw-refreeze cycles on human sperm motility and viability. Fertil Steril. 2001;75(6):1242–3.
28. Loi P, Matsukawa K, Ptak G, Clinton M, Fulka Jr J, Natan Y, Arav A. Freeze-dried somatic cells direct embryonic development after nuclear transfer. PLoS One. 2008;3(8):e2978.
29. Loi P, Matsukawa K, Ptak G, Nathan Y, Fulka Jr J, Arav A. Nuclear transfer of freeze dried somatic cells into enucleated sheep oocytes. Reprod Domest Anim. 2008;43 Suppl 2:417–22.
30. Natan D, Nagler A, Arav A. Freeze-drying of mononuclear cells derived from umbilical cord blood followed by colony formation. PLoS One. 2009;4(4):e5240.
31. Balasubramanian SK, Coger RN. Heat and mass transfer during the cryopreservation of a bioartificial liver device: a computational model. ASAIO J. 2005;51:184–93.
32. Fahy GM, MacFarlane DR, Angell CA, Meryman HT. Vitrification as an approach to cryopreservation. Cryobiology. 1984;21:407–26.
33. Baudot A, Courbiere B, Odagescu V, et al. Towards whole sheep ovary cryopreservation. Cryobiology. 2007;55:236–48.
34. Courbiere B, Massardier J, Salle B, et al. Follicular viability and histological assessment after cryopreservation of whole sheep ovaries with vascular pedicle by vitrification. Fertil Steril. 2005;84 Suppl 2:1065–71.
35. Fahy GM, Wowk B, Paynter S, 2004. Improved vitrification solutions based on the predictability of vitrification solution toxicity. Cryobiology. 2004;48(1):22–35. Erratum in: Cryobiology. 2004;48(3):365. Cryobiology. 2004;56(4):845.
36. Elami A, Gavish Z, Korach A, et al. Successful restoration of function of frozen/thawed isolated rat hearts. J Thorac Cardiovasc Surg. 2008;135:666–72.
37. Baird DT, Webb R, Campbell BK, Harkness LM, Gosden RG. Long-term ovarian function in sheep after ovariectomy and transplantation of autografts stored at -196 C. Endocrinology. 1999;140(1):462–71.
38. Silber SJ, DeRosa M, Pineda J, et al. A series of monozygotic twins discordant for ovarian failure: ovary transplantation (cortical versus microvascular) and cryopreservation. Hum Reprod. 2005;23:1531–7.
39. Silber S, Pineda J, DeRosa M, et al. Successful pregnancy after whole ovary microvascular transplantation. Fertil Steril. 2008;90 Suppl 1:S37–8.
40. de Souza CJ, Campbell BK, Baird DT. Incipient ovarian failure associated with raised levels of follicle stimulating hormone and reduced levels of inhibin A in older sheep. Hum Reprod. 1998;13:3016–22.
41. Arav A, Gavish Z, Elami A, Natan Y, Revel A, Silber S, Gosden RG, Patrizio P. Ovarian function 6 years after cryopreservation and transplantation of whole sheep ovaries. Reprod Biomed Online. 2010;20(1):48–52.
42. Martinez-Madrid B, Camboni A, Dolmans MM, et al. Apoptosis and ultrastructural assessment after cryopreservation of whole human ovaries with their vascular pedicle. Fertil Steril. 2007;87:1153–65.
43. Gavish Z, Ben-Haim M, Arav A. Cryopreservation of whole murine and porcine livers. Rejuvenation Res. 2008;11:765–72.
44. Norman S, Rzepakosky V, Brosh T, Salai M. Maintaining viability of osteochondral allografts for transplantation using directional freezing. J Bone Joint Surg Br. 2006;88-B Suppl 2:344.

Chapter 33
Ovarian Tissue Cryopreservation

Jennifer L. Kulp, J. Ryan Martin, and Pasquale Patrizio

As cancer survival improves, women of reproductive age need options to preserve their fertility. Oncology treatments may involve gonadotoxic levels of chemotherapy or radiotherapy [1–5]. Freezing embryos is a traditional method of fertility preservation. This method has a long track record of success, and women can expect excellent pregnancy rates from cryopreserved embryos, with success rates in the United States ranging from 19 to 36% depending on a woman's age at the time of embryo freezing. However, the disadvantage of this method is that a woman needs a husband, male partner, or donated sperm. For women wishing to preserve fertility but without a male partner or not interested in donor sperm, oocyte cryopreservation is a viable option. Pregnancy rates from cryopreserved oocytes are approaching that seen from cyropreserved embryos in some centers, and it is expected that soon this option will no longer be considered experimental [6].

This chapter will focus on the cryopreservation of ovarian tissue. While this method of fertility preservation is not as well established as embryo or oocyte freezing, it does offer some advantages. Contrary to embryo or oocyte cryopreservation, which requires synchrony with the follicular phase of the menstrual cycle and approximately 10 days of controlled ovarian hyperstimulation, resulting in high serum estradiol levels, ovarian tissue can be extracted and cryopreserved on short notice. It can be offered to women who need timely chemotherapy or who have an estrogen-responsive cancer such as some types of breast cancer. Ovarian tissue cryopreservation offers an advantage here as no pretreatment is needed, and a laparoscopy to harvest ovarian tissue can be performed at any point in a woman's

J.L. Kulp, MD • J.R. Martin, MD
Division of Reproductive Endocrinology and Infertility, Yale University School of Medicine, New Haven, CT, USA

P. Patrizio, MD, MBE, HCLD (✉)
Department of Obstetrics, Gynecology and Reproductive Sciences, Yale University School of Medicine, Yale Fertility Center, New Haven, CT, USA
e-mail: Pasquale.patrizio@yale.edu

Z.P. Nagy et al. (eds.), *Clinical Embryology: A Practical Guide*,
DOI 10.1007/978-1-4614-8376-2_33,

menstrual cycle. It can also be offered to children, who are increasingly surviving from childhood malignancies, yet they may lose their fertility as a result of their chemotherapy [7–10]. The ability to preserve future fertility is important for quality of life in cancer survivors. Ovarian tissue cryopreservation may be the only viable option for children with malignancies who need to undergo gonadotoxic treatment.

Cryopreservation of Cortical Strips

The ovarian cortex contains a multitude of primordial and immature follicles. Cryopreservation of the ovarian cortex containing these large numbers of follicles is an emerging area of fertility preservation. The primordial and immature follicles are undifferentiated and are not metabolically active [11, 12]. In addition, the small water content, the high surface to volume ratio, and the absence of the zona pellucida may mean that these follicles are less susceptible to damage during the process of cryopreservation [3]. Ovarian cortical strips can be obtained via a same-day laparoscopy. The ovarian cortex can be harvested during laparoscopy in thin 1–3-mm strips, by removing approximately half the ovary in a block of cortical tissue or by taking small 5-mm biopsies [13, 14]. The use of cautery is avoided during ovarian cortex harvesting. Due to the unpredictable assessment of the risk for gonadotoxicity, some women can be expected to have some ovarian function remaining after chemo or radiotherapy; therefore, it is prudent to leave behind some of the ovarian cortex. With an experienced surgeon, the median operating time is 30 min. The complications from harvesting ovarian cortical strips via laparoscopy are minimal and not different from any other laparoscopic ovarian surgery [15]. However, there are challenges to freezing and reimplanting ovarian cortical strips. These thin strips are subject to ischemic damage both during cryopreservation and retransplantation. There may be poor permeability of the cryoprotectants and resultant freezing damage to the follicles contained within the ovarian cortex. Also, as these strips are frozen without their vascular supply, they rely on neovascularization for their post-transplant survival. Further depletion of follicles in fact occurs when the ovarian graft is reimplanted until a new vascular supply (generally after 5 days to a week) is established to perfuse the graft [16–19].

Ovarian cortical strips can be cryopreserved using both slow freezing and vitrification methods. The methods appear to be comparable in terms of preserving the follicles [20]. Success with cryopreserving ovarian cortical strips and autotransplantation was first demonstrated using animal models. In sheep, fertility was preserved after castration by autotransplantation of cryopreserved strips of ovarian cortex. After ovariectomy and transplantation of frozen–thawed ovarian cortex, FSH and LH levels returned to near normal for 60 weeks and estrous cycles resumed. Yet, a minority of primordial follicles, only 28% survived the process [17]. In the early 1990s, the birth of a lamb resulting from ovulation from a frozen–thawed ovarian cortical graft was reported [11]. Births of lambs were also reported after autotransplantation of cryopreserved hemi-ovaries, but again, only few follicles were seen on histologic examination of the frozen–thawed ovaries [21].

In humans, cryopreservation of ovarian cortical strips as a method of fertility preservation has emerged over the last 10 years. Ovarian cortical strips have been autotransplanted either into the pelvis (orthotopic) or outside the pelvis (heterotopic) [13, 22–27]. Orthotopic autotransplantation involves transplanting the thawed ovarian cortex onto the remaining ovary or into a peritoneal window in the pelvis. The transplantation surgery can be done laparoscopically but has also been done via laparotomy. The first live birth after orthotopic transplantation of cryopreserved ovarian tissue was reported in 2004 [24]. A 25-year-old with stage IV Hodgkin's lymphoma underwent a laparoscopy to biopsy the cortex of the left ovary. Five biopsies were taken and then cryopreserved. The patient received chemotherapy and radiation and then became amenorrheic. Five years later, the ovarian cortex was thawed and then transplanted into a peritoneal window which had been created 7 days earlier to help promote angiogenesis. Eleven months after reimplantation of the ovarian cortex, an intrauterine pregnancy was documented, and the patient went on to deliver a healthy son.

When thawed ovarian cortex is transplanted onto a remaining ovary or on nearby peritoneum, there is not always need for follicular aspiration and assisted reproductive techniques, as the fallopian tube can pick up and transport the ovulated oocyte. However, if the ovarian cortex is transplanted elsewhere, then follicular aspiration and in vitro fertilization are required. Initially, controversy existed because it could not be proven in the cases of orthotopic transplantation that the live birth was not a result of residual ovarian function from the remaining ovary. However, this initial skepticism is subsiding as more live births from the procedure are reported in the literature.

Since this first described successful orthotopic transplantation of frozen–thawed ovarian cortex, many others have been reported. The second successful case involved a 28-year-old with non-Hodgkin's lymphoma and ovarian failure after chemotherapy. She became pregnant after IVF and had a live birth when her cryopreserved ovarian cortex was thawed after 2 years and reimplantated on her ovary [25]. Overall, at least 12 live births have been described after orthotopic transplantation of frozen–thawed ovarian cortex [16, 24–31]. The patients were all in their twenties at the time of ovarian cortex freezing, and the cortex was frozen for a duration of 1–6 years prior to reimplantation. Some of these live births were after spontaneous conception and others after in vitro fertilization. In 2010, Andersen et al. reported the first women to give birth to a second child after transplantation of frozen–thawed ovarian tissue. She conceived her first child after ovarian cortex reimplantation on her left ovary and delivered a healthy girl in 2007. She spontaneously conceived again that same year and went on to deliver a second healthy girl [32].

Heterotopic transplantation of ovarian cortex has also been described. In 2004, Oktay et al. described cryopreserving ovarian tissue from a 30-year-old woman with breast cancer prior to chemotherapy-induced menopause [23]. The cortex was then transplanted to the skin beneath her abdominal skin. After undergoing eight cycles of in vitro fertilization, one oocyte, out of 20 retrieved, fertilized normally and developed into a 4-cell embryo.

In 2006, a case was reported of a woman diagnosed with Hodgkin's lymphoma who had frozen–thawed ovarian tissue transplanted to a subperitoneal pocket on the lower abdominal wall. Twice an oocyte was retrieved from this location and fertilized by ICSI. After one of the embryo transfers, a biochemical pregnancy occurred [33]. Heterotopic transplantation of ovarian cortex tissue to other sites such as the forearm has also been described [13, 22, 23]. In monkeys, a successful heterotopic transplantation of fresh ovarian tissue, which has led to the birth of a healthy female after oocyte production, fertilization and transfer to a surrogate mother has been reported [34]. A live birth after heterotopic ovarian cortex transplantation has not yet been reported in humans, so this approach to ovarian tissue cryopreservation is nowadays rarely recommended.

Risks

One major concern of cryopreserving tissue from patients with a malignancy and then reimplanting this tissue is the risk of metastasis [35]. In one Danish study, in which females with leukemia had ovarian cortex cryopreservation, 6 of 8 patients had PCR evidence of the leukemic cells in the ovarian tissue [36]. Molecular markers of malignant cells allow detection of small numbers of cells by PCR which cannot be detected by histologic examination.

Another group examined ovarian cortex biopsies of a patient with CML and did not find evidence of malignant cells by routine histologic methods, but again, identified some evidence of malignant cells by PCR. It is unclear whether this PCR evidence of malignant cells came from the ovarian biopsies or from contaminating blood [35]. The viability of these malignant cells is unknown.

A study examined the presence of malignant cells in ovarian cortex of women with CML and ALL and found malignant cells present by PCR in 2 out of 6 patients with CML and 7 out of 10 patients with ALL. Further, when the ovarian cortex tissue of patients with ALL was xenografted into immunodeficient mice, the mice developed intraperitoneal leukemic masses [37]. These findings suggest that in patients with leukemia, reimplantation of ovarian cortex should not be recommended. Other malignancies seen in the reproductive years with a relatively high risk of ovarian metastasis are Burkitt's lymphoma and neuroblastoma. Reimplanting ovarian cortex may not be recommended in these malignancies [38, 39].

Advanced-stage breast cancer (stages III and IV) can metastasize to the ovary, and in patients with known metastatic breast cancer, it may be prudent not to cryopreserve and then reimplant cortical strips [14]. In contrast, more than 10 women with Hodgkin's lymphoma have received reimplanted ovarian cortex tissue, and no relapses have been documented so far [40–42]. All ovarian cortex tissue should be examined for malignant cells or minimal residual disease prior to being reimplanted [3, 43].

As ovarian tissue cryopreservation and reimplantation techniques are fairly new and not in widespread use as of this publication. The true long-term risk of metastasis in patients with malignancy who had ovarian cortex reimplanted remains to be seen.

Whole Ovary

Cryopreservation of ovarian cortical strips and then reimplantation lead to follicular loss secondary to ischemia. Transplantation of a whole ovary may result in less follicular loss as vascular supply to the tissue in theory can be more quickly established, decreasing follicular loss secondary to ischemia. The challenges of whole ovary cryopreservation include optimizing methods for cryopreservation of large organs such as the ovary, which can be difficult as cryoprotectants do not diffuse well into whole organs and intravascular ice formation can cause vascular injury. Also, the technical aspect of harvesting and reimplanting a whole ovary requires a skilled surgeon to preserve a long and intact vascular pedicle at the time of harvesting and then perform the vascular reanastomosis at the time of reimplantation.

Whole ovary autotransplantation was first described using fresh ovaries in various animal models, including rats, sheep, and monkeys. Some authors reported on sheep ovaries, which were autotransplanted into the abdominal wall with microsurgical vascular anastomosis of the ovarian to the inferior epigastric vessels. After 7 days, the ovaries were removed and noted to have surviving follicles [44].

In a rodent model, successful transplantation of ovaries, fallopian tubes, and the upper segment of the uterus en bloc after cryopreservation was reported in 2002. In four out of seven attempts at transplantation, the rat ovaries survived 60 days or more and one pregnancy resulted [45]. Recently, adult female sheep have become a standard model to study intact ovary cryopreservation [46, 47]. Arav et al. described transplantation of frozen–thawed intact ovaries in eight sheep by artery and vein anastomosis to the contralateral ovarian artery and vein. From 24 to 36 months after the ovary was reimplanted, progesterone activity was detected in three sheep. Oocyte retrieval was successful in two sheep, and in embryonic development up to the 8-cell stage was noted [48]. Bedaiwy et al. described restoration of ovarian function in frozen–thawed sheep ovaries reimplanted with microvascular anastomosis. Yet, 8 of 11 ovaries failed due to thrombosis at the pedicle site [49]. In 2006, a liveborn lamb was reported after orthotopic microvascular reanastomosis of a whole cryopreserved ovary [50]. Whole ovary cryopreservation in the sheep has been attempted through both slow-cooling and vitrification methodologies [47, 51–53]. Recently, ovarian function of cryopreserved and transplanted whole sheep ovaries has been demonstrated 6 years after transplantation. This is the longest reported ovarian function of frozen–thawed whole ovaries [54].

In humans, the first report of cryopreservation and then thawing of a whole ovary was described by Martinez-Madrid et al. in 2004. They found that the percentage of live follicles was 99.4% in fresh tissue, 98.1% after cryoprotectant exposure, and 75.1% after thawing, and they also reported high survival rates of stromal cells and small vessels after thawing [55]. Bedaiwy et al. have recently described that successful cryopreservation of the human ovary in two premenopausal women with overall viability of the primordial follicles was 75 and 78% in intact cryopreserved–thawed ovaries [49]. Further, Patrizio et al. reported on successful whole human ovary cryopreservation with the vascular pedicle utilizing a Multi-Thermal-Gradient device and a slow-cooling, rapid-thawing protocol (Fig. 33.1) [56]. The ovaries were thawed

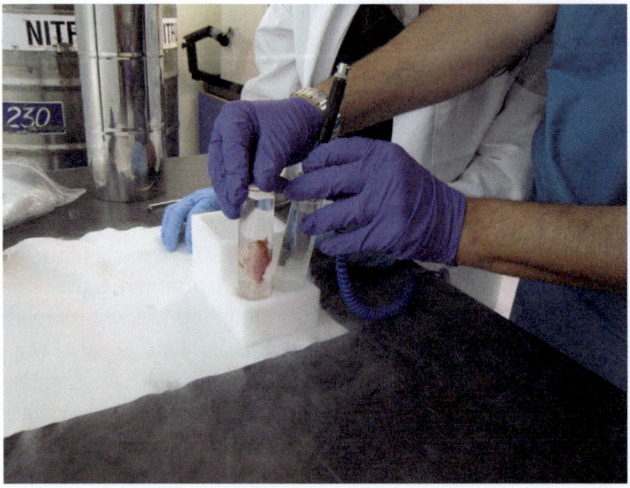

Fig. 33.1 Seeding of whole ovary in the glass tube prior to being loaded in the Multi-Thermal-Gradient device for cryopreservation

Table 33.1 A comparison of cryopreservation of cortical strips vs. whole ovaries

	Cortical strip	Whole ovary
Laparoscopic harvesting possible	Yes	Yes
Preserves ovarian stroma	No	Yes
Loss of follicles after cryopreservation	Yes	Yes
Loss of follicles due to ischemia	Yes	Yes
Microvascular anastomosis possible[a]	No	Yes
Short-term endocrine function	Yes	Yes
Long-term endocrine function	No	Yes

Adapted from Bromer and Patrizio [58], with permission

[a]In the event of anastomosis failure, the whole ovary will be lost. Cortical strips offer an advantage here because multiple strips are harvested and transplanted. If the loss of one cortical strip occurs, the others may remain viable

after cryopreservation for 2–4 days, and the frozen–thawed ovary was histologically similar to the fresh contralateral ovary used as a control and modest increase in markers of apoptosis. In three cases, the fallopian tube was cryopreserved along with the whole ovary, and after thawing, the histologic architecture was intact [57].

At the time of this writing, however, no cases of reimplanting a frozen–thawed whole ovary resulting in a live birth have been reported in humans. It is possible that the risks of whole ovary transplantation are greater than with ovarian cortical strips, as transplantation of a whole ovary may result in a higher risk of metastasis. Also, when transplanting organs such as a whole ovary, if the vascular anastomosis fails, then the whole ovary is lost. This compares to the transplantation of cortical strips which can be reimplanted in batches so that if the initial procedure fails, it can be repeated with the remaining cortical strips. See Table 33.1 for a comparison of the cryopreservation of whole ovaries vs. cortical strips.

Conclusions

There is a large need for fertility preservation options for cancer survivors, yet at this time, ovarian tissue cryopreservation for fertility preservation remains experimental. Ovarian cortex banking may be offered to patients undergoing gonadotoxic therapy under an approved experimental protocol when ovarian stimulation and in vitro fertilization is not an option. Cryopreservation and reimplantation of whole ovaries are areas where more research needs to be performed before it can be offered, even experimentally, to patients desiring fertility preservation. Future work will focus on clarifying patient selection for ovarian tissue cryopreservation. In addition, technical methods of cryopreservation of ovarian tissue should be optimized to enhance follicular survival. Lastly, surgical techniques for revascularization of thawed whole ovaries need to be perfected. The current outlook is hopeful that in the near future, ovarian tissue cryopreservation will be a viable treatment option for fertility preservation.

References

1. Chatterjee R, Goldstone AH. Gonadal damage and effects on fertility in adult patients with haematological malignancy undergoing stem cell transplantation. Bone Marrow Transplant. 1996;17(1):5–11.
2. Barlow DH. Premature ovarian failure. Baillieres Clin Obstet Gynaecol. 1996;10(3):361–84.
3. Sonmezer M, Oktay K. Fertility preservation in female patients. Hum Reprod Update. 2004; 10(3):251–66.
4. Sklar C. Reproductive physiology and treatment-related loss of sex hormone production. Med Pediatr Oncol. 1999;33(1):2–8.
5. Bakker B, Oostdijk W, Bresters D, Walenkamp MJ, Vossen JM, Wit JM. Disturbances of growth and endocrine function after busulphan-based conditioning for haematopoietic stem cell transplantation during infancy and childhood. Bone Marrow Transplant. 2004;33(10):1049–56.
6. Grifo JA, Noyes N. Delivery rate using cryopreserved oocytes is comparable to conventional in vitro fertilization using fresh oocytes: potential fertility preservation for female cancer patients. Fertil Steril. 2010;93(2):391–6.
7. Stillman RJ, Schinfeld JS, Schiff I, et al. Ovarian failure in long-term survivors of childhood malignancy. Am J Obstet Gynecol. 1981;139(1):62–6.
8. Byrne J. Infertility and premature menopause in childhood cancer survivors. Med Pediatr Oncol. 1999;33(1):24–8.
9. Afify Z, Shaw PJ, Clavano-Harding A, Cowell CT. Growth and endocrine function in children with acute myeloid leukaemia after bone marrow transplantation using busulfan/cyclophosphamide. Bone Marrow Transplant. 2000;25(10):1087–92.
10. Wallace WH, Shalet SM, Crowne EC, Morris-Jones PH, Gattamaneni HR. Ovarian failure following abdominal irradiation in childhood: natural history and prognosis. Clin Oncol (R Coll Radiol). 1989;1(2):75–9.
11. Gosden RG, Baird DT, Wade JC, Webb R. Restoration of fertility to oophorectomized sheep by ovarian autografts stored at -196 degrees C. Hum Reprod. 1994;9(4):597–603.
12. Nugent D, Meirow D, Brook PF, Aubard Y, Gosden RG. Transplantation in reproductive medicine: previous experience, present knowledge and future prospects. Hum Reprod Update. 1997;3(3):267–80.
13. Oktay K, Buyuk E, Rosenwaks Z, Rucinski J. A technique for transplantation of ovarian cortical strips to the forearm. Fertil Steril. 2003;80(1):193–8.

14. von Wolff M, Donnez J, Hovatta O, et al. Cryopreservation and autotransplantation of human ovarian tissue prior to cytotoxic therapy–a technique in its infancy but already successful in fertility preservation. Eur J Cancer. 2009;45(9):1547–53.
15. Mayerhofer K, Ott J, Nouri K, et al. Laparoscopic ovarian tissue harvesting for cryopreservation: an effective and safe procedure for fertility preservation. Eur J Obstet Gynecol Reprod Biol. 2010;152(1):68–72.
16. Silber SJ, DeRosa M, Pineda J, et al. A series of monozygotic twins discordant for ovarian failure: ovary transplantation (cortical versus microvascular) and cryopreservation. Hum Reprod. 2008;23(7): 1531–7.
17. Baird DT, Webb R, Campbell BK, Harkness LM, Gosden RG. Long-term ovarian function in sheep after ovariectomy and transplantation of autografts stored at -196°C. Endocrinology. 1999;140(1):462–71.
18. Liu J, Van der Elst J, Van den Broecke R, Dhont M. Early massive follicle loss and apoptosis in heterotopically grafted newborn mouse ovaries. Hum Reprod. 2002;17(3):605–11.
19. Nisolle M, Casanas-Roux F, Qu J, Motta P, Donnez J. Histologic and ultrastructural evaluation of fresh and frozen-thawed human ovarian xenografts in nude mice. Fertil Steril. 2000;74(1): 122–9.
20. Keros V, Xella S, Hultenby K, et al. Vitrification versus controlled-rate freezing in cryopreservation of human ovarian tissue. Hum Reprod. 2009;24(7):1670–83.
21. Salle B, Demirci B, Franck M, Rudigoz RC, Guerin JF, Lornage J. Normal pregnancies and live births after autograft of frozen-thawed hemi-ovaries into ewes. Fertil Steril. 2002;77(2): 403–8.
22. Oktay K, Economos K, Kan M, Rucinski J, Veeck L, Rosenwaks Z. Endocrine function and oocyte retrieval after autologous transplantation of ovarian cortical strips to the forearm. JAMA. 2001;286(12):1490–3.
23. Oktay K, Buyuk E, Veeck L, et al. Embryo development after heterotopic transplantation of cryopreserved ovarian tissue. Lancet. 2004;363(9412):837–40.
24. Donnez J, Dolmans MM, Demylle D, et al. Livebirth after orthotopic transplantation of cryopreserved ovarian tissue. Lancet. 2004;364(9443):1405–10.
25. Meirow D, Levron J, Eldar-Geva T, et al. Pregnancy after transplantation of cryopreserved ovarian tissue in a patient with ovarian failure after chemotherapy. N Engl J Med. 2005;353(3): 318–21.
26. Demeestere I, Simon P, Emiliani S, Delbaere A, Englert Y. Fertility preservation: successful transplantation of cryopreserved ovarian tissue in a young patient previously treated for Hodgkin's disease. Oncologist. 2007;12(12):1437–42.
27. Andersen CY, Rosendahl M, Byskov AG, et al. Two successful pregnancies following autotransplantation of frozen/thawed ovarian tissue. Hum Reprod. 2008;23:2266–72.
28. Sanchez-Serrano M, Crespo J, Mirabet V, et al. Twins born after transplantation of ovarian cortical tissue and oocyte vitrification. Fertil Steril. 2010;93:268.e11–3.
29. Roux C, Amiot C, Agnani G, Aubard Y, Rohrlich PS, Piver P. Live birth after ovarian tissue autograft in a patient with sickle cell disease treated by allogeneic bone marrow transplantation. Fertil Steril. 2010;93(7):2413.e15–19.
30. Silber S, Kagawa N, Kuwayama M, Gosden R. Duration of fertility after fresh and frozen ovary transplantation. Fertil Steril. 2010;94:2191–6.
31. Demeestere I, Simon P, Buxant F, et al. Ovarian function and spontaneous pregnancy after combined heterotopic and orthotopic cryopreserved ovarian tissue transplantation in a patient previously treated with bone marrow transplantation: case report. Hum Reprod. 2006;21(8): 2010–4.
32. Ernst E, Bergholdt S, Jorgensen JS, Andersen CY. The first woman to give birth to two children following transplantation of frozen/thawed ovarian tissue. Hum Reprod. 2010;25(5):1280–1.
33. Rosendahl M, Loft A, Byskov AG, et al. Biochemical pregnancy after fertilization of an oocyte aspirated from a heterotopic autotransplant of cryopreserved ovarian tissue: case report. Hum Reprod. 2006;21(8):2006–9.

34. Lee DM, Yeoman RR, Battaglia DE, et al. Live birth after ovarian tissue transplant. Nature. 2004;428(6979):137–8.
35. Courbiere B, Prebet T, Mozziconacci MJ, Metzler-Guillemain C, Saias-Magnan J, Gamerre M. Tumor cell contamination in ovarian tissue cryopreserved before gonadotoxic treatment: should we systematically exclude ovarian autograft in a cancer survivor? Bone Marrow Transplant. 2010;45(7):1247–8.
36. Rosendahl M, Andersen MT, Ralfkiaer E, Kjeldsen L, Andersen MK, Andersen CY. Evidence of residual disease in cryopreserved ovarian cortex from female patients with leukemia. Fertil Steril. 2010;94:2186–90.
37. Dolmans MM, Marinescu C, Saussoy P, Van Langendonckt A, Amorim C, Donnez J. Reimplantation of cryopreserved ovarian tissue from patients with acute lymphoblastic leukemia is potentially unsafe. Blood. 2010;116:2908–14.
38. Meirow D, Hardan I, Dor J, et al. Searching for evidence of disease and malignant cell contamination in ovarian tissue stored from hematologic cancer patients. Hum Reprod. 2008;23(5): 1007–13.
39. Sonmezer M, Oktay K. Orthotopic and heterotopic ovarian tissue transplantation. Best Pract Res Clin Obstet Gynaecol. 2010;24(1):113–26.
40. Meirow D, Ben Yehuda D, Prus D, et al. Ovarian tissue banking in patients with Hodgkin's disease: is it safe? Fertil Steril. 1998; 69(6):996–8.
41. Seshadri T, Gook D, Lade S, et al. Lack of evidence of disease contamination in ovarian tissue harvested for cryopreservation from patients with Hodgkin lymphoma and analysis of factors predictive of oocyte yield. Br J Cancer. 2006;94(7):1007–10.
42. Wallace WH, Anderson RA, Irvine DS. Fertility preservation for young patients with cancer: who is at risk and what can be offered? Lancet Oncol. 2005;6(4):209–18.
43. Blumenfeld Z. Gynaecologic concerns for young women exposed to gonadotoxic chemotherapy. Curr Opin Obstet Gynecol. 2003; 15(5):359–70.
44. Jeremias E, Bedaiwy MA, Gurunluoglu R, Biscotti CV, Siemionow M, Falcone T. Heterotopic autotransplantation of the ovary with microvascular anastomosis: a novel surgical technique. Fertil Steril. 2002;77(6):1278–82.
45. Wang X, Chen H, Yin H, Kim SS, Lin Tan S, Gosden RG. Fertility after intact ovary transplantation. Nature. 2002;415(6870):385.
46. Bedaiwy MA, Jeremias E, Gurunluoglu R, et al. Restoration of ovarian function after autotransplantation of intact frozen-thawed sheep ovaries with microvascular anastomosis. Fertil Steril. 2003;79(3):594–602.
47. Revel A, Elami A, Bor A, Yavin S, Natan Y, Arav A. Whole sheep ovary cryopreservation and transplantation. Fertil Steril. 2004; 82(6):1714–5.
48. Arav A, Revel A, Nathan Y, et al. Oocyte recovery, embryo development and ovarian function after cryopreservation and transplantation of whole sheep ovary. Hum Reprod. 2005;20(12): 3554–9.
49. Bedaiwy MA, Hussein MR, Biscotti C, Falcone T. Cryopreservation of intact human ovary with its vascular pedicle. Hum Reprod. 2006;21(12):3258–69.
50. Imhof M, Bergmeister H, Lipovac M, Rudas M, Hofstetter G, Huber J. Orthotopic microvascular reanastomosis of whole cryopreserved ovine ovaries resulting in pregnancy and live birth. Fertil Steril. 2006;85 Suppl 1:1208–15.
51. Courbiere B, Massardier J, Salle B, Mazoyer C, Guerin JF, Lornage J. Follicular viability and histological assessment after cryopreservation of whole sheep ovaries with vascular pedicle by vitrification. Fertil Steril. 2005;84 Suppl 2:1065–71.
52. Imhof M, Hofstetter G, Bergmeister H, et al. Cryopreservation of a whole ovary as a strategy for restoring ovarian function. J Assist Reprod Genet. 2004;21(12):459–65.
53. Fahy GM, Wowk B, Wu J, et al. Cryopreservation of organs by vitrification: perspectives and recent advances. Cryobiology. 2004;48(2):157–78.
54. Arav A, Gavish Z, Elami A, Natan Y, Revel A, Silber S, Patrizio P. Ovarian function 6 years after cryopreservation and transplantation of whole sheep ovaries. Reprod Biomed Online. 2010;20: 48–52.

55. Martinez-Madrid B, Dolmans MM, Van Langendonckt A, Defrere S, Donnez J. Freeze-thawing intact human ovary with its vascular pedicle with a passive cooling device. Fertil Steril. 2004; 82(5):1390–4.
56. Patrizio P, Gavish Z, Martel M, Azodi M, Silber S, Arav A. Whole ovary cryopreservation using a novel multi-gradient freezing device. Presented at the 63rd annual meeting of the American Society of Reproductive Medicine, Washington; 2007.
57. Patrizio P, Arav A, Bromer JG, Martel M, Azodi M, Siber S. Cryopreservation of whole human ovaries together with fallopian tubes. Presented at the 64th annual meeting of the American Society of Reproductive Medicine, San Francisco; 2008.
58. Bromer J, Patrizio P. Fertility preservation: the rationale for cryopreservation of the whole ovary. Semin Reprod Med. 2009;27(6): 465–71.

Part VII
Embryo Transfer

Chapter 34
Assessment of Uterine Receptivity

Hakan Cakmak and Hugh S. Taylor

Embryo implantation represents the most critical step of the reproductive process and consists of a unique biological phenomenon. The blastocyst comes into intimate contact with the endometrium and forms the placenta that will provide an interface between the growing fetus and the maternal circulation. Successful implantation requires a receptive endometrium, a viable embryo at the blastocyst stage, and a synchronized dialogue between maternal and embryonic tissues [1].

The human endometrium undergoes a complex series of organized proliferative and secretory changes in each menstrual cycle and exhibits only a short period of receptivity, known as the "window of implantation" [2]. In humans, during a natural cycle, the embryo enters the uterine cavity 4 days after ovulation. The endometrium becomes receptive to blastocyst implantation approximately 6 days after ovulation and remains receptive for 4 days (cycle days 20–24) [3]. When implantation does not occur, a timely destruction of the fully developed endometrium leads to menstruation. However, if implantation occurs, the endometrium continues to grow and undergoes further morphological and molecular changes to support the growing embryo [2].

Implantation has three stages: apposition, adhesion, and penetration. Apposition is the unstable adhesion of the blastocyst to the endometrial surface. During this stage, the trophoblast becomes closely apposed to the luminal epithelium [4]. This is followed by the adhesion stage in which the association of the trophoblast and the luminal epithelium is strong enough to resist dislocation of the blastocyst by flushing the uterine lumen. This stage occurs on day 20–21 in humans and coincides with a localized increase in the vascular permeability at the site of blastocyst attachment.

H. Cakmak, MD (✉)
Department of Obstetrics, Gynecology and Reproductive Sciences,
Yale-New Haven Hospital, New Haven, CT, USA
e-mail: Hakan.cakmak@yale.edu

H.S. Taylor, MD
Section of Reproductive Endocrinology and Infertility, Department of Obstetrics,
Gynecology and Reproductive Sciences, Yale University School of Medicine,
New Haven, CT, USA

Z.P. Nagy et al. (eds.), *Clinical Embryology: A Practical Guide*,
DOI 10.1007/978-1-4614-8376-2_34, © Springer Science+Business Media New York 2013

Local paracrine signaling between the embryo and endometrium triggers a stronger attachment [5]. Following adhesion, the embryo invades through the luminal epithelium into the stroma to establish a vascular connection with the mother, and this process is mainly controlled by trophoblasts; however, the decidua also limits the extent of invasion [5]. In response to this invasion and progesterone, the endometrial stromal cells and extracellular matrix undergo decidualization that is essential for the viability of the pregnancy.

Uterine receptivity plays a key role in establishment of successful pregnancies, and its impairment may limit assisted reproductive technologies (ART) success and contribute to the subfertility in several benign gynecologic disorders including endometriosis, hydrosalpinx, leiomyoma, endometrial polyp, adenomyosis, endometritis, and polycystic ovarian syndrome [6]. ART tools are now available that enable the selection of high-quality embryos, and protocols continue to evolve with the aim of achieving higher pregnancy rates, fewer multiple births, as well as healthy babies from genetically affected progenitors. However, despite these advances, implantation rates are still relatively low and have not increased sufficiently in the last decade to allow widespread adoption of single embryo transfer [7].

From a clinical point of view, practitioners need to have objective measurements to determine the probability for a healthy pregnancy, evaluating aspects of both embryo and endometrium, in a given menstrual cycle. This chapter aims to summarize the current knowledge about the available assessment methods of uterine receptivity.

Histological Assessment of the Endometrium

Histological analysis of the endometrium during the implantation window is limited by methodological issues, and there is no strong data to support the link between the endometrial receptivity and morphology within the same cycle.

Prerequisites for an adequate histological evaluation are exact timing of the biopsy within the cycle, selection of representative tissue of the functional endometrial layers, and optimal fixation and processing of the specimen. Timing of the endometrial biopsy must be synchronized to the LH surge, preferentially measured in serum.

Endometrium is a morphologically complex organ, encompassing several functional compartments with cellular heterogeneity that undergoes profound cyclic variations. In vivo studies are performed almost exclusively in nonconceptual cycles, and the quantification of profound cyclic variations in a reproducible manner is difficult. Noyes and coworkers examined the histological features of endometrial biopsies taken during 8,000 spontaneous cycles in 300 women and created the criteria for endometrial dating that previously accepted as gold standard approach for evaluating endometrial responsiveness and detecting endometrial abnormalities [8]. However, a number of weaknesses in Noyes' approach have been identified. Dating is most accurate in the early and late luteal phase, but not in the implantation window as very few histological parameters allow differentiation within the time span of the receptive endometrium [9]. The most notable weakness is high intra- and interobserver variability. Intraobserver variability has been shown to be highest among infertile women during the implantation window [9, 10]. Furthermore, ovarian stimulation in artificial cycles may lead to differences in the timing of endometrial maturation compared with natural cycles [11]. Additionally, histological dating does not discriminate between women of fertile and infertile couples and is therefore not a valid tool in routine evaluation of infertility or implantation failure [12].

Endometrial biopsy has proven to be useful for the diagnosis of intrauterine inflammatory states. Chronic endometritis has been associated with infertility and implantation failure because of the possible action of microbial products on the endometrial receptivity [13]. Patients with chronic endometritis have significantly lower clinical pregnancy and implantation rates (11 and 8%) compared with patients with negative biopsies (58 and 31%) [14]. Endometritis has been described in approximately 15% of patients undergoing a hysteroscopic workup before IVF and intracytoplasmic sperm injection and in up to 42% of patients with repeated IVF failure [15]. Moreover, a significant increase in pregnancy rates in subsequent IVF cycle was reported on completion of antibiotic treatment [14, 15].

Ultrastructural Assessment of Endometrium

Ultrastructural changes in endometrial epithelial morphology, characterized by the appearance of membrane projections called pinopodes, have been observed during the implantation window [16]. Pinopodes are progesterone-dependent organelles, appearing as apical cellular protrusions that become visible between days 20 and 21 of the natural menstrual cycle, as shown by scanning electron microscopy in sequential endometrial biopsies [17]. Moreover, HOXA10, a homeobox gene whose expression is necessary for endometrial receptivity to blastocyst implantation, has an essential role in pinopod development. Indeed, blocking HOXA10 expression dramatically decreases the number of pinopods [18]. Although the mechanisms of action of pinopodes are still unclear, blastocyst attachment has been shown to occur at the top of endometrial pinopods [19]. Hypothetically, the receptors required for blastocyst adhesion may be located on the pinopod surface.

The clinical use of pinopod expression as a marker endometrial receptivity was supported by a study in which two consecutive endometrial biopsies were obtained during IVF mock cycles on days 6 and 8 of progesterone administration. The day of maximal receptivity, as established by the day on which mature pinopodes were detected, was determined for each woman [20]. In three-fourths of the patients, a new ideal embryo transfer day was determined and used in a subsequent transfer cycle. Of these women, 67% delivered a healthy baby. For one-fourth of women with no indication for modification to their transfer protocol, take-home baby rate was only 25%. However, the reproducibility and reliability of pinopod expression for testing endometrial receptivity was challenged by other studies. Poor intrapatient consistency in pinopode scores of postovulatory day 7 endometrial samples at consecutive cycles was demonstrated among infertile women [21]. Pinopode expression was not limited to the window of implantation but persists through to the end of the luteal phase [21, 22]. Another intriguing observation was that infertile women exhibit equivalent number of pinopodes as fertile controls at the time of implantation window [21–23]. Overall, there are mixed reports about the use of pinopods as an implantation marker in human; therefore, it should not be used as a predictor of the most receptive day of the cycle in clinical practice.

Functional Assessment of Endometrium

Implantation involves a complex sequence of signaling events that are crucial to the establishment of pregnancy. A number of molecular mediators, which are regulated with highest levels in the mid-secretory phase under the influence of ovarian hormones, have been postulated to be involved in this early feto–maternal interaction. These mediators embrace a large variety of interrelated molecules including adhesion molecules, cytokines, growth factors, and homeobox genes. The use of some of these molecules (such as αvβ3 integrin, MUC1, LIF, and HOXA10) has been investigated in order to identify a marker to better assess endometrial receptivity [24–27].

The Endometrial Function Test® (EFT) involves immunohistochemically staining of the endometrium with markers for the mitotic regulators cyclin E (the rate-limiting activator of the mitotic G1 to S phase transition) and p27 (an inhibitor of cyclin E) [28]. However, the use of endometrial receptivity markers has not been widely adopted clinically. αvβ3 integrin testing and the EFT are the only commercially available methods, and their clinical use has not yet been shown to improve pregnancy outcomes. Moreover, immunohistochemistry is subject to the same restrictions of histological assessment such as adequate timing of the endometrial biopsy and sampling accuracy. Overall, there is no perfect clinical assay to detect implantation defect so far.

Since morphological and single-gene approaches have failed to identify a marker that could be used in a clinical assay, research is now shifting toward microarray or global gene analysis [29]. DNA microarrays enable analysis of the simultaneous expression of thousands of genes in a single sample. Gene expression is a better marker of the biological phases and is likely a more reliable predictor of endometrial receptivity than morphology. A number of microarray studies have been performed during the implantation window, and all have reported genes that are strongly up- or downregulated when the endometrium is receptive [30–34]. The information obtained from microarray studies is currently being used to form databases against which future biopsies can hopefully be compared to assist in patient management. The use of genome-wide arrays should eventually enable the verification of a cassette of genes that reliably predict or reflect endometrial receptivity as opposed to a single marker. As well as array technologies being used to study gene expression, methods are also being developed to study proteomic changes occurring during implantation. Endometrial secretion aspiration is one such approach and enables the measurement of protein changes in the uterine lumen during treatment cycles [35].

Morphological Assessment of the Endometrium

Ultrasonography

Ideally, a technique to assess endometrium and thereby predict endometrial receptivity must be easily performable within the daily clinical routine and would preferably be noninvasive. These requirements are met by ultrasonographic evaluation of endometrium.

Endometrial thickness is defined as the minimal distance between the echogenic interfaces of myometrium and endometrium, measured in the plane through the central longitudinal axis of the uterine body. Endometrial thickness is a relatively easily obtained and objective measurement with low intraobserver and interobserver variability [36]. In premenopausal women, the endometrium is thinnest at the end of menstruation and appears as a single thin, well-defined line. The endometrial lining then expands under the influence of estrogen in the follicular phase of the cycle to the typical trilaminar hypoechoic appearance that measures typically between 6 and 10 mm in thickness [37]. After ovulation, the endometrium thickens to a diameter of 7–14 mm and becomes homogeneously echogenic under the influence of progesterone.

Compared with the natural cycle, sonographic endometrial lining is slightly thicker in patients receiving gonadotropin injections for infertility, and the thickness of the endometrium correlates with serum estradiol concentration [38]. The presence of endometrial polyps or intracavitary fibroids can falsely elevate the apparent endometrial thickness. Diethylstilbestrol (DES) exposure and intrauterine adhesions (Asherman's syndrome) will decrease the endometrial thickness.

Pregnancy rates after IVF are influenced only marginally by the endometrial thickness [38, 39]. Endometrial thickness has poor specificity and positive predictive value of 21 and 45%, respectively. In other words, many women with a normal endometrial thickness will still not be pregnant after transfer of embryos. The data extracted from the donor oocyte programs suggest that a pregnancy cannot be achieved if the endometrium thickness is below a certain critical cutoff limit. Although there are studies revealing that the thickness of endometrium for a successful implantation can be as thin as 4 mm [40–42] for the majority of the cases, at least 6 mm thickness of endometrium should be set forth as the prerequisite for a successful implantation [43, 44]. However, no correlation was demonstrated between endometrial histology and endometrial thickness either in spontaneous ovulatory cycles or in IVF patients [45, 46]. Fortunately, the proportion of patients with an unusually thin endometrium is low. If a pregnancy does not occur in a woman found to have a thin endometrium, then she should be assessed after the cycle for intrauterine pathology including Asherman's syndrome.

There is no consensus regarding the effect of abnormally thick endometrium on pregnancy rates during IVF cycles. Poor pregnancy and implantation rates were reported when the endometrial thickness was >14 mm on the day of hCG administration, or >15 mm on the day of embryo transfer, and >16 mm on the day of oocyte retrieval [47–49]. In contrast, others have found no effect of an increased thickness on pregnancy rates [50].

The ultrasonographic texture of the endometrium may have a prognostic value for implantation. In gonadotropin-stimulated cycles, echogenicity is usually assessed on the day of hCG administration. The "optimal" pattern is characterized by a multilayered hypoechogenic triple line pattern, but a hyperechogenic, homogenous solid pattern has also been described. Significantly reduced clinical pregnancy rate was demonstrated in patients with a solid endometrial pattern (34%) compared to those with a trilaminar pattern (47%) [41]. The interpretation of these findings is probably that an early luteal appearance is a sign of early progesterone production rather than any inherent fault with endometrial development. Hypoechogenic triple line pattern has a low positive predictive value (32%) for clinical pregnancy after assisted reproduction treatment [39]. In contrast, a hyperechogenic solid pattern has a reasonably high negative predictive value for pregnancy (75–89%) [39]. However, homogenously solid pattern should not be used an indication to cancel embryo transfers since patients with this endometrial pattern still have acceptable pregnancy rates after embryo transfer.

Transvaginal ultrasonography, especially when performed during the late follicular phase, provides excellent imaging of the uterus and of endometrial abnormalities that may affect the endometrial receptivity including endometrial polyps, leiomyoma, and adenomyosis.

Uterine fibroids can be detected by transvaginal ultrasound with great sensitivity. Leiomyomas are present in approximately 5–10% of women with infertility and are the sole factor identified in 1–2.4% [51]. Intramural and submucosal leiomyomas can distort the uterine cavity or obstruct the tubal ostia or cervical canal and, thus, may affect fertility [52]. Recent studies demonstrated that leiomyomas may also adversely affect the overlying endometrium and globally impair endometrial receptivity [53, 54]. Moreover, in the setting of a distorted uterine cavity caused by leiomyomas, significantly lower IVF pregnancy rates were identified [52, 55]. When myomectomies have been performed on women with otherwise unexplained infertility, the subsequent pregnancy rates have been reported to be 40–60% after 1–2 years [56, 57].

When evaluating the endometrium, endometrial polyps are not uncommonly found in infertile women. Endometrial polyps are identified by hysteroscopy in 16–26% of women with otherwise unexplained infertility, and the rate is much higher (46%) in infertile women with endometriosis [58, 59]. Endometrial polyps can be suggested by irregularities within the endometrial echo on traditional transvaginal ultrasound. Polyps are best detected by either saline infusion sonohysterography (SIS) or hysteroscopy as these have approximately equal sensitivity and specificity. The mechanism by which polyps may adversely affect fertility is also poorly understood but may be related to mechanical interference with sperm transport or embryo implantation. The only randomized trial examining the effect of polypectomy on pregnancy rate after intrauterine insemination demonstrated a statistically significant improvement in pregnancy rate in women who underwent hysteroscopic polypectomy compared with those who did not undergo polypectomy (63% vs. 28%) [60]. Three nonrandomized studies also found an association between polypectomy and improved spontaneous pregnancy rates [61–63]. The effect of endometrial polyps on IVF remains unclear. Further, endometrial polyps <2 cm in size do not appear to impact IVF outcome.

A pathologic finding that can be mistaken for leiomyoma on ultrasound is adenomyosis. It is characterized by the presence of heterotopic endometrial glands and stroma in the myometrium with adjacent smooth muscle hyperplasia. Common ultrasound findings of adenomyosis include an enlarged uterus, poor definition of the endomyometrial junction, and the presence of myometrial cysts. Compared with fibroids, adenomyosis is characterized by more variable echogenicity and by a poorly defined lesion border. Ultrasound lacks adequate sensitivity and specificity identify adenomyosis. Magnetic resonance imaging using a T2-weighted image has improved test characteristics, but even MRI lacks both sensitivity and specificity to make it an ideal test for adenomyosis. An association between adenomyosis and subfertility has not been fully established. The presenting symptoms include a soft and diffusely enlarged uterus with menorrhagia, dysmenorrhoea, and metrorrhagia. Infertility is a less frequent complaint, since uterine adenomyosis is usually diagnosed in the fourth and fifth decade of life. However, when adenomyosis is encountered in younger reproductive age women, it is likely to reduce endometrial receptivity.

Transvaginal ultrasound may also be used to diagnose hydrosalpinges that are described as distally blocked, dilated, fluid-filled fallopian tubes with a heterogeneous spectrum of pathology. Two meta-analyses have shown that women with hydrosalpinx have lower implantation, pregnancy and delivery rates, and a higher incidence of spontaneous abortion after IVF-embryo transfer compared with women with tubal infertility of other causes [64, 65]. Furthermore, a prospective randomized clinical trial and a Cochrane review have demonstrated improved pregnancy and delivery rates with laparoscopic salpingectomy for hydrosalpinges prior to IVF, and the greatest beneficial effect was seen in women in whom the hydrosalpinges were both bilateral and visible by ultrasound [66, 67]. These findings suggest that, besides occluding the fallopian tubes, hydrosalpinx may also affect infertility through other mechanisms such as the impairment of endometrial receptivity by decreasing the expression of specific factors including $\alpha v\beta 3$ integrin, LIF, and HOXA10 [68–70]. Furthermore, if the hydrosalpinges are removed, the expression of these markers returns to normal physiological levels in these patients [68–71].

Saline Infusion Sonohysterography

SIS is a procedure in which warm saline is instilled into the uterine cavity to provide enhanced endometrial visualization during transvaginal ultrasound. This technique improves detection of potential anatomic causes of reduced fertility, such as submucosal myomas, endometrial polyps, and intrauterine adhesions. The sensitivity, specificity, positive predictive value, and negative predictive value of SIS have been reported to be 98, 94, 95, and 98%, respectively [72]. In addition, it helps avoid invasive diagnostic procedures as well as optimize the preoperative triage process for women requiring therapeutic intervention. It is typically scheduled early in the follicular phase of the menstrual cycle, after cessation of menstrual flow and before day 10, as the endometrium is thin at this point in the cycle. Later in the cycle, focal contour irregularities of the endometrium may be mistaken for small polyps or focal areas of endometrial hyperplasia. Sonohysterography usually depicts leiomyomas and accurately assesses their location, size, and degree of intramural extension. It has added advantage of better estimation of the percentage circumference projecting into the endometrial cavity. This is important because if removal is planned, a greater than 50% projection of the leiomyoma into the uterine cavity suggests that hysteroscopic removal, instead of open removal, can be performed [73]. Therefore, in experienced hands, SIS may be an easy, safe, and well-tolerated alternative to diagnostic hysteroscopy in the initial evaluation of the uterine cavity.

Hysteroscopy

Hysteroscopy is considered to be the gold standard in the diagnosis of intrauterine pathology, including endometrial polyp, submucous leiomyoma, and intrauterine adhesions. Hysteroscopy can be performed without general anesthesia in an ambulatory setting with low cost, minimal morbidity, and inconvenience to the patient [74]. Furthermore, it gives the opportunity to correct the majority of the pathologies at the same time. There is no doubt that hysteroscopy should be performed when there is suspicion of intrauterine pathology at transvaginal ultrasonography or SIS. However, even when no abnormality is detected with these tools, subtle intrauterine pathologies have been noted in 18–50% of patients undergoing IVF at hysteroscopy [75]. In patients with at least two failed IVF or ICSI attempts, simple diagnostic or operative hysteroscopy before a subsequent IVF or ICSI treatment has shown to improve reproductive outcome [76, 77]. The higher pregnancy rates after hysteroscopy even in the absence of intrauterine pathology are a somewhat unexpected but biologically plausible observation. It is possible that cervical dilatation and/or an immunological mechanism triggered by the hysteroscopic manipulation or by the effect of the distension medium on the endometrium might play a role [78].

Conclusions

Receptive endometrium is indispensable for a successful pregnancy in ART cycles. Unfortunately, endometrial biopsy is invasive, and current histological dating and markers of endometrial receptivity are poor predictors of pregnancy. Evaluation using endometrial biopsy has not been shown to improve pregnancy outcomes. The need to evaluate endometrial development encouraged the use of ultrasonography as an alternative noninvasive method of assessment for uterine receptivity. Ultrasonographic endometrial thickness measurement and endometrial pattern determination were utilized to assess uterine receptivity and consequently to better predict pregnancy outcome in ART cycles. However, the endometrial sonographic parameters used to evaluate uterine receptivity still lack specificity, and its prognostic value in determining pregnancy rate is low. In contrast, endometrial biopsy and ultrasonography can be used efficiently to diagnose gynecologic disease that may affect uterine receptivity. Although hysteroscopy is the gold standard to evaluate endometrial lining and has been shown to improve pregnancy outcomes after failed IVF cycles, it should not be offered as a first-line investigation in all subfertile women.

In summary, there is no perfect diagnostic tool to assess endometrial receptivity. However, ultrasonography should be the first-line modality in detection of various endometrial pathologies, and efforts to optimize implantation should be directed to the treatment of possible underlying gynecologic condition disrupting endometrial receptivity.

References

1. Simon C, Martin JC, Pellicer A. Paracrine regulators of implantation. Baillieres Best Pract Res Clin Obstet Gynaecol. 2000;14:815–26.
2. Strowitzki T, Germeyer A, Popovici R, et al. The human endometrium as a fertility-determining factor. Hum Reprod Update. 2006;12:617–30.
3. Bergh PA, Navot D. The impact of embryonic development and endometrial maturity on the timing of implantation. Fertil Steril. 1992;58:537–42.
4. Tabibzadeh S, Babaknia A. The signals and molecular pathways involved in implantation, a symbiotic interaction between blastocyst and endometrium involving adhesion and tissue invasion. Hum Reprod. 1995;10:1579–602.
5. Sharkey AM, Smith SK. The endometrium as a cause of implantation failure. Best Pract Res Clin Obstet Gynaecol. 2003;17:289–307.
6. Donaghay M, Lessey BA. Uterine receptivity: alterations associated with benign gynecological disease. Semin Reprod Med. 2007;25:461–75.
7. Andersen AN, Gianaroli L, Felberbaum R, et al. Assisted reproductive technology in Europe, 2001. Results generated from European registers by ESHRE. Hum Reprod. 2005;20: 1158–76.
8. Noyes RW, Hertig AT, Rock J. Dating the endometrial biopsy. Am J Obstet Gynecol. 1975;122: 262–3.
9. Myers ER, Silva S, Barnhart K, et al. Interobserver and intraobserver variability in the histological dating of the endometrium in fertile and infertile women. Fertil Steril. 2004;82: 1278–82.

10. Murray MJ, Meyer WR, Zaino RJ, et al. A critical analysis of the accuracy, reproducibility, and clinical utility of histologic endometrial dating in fertile women. Fertil Steril. 2004;81: 1333–43.
11. Papanikolaou EG, Bourgain C, Kolibianakis E, et al. Steroid receptor expression in late follicular phase endometrium in GnRH antagonist IVF cycles is already altered, indicating initiation of early luteal phase transformation in the absence of secretory changes. Hum Reprod. 2005;20:1541–7.
12. Coutifaris C, Myers ER, Guzick DS, et al. Histological dating of timed endometrial biopsy tissue is not related to fertility status. Fertil Steril. 2004;82:1264–72.
13. Devi Wold AS, Pham N, Arici A. Anatomic factors in recurrent pregnancy loss. Semin Reprod Med. 2006;24:25–32.
14. Romero R, Espinoza J, Mazor M. Can endometrial infection/inflammation explain implantation failure, spontaneous abortion, and preterm birth after in vitro fertilization? Fertil Steril. 2004;82:799–804.
15. Feghali J, Bakar J, Mayenga JM, et al. [Systematic hysteroscopy prior to in vitro fertilization]. Gynecol Obstet Fertil. 2003;31: 127–31.
16. Nikas G. Pinopodes as markers of endometrial receptivity in clinical practice. Hum Reprod. 1999;14 Suppl 2:99–106.
17. Nikas G, Aghajanova L. Endometrial pinopodes: some more understanding on human implantation? Reprod Biomed Online. 2002;4 Suppl 3:18–23.
18. Bagot CN, Kliman HJ, Taylor HS. Maternal Hoxa10 is required for pinopod formation in the development of mouse uterine receptivity to embryo implantation. Dev Dyn. 2001;222: 538–44.
19. Bentin-Ley U, Sjogren A, Nilsson L, et al. Presence of uterine pinopodes at the embryo-endometrial interface during human implantation in vitro. Hum Reprod. 1999;14:515–20.
20. Pantos K, Nikas G, Makrakis E, et al. Clinical value of endometrial pinopodes detection in artificial donation cycles. Reprod Biomed Online. 2004;9:86–90.
21. Ordi J, Creus M, Quinto L, et al. Within-subject between-cycle variability of histological dating, alpha v beta 3 integrin expression, and pinopod formation in the human endometrium. J Clin Endocrinol Metab. 2003;88:2119–25.
22. Quinn C, Ryan E, Claessens EA, et al. The presence of pinopodes in the human endometrium does not delineate the implantation window. Fertil Steril. 2007;87:1015–21.
23. Creus M, Ordi J, Fabregues F, et al. alphavbeta3 integrin expression and pinopod formation in normal and out-of-phase endometria of fertile and infertile women. Hum Reprod. 2002;17: 2279–86.
24. Lessey BA, Castelbaum AJ, Wolf L, et al. Use of integrins to date the endometrium. Fertil Steril. 2000;73:779–87.
25. Aplin JD, Hey NA, Li TC. MUC1 as a cell surface and secretory component of endometrial epithelium: reduced levels in recurrent miscarriage. Am J Reprod Immunol. 1996;35:261–6.
26. Arici A, Engin O, Attar E, et al. Modulation of leukemia inhibitory factor gene expression and protein biosynthesis in human endometrium. J Clin Endocrinol Metab. 1995;80:1908–15.
27. Taylor HS, Arici A, Olive D, et al. HOXA10 is expressed in response to sex steroids at the time of implantation in the human endometrium. J Clin Invest. 1998;101:1379–84.
28. Dubowy RL, Feinberg RF, Keefe DL, et al. Improved endometrial assessment using cyclin E and p27. Fertil Steril. 2003;80:146–56.
29. Horcajadas JA, Pellicer A, Simon C. Wide genomic analysis of human endometrial receptivity: new times, new opportunities. Hum Reprod Update. 2007;13:77–86.
30. Borthwick JM, Charnock-Jones DS, Tom BD, et al. Determination of the transcript profile of human endometrium. Mol Hum Reprod. 2003;9:19–33.
31. Carson DD, Lagow E, Thathiah A, et al. Changes in gene expression during the early to mid-luteal (receptive phase) transition in human endometrium detected by high-density microarray screening. Mol Hum Reprod. 2002;8:871–9.
32. Kao LC, Tulac S, Lobo S, et al. Global gene profiling in human endometrium during the window of implantation. Endocrinology. 2002;143:2119–38.

33. Mirkin S, Arslan M, Churikov D, et al. In search of candidate genes critically expressed in the human endometrium during the window of implantation. Hum Reprod. 2005;20:2104–17.
34. Riesewijk A, Martin J, van Os R, et al. Gene expression profiling of human endometrial receptivity on days LH+2 versus LH+7 by microarray technology. Mol Hum Reprod. 2003;9: 253–64.
35. van der Gaast MH, Beier-Hellwig K, Fauser BC, et al. Endometrial secretion aspiration prior to embryo transfer does not reduce implantation rates. Reprod Biomed Online. 2003;7:105–9.
36. Spandorfer SD, Arrendondo-Soberon F, Loret de Mola JR, et al. Reliability of intraobserver and interobserver sonographic endometrial stripe thickness measurements. Fertil Steril. 1998;70:152–4.
37. Bromer JG, Aldad TS, Taylor HS. Defining the proliferative phase endometrial defect. Fertil Steril. 2009;91:698–704.
38. De Geyter C, Schmitter M, De Geyter M, et al. Prospective evaluation of the ultrasound appearance of the endometrium in a cohort of 1,186 infertile women. Fertil Steril. 2000;73: 106–13.
39. Friedler S, Schenker JG, Herman A, et al. The role of ultrasonography in the evaluation of endometrial receptivity following assisted reproductive treatments: a critical review. Hum Reprod Update. 1996;2:323–35.
40. Check JH, Dietterich C, Check ML, et al. Successful delivery despite conception with a maximal endometrial thickness of 4 mm. Clin Exp Obstet Gynecol. 2003;30:93–4.
41. Noyes N, Liu HC, Sultan K, et al. Endometrial thickness appears to be a significant factor in embryo implantation in in-vitro fertilization. Hum Reprod. 1995;10:919–22.
42. Sundstrom P. Establishment of a successful pregnancy following in-vitro fertilization with an endometrial thickness of no more than 4 mm. Hum Reprod. 1998;13:1550–2.
43. Alam V, Bernardini L, Gonzales J, et al. A prospective study of echographic endometrial characteristics and pregnancy rates during hormonal replacement cycles. J Assist Reprod Genet. 1993;10:215–9.
44. Coulam CB, Bustillo M, Soenksen DM, et al. Ultrasonographic predictors of implantation after assisted reproduction. Fertil Steril. 1994;62:1004–10.
45. Sterzik K, Abt M, Grab D, et al. Predicting the histologic dating of an endometrial biopsy specimen with the use of Doppler ultrasonography and hormone measurements in patients undergoing spontaneous ovulatory cycles. Fertil Steril. 2000;73:94–8.
46. Sterzik K, Grab D, Schneider V, et al. Lack of correlation between ultrasonography and histologic staging of the endometrium in in vitro fertilization (IVF) patients. Ultrasound Med Biol. 1997;23:165–70.
47. Kupesic S, Bekavac I, Bjelos D, et al. Assessment of endometrial receptivity by transvaginal color Doppler and three-dimensional power Doppler ultrasonography in patients undergoing in vitro fertilization procedures. J Ultrasound Med. 2001;20:125–34.
48. Schild RL, Indefrei D, Eschweiler S, et al. Three-dimensional endometrial volume calculation and pregnancy rate in an in-vitro fertilization programme. Hum Reprod. 1999;14:1255–8.
49. Weissman A, Gotlieb L, Casper RF. The detrimental effect of increased endometrial thickness on implantation and pregnancy rates and outcome in an in vitro fertilization program. Fertil Steril. 1999;71:147–9.
50. Dietterich C, Check JH, Choe JK, et al. Increased endometrial thickness on the day of human chorionic gonadotropin injection does not adversely affect pregnancy or implantation rates following in vitro fertilization-embryo transfer. Fertil Steril. 2002;77:781–6.
51. Donnez J, Jadoul P. What are the implications of myomas on fertility? A need for a debate? Hum Reprod. 2002;17:1424–30.
52. Pritts EA. Fibroids and infertility: a systematic review of the evidence. Obstet Gynecol Surv. 2001;56:483–91.
53. Matsuzaki S, Canis M, Darcha C, et al. HOXA-10 expression in the mid-secretory endometrium of infertile patients with either endometriosis, uterine fibromas or unexplained infertility. Hum Reprod. 2009;24:3180–7.

54. Rackow BW, Taylor HS. Submucosal uterine leiomyomas have a global effect on molecular determinants of endometrial receptivity. Fertil Steril. 2010;93:2027–34.
55. Surrey ES, Lietz AK, Schoolcraft WB. Impact of intramural leiomyomata in patients with a normal endometrial cavity on in vitro fertilization-embryo transfer cycle outcome. Fertil Steril. 2001;75:405–10.
56. Campo S, Campo V, Gambadauro P. Reproductive outcome before and after laparoscopic or abdominal myomectomy for subserous or intramural myomas. Eur J Obstet Gynecol Reprod Biol. 2003; 110:215–9.
57. Sudik R, Husch K, Steller J, et al. Fertility and pregnancy outcome after myomectomy in sterility patients. Eur J Obstet Gynecol Reprod Biol. 1996;65:209–14.
58. de Sa Rosa e de Silva AC, Rosa e Silva JC, Candido dos Reis FJ, et al. Routine office hysteroscopy in the investigation of infertile couples before assisted reproduction. J Reprod Med. 2005;50:501–6.
59. Kim MR, Kim YA, Jo MY, et al. High frequency of endometrial polyps in endometriosis. J Am Assoc Gynecol Laparosc. 2003; 10:46–8.
60. Perez-Medina T, Bajo-Arenas J, Salazar F, et al. Endometrial polyps and their implication in the pregnancy rates of patients undergoing intrauterine insemination: a prospective, randomized study. Hum Reprod. 2005;20:1632–5.
61. Shokeir TA, Shalan HM, El-Shafei MM. Significance of endometrial polyps detected hysteroscopically in eumenorrheic infertile women. J Obstet Gynaecol Res. 2004;30:84–9.
62. Spiewankiewicz B, Stelmachow J, Sawicki W, et al. The effectiveness of hysteroscopic polypectomy in cases of female infertility. Clin Exp Obstet Gynecol. 2003;30:23–5.
63. Varasteh NN, Neuwirth RS, Levin B, et al. Pregnancy rates after hysteroscopic polypectomy and myomectomy in infertile women. Obstet Gynecol. 1999;94:168–71.
64. Camus E, Poncelet C, Goffinet F, et al. Pregnancy rates after in-vitro fertilization in cases of tubal infertility with and without hydrosalpinx: a meta-analysis of published comparative studies. Hum Reprod. 1999;14:1243–9.
65. Zeyneloglu HB, Arici A, Olive DL. Adverse effects of hydrosalpinx on pregnancy rates after in vitro fertilization-embryo transfer. Fertil Steril. 1998;70:492–9.
66. Johnson NP, Mak W, Sowter MC. Laparoscopic salpingectomy for women with hydrosalpinges enhances the success of IVF: a Cochrane review. Hum Reprod. 2002;17:543–8.
67. Strandell A, Lindhard A, Waldenstrom U, et al. Hydrosalpinx and IVF outcome: cumulative results after salpingectomy in a randomized controlled trial. Hum Reprod. 2001;16:2403–10.
68. Bildirici I, Bukulmez O, Ensari A, et al. A prospective evaluation of the effect of salpingectomy on endometrial receptivity in cases of women with communicating hydrosalpinges. Hum Reprod. 2001;16:2422–6.
69. Seli E, Kayisli UA, Cakmak H, et al. Removal of hydrosalpinges increases endometrial leukaemia inhibitory factor (LIF) expression at the time of the implantation window. Hum Reprod. 2005;20:3012–7.
70. Daftary GS, Taylor HS. Hydrosalpinx fluid diminishes endometrial cell HOXA10 expression. Fertil Steril. 2002;78:577–80.
71. Daftary GS, Kayisili U, Seli E, Bukulmez O, Arici A, Taylor HS. Peri-implantation endometrial HOXA10 expression is increased in patients with hydrosalpinx and improved by salpingectomy. Fertil Steril. 2007;87:367–72.
72. Ragni G, Diaferia D, Vegetti W, et al. Effectiveness of sonohysterography in infertile patient work-up: a comparison with transvaginal ultrasonography and hysteroscopy. Gynecol Obstet Invest. 2005;59:184–8.
73. Elsayes KM, Pandya A, Platt JF, et al. Technique and diagnostic utility of saline infusion sonohysterography. Int J Gynaecol Obstet. 2009;105:5–9.
74. Bosteels J, Weyers S, Puttemans P, et al. The effectiveness of hysteroscopy in improving pregnancy rates in subfertile women without other gynaecological symptoms: a systematic review. Hum Reprod Update. 2010;16:1–11.
75. Doldi N, Persico P, Di Sebastiano F, et al. Pathologic findings in hysteroscopy before in vitro fertilization-embryo transfer (IVF-ET). Gynecol Endocrinol. 2005;21:235–7.

76. Demirol A, Gurgan T. Effect of treatment of intrauterine pathologies with office hysteroscopy in patients with recurrent IVF failure. Reprod Biomed Online. 2004;8:590–4.
77. Rama Raju GA, Shashi Kumari G, Krishna KM, et al. Assessment of uterine cavity by hysteroscopy in assisted reproduction programme and its influence on pregnancy outcome. Arch Gynecol Obstet. 2006;274:160–4.
78. Mansour RT, Aboulghar MA. Optimizing the embryo transfer technique. Hum Reprod. 2002; 17:1149–53.

Chapter 35
Single Embryo Transfer

Thorir Hardarson and Matts Wikland

Assisted reproduction technology (ART) is the single most effective method to treat infertility [1]. This high success rate has generally been achieved through replacement of multiple embryos resulting in an increased number of multiple births, being 30% of all ART live births in the United States in 2006 [2]. In the United States, the *ASRM practice committee* [3] recommended that between one and five embryos be replaced depending on the maternal age and/or the prognosis. It has been advocated that it should be up to the infertile couple and their physician to decide how many embryos should be transferred. In contrast, other countries like Sweden, Finland, Belgium, and recently Turkey have promoted a stricter line in the form of legislation/recommendations greatly restricting the use of multiple embryo replacement. In those countries, the trend has been steadily toward reducing multiple pregnancies through the use of single embryo transfer (SET). Globally, however, there are a large variations between how SET has been implemented ranging from 2.8% in USA to 69.4% in Sweden [4]. These variations are likely to persist unless there are major changes in the way ART is viewed, funded, and legislated.

Multiple Pregnancies

The most important reason for decreasing the number of replaced embryos is the need to decrease the high incidence of multiple gestation and multiple birth rates (MBRs) produced through ART. In the USA, it has been estimated although ART only accounts for 1% of all births, ART births are 18% of all multiple births [5]. Despite that the majority of children born after multiple pregnancies are healthy,

T. Hardarson, PhD (✉)
Fertility Center Scandinavia, Gothenburg, Sweden
e-mail: thorir.hardarson@fcivf.com

M. Wikland, PhD
Department of Obstetrics and Gynaecology, University of Göteborg, Gothenburg, Sweden

Z.P. Nagy et al. (eds.), *Clinical Embryology: A Practical Guide*,
DOI 10.1007/978-1-4614-8376-2_35, © Springer Science+Business Media New York 2013

there are significant problems linked to multiple births both obstetrical and neonatal [6]. The obstetrical risks include hypertension, preeclampsia, preterm labor, anemia, and an increased Cesarean section rate. The neonatal risks include increased mortality, lower gestational age, low birth weight, and respiratory distress syndrome along with numerous other complications associated with preterm birth. In addition, long-term neurological complications have been associated with preterm birth along with the strain such a birth puts on the family both psychologically and financially.

Multiple births are associated with increased costs for the society compared to singletons. It has been estimated that the total cost of ART-associated preterm deliveries in USA to be approximately one billion dollars annually [2]. In the Netherlands, it has been estimated that lifetime extra healthcare costs of a twin pregnancy add up to 30,000€ [7].

What can be done to reduce MBR in relation to IVF? Embryo reduction has been used to escape the complications associated with higher order of multiple pregnancies. Although embryo reduction is a relatively safe method, it however is not a solution for the quantitatively largest problem of twins, which are normally not reduced to singletons.

The only realistic way of avoiding multiple pregnancies in IVF is to reduce the number of embryos replaced. The problem with this approach is that in order to really reduce the multiple pregnancies, only one embryo should be transferred. By doing so, the total delivery rate will be affected negatively [8]. The question is then what is an acceptable delivery rate per transfer or started cycle? The attitude among patients as well doctors working with IVF is that the delivery rate should be as high as possible. With such an attitude, more than one embryo should be transferred. However, growing evidence indicates that by doing so, the problem with the high MBR in IVF will never be solved.

Pregnancy Results After SET

Pregnancy rates calculated per transfer are understandably the golden standard on success as it relates to an output parameter that is easily understood, gives fast feedback to the clinic on its performance, and relates the fresh cycle most commonly performed in IVF. There are of course many ways of comparing results and success. One other way of determining success is to calculate the cumulative birth rate per oocyte retrieval. Such an approach decreases the emphasis on the fresh transfer adding the increasingly important factor of cryopreservation of human embryos.

Results from Studies Comparing SET and Double Embryo Transfer (DET)

Comparing pregnancy results of SET contra multiple replacements has been reported in numerous randomized prospective trials [9–15]. The RCT studies show a clear advantage of transferring two embryos as compared to one. DET produces a significantly higher ongoing clinical pregnancy rate (44.5%) than SET (28.3%) [8].

Several studies show, however, that a comparable ongoing clinical pregnancy rates can be achieved by transferring two embryos, one at a time [12, 13, 16]. However, such an approach requires a very good cryopreservation programs. Improved techniques for cryopreservation have dramatically increased both the survival rates as well as the ongoing pregnancy rates.

Generally, RCTs are very valuable in clinical research, as their study design results in a similar distribution of confounding variables over the study arms. However, the normal IVF clinic cannot be a never-ending RCT study; it is a mixture of many different embryo transfer regimes that have been established over time. Those cohort studies that have been published reflect this reality [17–20]. They have compared SET vs. DET and show no significant difference in the ongoing pregnancy rate while there is a 30-fold decrease in the twinning rate in the SET group.

The Swedish Experience of SET

Due to the high MBR, resulting in criticism from obstetricians and neonatologists, Swedish IVF clinics already in 1993 on their own initiative started to reduce the number of transferred embryos from three to two. This resulted, as expected, in a dramatic drop in triplets, whereas the twinning rate remained unchanged at around 20%. Due to the known less favorable outcome for twins as compared singletons shown in a large follow-up studies of all IVF children born in Sweden between 1982 and 1995 [21], voices were raised that only one embryo should be transferred in the majority of cycles. Due to the debate concerning the high MBR clearly related to the number of transferred embryos and unchanged twinning rate, a multicenter randomized controlled trial was set up in Scandinavia by a group in Sweden [12]. The aim of the study was to compare one fresh embryo and if no live birth occurred, adding another embryo transfer from the frozen thawed embryo, with transfer of two fresh embryos. The results did not show any difference in pregnancy rates between the groups with one fresh plus one frozen/thawed, as compared to the DET group. However, the twinning rate was 0.8 and 33%, respectively [12]. Without waiting for the final result from the abovementioned study, the Swedish IVF legislation was revised with regard to the number of embryos that could be transferred. Thus, the Swedish National Board of Health and Welfare in their new guidelines in 2003 stated that only one embryo be replaced in the majority of cases. However, the guidelines did not state in which situation only one embryo was allowed to replace. A detailed guideline was left to the profession to outline. The Swedish IVF clinics today, thus, recommend that only one embryo shall be transferred in the first two cycles in women under the age of 38 years. With this recommendation, almost 70% of the transfers performed in Sweden between 2003 and 2008 utilized only one embryo (Fig. 35.1). During the same period, the delivery rate per transfer has remained stable around 26%. The MBR has, during the same period, dropped from

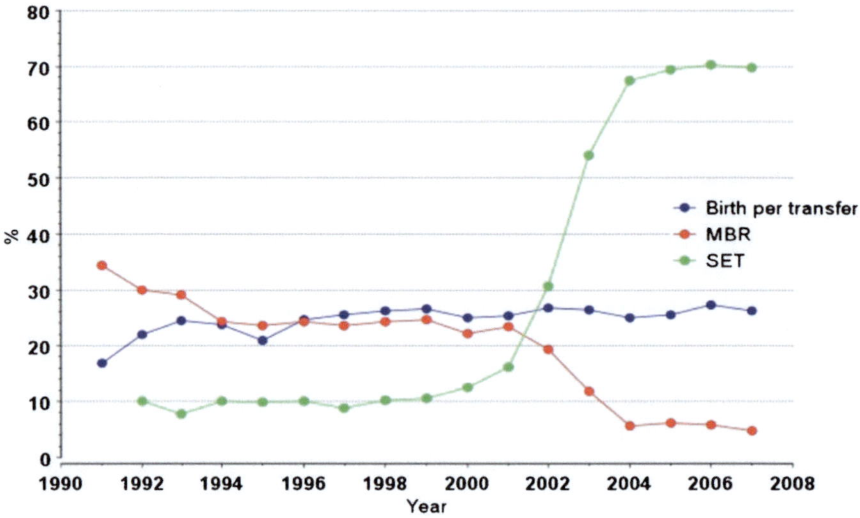

Fig. 35.1 Birth per transfer (standard IVF and ICSI), multiple birth rate (MBR), and single embryo transfer in Sweden in 1991–2007

25 to 5.7%. Data from our own clinic also show that the overall pregnancy results are not affected by increasing the proportion of SET below 10% in 1998 to 86% in 2010 (Fig. 35.2). It is also interesting to notice that in women, 40 years or younger, the birth rate remained stable, while a dramatic decrease in MBR occurred [22]. Comparing the Swedish results with USA shows a continuous increase in delivery rate to 35%; however, the MBR is still around 30% (The Society for Assisted Reproductive Technology. National data summary. 2008 [30 October, 2010]; available from: www.sart.org).

The significant health consequences of such high MBR are obvious, and the cost for the American society is very high [2].

If Sweden had continued to transfer two embryos in the majority of patients, one could have expected an increase in the delivery rate similar to USA. However, considering the unchanged delivery rate at an acceptable level and the dramatic decrease in the MBR with decreased risks for the IVF children, SET seems preferable, both from the patient's and society's point of view.

Result from Sweden, with an overall SET frequency of almost 70% resulting in a multiple birth of less than 6% without reducing the overall birth rate, as well as published cohort studies, indicates how important it is to choose the correct embryo when implementing SET. This is because SET often is performed when a good quality embryo is available from a cohort of embryos. DET is, therefore, only used on patients who have a worse embryo quality, are older, and/or have many previous failed cycles. By using SET on patients that run a high risk of a multiple pregnancy, you, therefore, reduce this risk significantly. Methods for embryo selection have

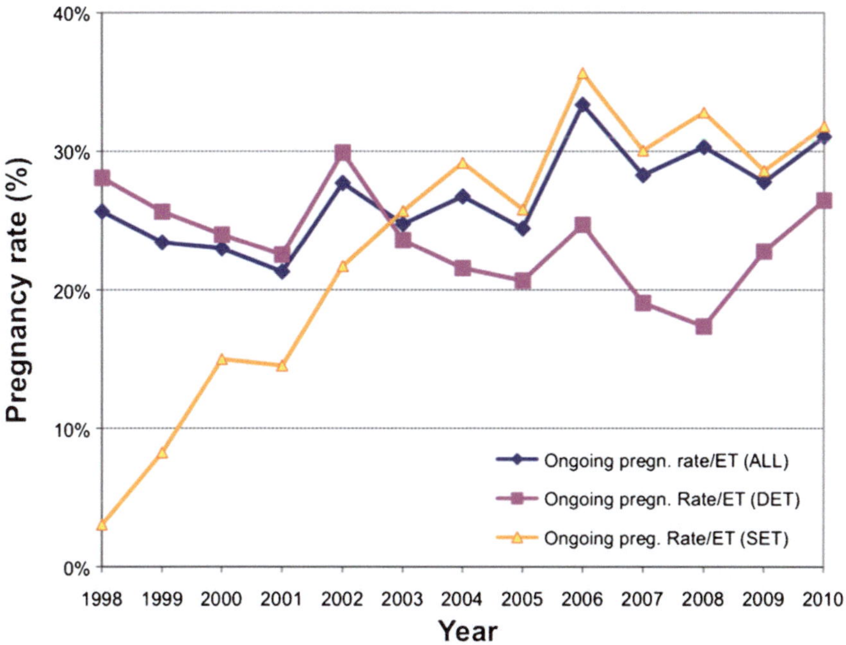

Fig. 35.2 Ongoing pregnancy rate after SET and DET at Fertilitetscentrum, Gothenburg, Sweden, during a 12-year period

improved during the last decade or so using mainly morphological markers to increase the power of the embryo selection. Although improved embryo selection has been pivotal in maintaining a high pregnancy rate despite introducing SET, improved embryo culture media, blastocyst culture, and general improvement within the IVF clinics have also played a big part.

Conclusion

At the end of the day, SET is not a big technical innovation, but rather more of an ideology, another way of defining success, not only through pregnancy rates in the fresh cycle. Successful implementation of SET requires that everybody involved in the IVF treatment perform at their best, and some authors claim that the degree of SET performed at a particular center is the best measure for performance of that center [23]. Given that there are both pros and cons with SET, it is, however, likely that it will become more and more utilized as both patients and society realize the risk even with twins.

References

1. Collins J. Cost-effectiveness of in vitro fertilization. Semin Reprod Med. 2001;19(3):279–89.
2. Bromer JG, et al. Preterm deliveries that result from multiple pregnancies associated with assisted reproductive technologies in the United States: a cost analysis. Curr Opin Obstet Gynecol. 2011;23:168–73.
3. American Society for Reproductive Medicine and Society for Assisted Reproductive Technology. Guidelines on number of embryos transferred. Fertil Steril. 2009;92(5):1518–9.
4. Maheshwari A, Griffiths S, Bhattacharya S. Global variations in the uptake of single embryo transfer. Hum Reprod Update. 2011;17(1): 107–20.
5. Sunderam S, et al. Assisted reproductive technology surveillance–United States, 2006. MMWR Surveill Summ. 2009;58(5):1–25.
6. Gerris JM. Single embryo transfer and IVF/ICSI outcome: a balanced appraisal. Hum Reprod Update. 2005;11(2):105–21.
7. van Heesch MM, et al. Long term costs and effects of reducing the number of twin pregnancies in IVF by single embryo transfer: the TwinSing study. BMC Pediatr. 2010;10:75.
8. Baruffi RL, et al. Single-embryo transfer reduces clinical pregnancy rates and live births in fresh IVF and intracytoplasmic sperm injection (ICSI) cycles: a meta-analysis. Reprod Biol Endocrinol. 2009;7:36.
9. Gerris J, et al. Prevention of twin pregnancy after in-vitro fertilization or intracytoplasmic sperm injection based on strict embryo criteria: a prospective randomized clinical trial. Hum Reprod. 1999;14(10):2581–7.
10. Martikainen H, et al. One versus two embryo transfer after IVF and ICSI: a randomized study. Hum Reprod. 2001;16(9):1900–3.
11. Gardner DK, et al. Single blastocyst transfer: a prospective randomized trial. Fertil Steril. 2004;81(3):551–5.
12. Thurin A, et al. Elective single-embryo transfer versus double-embryo transfer in in vitro fertilization. N Engl J Med. 2004; 351(23):2392–402.
13. Lukassen HG, et al. Two cycles with single embryo transfer versus one cycle with double embryo transfer: a randomized controlled trial. Hum Reprod. 2005;20(3):702–8.
14. van Montfoort AP, et al. In unselected patients, elective single embryo transfer prevents all multiples, but results in significantly lower pregnancy rates compared with double embryo transfer: a randomized controlled trial. Hum Reprod. 2006;21(2):338–43.
15. Moustafa MK, Sheded SA, El Aziz Mousta MA. Elective single embryo transfer versus double embryo transfer in assisted reproduction. Reprod Biomed Online. 2008;17(1):82–7.
16. Leniaud L, et al. [Prospective evaluation of elective single-embryo transfer versus double-embryo transfer following in vitro fertilization: a two-year French hospital experience]. Gynecol Obstet Fertil. 2008;36(2):159–65.
17. Gerris J, et al. Elective single day 3 embryo transfer halves the twinning rate without decrease in the ongoing pregnancy rate of an IVF/ICSI programme. Hum Reprod. 2002;17(10):2626–31.
18. Catt J, et al. Single embryo transfer in IVF to prevent multiple pregnancies. Twin Res. 2003; 6(6):536–9.
19. Tiitinen A, et al. Impact of elective single embryo transfer on the twin pregnancy rate. Hum Reprod. 2003;18(7):1449–53.
20. Martikainen H, et al. Day 2 elective single embryo transfer in clinical practice: better outcome in ICSI cycles. Hum Reprod. 2004;19(6):1364–6.
21. Bergh T, et al. Deliveries and children born after in-vitro fertilisation in Sweden 1982-95: a retrospective cohort study. Lancet. 1999;354(9190):1579–85.
22. Karlstrom PO, Bergh C. Reducing the number of embryos transferred in Sweden-impact on delivery and multiple birth rates. Hum Reprod. 2007;22(8):2202–7.
23. Land JA, Evers JL. What is the most relevant standard of success in assisted reproduction? Defining outcome in ART: a Gordian knot of safety, efficacy and quality. Hum Reprod. 2004; 19(5):1046–8.

Chapter 36
Ultrasound-Guided Embryo Transfer (Abdominal/Vaginal): An Evidence-Based Evaluation

Ahmed M. Abou-Setta

Throughout time, fertility has been one of the most sought after aspects in societies. In addition to the natural wish to procreate, pregnancy and childbirth have been a highly sought after character in women of all walks of life. In ancient Egypt, women were graded according to potential fertility rather than their physical beauty, with the most attractive women being the fertile ones. In ancient Rome, fertility was such a key factor in the preservation of society that pregnancy and fertility were gracefully depicted on coins from the Roman Empire, a means to encourage fertility among couples.

Modern fertility practices can be traced back to the revolutionary work performed by Edwards and Steptoe in the 1970s. With the birth of the first baby in vitro, a new era was ushered in that was built on scientific discoveries and evidence-based decision making. Since their initial discoveries, major advancements have been made in ovarian stimulation protocols, embryo manipulation techniques, and in vitro embryo development. The result has been an increased probability of a live birth following embryo transfer from close to nil to over 25%. Even so, there has been a noticeable ceiling effect to success rates that does not seem to be related to the number or quality of embryos produced through in vitro fertilization since most women today will reach the embryo transfer stage with an adequate number of high-quality embryos. Therefore, the culprit preventing these healthy embryos from developing inside the maternal womb must lie later down the IVF chain. This weak link (embryo implantation) may be related to the technique used for embryo transfer and remains the rate-limiting step in the success of this form of therapy. It is estimated that up to 85% of the embryos replaced into the uterine cavity will fail to implant [1]. This makes the embryo transfer procedure a highly vital and, at the same time, highly inefficient step in IVF.

A.M. Abou-Setta, MD, PhD (✉)
George & Fay Yee Centre for Healthcare Innovation, University of Manitoba/Winnipeg Regional Health Authority, Winnipeg, MB, Canada R3A 1R9
e-mail: ahmedabou-setta@umanitoba.ca

Z.P. Nagy et al. (eds.), *Clinical Embryology: A Practical Guide*, 567
DOI 10.1007/978-1-4614-8376-2_36,

The pregnancy rate following embryo transfer is dependent upon multiple factors including embryo quality, endometrial receptivity, and the technique of the embryo transfer itself [2]. The aim of the embryo transfer procedure is to atraumatically and accurately place embryos within the uterus, in order to allow for proper implantation and fetal development. Years of experience and research have shown us that neither one of these goals are a given must during the transfer procedure. In addition, it is important to prevent iatrogenic complications of embryo transfer, such as vaginal bleeding and ectopic pregnancies. Ironically, just as Steptoe and Edwards were the first to describe a live birth following embryo transfer, they were also the first to describe an ectopic pregnancy following embryo transfer [3].

In recent years, the revelation of the importance of this stage of the IVF process has reflected in more research into ways of optimizing and standardizing the embryo transfer technique. Factors such as ease of the procedure [4], catheter choice [5], and dummy embryo transfer [6] have proven to improve the clinical outcomes, but nothing seems to have had such a major impact as the introduction of ultrasound guidance during embryo transfer.

The first reports of the beneficial effect of ultrasound guidance during the "blind" embryo transfer procedure were published over 20 years ago [7, 8]. Today, many centers and clinicians worldwide routinely perform all embryo transfer with the assistance of ultrasound imaging. Having said that, not all clinicians are believers, and there are a lot of skeptics over the true benefit of using ultrasound guidance during embryo transfer. This has been fueled by conflicting results from published clinical trials, with the majority concluding that ultrasound guidance improves the clinical pregnancy, and implantation rates, while some reports have shown no such improvement. In light of this controversy, it is important to critically view the relative efficacy of ultrasound guidance in an evidence-based fashion in order to appraise the best available evidence today for the use of ultrasonography during embryo transfer.

Abdominal Ultrasound-Guided Embryo Transfer

Two-dimensional (2D) transabdominal ultrasound is the most commonly used form of ultrasound guidance during embryo transfer. Even so, three-dimensional (3D) and four-dimensional (4D) ultrasound-guided embryo transfers have been reported [9]. Nonetheless, it is important to mention that the majority of the evidence in the medical literature relates to comparing to use of the 2D US-guided method.

All the preparatory steps (e.g., removing cervical mucus) before embryo transfer are performed just as with the clinical touch embryo transfer. Additionally, the woman is asked to fill the bladder to allow for proper visualization of the cervico-uterine axis. Once the clinician is ready to perform the actual transfer, a transabdominal ultrasound probe is placed on the lower part of the abdomen and adjusted by an ultrasonographer until a clear view of the reproductive path is evident. The clinician is therefore able to visualize the embryo transfer catheter as it traverses the cervical canal, internal os, and enters the uterine cavity. Once in the cavity, the embryos can be deposited as a specific distance from the uterine fundus. Moreover, the use of air bubbles to bracket the embryo containing media can give both the clinician and patient an accurate visualization of the final site of the embryos in the uterine cavity after the transfer catheter is removed.

Vaginal Ultrasound-Guided Embryo Transfer

Vaginal ultrasound-guided embryo transfer has been described in the literature but less frequently than with the use of abdominal ultrasonography [10, 11]. With the use of vaginal ultrasonography, the embryo transfer catheter is threaded through the external os into the cervical canal before the vaginal ultrasound probe is introduced. Further advancement of the catheter is then performed under ultrasound guidance.

The main advantage of this technique is that it allows the clinician to perform this procedure without the assistance an ultrasonographer, as opposed to the abdominal ultrasound. Additionally, the patient does not have to fill the bladder, not micturate immediately following the procedure. Advocates of this form of ultrasound-guided transfer claim that it is therefore more patient friendly by removing some of the discomfort associated with a full bladder.

Evidence-Based Evaluation on the Benefits and Drawbacks of Ultrasound-Guided Embryo Transfer

Systematic reviews and meta-analysis of randomized controlled trials have proven to be the highest level of evidence in the hierarchy of medical knowledge. The transparent nature and comprehensive coverage of a topic have made this form of research the most fundamental building block in search for the truth. There is an almost exponential growth in the number of published systematic reviews in the medical literature, reflecting the growing recognition among clinicians and researchers of their importance for improving our understanding of health-related topics.

On the topic of ultrasonography during embryo transfer, there are several published systematic reviews of the evidence [12–16]. All the reviews were attempting to quantify the relative efficacy of ultrasound-guided embryo transfer compared with the standard "clinical touch" embryo transfer. Even so, it should be noted that the individual clinical queries were not precisely the same, neither were their search strategies nor inclusion criteria. Nevertheless, regardless of the differing methodologies, all the reviews came to the same final conclusion that there is adequate evidence to support the use of ultrasound guidance during embryo transfer.

The first systematic reviews using similar accepted methodologies identified eight prospective trials (four properly randomized and four quasi-randomized trials) comparing abdominal ultrasound-guided embryo transfer to clinical touch embryo transfer were published in late 2003 [12, 13]. The trials brought together data from 8,392 embryo transfer cycles (2,145 with ultrasound guidance and 2,051 without ultrasound guidance). The combined results showed that the clinical pregnancy rate was at least 17–32% better with ultrasound guidance than without. Additionally, the ongoing pregnancy rates were similar higher with ultrasound than without (22%). Even so, the multiple pregnancy, miscarriage, and ectopic pregnancy rates were found to be similar in the two groups. On the bright side, the incidence of difficult embryo transfers was found to be lower with ultrasound guidance (9.1% compared with 15.1%).

It was several years later before the next systematic review on this topic was performed by our team in 2007 [14]. Again the methodology was built on well-defined and accepted practices in evidence-based medicine but differed slightly from the two previous reviews. We were able to include 20 randomized trials (5,968 embryo transfer cycles) in women undergoing ultrasound-guided (2,941 cycles) compared with clinical touch (3,027 cycles) embryo transfers. There was a general trend toward better results with ultrasound guidance, with only a limited number of studies demonstrating equivocal or better results than clinical touch method. It may be assumed that studies with equivocal results demonstrate that some clinicians have excellent clinical sense and therefore nullifying any extra advantage provided by sonographic visualization. The pooled results from the properly randomized trials still demonstrated at least a 23% improvement in clinical pregnancy rates with the use of ultrasound guidance, with the number needed to treat (NNT) to obtain one additional clinical pregnancy using ultrasound guidance calculated to be 13 (95% CI = 10–19).

As with the previous reviews, the multiple pregnancy, miscarriage, and ectopic pregnancy rates were found to be similar in the two groups. Furthermore, the incidence of difficult embryo transfers and the need for instrumental assistance during transfer were confirmed to be lower with ultrasound guidance. Additionally, for the first time, the live birth rates were shown to be also improved with ultrasound usage. This is of importance since outcomes like the clinical pregnancy rates are only surrogate outcomes and not the final primary outcome in assisted reproduction.

One of the major points of concern in clinical trials and systematic reviews is the issue of sample sizes. It is theorized that smaller trials might not have a sufficient sample size to detect minor differences between the study groups (type II error) and will therefore present false equivocal results. The largest included trial (n = 800) in this review had enough power to detect an 8% difference in clinical pregnancy rates [17], while the overall review could detect an absolute difference of 3.3%.

In 2007, the first Cochrane systematic review [15] on the topic was published. This review included 13 truly randomized trials (2,714 women) comparing women randomized to ultrasound guidance (1,376 women) with clinical touch only (1,338 women) for catheter guidance during embryo transfer. This review was later updated in 2010 to reflect the most up-to-date information on the topic. The updated review [16] included 17 truly randomized trials (2,714 women) comparing women randomized to ultrasound guidance (1,254 women) with clinical touch only (1,218 women) for catheter guidance during embryo transfer.

Both the original and the updated reviews were performed according to the highest standards of evidence-based medicine and in accordance with the practice guidelines of the international Cochrane Collaboration. The results of the most recent update still demonstrate significantly higher incidences of pregnancy with ultrasound guidance, but no evidence of a significant difference in live birth rates was noted. Even so, the authors declare that the results from the trials were not homogenous and therefore should be interpreted with caution. Additionally, as with the previous reviews, the multiple pregnancy, miscarriage, and ectopic pregnancy rates were found to be similar in the two groups

Clinical Discussion

It is evident from the aforementioned evidence that the literature generally supports the use of ultrasound guidance to assist clinicians during embryo transfer. However, the exact mechanism(s) whereby ultrasound-guided embryo transfer improves pregnancy rates remains unclear. Several theories have been proposed including (1) confirming the position of the tip of the embryo transfer catheter within the uterine cavity, (2) accurately determining the site of embryo deposition, (3) increasing the frequency of "easy" embryo transfers, and (4) avoiding endometrial indentation.

Nevertheless, some clinicians might argue that the actual benefit of using ultrasound during embryo transfer is the ability to visualize the pelvic structures in real time. Distorted pelvic anatomy, whether congenital or iatrogenic following surgery, can confuse the clinician into depositing the embryos at an improper site in the female reproductive tract. Furthermore, some clinicians have abandoned using measurements or information from dummy embryo transfers with the ultrasound guidance during embryo transfer. The reasoning is that the characteristics of pelvic structures tend to slightly change following ovarian stimulations, and therefore, any information passed on from the earlier stages of IVF may not be as accurate on the day of embryo transfer.

Others have been skeptical about the beneficial attributes of using ultrasonography during the transfer procedure. The argument is that experienced professionals have a strong clinical sense and therefore do not need to visualize the structures during embryo transfer. Additionally, the time to perform the transfer procedure is both increased and, in the case of abdominal ultrasonography, there is a need for additional participant in order to perform the transfer procedure.

Whatever the underlying mechanism, or criticism of the procedure, the overall conclusion is that with most clinicians, using ultrasound will significantly improve their patients' pregnancy rates. Coupled with the fact that no study to date has shown any negative adverse events to the use of ultrasonographic guidance during embryo transfer, this technique has gained enormous popularity in the world of assisted reproduction.

References

1. Edwards RG. Clinical approaches to increasing uterine receptivity during human implantation. Hum Reprod. 1995;10 Suppl 2:60–6.
2. Mansour RT, Aboulghar MA. Optimizing the embryo transfer technique. Hum Reprod. 2002; 17(5):1149–53.
3. Steptoe PC, Edwards RG. Reimplantation of a human embryo with subsequent tubal pregnancy. Lancet. 1976;1(7965):880–2.
4. Lesny P, Killick SR, Tetlow RL, Robinson J, Maguiness SD. Embryo transfer–can we learn anything new from the observation of junctional zone contractions? Hum Reprod. 1998;13(6): 1540–6.
5. Abou-Setta AM, Al-Inany HG, Mansour RT, Serour GI, Aboulghar MA. Soft versus firm embryo transfer catheters for assisted reproduction: a systematic review and meta-analysis. Hum Reprod. 2005;20(11):3114–21.
6. Mansour R, Aboulghar M, Serour G. Dummy embryo transfer: a technique that minimizes the problems of embryo transfer and improves the pregnancy rate in human in vitro fertilization. Fertil Steril. 1990;54(4):678–81.
7. Strickler RC, Christianson C, Crane JP, Curato A, Knight AB, Yang V. Ultrasound guidance for human embryo transfer. Fertil Steril. 1985;43(1):54–61.
8. Leong M, Leung C, Tucker M, Wong C, Chan H. Ultrasound-assisted embryo transfer. J In Vitro Fert Embryo Transf. 1986;3(6):383–5.
9. Baba K, Ishihara O, Hayashi N, Saitoh M, Taya J, Kinoshita K. Three-dimensional ultrasound in embryo transfer. Ultrasound Obstet Gynecol. 2000;16(4):372–3.
10. Woolcott R, Stanger J. Ultrasound tracking of the movement of embryo-associated air bubbles on standing after transfer. Hum Reprod. 1998;13(8):2107–9.
11. Kojima K, Nomiyama M, Kumamoto T, Matsumoto Y, Iwasaka T. Transvaginal ultrasound-guided embryo transfer improves pregnancy and implantation rates after IVF. Hum Reprod. 2001; 16(12):2578–82.
12. Buckett WM. A meta-analysis of ultrasound-guided versus clinical touch embryo transfer. Fertil Steril. 2003;80(4):1037–41.
13. Sallam HN, Sadek SS. Ultrasound-guided embryo transfer: a meta-analysis of randomized controlled trials. Fertil Steril. 2003;80(4):1042–6.
14. Abou-Setta AM, Mansour RT, Al-Inany HG, Aboulghar MM, Aboulghar MA, Serour GI. Among women undergoing embryo transfer, is the probability of pregnancy and live birth improved with ultrasound guidance over clinical touch alone? A systemic review and meta-analysis of prospective randomized trials. Fertil Steril. 2007;88(2):333–41.
15. Brown JA, Buckingham K, Abou-Setta A, Buckett W. Ultrasound versus 'clinical touch' for catheter guidance during embryo transfer in women. Cochrane Database Syst Rev. 2007; (1):CD006107.
16. Brown J, Buckingham K, Abou-Setta AM, Buckett W. Ultrasound versus 'clinical touch' for catheter guidance during embryo transfer in women. Cochrane Database Syst Rev. 2010;(1): CD006107.
17. Tang OS, Ng EH, So WW, Ho PC. Ultrasound-guided embryo transfer: a prospective randomized controlled trial. Hum Reprod. 2001;16(11):2310–5.

Index

DOI 10.1007/978-1-4614-8376-2, © Springer Science+Business Media New York 2013

D

P

R

MIX
Papier aus verantwortungsvollen Quellen
Paper from responsible sources
FSC® C105338

If you have any concerns about our products,
you can contact us on
ProductSafety@springernature.com

In case Publisher is established outside the EU,
the EU authorized representative is:
Springer Nature Customer Service Center GmbH
Europaplatz 3, 69115 Heidelberg, Germany

Printed by Libri Plureos GmbH
in Hamburg, Germany